Lecture Notes in Electrical Engineering

Volume 796

The book series *Lecture Notes in Electrical Engineering* (LNEE) publishes the latest developments in Electrical Engineering - quickly, informally and in high quality. While original research reported in proceedings and monographs has traditionally formed the core of LNEE, we also encourage authors to submit books devoted to supporting student education and professional training in the various fields and applications areas of electrical engineering. The series cover classical and emerging topics concerning:

- Communication Engineering, Information Theory and Networks
- Electronics Engineering and Microelectronics
- Signal, Image and Speech Processing
- Wireless and Mobile Communication
- Circuits and Systems
- Energy Systems, Power Electronics and Electrical Machines
- Electro-optical Engineering
- Instrumentation Engineering
- Avionics Engineering
- Control Systems
- Internet-of-Things and Cybersecurity
- Biomedical Devices, MEMS and NEMS

For general information about this book series, comments or suggestions, please contact leontina.dicecco@springer.com.

To submit a proposal or request further information, please contact the Publishing Editor in your country:

China

Jasmine Dou, Editor (jasmine.dou@springer.com)

India, Japan, Rest of Asia

Swati Meherishi, Editorial Director (Swati.Meherishi@springer.com)

Southeast Asia, Australia, New Zealand

Ramesh Nath Premnath, Editor (ramesh.premnath@springernature.com)

USA, Canada:

Michael Luby, Senior Editor (michael.luby@springer.com)

All other Countries:

Leontina Di Cecco, Senior Editor (leontina.dicecco@springer.com)

** This series is indexed by EI Compendex and Scopus databases. **

More information about this series at https://link.springer.com/bookseries/7818

Manish Kumar Bajpai · Koushlendra Kumar Singh ·
George Giakos
Editors

Machine Vision and Augmented Intelligence—Theory and Applications

Select Proceedings of MAI 2021

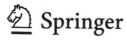 Springer

Editors
Manish Kumar Bajpai
Department of Computer Science
and Engineering
IIITDM Jabalpur
Jabalpur, India

Koushlendra Kumar Singh
Department of Computer Science
and Engineering
National Institute of Technology
Jamshedpur
Jamshedpur, India

George Giakos
Department of Electrical and Computer
Engineering
Manhattan College
New York, NY, USA

ISSN 1876-1100   ISSN 1876-1119 (electronic)
Lecture Notes in Electrical Engineering
ISBN 978-981-16-5080-2   ISBN 978-981-16-5078-9 (eBook)
https://doi.org/10.1007/978-981-16-5078-9

This Springer imprint is published by the registered company Springer Nature Singapore Pte Ltd.
The registered company address is: 152 Beach Road, #21-01/04 Gateway East, Singapore 189721,
Singapore

Preface

Machine Vision and Augmented Intelligence—Theory and Applications: Selected Proceedings of MAI 2021 brings together academicians, researchers, industry people, and students to come together and discuss the current state-of-the-art developments in their fields. The book had provided a benchmark and platform to the "AATM NIRBHAR BHARAT" by using modern augmented intelligence. The theme of the book encompasses all industrial and non-industrial applications in which a combination of hardware and software provides operational guidance to devices in the execution of their functions based on the capture and processing of images. Today, manufacturers are using machine vision and Augmented Intelligence-based metrology to improve their productivity and reduce costs. Machine vision and Augmented Intelligence integrates optical components with computerized control systems to achieve greater productivity from existing automated manufacturing equipment. This will become very useful to improve the efficiency in different fields like security, crime detection, forensic, Inventory control, etc.

Jabalpur, India
2021

Manish Kumar Bajpai
Koushlendra Kumar Singh
George Giakos

Contents

About the Editors

Manish Kumar Bajpai is an assistant professor in the Department of Computer Science and Engineering at the Indian Institute of Information Technology Design and Manufacturing, Jabalpur, India. He completed his Ph.D. from IIT Kanpur in the area of image reconstruction and parallel algorithm design. Dr. Bajpai has published over 50 publications in international journals and conferences. He has several sponsored research and consultancy projects funded by agencies such as SPARC, MHRD, DST, USIEF, ATAL, BRNS, and NVIDIA. 11 students have completed/pursuing their Ph.D. under his supervision. His areas of research are augmented intelligence, machine vision, brain-computer interface, medical imaging, and parallel algorithms design. Dr. Bajpai is a senior member of IEEE and a life member of the Indian Science Congress and Indian Nuclear Society.

Koushlendra Kumar Singh is currently working as an assistant professor in the Department of Computer Science and Engineering at the National Institute of Technology, Jamshedpur, India. He completed his doctoral degree and master's program from the Indian Institute of Information Technology, Design, and Manufacturing, Jabalpur, India, in 2016 and 2011, respectively. Dr. Singh graduated in computer science and engineering from Bhagalpur College of Engineering, Bhagalpur, in 2008. He has published several papers in international refereed journals and conferences. His current research interest areas are image processing, biometrics, and different applications of fractional derivatives, computational modeling, epidemic forecasting, etc.

George Giakos is a professor and chair in the Department of Electrical and Computer Engineering at Manhattan College, NY, USA. His research is articulated in technology innovation through the integration of physics, engineering, and artificial intelligence. He is a founding director of the Laboratory for Quantum Cognitive Imaging and Neuromorphic Engineering (CINE), Augmented Intelligence, and Bioinspired Vision Systems at Manhattan College. He has more than 20 US and foreign patents,

350 peer-reviewed published papers. He got extensive training in the design of innovative bioinspired electro-optical imaging sensor systems, by serving as a contractor at NASA, US Air Force Laboratories (AFRL), and Office of Naval Research. He is the recipient of the Fulbright Award to India, granted by the US Department of State, 2019–2020. Dr. Giakos has been recognized for his leadership efforts in advancing the professional goals of IEEE by receiving the 2014 IEEE-USA Professional Achievement Award in recognition of his efforts in strengthening links between industry, government, and academia.

Stock Market Predictions Using FastRNN, CNN, and Bi-LSTM-Based Hybrid Model

Konark Yadav, Milind Yadav, and Sandeep Saini

1 Introduction

Forecasting is the process of predicting the future value of any series by considering the previous patterns or long historical data. For example, if the price of gold is increasing every year at Christmas time, then we can predict a similar trend for the current year as well and plan the purchase well in advance to avoid the high rates at Christmas time. Similarly, computational models can help us in predicting the weather for the next day, week, or month as well. With the high volume of money involved, stock market values have attracted the attention of computer scientists as well to design models and architectures for precise stock value prediction. A lot of such systems have been developed with high accuracies during the past decades as well.

Stock values are not a simple time series with only one factor affecting the outcome. These can either be univariate or multivariate. Univariate stocks are rare and they are dependent on only one factor or only one company's performance. With the emerging partnerships and dependence of every big company on its partner's stocks, the second type of stock, i.e., multivariate is more common now. So in such cases, the prediction of exact future stock values can help a lot of investors and stakeholders. This is the motivation behind our proposed model.

One of the first computational models to predict the outcome of a time series was first proposed by Ahmed and Cook [1] in 1979. In this work, Auto Regressive

K. Yadav · S. Saini (✉)
Department of Electronics and Communication Engineering, The LNM Institute of Information Technology, Jaipur 302031, India
e-mail: sandeep.saini@lnmiit.ac.in

M. Yadav
Department of Computer Science and Engineering, Rajasthan Technical University, Akelgarh, Kota, Rajasthan, India

Integrated Moving Average (ARIMA) model was introduced which is one of the most trusted models for time-series forecasting even now. This is also a reason behind the fact that a lot of conventional models are based on Auto Regression (AR) and Moving Average (MA) and exponential smoothing [2].

In this decade, the focus has shifted to deep learning-based models. Ding et al. [3] developed an event-driven deep learning model. In this model, a variant of Convolutional Neural Network (CNN), i.e., Deep CNN was used to predict the stock values. The events are extracted from the news articles and stored as dense vectors, trained using a novel neural tensor network. This dense network was trained using the Deep CNN. Akita et al. [4] applied deep learning models Paragraph Vector, and Long Short-Term Memory (LSTM), to financial time-series forecasting. The model also utilized the news article data and converted those into the Paragraph vector which was then fed to LSTM to foretell the stock prices. This model was texted on the Tokyo Stock Exchange. Fischer et al. [5] also proposed a similar LSTM based architecture. The model outperformed a deep neural net (DNN), a logistic regression classifier (LOG), and a random forest-based model. Convolutional Neural Network (CNN) has been used by several researchers for the problem. Hoseinzade et al. [6] proposed CNNpred, which was a CNN-based model for establishing the relations between different stock markets across the globe and showed the positive correlation between the trends across the global stock exchanges. Eapen et al. [7] presented a hybrid model that was made using CNN and Bidirectional LSTM (Bi-LSTM) [8, 9]. The proposed model was 9% better than a single network-based model.

After considering the shortcomings in terms of their computational time and RMSE values, we have proposed the hybrid model in this work. We have focused on two performance parameters, i.e., execution time and RMSE. A model can be very accurate in prediction but very slow in computing the output. Such a model cannot be applied for live stock value prediction, but is very useful for long-term predictions. On the other hand, a faster model with acceptable RMSE can be utilized for live predictions as well. The proposed model is designed by considering a better performance in both these aspects.

2   Proposed Model

In designing a stock market price prediction model, the most important obligation is the accessibility of a suitable dataset. We have considered four companies for our study and those are Facebook Inc., Uber Inc., Apple Inc., and Nike Inc. from the New York Stock Exchange (NYSE). We have obtained the stock values from Yahoo finance.[1] The dataset includes information about day stamp, time stamp, transaction id, the stock price (open and close), and volume of stock sold in each minute interval. In our model, we have used the close price for each stock. Our work also aims on creating a prototype for live prediction. We consider a working duration of 8 h and

---

[1] https://finance.yahoo.com.

divide those hours into training and testing time. We are predicting the future prices of each minute for the next 50 min by keeping the initial 7 h 10 min data in training. The most suitable window size was picked out by calculating the root mean squared error for various window dimensions.

We kept the size of the data the same for all the stocks, i.e., each stock has 430 rows and trained the model on 40 epochs. We have considered the error and computation time of each model for our study. If the loss (mean squared error) for the current epoch is lesser than the value procured from the previous epoch, the weight matrix for that particular epoch is stored. After the completion of the training process, each of these models was tested on the remaining 50 values. In this process, the model with the least RMSE (Root Mean Squared Error) is taken as the final model for prediction.

To compare our model with existing similar models, we have initially considered a few baseline models and then the advanced models. These baseline models have their advantages and disadvantages. For example, FBProphet is the fastest model but under-performs in terms of error. Similarly, the hybrid model based on CNN and LSTM provides very little error but takes more time in predictions. A single neural network-based model performs well on one aspect of the problem while lags behind on the other front. Thus, we decided to exploit the good features of multiple networks.

2.1 FastRNN + CNN + Bi-LSTM-Based Hybrid Model

We aim to maintain the fast computation with improved accuracy for the live stock values predictions. In this direction, we propose a hybrid model that exploits the good features of multiple networks. We use FastRNN as our first network that will provide faster results and augment it with CNN and Bi-LSTM networks to enhance the accuracy of the forecast. Bi-LSTM was proposed in 1997 [10]. This model is designed to learn in both directions and is one of the best-suited models for a sequence to sequence learning. For time-series forecasting as well, the model has been proven to be a good fit. The encouraging results from these recent works have inspired us to consider Bi-LSTM as our last network. We have taken the conventional CNN in between FastRNN and Bi-LSTM to stabilize the network. A convolutional neural network (CNN) has similarities with an artificial neural network (ANN) but it takes specific suppositions about the input data which lets it achieve higher invariance when encoding properties of input data into the network. CNN needs to be trained on large training data to create deep learning models that achieve higher generalization accuracy. The proposed architecture of the hybrid model is shown in Fig. 1.

In the suggested model, we have taken a 3-stage pipeline consisting of FastRNN, CNN, and Bi-LSTM. In the first model, we have explained the added advantages of FastRNN for time-series forecasting. The CNN layer is one-dimensional in nature with a ReLU activation function. The kernel size is kept as 3 and keeping padding as "same" followed by Maxpooling. 1-D CNN is used to take out the higher-level

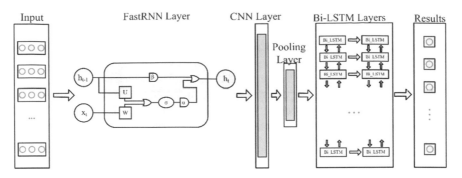

Fig. 1 FastRNN, CNN, and Bi-LSTM-based hybrid model for higher accuracy stock market predictions

features only. These take out features are nourished to the final stage, i.e., Bi-LSTM network. Bi-LSTM is followed by 2 dense layers. In the proposed model, the Bi-LSTM unit learns from both the backward and forward sequence of data and uses concatenation to merge the two sequence outputs. There was no over-fitting observed, that is why we haven't added a dropout layer. Here, using Bi-LSTM also prevented us from the vanishing gradient problem.

2.1.1 Network Parameters

As mentioned before, we as using 430 stock values as input, and the 1-D CNN layers use 3-kernel windows to return another sequence of smaller size. The output from the 1-D CNN is then fed into the Bi-directional LSTM layer group and is giving an output sequence of length 50. The output of this group is then fed to a dropout layer which gives 25 units and 1 unit output, respectively. As it can be considered as a classic regression problem, we have taken into account root mean squared error (RMSE) as the loss function to calculate the error in the forecasted versus actual data. We have to keep input and output rates identical and are critical for time-series forecasting.

Let us assume that $x = x_1, x_2, x_3, \ldots x_n$ is the one-dimensional input for the 1-D CNN layer. The equation makes a feature map after it gets convoluted with the convolution operator and is passed through a filter $W \in Rf_d$, where f denotes the inherent features from the input data producing as its output. A new feature set f_m from the set of features f is represented in the following equation:

$$hl_i^{fm} = \tanh\left(w^{fm} x_{i:i+f-1} + b\right) \tag{1}$$

Every set of features f uses the filter hl in the input defined by $\left[x_{1-f}, x_{2-f+1}, \ldots, x_{n-f+1}\right]$. This operation generates a feature map denoted by $\left[hl_1, hl_2, \cdots, hl_{n-f+1}\right]$.

Convolution layer outputs are obtained as a sum of weighted inputs after multiple linear transformations. For a non-linear feature extraction problem, linear transformations do not perform with satisfactory success, and thus we have to add non-linear activation functions. In this model, we have chosen the Rectified Linear Unit (ReLU) activation function which applies $\max(0, x)$ on each input. The output is down-sampled in the next step to reduce the information so that computation time can be improved. In our model, we have used max-pooling for that which is represented by $hl = \max(hl)$. Here, pooling helps the model to select the most relevant information and the output of the max-pooling layer can be denoted as follows:

$$x_i' = CNN(x_i) \tag{2}$$

where x_i is the input data vector to the CNN network and x_i' is the output of the CNN network which will be further passed to the Bi-LSTM network. To understand Bi-LSTM, we introduce the LSTM with the forget gate structure. The formulation is denoted by

$$i_t = \sigma\left(W_i[x_t, y_{t-1}]\right) \tag{3}$$

$$f_t = \sigma\left(W_f([x_t, y_{t-1}])\right) \tag{4}$$

$$o_t = \sigma\left(W_o([x_t, y_{t-1})]\right) \tag{5}$$

$$g_t = \tanh\left(W_g([x_t, y_{t-1}])\right) \tag{6}$$

$$c_t = f \odot c_{t-1} + i \odot g \tag{7}$$

$$y_t = o \odot \tanh(c_t) \tag{8}$$

where i, f, o, g and c are input, forget, output and input modulation gate, respectively. Keep in mind that these are in n-dimensional real vectors. In Eqs. (6–8), the σ is a sigmoid function and W_i, W_f, W_o, and W_g are fully connected neural networks for the input, forget, output, and input modulation gates, respectively. The issue with the LSTM model is that it only takes into account one-directional information on a sequence which leads to the reduction of the potency of the LSTM model. Besides, multi-directional information on the sequence can have valuable information. Therefore, bi-directional long short-term memory (Bi-LSTM) was developed which joins backward and forward directions in the series.

The order for the forward LSTM is $[x_1, x_2, \ldots .x_n]$ while for the backward LSTM is $[x_n, x_{n-1}, \ldots x_1]$. After training both backward and the forward LSTMs separately, they are unified by fusing their outputs in the previous step which is denoted in Eq. 9 as

$$y_t = y_F(t)y_B(n - t + 1) \tag{9}$$

where y_F and y_B are the outputs of the forward and backward LSTMs, respectively. The proposed model is developed on Google Colab. Details of the experimental setup and results are provided in the next section.

3 Experimental Results and Discussions

3.1 Experimental Setup

We have used a free version of Google Colab with AMD EPYC 7B12 CPU as our execution environment with 12 GB (adjustable) assigned RAM, with one socket, two threads per core, 13684 K of L3 cache, CPU of around 2250 MHz, and with No Power level. We have created our proposed model using the Python programming language (Python 3.5). We used Keras (with Tensorflow backend) library for making our deep learning models. For making the data into a suitable format, we have used Pandas, and for dividing our data into test and train, we have used Numpy. For visualization, we have the matplotlib library. The dataset and the corresponding codes are available at GitHub.[2]

3.2 Results

We have used 430 stock values for training and 70 for testing. We have tested our models on the stock values of 4 companies, i.e., Apple, Facebook, Nike, and Uber. These proposed models are compared with 9 other advanced models. We have trained the models for 40 epochs. The RMSE values and the computation time for each of the 9 models along with 2 proposed models for 4 companies, i.e., Apple, Facebook, Nike, and Uber are shown in Table 1.

The training process is fast and could be carried out on a CPU because the data size was not very high. The values of loss functions for each of the 4 companies' data training are shown in the graphical form in Fig. 2.

---

[2] https://github.com/MilindYadav-97/Hybrid_FastRNN-for-stock-predictions.git.

Table 1 Root mean square error (RMSE) and computation time calculated for the state-of-the-art and proposed models for apple, facebook, nike, and uber stock values

Model Name	Apple		Facebook		Nike		Uber	
	RMSE	Time(S)	RMSE	Time(S)	RMSE	Time(S)	RMSE	Time(S)
ARIMA [11]	0.1639	–	0.8666	–	0.4658	–	0.1639	–
CNN_2_LSTM_2 [12]	0.0258	17.8949	0.1699	17.2931	0.0718	18.3898	0.0258	17.8949
CNN_Bi-LSTM [7]	0.0214	17.2251	0.1710	17.2284	0.0529	18.3757	0.0214	17.2251
FBProphet [13]	0.0640	**0.5428**	1.5905	**0.4136**	0.5509	**0.5437**	0.0640	**0.5428**
LSTM (1 Unit) [14]	0.0226	6.9058	0.1767	6.9554	0.0442	8.0340	0.0226	6.9058
LSTM (50 Units) [14]	0.0227	**7.4888**	0.1616	**7.8642**	0.0455	**7.8041**	0.0227	**7.4888**
LSTM_Attention [15]	0.0214	17.2251	0.1710	17.2284	0.0529	18.3757	0.0214	17.2251
LSTM_CNN [16]	0.0300	12.5301	0.1644	9.3029	0.0488	14.1855	0.0300	12.5301
Proposed	**0.0213**	**11.7473**	**0.1492**	**11.9100**	**0.0421**	**11.8980**	**0.0213**	**11.7473**

From Table 1, it can be observed that the proposed models, not only have lesser RMSE, but also they perform better in terms of their computation speed, which gives a clear indication that these models can be useful for making live next minute predictions of a stock price which will help the investor to buy stocks more wisely as the market can crash anytime due to any reason. The proposed models work best on multiple stocks, which can be seen in the mentioned tables that proposed models have outperformed other classical and hybrid models in terms of both RMSE and computation time. There is a visualized comparative study in Fig. 2, which shows how the validation loss (Mean Square Error) on the validation dataset is improving after each epoch for all the studied stocks. Figure 3 shows the comparative study of the actual and predicted values of the baseline model and our proposed models for the next 20 min and it can be observed that the proposed models' predictions were closer than the actual stock values for each of the visualized stocks.

4   Conclusion

Financial data prediction can be very beneficial for companies and investors. Deep learning-based models have been quietly effective for such predictions in recent years. In this work, we have proposed two models for this purpose.

The first model that is based on FastRNN, can provide faster predictions when they are out in comparison with other state-of-the-art models (except ARIMA and FBProphet). While improving the speed of prediction, it also provides better or at

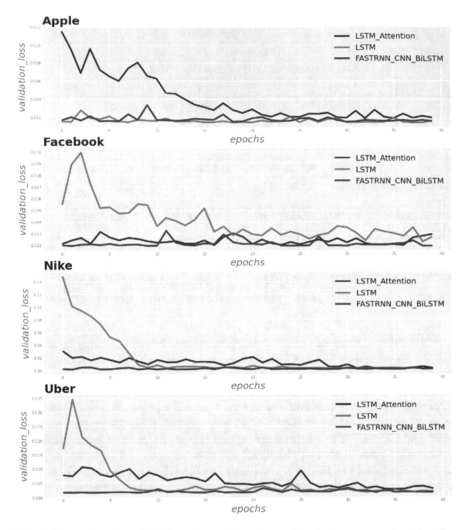

Fig. 2 Comparison plots of validation losses (Mean Square Error) of our proposed and baseline models at each epoch for all the studied stocks

par RMSE values as well. Thus, compared to FBProphet and ARIMA, this is a better choice for a reliable model. The second model improves the first proposed model while keeping the speed almost the same. It compromises a bit on the speed of perdition but improves the RMSE values. In the future, these models can be used with other time-series prediction problems as well.

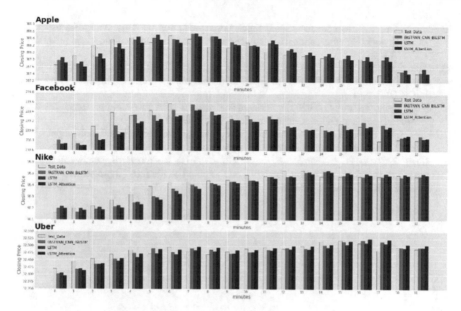

Fig. 3 Predicted stock values with the proposed model and baseline models

References

1. Ahmed MS, Cook AR (1979) Analysis of freeway traffic time-series data by using Box-Jenkins techniques, no. 722. Transport Res Board
2. Huang S-J, Shih K-R (2003) Short-term load forecasting via ARMA model identification including non-Gaussian process considerations. IEEE Trans power Syst 18(2):673–679
3. Ding X, Zhang Y, Liu T, Duan J (2015) Deep learning for event-driven stock prediction.
4. Akita R, Yoshihara A, Matsubara T, Uehara K (2016) Deep learning for stock prediction using numerical and textual information. In: 2016 IEEE/ACIS 15th international conference on computer and information science (ICIS). pp 1–6
5. Fischer T, Krauss C (2018) Deep learning with long short-term memory networks for financial market predictions. Eur J Oper Res 270(2):654–669
6. Hoseinzade E, Haratizadeh S (2019) CNNpred: CNN-based stock market prediction using a diverse set of variables. Expert Syst Appl 129:273–285
7. Eapen J, Bein D, Verma A (2019) Novel deep learning model with CNN and bi-directional LSTM for improved stock market index prediction. In 2019 IEEE 9th annual computing and communication workshop and conference (CCWC). pp 264–270
8. Yadav K, Lamba A, Gupta D, Gupta A, Karmakar P, Saini S (2020) "Bilingual Sentiment Analysis for a Code-mixed Punjabi English Social Media Text. In: 2020 5th international conference on computing, communication and security (ICCCS). pp 1–5
9. Jain M, Saini S, Kant V (2017) A hybrid approach to emotion recognition system using multi-discriminant analysis & k-nearest neighbor. In: 2017 international conference on advances in computing, communications and informatics (ICACCI). pp 2251–2256
10. Schuster M, Paliwal KK (1997) Bidirectional recurrent neural networks. IEEE Trans Signal Process 45(11):2673–2681
11. Ariyo AA, Adewumi AO, Ayo CK (2014) Stock price prediction using the ARIMA model. In: 2014 UKSim-AMSS 16th international conference on computer modelling and simulation. pp 106–112

12. Jain S, Gupta R, Moghe AA (2018) Stock price prediction on daily stock data using deep neural networks. In: International conference on advanced computation and telecommunication (ICACAT). pp 1–13
13. Chikkakrishna NK, Hardik C, Deepika K, Sparsha N (2019) Short-term traffic prediction using sarima and FbPROPHET. In: 2019 IEEE 16th India Council International Conference (INDICON). pp 1–4
14. Qiu J, Wang B, Zhou C (2020) Forecasting stock prices with long-short term memory neural network based on attention mechanism. PLoS One 15:e0227222.
15. Li H, Shen Y, Zhu Y (2018) Stock price prediction using attention-based multi-input LSTM. In Asian conference on machine learning. pp 454–469
16. Zheng S, Ristovski K, Farahat A, Gupta C (2017) Long short-term memory network for remaining useful life estimation. In: IEEE international conference on prognostics and health management (ICPHM). pp 88–95

Feature Extraction and Comparison of EEG-Based Brain Connectivity Networks Using Graph Metrics

Mangesh Ramaji Kose, Mithilesh Atulkar, and Mitul Kumar Ahirwal

1 Introduction

The human brain is responsible for controlling the cognitive as well as physsical activities of a person [1]. Various disorders cause degradation in brain functionality. Epilepsy is one of the most common neurological disorders characterized by seizures causing abnormal functioning of the brain. About 37 million people around the world are suffering from epilepsy disorder [2]. The traditional approach for EEG-based epilepsy diagnosis includes two steps: (1) extracting features from time-series signal using signal processing technique and (2) applying classification algorithms to the extracted features for predicting whether the disorder is present or not. Many authors have applied this technique for the automated diagnosis of epilepsy disorder [3].

Antonio Quintero-Rincón et al. proposed a technique for the classification of epileptic EEG signals based on a Fast statistical model. The purpose of this technique is to identify the frequency band of the EEG signal where the epileptic seizure occurs and the classification of an epileptic seizure. They divided the EEG signals into different frequency bands and applied feature extraction and classification on different bands simultaneously [4]. Deriche et al. proposed a new feature extraction algorithm based on eigenspace time–frequency for epileptic seizure detection using EEG signals. The extracted features are classified using different classifiers and achieved an accuracy of 99.5% accuracy using a decision tree classifier [5]. Sharaf et al. [6] have introduced a novel approach for classifying the epileptic seizure and seizure-free EEG signals based on tunable Q-wavelet and firefly feature selection

M. R. Kose (✉) · M. Atulkar
National Institute of Technology, Raipur, India

M. Atulkar
e-mail: matulkar.mca@nitrr.ac.in

M. K. Ahirwal
Maulana Azad National Institute of Technology, Bhopal, India

© The Author(s), under exclusive license to Springer Nature Singapore Pte Ltd. 2021   11
M. K. Bajpai et al. (eds.), *Machine Vision and Augmented Intelligence—Theory and Applications*, Lecture Notes in Electrical Engineering 796,
https://doi.org/10.1007/978-981-16-5078-9_2

algorithm. The firefly algorithm is used to reduce the dimension of extracted features. After applying the random forest classification algorithm, 98% accuracy is obtained.

The feature-based techniques ignore the basic fact that the human brain is composed of different functional regions that work together to perform some task. In order to diagnose epilepsy, a functional connectivity network (FCN) of the whole brain needs to be considered. FCN defines the pattern of connection between different functionally characterized brain regions [7]. The connectivity of different functionally characterized brain regions is modeled using a graph also called network [8], henceforth, the terms network and graph will appear interchangeably. Applying graph-based approach to the field provides a systematic framework for comparing FCN related to different brain conditions.

This study focuses on the selection of graph-based metrics for comparing BCN corresponding to different brain conditions. The choice of graph theory-based measure varies for comparing the BCN having the same number of vertices and BCNs having different numbers of vertices. For comparing the BCNs having the same number of vertices, vertices/node-dependent graph metrics can be calculated, whereas for comparing the BCNs with different numbers of vertices, graph metrics independent of the number of vertices/nodes are calculated. The paper is arranged as follows: Sect. 1 presents the introduction of the study; Sect. 2 describes the methods and materials used; Sect. 3 presents the result and observations; and Sect. 4 is dedicated to conclusion and future scope.

2 Methodology

Initially, the section describes the dataset used for the study. After that, the BCN construction process is described in detail followed by graph metrics that can be extracted.

2.1 Dataset

TUH EEG epileptic dataset can be freely downloaded from [9]. TUH EEG epilepsy database consists of 1,648 EEG signal records, where 1,360 records are obtained from 133 subjects with epileptic seizure and 288 records are obtained from 104 healthy subjects. The majority of the EEG data was sampled at 250 Hz frequency. To generate a brain connectivity network and extract a graph matrix for both the epileptic and non-epileptic signals, channels other than EEG have been removed from the record, so that each record will have only EEG-related channels. The EEG signals were filtered using an FIR bandpass filter with a bandpass frequency range 1–45 Hz. The final database contains 19-channel EEG signals from a total of 28 participants including 14 epilepsy patients and 14 healthy participants. The 19 channels include Fp1, Fp2, F3, F4, C3, C4, P3, P4, O1, O2, F7, F8, T3, T4, T5, T6, Fz, Cz, and Pz [10].

2.2 Brain Connectivity Network

The BCN represents the association between functionally characterized brain regions. The process of constructing a functional brain connectivity network includes the following steps:

Define vertices/nodes of the BCN: In the case of EEG-based brain connectivity network, vertices are nothing but the channels used to record EEG signals. Hence, the location of vertices in the network is defined based on the location of the scalp used while recording the EEG data. The number of vertices in the functional brain connectivity network is equal to the number of EEG channels. Figure 1 represents node placement for brain connectivity network using 19-channel EEG signals record. Each blue filled circle represents one of the 19 channels of the EEG signal record, considered as the node for the brain connectivity network.

Calculating similarity measure between each pair of nodes: After defining the vertices of the brain connectivity network, the next step is to find the link between the pair of vertices. To connect the pair of nodes using the link, they must share some similar properties. In another way, if the pair of nodes is related to each other, the link will exist between those vertices; otherwise, the link will not exist. There are various connectivity/similarity measures available in the literature to evaluate the similarity between pair of vertices. In this study, the correlation coefficient is used as a similarity measure for identifying the correlation between pair of nodes [11]. The correlation coefficient (ρ_{XY}) is the measure of similarity between pair of EEG signals in time domain [12]. The correlation between channels X and Y is calculated using Eq. (1) [13] as follows:

$$\rho_{XY} = \frac{1}{M} \sum_{m=1}^{M} \frac{(X(m) - \phi_X)(Y(m) - \phi_Y)}{\Gamma_X \Gamma_Y} \tag{1}$$

Fig.1 Defining nodes for 19-channel EEG signal-based brain connectivity network

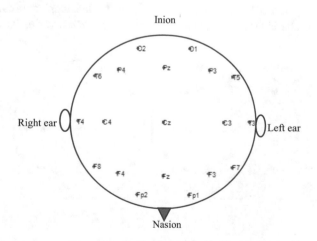

Here, M is the length of the signal; ϕ_X and ϕ_Y are the mean value of signals X and Y, respectively; and Γ_X and Γ_X are the standard deviation from signal X and Y, respectively. The range of the correlation coefficient is -1 to $+1$. The value of $+1$ means that the signals are positively correlated and -1 means the signals are negatively correlated. A value of 0 means the signals are not correlated.

Establishing a link between pair of vertices based on threshold value: After calculating the correlation between all the possible pairs of EEG channels, the next step is to establish a link between pair of vertices. The threshold value θ is required to put a lower limit on correlation value for establishing the link. The pair of nodes with a correlation value greater than chosen threshold value θ will have a link between them; otherwise, no link will be established. Equation (2) interprets the logic of deciding whether the link should be present or not based on the threshold value. The value of threshold θ must be chosen wisely [14]. The lower value of threshold results in a denser brain connectivity graph and a large value of threshold will produce a sparser network.

$$\left.\begin{array}{c} If \ \rho_{XY} \geq \theta, \ then \ link \ will \ be \ established \\ Otherwise, \ no \ link \ will \ be \ established \end{array}\right\} \qquad (2)$$

There is no standard value for the threshold mentioned in the literature. Following Fig. 2a, and c represents the effect of threshold on brain connectivity network from EEG signals of subject no. 1 from the healthy category of the used database. In this study, the correlation value 0.8 is considered as the threshold value θ.

After constructing the brain connectivity network, the next step is to compare the networks obtained from different categories of EEG signals (i.e. epileptic and normal). Comparison of brain connectivity networks can be performed on the basis of structural or/and quantitative analysis. Structural analysis is nothing but, identifying the topological patterns of the FCN. On the other hand, in the case of quantitative analysis, the graph-based measures are extracted from the FCN. There are various graph-based measures available in the literature that can be extracted from FCN. The choice of graph measures to be extracted varies based on whether the number

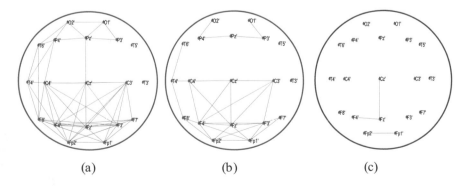

      (a)   (b)   (c)

Fig.2 Brain connectivity network for threshold value **a** 0.4, **b** 0.6, and **c** 0.8 of correlation coefficient

of nodes in all of the FCNs is equal or not. The following section describes different graph-based measures according to their dependency on the number of nodes.

2.3 Graph-Based Measures/metrics

As the brain connectivity is modeled as a graph, various graph-based measures need to be calculated for the purpose of comparing different brain networks based on quantitative analysis. The graph-based measures are categorized as (A) node-dependent measures and (B) node-independent measures. These different types of graph measures are discussed below in detail.

Node-independent graph measures (Network-level measures): For comparing the FCNs having a variable number of nodes, this category of measures was extracted. This category includes the following graph measures:

Characteristic path length: Integration is an important characteristic of a network. It represents the ability of a network to become interconnected and exchange information. This ability of the network is quantified using characteristic path length [15]. The characteristic path length is calculated using Eq. (3).

$$L = \frac{1}{N} \sum_{i=1}^{N} l_i \tag{3}$$

where l_i is the average shortest path length between node i and every other node, and it is calculated using Eq. (4).

$$l_i = \frac{1}{N-1} \sum_{i \neq j} l_{ij} \tag{4}$$

Here, l_{ij} is path length from node i to node j and N is the number of nodes in the network.

Assortativity coefficient [16, 17]: This is an important measure also called as the degree of correlation. It represents the tendency of a node with many connections in the network to connect to the other nodes with many connections and vice versa. The value of the assortativity coefficient (r) lies between -1 and $+ 1$, where -1 means the network is disassortative and $+ 1$ means the network is fully assortative. The assortative coefficient of the network can be calculated using Eq. (5).

$$r = \frac{l^{-1}\sum_{(i,j)\in L} k_i k_j - \left[l^{-1}\sum_{(i,j)\in L} \frac{1}{2}(k_i + k_j)\right]^2}{l^{-1}\sum_{(i,j)\in L} \frac{1}{2}(k_i^2 + k_j^2) - \left[l^{-1}\sum_{(i,j)\in L} \frac{1}{2}(k_i + k_j)\right]^2} \tag{5}$$

where k_i is the degree of node i, L is the characteristic path length, and l is the number of edges with a degree greater than k.

Modularity [18, 19]: It is the measure of segregation of the network. Modularity represents the measure of the ability of the network to get divided into modules, where the module is nothing but the collection of nodes having denser internal connections and sparser external connections. The modularity of the network with nodes N is calculated using Eq. (6).

$$Q = \frac{1}{2N(N-1)} \sum_{xy} \left(A_{xy} - \frac{K_x K_y}{N(N-1)} \right) \delta(\omega_x \omega_y) \qquad (6)$$

Here, ω_x and ω_y are the different modules containing node x and node y, respectively. A_{xy} is connectivity matrix having value 1 if there is a link between node x and y, otherwise 0. K_x is the degree of node x and K_y is the degree of node y.

Link density [20]: It is also called as connectivity density, which represents the ability of the network to resist connection failure. It is defined as the ratio of the number of edges present to the maximum possible number of edges that can be present in the network. It can be calculated using Eq. (7).

$$L = \frac{2E}{N(N-1)} \qquad (7)$$

where N is the number of nodes in the network and E is the number of edges/links available in the network.

Network transitivity [21, 22]: It is the variant of the classical clustering coefficient. It reflects the connectivity of a specialized region to its neighbors. This measure represents the ability of the brain to segregate into independent, local neighborhoods. Network transitivity can be calculated using Eq. (8).

$$T = \frac{\sum_{i \in N} 2t_i}{\sum_{i \in N} K_i(K_i - 1)} \qquad (8)$$

where t_i is the number of triangles around node I and K_i is the degree of node i.

Node-dependent graph measures: To extract these measures, FCNs must have the same number of nodes; otherwise, the obtained results will be biased. The node-independent graph measures are as follows:

Node degree [7, 23]: It is an important elementary measure of brain connectivity network. The degree of a node represents the number of links connecting that node to all the other nodes. It is used to show whether the node is important in the network or not, i.e. a node having a maximum degree is more important in the network. The node degree for node i can be calculated using Eq. (9).

$$K_i = \sum_{i \neq j} A_{ij} \qquad (9)$$

Here, A is the adjacency matrix. $'A'_{ij}$ will have value 1 if there is a link between node i and j, otherwise 0.

Betweenness centrality [7]: This graph-based measure represents the impact of a particular region in information flow over the brain network. It counts that how many times a particular node acts as a bridge along the shortest path of two other nodes. The betweenness centrality for ith node can be calculated using Eq. (10).

$$C_b(i) = \frac{2}{(N-1)(N-2)} \sum_{j \neq h \neq i} \frac{n_{hj}(i)}{n_{hj}} \tag{10}$$

Here, $n_{hj}(i)$ is the number of shortest paths between node h and j that pass through node i. n_{hj} represents the total number of shortest paths between node h and j.

Closeness centrality [24]: It is the most important measure of centrality; it measures the closeness of a node with all the other nodes. The closer to all the other nodes will have higher closeness centrality. This measure represents the indirect impact of the brain region over other brain regions. It is calculated using Eq. (11).

$$C_c(i) = \frac{N-1}{\sum_{i \neq j} l_{ij}} \tag{11}$$

Here, l_{ij} is the shortest path length between node i and j. N is the total number of nodes.

Participation coefficient [25]: Participation coefficient is an important measure that represents the edge distribution of the node. The node having the same number of links to all the modules in the network will have participation coefficient 1. The node having all the links within its own model will have a participation coefficient equal to 0. The participation coefficient for node i from module μ in the network having total C modules can be calculated using Eq. (12).

$$PC_i = 1 - \sum_{\mu=1}^{C} \left(\frac{K_{i,\mu}}{K_i} \right) \tag{12}$$

Here, $K_{i,\mu}$ represents the degree of ith node within module μ.

Within module degree(Z-score) [25]: The Z-score represents the strength of connectivity of a node in a module, i.e. how well a node i is connected to the other nodes in the same module. The Z-score of a node can be calculated using Eq. (13) as follows.

$$Z_i = \frac{K_i - K_\mu}{\Gamma_{K_\mu}} \tag{13}$$

Here, K_i is the degree of node i in module μ, K_μ is the average degree of all the nodes in module μ, and Γ_{K_μ} represents the standard deviation of K.

3 Results

After calculating graph measures mentioned in the above section, from epileptic and non-epileptic EEG signal-based brain connectivity network, the significance of each of the features is calculated. Classification and regression tree (CART) provides an approach for assigning the importance score for the input features depending on their ability to predict the class label. The CART represents the simple but very powerful approach for prediction. The differentiating factor from the linear regression approach is that it does not develop any predictive equation. The input data get divided into subsets, and the whole process is represented by a decision tree [26]. Detailed information and related mathematical expressions regarding decision tree regressor are available in [27].

Table 1 represents the individual as well as the average importance score assigned to each of the node-dependent features calculated from BCN. From the table, it is observed that, among all the node-dependent features, participation coefficient assigned the maximum individual as well as average importance score.

Table 2 lists the importance score assigned to each of the node-independent features calculated from BCN. The importance score for the features varies for each trial hence, the average importance score from each of the 10 trials is considered to identify the most important feature. From Table 2, it is observed that among the node-independent features, the network transitivity achieves maximum importance. Finally, comparing Tables 1 and 2, it is observed that the node-dependent feature participation coefficient is the most important feature obtained for BCN corresponding to epilepsy diseased and healthy subjects [25].

The results presented in Tables 1 and 2 are the importance score assigned to the respective features/graph metrics. Table 1 presents the 10 trials of importance score,

Table 1 Importance score for node-dependent features

| Trial | Node-dependent features | | | | |
	Node degree	Betweenness centrality	Closeness centrality	Participation coefficient	Within module degree
1	0.17	0.00	0.12	0.42	0.29
2	0.00	0.27	0.07	0.42	0.24
3	0.00	0.00	0.07	0.59	0.34
4	0.00	0.07	0.10	0.47	0.36
5	0.07	0.12	0.10	0.49	0.22
6	0.00	0.10	0.17	0.42	0.31
7	0.05	0.19	0.00	0.59	0.17
8	0.05	0.10	0.07	0.47	0.31
9	0.07	0.10	0.05	0.49	0.29
10	0.00	0.15	0.07	0.42	0.36
Average	0.04	0.11	0.08	0.48	0.29

Table 2 Importance score for node-independent features

Trial	Node-independent features				
	Characteristic path length	Assortativity coefficient	Modularity	Link density	Network transitivity
1	0.20	0.22	0.18	0.11	0.29
2	0.32	0.12	0.08	0.33	0.15
3	0.20	0.03	0.18	0.33	0.26
4	0.14	0.09	0.31	0.03	0.43
5	0.11	0.10	0.30	0.24	0.26
6	0.20	0.11	0.30	0.10	0.29
7	0.20	0.03	0.30	0.21	0.26
8	0.11	0.11	0.40	0.13	0.26
9	0.25	0.22	0.29	0.00	0.24
10	0.21	0.25	0.08	0.11	0.36
Average	0.20	0.13	0.24	0.16	0.28

i.e. the value of importance score varies each time, hence the average value of importance score for each of the graph metrics is considered for final comparison among all the graph metrics. The average importance score from node-dependent graph metrics is presented in Table 1. Observing Table 1, it is found that the maximum importance score is assigned to the participation coefficient and the minimum importance score is assigned to the node degree metrics. The participation coefficient is more effective for categorizing the networks belonging to different groups.

Similarly, observing Table 2, it is found that among the graph metrics, independent of the number of nodes in the network, the maximum importance score is assigned to the network transitivity and the minimum importance score is assigned to the assortativity coefficient. That means that the network transitivity graph metrics of the node-independent graph metrics gives more effective differentiation between diseased and healthy subject. Now, comparing Table 1 with Table 2, it is found that among all the types of graph metrics, with maximum importance score the participation coefficient is the most significant feature for brain disorder detection. Finally, the minimum importance score is assigned to the node degree.

4 Conclusion and Future Scope

This study implements an advanced approach for brain functionality analysis. The EEG signal-based BCN is constructed corresponding to epilepsy diseased as well as healthy subjects. To perform the analysis of the BCN, the graph metrics which can be used as features for classification tasks are calculated. The calculated features are of two types of graph-based metrics, i.e. the node-dependent metrics which are calculated when all the EEG records in the dataset have the same number of channels. On the other hand, the node-independent metrics are calculated, if the EEG datasets used for constructing BCN have different numbers of channels for different EEG records. This study compares these two types of features and finds the most important feature using the decision tree regressor-based importance score assigned to each feature. From the obtained results, it is observed that the node-dependent feature participation coefficient assigned the maximum importance score among all the features.

The study can be further extended by applying various classification algorithms on the most important features selected based on importance score and comparing the performance of classification algorithms. Instead of considering binary graphs the weighted graph-based features might provide more descriptive BCNs.

References

1. Mohammadi Z, Frounchi J, Amiri M (2017) Wavelet-based emotion recognition system using EEG signal. Neural Comput Appl 28:1985–1990. https://doi.org/10.1007/s00521-015-2149-8
2. Hassan M, Chaton L, Benquet P, Delval A, Leroy C, Plomhause L, Moonen AJH, Duits AA, Leentjens AFG, van Kranen-Mastenbroek V, Defebvre L, Derambure P, Wendling F, Dujardin K (2017) Functional connectivity disruptions correlate with cognitive phenotypes in Parkinson's disease. NeuroImage: Clinical 14:591–601. https://doi.org/10.1016/j.nicl.2017.03.002
3. Ullah I, Hussain M, Qazi E-H, Aboalsamh H (2018) An automated system for epilepsy detection using EEG brain signals based on deep learning approach. Expert Syst Appl 107:61–71. https://doi.org/10.1016/j.eswa.2018.04.021
4. Quintero-rincón A, Pereyra M, Giano CD, Risk M, Batatia H (2018) Science direct fast statistical model-based classification of epileptic EEG signals. Integr Med Res 38:877–889. https://doi.org/10.1016/j.bbe.2018.08.002
5. Deriche M, Arafat S, Siddiqui M (2019) Eigenspace time frequency based features for accurate seizure detection from EEG data. IRBM 40:122–132. https://doi.org/10.1016/j.irbm.2019.02.002
6. Sharaf AI, El-soud MA, El-henawy IM (2018) An automated approach for epilepsy detection based on tunable Q -wavelet and firefly feature selection algorithm. https://doi.org/10.1155/2018/5812872.
7. Liu J, Li M, Pan Y, Lan W, Zheng R, Wu F, Wang J (2017) Complex brain network analysis and its applications to brain disorders : a survey.
8. Ahirwal MK, Kumar A, Londhe ND, Bikrol H (2016) Scalp connectivity networks for analysis of EEG signal during emotional stimulation. In: International conference on communication and signal processing, ICCSP 2016. IEEE, pp 592–596. https://doi.org/10.1109/ICCSP.2016.7754208
9. Picone Joseph: Temple University EEG Corpus, https://www.isip.piconepress.com/projects/tuh_eeg/index.shtml., last accessed 2019/06/14.
10. Golmohammadi M, Ziyabari S, Shah V, Von Weltin E, Campbell C, Obeid I, Picone J (2018) Gated recurrent networks for seizure detection. In: 2017 IEEE signal processing in medicine and biology symposium, SPMB 2017—proceedings, pp 1–5, Jan 2018. https://doi.org/10.1109/SPMB.2017.8257020
11. Jalili M (2016) Functional brain networks: does the choice of dependency estimator and binarization method matter? Sci Rep 6:29780. https://doi.org/10.1038/srep29780
12. Ahirwal MK, Kose MR (2020) Audio-visual stimulation based emotion classification by correlated EEG channels. Heal Technol 10:7–23. https://doi.org/10.1007/s12553-019-00394-5

13. van Mierlo P, Papadopoulou M, Carrette E, Boon P, Vandenberghe S, Vonck K, Marinazzo D (2014) Functional brain connectivity from EEG in epilepsy: Seizure prediction and epileptogenic focus localization. https://doi.org/10.1016/j.pneurobio.2014.06.004.
14. Van Diessen E, Zweiphenning WJEM, Jansen FE, Stam CJ, Braun KPJ, Otte WM (2014) Brain network organization in focal epilepsy: a systematic review and meta-analysis. PLoS ONE 9:1–21. https://doi.org/10.1371/journal.pone.0114606
15. Rossini PM, Di Iorio R, Bentivoglio M, Bertini G, Ferreri F, Gerloff C, Ilmoniemi RJ, Miraglia F, Nitsche MA, Pestilli F, Rosanova M, Shirota Y, Tesoriero C, Ugawa Y, Vecchio ZU, Hallett M (2019) Methods for analysis of brain connectivity: an IFCN-sponsored review. Clin Neurophysi. https://doi.org/10.1016/j.clinph.2019.06.006.
16. Rocca MA, Valsasina P, Meani A, Falini A, Comi G, Filippi M (2016) Impaired functional integration in multiple sclerosis: a graph theory study. Brain Struct Funct 221:115–131. https://doi.org/10.1007/s00429-014-0896-4
17. Rubinov M, Sporns O (2010) NeuroImage Complex network measures of brain connectivity : uses and interpretations. 52:1059–1069. https://doi.org/10.1016/j.neuroimage.2009.10.003
18. Liu J, Li M, Pan Y, Lan W, Zheng R, Wu FX, Wang J (2017) Complex brain network analysis and its applications to brain disorders: a survey. Complexity 2017:1–27. https://doi.org/10.1155/2017/8362741
19. Brier MR, Thomas JB, Fagan AM, Hassenstab J, Holtzman DM, Benzinger TL, Morris JC, Ances BM (2014) Functional connectivity and graph theory in preclinical Alzheimer's disease. Neurobiol Aging 35:757–768. https://doi.org/10.1016/j.neurobiolaging.2013.10.081
20. Matrix THEC (2016) Connectivity matrices and brain graphs. Fundamentals of brain network analysis, pp 89–113. https://doi.org/10.1016/b978-0-12-407908-3.00003-0
21. Paldino MJ, Zhang W, Chu ZD, Golriz F (2017) NeuroImage : clinical metrics of brain network architecture capture the impact of disease in children with epilepsy. NeuroImage: Clinical 13:201–208. https://doi.org/10.1016/j.nicl.2016.12.005
22. Chen H, Song Y, Li X (2019) A deep learning framework for identifying children with ADHD using an EEG-based brain network. Neurocomputing 356:83–96. https://doi.org/10.1016/j.neucom.2019.04.058
23. Lee H, Golkowski D, Jordan D, Berger S, Ilg R, Lee J, Mashour GA, Lee U, Avidan MS, Blain-moraes S, Golmirzaie G, Hardie R, Hogg R, Janke E, Kelz MB, Maier K, Mashour GA, Maybrier H, Mckinstry-wu A, Muench M (2019) Relationship of critical dynamics, functional connectivity, and states of consciousness in large-scale human brain networks. NeuroImage 188:228–238
24. Opsahl T, Agneessens F, Skvoretz J (2010) Node centrality in weighted networks: generalizing degree and shortest paths. Soc Netw 32:245–251. https://doi.org/10.1016/j.socnet.2010.03.006
25. Aggarwal P, Gupta A (2019) Multivariate graph learning for detecting aberrant connectivity of dynamic brain networks in autism. Med Image Anal 56:11–25. https://doi.org/10.1016/j.media.2019.05.007
26. Regression Tree (2013). https://doi.org/10.1007/978-1-4419-9863-7_101273
27. Sklearn tree. Decision Tree Regressor—scikit-learn 0.15-git documentation. https://scikit-learn.org/0.15/modules/generated/sklearn.tree.DecisionTreeRegressor.html#examples-using-sklearn-tree-decisiontreeregressor. Accessed 12 Oct 2020

Mathematical Model with Social Distancing Parameter for Early Estimation of COVID-19 Spread

Saroj Kumar Chandra, Avaneesh Singh, and Manish Kumar Bajpai

1 Introduction

COVID-19 has emerged as a life-threatening outbreak disease. World Health Organization has declared COVID-19 as a pandemic in January 2020 [1]. The first case has been reported in Wuhan city of Hubei Province in South China on 31, December 2019 as unidentified pneumonia [2, 3]. COVID-19 disease has been identified as a member of the Severe Acute Respiratory Syndrome (SARS) that outbroke also in South China in 2002–2003 [4]. This disease is developed in the human body in the presence of a coronavirus. Tyrell and Bynoe have described the coronavirus in 1966 [5]. The virus is divided into four categories namely alpha, beta, gamma, and delta. Bats are a major source of alpha and beta virus category of the coronavirus. While gamma and delta originate from pigs and birds. Among these viruses, beta can infect human beings. The most common symptoms of COVID-19 are fever, tiredness, and dry cough. Some patients may have aches and pains, nasal congestion, runny nose, sore throat, or diarrhea. Around 1 out of every 6 people who get COVID-19 becomes seriously ill and develops difficulty breathing [6]. COVID-19 is a transmissible disease. Hence, people get infected with coronavirus from others (COVID patients) by coughs or sneezing [7]. No vaccine or antiviral treatment is available until now. The mortality rate is increasing day by day. The rapid spread of

S. K. Chandra
School of Computing Science and Engineering, Galgotias University, Uttar Pradesh, Gautam Budhha Nagar, Greater Noida, India

A. Singh (✉) · M. K. Bajpai
Department of Computer Science and Engineering, PDPM Indian Institute of Information Technology, Design and Manufacturing, Jabalpur, India
e-mail: avaneesh.singh@iiitdmj.ac.in

M. K. Bajpai
e-mail: mkbajpai@iiitdmj.ac.in

© The Author(s), under exclusive license to Springer Nature Singapore Pte Ltd. 2021
M. K. Bajpai et al. (eds.), *Machine Vision and Augmented Intelligence—Theory and Applications*, Lecture Notes in Electrical Engineering 796,
https://doi.org/10.1007/978-981-16-5078-9_3

the COVID-19 may be due to multiple causes. One cause is the lacking of information transparency at the early stage of the epidemic outbreak. Releasing the epidemic information in a timely and accurate way is extremely important for the anti-epidemic response of the public. The authentic and transparent information could have prohibited the spread of the COVID-19 at the early stage. The other cause is the lacking of the scientific diagnostic criterion for the COVID-19. As preventive measures, all the major countries have canceled events and classes in schools and colleges, and businesses have pushed work from home policies. All of these measures are adopted to slow the spread of the disease. These measures are broadly referred to as social distancing. In the present manuscript, a mathematical model is being developed for estimating COVID-19 disease. In addition, the proposed model incorporates the social distancing parameter for better spread estimation.

Mathematical modeling has gained more attention and awareness in epidemiology and the medical sciences [8–11]. It has been used for cancer detection, segmentation, and classification [12, 13]. These models are useful in cases where disease dynamics are not unclear. It estimates the number of cases in worst and best-case scenarios. Susceptible-Infected-Removed (SIR) and Susceptible-Exposed-Infected-Removed (SEIR) models are the most studied and used models to estimate disease spread. These models are helpful in estimating the effect of preventive measures on disease spread. The SIR model originated from the study of the plague almost one hundred years ago. This model estimates spread by using contact rate and infection period only. It has been observed that this model is not suitable for estimating the spread in which the incubation period is involved such as COVID-19. Hence, the SEIR model is a suitable model for estimating COVID-19 spread since it incorporates the incubation period. However, the SEIR model failed to estimate the spread where preventive measures are adopted such as social distancing. In the present manuscript, a modified SEIR model is presented estimating COVID-19 spread. The proposed model has incorporated the social distancing parameter for a more accurate estimation of COVID-19 disease. Our main contribution is to include the social distancing parameter and to analyze the spread scenario and its effect. The novelty of current work is to include the social distancing parameter in two scenarios: first, before lockdown, and second, after lockdown.

The present work is organized as follows. The mathematical model for COVID-19 spread estimation is presented in Sect. 2. Section 3 discusses the results obtained by the proposed mathematical model.

2   Proposed Methodology with Social Distancing

In this section, a modified SEIR mathematical model is being presented for estimating COVID-19 spread. The proposed model uses the basic SEIR model to design a novel mathematical model. The SEIR model is a compartmental model for estimating disease spread in the population. It's an acronym for Susceptible, Exposed, Infected, and Recovered. When a disease is introduced to a population, the people move from one compartment to another compartment. When people has reached to R state, then the people either survived the disease or out of the population. The classical SEIR is defined by the following equations:

$$\frac{ds}{dt} = -\beta \times S \times I \tag{1}$$

$$\frac{dE}{dt} + \beta \times S \times I - \alpha \times E \tag{2}$$

$$\frac{dI}{dt} = \alpha \times E - \gamma \times I \tag{3}$$

$$\frac{dR}{dt} = \gamma \times I \tag{4}$$

Here, Eqs. (1), (2), (3), and (4) represent four Ordinary Differential Equations (ODEs). The three parameters are α, β, and γ. These are defined as follows:

α is the inverse of the incubation period.
β is the average contact rate in the population.
γ is the inverse of the mean infectious period.

Equation (1) is the change in people susceptible to the disease and is moderated by the number of infected people and their contact with the infected. Equation (2) gives the people who have been exposed to the disease. It grows based on the contact rate and decreases based on the incubation period whereby people then become infected. Equation (3) gives us the change in infected people based on the exposed population and the incubation period. It decreases based on the infectious period, so the higher γ is, the more quickly people die/recover and move on to the final stage in Eq. (4). The proposed mathematical model is shown in Fig. 1.

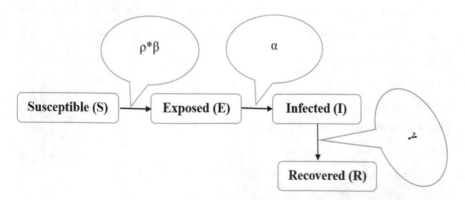

Fig. 1 Proposed mathematical model with social distancing

In the proposed model, a novel factor ρ has been introduced as a social distancing parameter. Social distancing is maintained in transmissible diseases like COVID-19. It includes avoiding large gatherings, physical contact, and other efforts to mitigate the spread of infectious diseases. This parameter controls contact rate, β. The social distancing parameter ρ lies in the range 0 and 1, where 0 indicates everyone is locked down and quarantined while 1 is equivalent to our base case above. Equations (1) and (2) are being multiplied with a parameter to have a social distancing effect. The modified equations are defined as follows:

$$\frac{dS}{dt} = -\rho \times \beta \times S \times I \tag{5}$$

$$\frac{dE}{dt} = \rho \times \beta \times S \times I - \alpha \times E \tag{6}$$

3 Results and Discussion

All the experimental studies have been performed on PYTHON. The machine used for performing simulation work has CPU clock speed 1.60 GHz, 8 GB RAM, 256 KB L1 cache, 1.0 MB L2 cache, and 6.0 MB L3 cache hardware configuration. The proposed mathematical model has been validated in cases of COVID-19 in India [14]. The day-wise COVID-19 cases are shown in Fig. 2. The state-wise active COVID-19 cases in India are shown in Fig. 2 [15]. It can be analyzed from Fig. 2 that COVID-19 cases are increasing day by day.

The state-wise COVID-19 cases are Tabulated in Table 1. It can be easily analyzed from Table 1 that Maharashtra, Delhi, Tamil Nadu, Uttar Pradesh, Madhya

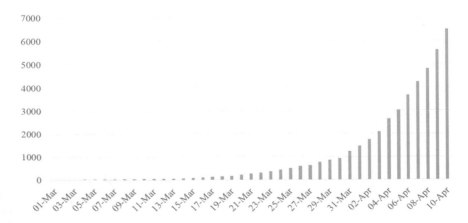

Fig. 2 Day-wise active COVID-19 cases in India

Table 1 Total number of confirmed state-wise cases in India till 17-March-2020

Name of state/ UT	Total confirmed cases	Cured/ discharged	Death
Andaman and Nicobar Islands	11	10	0
Andhra Pradesh	534	20	14
Arunachal Pradesh	1	0	0
Assam	35	5	1
Bihar	74	29	1
Chandigarh	21	7	0
Chhattisgarh	33	17	0
Delhi	1578	42	32
Goa	7	5	0
Gujarat	871	64	36
Haryana	205	43	3
Himachal Pradesh	35	16	1
Jammu and Kashmir	300	36	4
Jharkhand	28	0	2
Karnataka	315	82	13
Kerala	388	218	3
Ladakh	17	10	0
Madhya Pradesh	1120	64	53
Maharashtra	2919	295	187
Manipur	2	1	0
Meghalaya	7	0	1
Mizoram	1	0	0
Nagaland	0	0	0
Odisha	60	18	1
Puducherry	7	1	0
Punjab	18	27	13
Rajasthan	1023	147	3
Tamil Nadu	1242	118	14
Telangana	698	120	18
Tripura	2	1	0
Uttarakhand	37	9	0
Uttar Pradesh	773	68	13
West Bengal	231	42	7

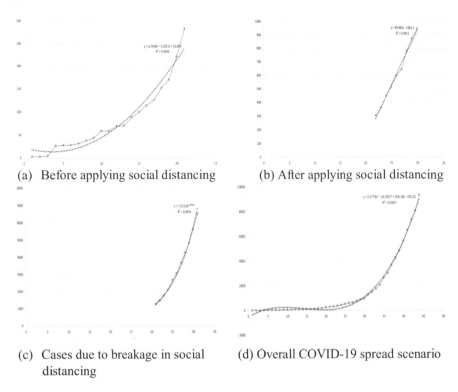

(a) Before applying social distancing   (b) After applying social distancing

(c) Cases due to breakage in social   (d) Overall COVID-19 spread scenario
    distancing

Fig. 3 Active COVID-19 cases spread scenarios in India

Pradesh, Telangana, and Rajasthan are major affected states with COVID-19 diseases. The COVID-19 spread behavior with different measurements such as before and after applying social distancing and spread due to breakage in maintaining social distancing have been shown in Fig. 3.

Figure 3a shows polynomial spread behavior with degree 2 before applying social distancing. The effect of social distancing can be seen in Fig. 3b which shows a reduction of spread behavior from polynomial to linear. Exponential behavior has been analyzed by breaking the social distancing as can be seen in Fig. 3c. The overall spread behavior up to 10 April 2020 is shown in Fig. 3d. Figure 3d shows how spread behavior has been changed from polynomial of degree 2 to polynomial of degree 3. The overall population has been considered as susceptible cases. The experimental studies have been performed on 10,000 population. The cases which do not belong to susceptible cases either belong to exposed, infected, or recovered. The people who have contacted recently infected people move to exposed cases. The exposed cases move to infected after completion of the incubation period. The infected people's moves recover cases after successful completion of coronavirus cycle, clinical process, or death.

The value of incubation period α has been fixed with 0.2, and an infection period of 0.5 days has been considered in all modes for validating the proposed methodology

[16, 17]. The performance of the proposed mathematical model works in two different modes. The first mode works on the classical SEIR model in which the value of the social distancing rate ρ is fixed to 1. In this mode, the spread of disease depends only on the contact rate β. The result obtained by the proposed mathematical model with $\rho = 1$ and $\beta = 1.5$, $\beta = 1.75$, and $\beta = 2.0$ has been shown in Fig. 4. The green line shows COVID-19 spread with $\beta = 1.5$, similarly red and blue line shows spread with $\beta = 1.75$ and $\beta = 2.0$, respectively. It can be easily analyzed from the green dotted line that spread is about 3% in 21 day, which is approximately the same as COVID-19 disease spread before applying social distancing in India. It can be also analyzed that if this spread has been followed, then the maximum 35% population could have been suffered from COVID-19 disease in 30 days.

The second mode is with different social distancing rates. The results obtained have been shown in Fig. 5. It has been analyzed with about 300 active cases. It can be easily analyzed from the green dotted line that spread is about 10% in 10 days, which is approximately the same as COVID-19 disease spread after applying social distancing in India. Hence, it can be also analyzed that spread behavior is linear in nature. In addition, it can be said that if this spread has been followed, then the

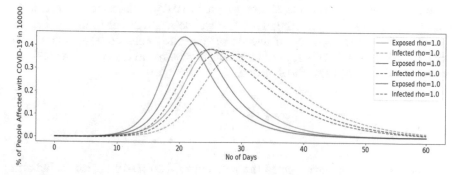

Fig. 4 COVID-19 Spread before applying social distancing with $\rho = 1$

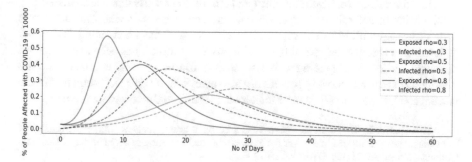

Fig. 5 COVID-19 spread after applying different social distancing rates

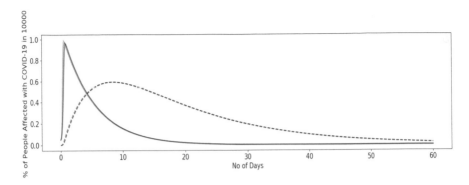

Fig. 6 COVID-19 spread due to breakage in social distancing

maximum 30% population could have been suffered from COVID-19 disease in 30 days.

The sudden increase has been analyzed after 30 March 2020. This is due to the breakage of social distancing as a gathering of people. It can be easily observed from Fig. 6 that spread is about to 60% people in 10 days which closely resembles COVID-19 spread after gathering. Hence, it can be said that due to this gathering, the spreading behavior has been changed from linear to a polynomial of degree 3. In addition, it is found that 60 days of lockdown is required in the current scenario to complete recovery of COVID-19 disease.

4 Conclusion

The present work has investigated the problem of COVID-19 spread in India in current scenarios. A mathematical model has been established, which follows the actual data trend of COVID-19 spread in India. It has been proved from analytical (based on mathematical modeling) and simulation results that social distancing plays an important role in spread estimation. The effect of social distancing has been discussed with different social distancing rates. It has been found that social distancing can reduce the spread from polynomial to linear. It has been also observed breakage in social distancing can rise spread from linear to exponential. The maximum cases and recovery periods are also analyzed. It has been found that in the current spread scenario 60 days of lockdown is required for complete recovery.

Acknowledgements The work has been supported by a grant received from the Ministry of Education, Government of India under the Scheme for the Promotion of Academic and Research Collaboration (SPARC) (ID: SPARC/2019/1396).

References

1. Organization WH (2020) Novel coronavirus (2019-nCoV) advice for the public. https://www.who.int/emergencies/diseases/novel-coronavirus-2019/advice-for-public
2. Hongzhou Lu1 CWS, Tang Y (2020) Outbreak of pneumonia of unknown etiology in Wuhan, China: the mystery and the miracle. J Med Virol 401–402
3. Zhong L, Mu L, Li J, Wang J, Yin Z, Liu D (2020) Early prediction of the 2019 novel coronavirus outbreak in the mainland china based on simple mathematical model IEEE access 8 2020, pp 51761–51769. https://doi.org/10.1109/ACCESS.2020.2979599
4. Haung M, Zou L, Ruan Γ (2020) Sars-cov-2 viral load in upper respiratory specimens of infected patients, N Engl J Med 382:1177–1179.
5. Williamson G (2020) Covid-19 epidemic editorial. The open Nurs J 14:37–38. https://doi.org/10.2174/1874434602014010037
6. Zarebski A, Mizumoto K, Kagaya K (2020) Estimating the asymptomatic proportion of coronavirus disease 2019 (covid-19) cases on board the diamond princess cruise ship, yokohama, japan, 2020. Eeurosurveillance, Epub ahead of print 25
7. Kwok K, Lai F, Wei W, Wong S, Tang J. Herd immunity estimating the level required to halt the covid-19 epidemics in affected countries J Infect. https://doi.org/10.1016/j.jinf.2020.03.027.
8. Blackwood JC, Childs L (2018) An introduction to compartmental modeling for the budding infectious disease modeler. Lett Biomath 5:195–221
9. Huppert A, Katriel G (2013) Mathematical modelling and prediction in infectious disease epidemiology. Clin Microbiolog Infect 19(11):999–1005. https://doi.org/10.1111/1469-0691.12308. http://www.sciencedirect.com/science/article/pii/S1198743X14630019
10. Lizarralde-Bejarano DP, Arboleda-Snchez S, Puerta-Yepes ME (2017) Understanding epidemics from mathematical models: details of the 2010 dengue epidemic in bello (antioquia, colombia). Appl Math Modell 43:566–578. https://doi.org/10.1016/j.apm.2016.11.022. http://www.sciencedirect.com/science/article/pii/S0307904X16306278
11. Longini IM (1988) A mathematical model for predicting the geographic spread of new infectious agents. Math Biosci 90(1):367–383. https://doi.org/10.1016/0025-5564(88)90075-2. http://www.sciencedirect.com/science/article/pii/0025556488900752
12. Chandra SK, Bajpai MK (2019) Mesh free alternate directional implicit method based three dimensional super-diffusive model for benign brain tumor segmentation. Comput Math Appl. https://doi.org/10.1016/j.camwa.2019.02.009. http://www.sciencedirect.com/science/article/pii/S089812211930077X
13. Chandra SK, Bajpai MK (2020) Fractional mesh-free linear diffusion method for image enhancement and segmentation for automatic tumor classification. Biomed Sign Process Control 58. https://doi.org/10.1016/j.bspc.2019.101841. http://www.sciencedirect.com/science/article/pii/S1746809419304227
14. Worldometer, Coronavirus Update (Live): 1,521,090 cases, 88,565 deaths and 331,354 recovered cases from COVID-19 virus outbreak. https://www.worldometers.info/coronavirus/
15. Ministry of health and family welfare: Goverment of India. https://www.mohfw.gov.in/
16. Hellewell J et al (2020) Feasibility of controlling covid-19 outbreaks by isolation of cases and contacts. Lancet Glob Health 8(4):488–496
17. Liangrong P, Yang W, Zhang D, Zhuge C, Hong L (2020) Epidemic analysis of covid-19 in china by dynamical modelingdoi. https://doi.org/10.1101/2020.02.16.20023465

NVM Device-Based Deep Inference Architecture Using Self-gated Activation Functions (Swish)

Afroz Fatima and Abhijit Pethe

1 Introduction

Neural-inspired computing has become a compelling area of research in the past decade with applications in varied field such as robotics, image, speech and video recognition, cyber security [1]. The implementation of neurons and synapses in the conventional neuromorphic processors had been in the CMOS process and the more recent ones have been designed using memristors and hybrid technology (CMOS with memristors) due to the scaling limits of transistors. Resistive Random-Access Memory (RRAM) have been proven suitable candidate for designing both the neuron circuits and electronic synapses. The RRAM devices generally consume low power, have better data density than DRAM, perform faster than FLASH memory, and are reliable and resilient in nature [2]. When an input arrives at the pre-neuron circuit, it gets combined with their respective synaptic weights and fires an action potential signal to the post-neuron circuit. This process continues depending upon the number of input neurons and synapses considered. A typical structure of neuron and synapse is shown in Fig. 1.

The neuron function (independent of bias) can be expressed as

$$\text{Output Neuron} = f(w_1x_1 + w_2x_2 + \ldots + w_nx_n) \tag{1}$$

where 'f' is the non-linear activation function; w_1, $w_2 \ldots w_n$ are weights; and x_1, $x_2 \ldots x_n$ are inputs.

A. Fatima (✉) · A. Pethe
Electrical and Electronics Engineering Department, Birla Institute of Technology and Science Pilani, K K Birla Goa Campus, Goa 403726, India
e-mail: p20180404@goa.bits-pilani.ac.in

A. Pethe
e-mail: abhijitp@goa.bits-pilani.ac.in

© The Author(s), under exclusive license to Springer Nature Singapore Pte Ltd. 2021
M. K. Bajpai et al. (eds.), *Machine Vision and Augmented Intelligence—Theory and Applications*, Lecture Notes in Electrical Engineering 796,
https://doi.org/10.1007/978-981-16-5078-9_4

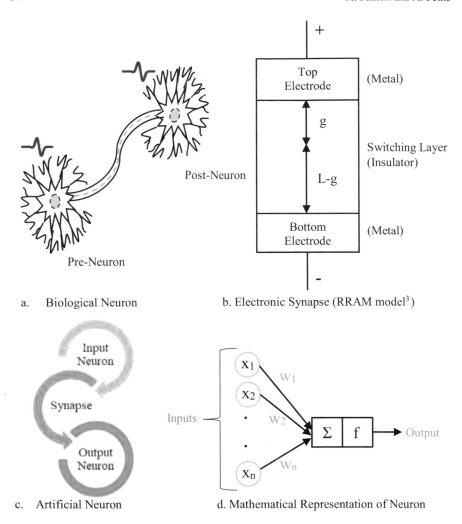

Fig. 1 Neuron-synapse structure

Typically, a linear function is not conducive in solving complex problems in deep neural networks as linear activation function in the hidden layer outputs only a linear function of the inputs and this keeps happening, no matter how much deep the neural network is [4]. Consequently, a non-linearity is added at the end of the output to provide a constructive solution for deep neural networks. A substantial list of activation functions had been demonstrated in software for machine learning applications, whereas the hardware implementations of the activation functions have been sub-ordinate in literature. In this paper, we present the design of non-linear Self-Gated Activation Function (Swish) [5] for analog hardware applications using the RRAM devices [3]. The electronic synapse has been implemented using the

1T-1RRAM crossbar structure. This design speeds up the dot-product operation, is energy efficient and has low latency counts [6]. The main aspect of RRAM is its nature of changing the conductance state when a positive or negative voltage is applied. The switching of conductance state signifies that the weights have been applied to the neural network. RRAM is a 2-terminal device with Metal–Insulator-Metal stack as depicted in Fig. 1b. The model consists of metal-oxide-based RRAM devices with bipolar switching characteristics.

This paper exhibits key aspects of artificial neural networks such as suitable activation functions for NVM applications, details on how the deep neural architecture is designed and implemented for inference of the neural network across three datasets. The paper is further organized as Sect. 2 presents the background about the inference architecture by highlighting some recent neuromorphic processors that has proven NVM technology as a viable solution to replace CMOS, Sect. 3 discusses the importance of non-linear activation functions in neural networks and compares the proposed Swish Activation Function using RRAM to the existing Activation Functions from literature, Sect. 4 details on the implementation methodology of the deep inference architecture using RRAM and showcases the datasets being employed for classification tasks, Sect. 5 gives comprehensive details on the results obtained and Sect. 6 concludes the paper.

2 Background

Different classes of NVM technologies such as Resistive Random-Access Memory (RRAM), Phase Change Memory (PCM), Spin Transfer Torque-Magnetic RAM (STT-MRAM) have been extensively used for the design of neural crossbar architectures for performing dedicated tasks of inferring and training the deep neural network in order to further propose unique circuit-level solutions [7, 8]. Recent results show that the semiconductor industry has heavily invested in NVM technologies with their fabricated process being commercially available to the market, some examples include TSMC's 40 nm RRAM, Intel's 22 nm RRAM, TSMC's 40 nm PCM, Intel's 22 nm STT-MRAM, Samsung's 28 nm STT-MRAM, and an emerging 22 nm FeFET from Global Foundries [9, 10]. Besides the above, the recent prototype chips relying on the NVM technologies include IBM's PCM, UMass and UMich's RRAM for 'training' and Panasonic, NTHU and ASU/ GaTech's RRAM for 'inference' of the deep neural network architectures [9, 10]. RRAMs have been preferred in this paper due to its advantages such as high density, low leakage power, non-volatility, parallel-readout operation multi-level programming, fast switching (sub-ns), good retention (>10 years), and high endurance (>Megacycles) [11, 12]. Another important consideration while designing the neural network is the 'activation function' as this helps in generating the action potential or spike from the present layer and transmit it to the next layer. The name itself signifies that it activates the circuit for firing a signal. Recently, the Swish Activation Function from Google Brain has been proven successful across a number of datasets as it improves top-1 classification accuracy on ImageNet by 0.9% for Mobile NASNet-A and 0.6% for Inception-ResNet-v2 [5]. However, only ReLU and Sigmoid function have been investigated for analog circuits using memristors. In this paper, we have considered the Swish Activation function using RRAMs for the task of classification using the deep neural network across multiple datasets.

3 Activation Functions

3.1 Role of Activation Functions in Neural Networks

Activation Functions generally represent the rate of firing a signal depending upon the input applied. The rate at which the signal is fired is called as firing potential or action potential signifying the potentiation (Na^+) and depression (K^+) in the form of a spike signal activity. In biology, these action potentials are abstracted when the neurotransmitters release the Ca^{2+} and Mg^{2+} ions by opening their voltage-gated channels and fire an activation signal at the output and this activity lasts for a few milli-seconds in the brain. The action potentials can be controlled by increasing or decreasing the input current.

Activation functions may be linear or non-linear. Linear activation functions mostly fail in complex neural networks, if we compute two linear functions then, the result would be linear itself which is inappropriate in deep neural networks. The non-linear functions are responsible for the mappings between the inputs and response variables with the main aim to convert an input signal of a node in a neural network to an output signal which will be used as an input in the next layer in the stack. Unless we add some non-linearity in the deep neural network, the system will not produce accurate results as it is same as not having a network deep enough or having just a shallow network, because using a linear activation function would only lead to producing outputs which are again linear in nature. Due to the limitations of linear activation functions, it is rarely used except in some circumstances like prediction of house prices [4]. Non-linear activation functions are considered good at performing complex tasks when the network is deep with many hidden layers.

There is a diverse list of activation functions in neural networks having specific working range and mathematical property of a function. Some of the most widely used activation functions in machine learning applications are Sigmoid, TanH, Rectified Linear Unit (ReLU), Exponential Linear Unit (ELU), Gaussian Error Linear Unit (GELU), Sigmoid Linear Unit (SiLU/Swish), Sinusoid, etc., having different mathematical property and range of operation. The above functions have been widely adopted in the software for machine learning applications, whereas only a few have been investigated using hardware circuits. In this paper, we have considered the Sigmoid Linear Unit or Self-Gated Activation Function (Swish) for the implementation of deep inference architecture using the 1T-1RRAM crossbars.

3.2 Implementation of Self-Gated Activation Function (Swish) Using Resistive Random-Access Memory (RRAM)

Swish is a smooth, non-monotonic function with one-sided boundedness at zero. Swish was initially designed to improve the performance characteristics of ReLU function for deep models and challenging datasets. Experimental results show that Swish outperforms ReLU for deep neural networks for applications such as image classification and machine translation [5].

Swish activation function is defined as [5],

$$f(x) = \frac{x}{1 + e^{-x}} \tag{2}$$

where 'x' is the input and '$f(x)$' is the output.

Besides being smooth and non-monotonic, swish is unbounded above and bounded below and this makes it different from the other activation functions [5].

3.2.1 Working Principle

Swish activation function has been designed using 5 pairs of CMOS transistors of Length = 180 nM and Total Width = 2 uM each, 2 RRAM devices and a 2-input multiplier circuit as defined in (2) and shown in Fig. 2. The circuit is controlled by a dc voltage and the bias voltages ($\pm V_\beta$) from T_1-T_2 are used to turn 'ON/OFF' the transistors T_3-T_{10}. Initially when a high voltage is given to the input 'x', i.e., the

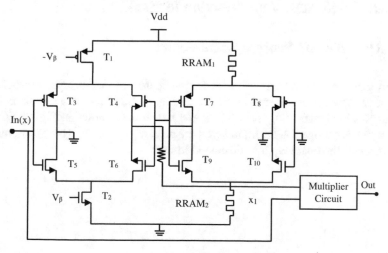

Fig. 2 Design of self-gated activation function (Swish) using RRAM

Table 1 Comparison of NVM device-based activation functions in analog circuits

Parameters	Sigmoid [13]	ReLU [14]	Swish [This work]
Cell structure	10 T-2 M	1Comparator-2 M	10 T-2RRAM-1Multiplier
Device	Memristor	Memristor	RRAM
Operating voltage	± 3 V	-	1.2 V
Total power	3 mW	-	498 uW (peak)
Ron	-	125 kΩ	267.8 kΩ
Roff	-	125 MΩ	11.4 kΩ
On/Off ratio	-	10^6	23.49

gates of the transistors T_3 and T_5, it will cause the 'nmos' to conduct and 'pmos' not to conduct, while a low voltage on the input will cause it to reverse and causes the $RRAM_1$ and $RRAM_2$ to switch their state from High Resistance State (HRS) to Low Resistance State (LRS) (the set process) and LRS to HRS (the reset process) by making both the 'nmos' and 'pmos' transistors to conduct briefly during the switching period thereby inducing a signal at 'x_1' of the multiplier circuit. The signal 'x_1'drives the output for sigmoid equation $(1/(1 + e^{-x}))$ and this signal is combined with the initial input 'x' using the multiplier circuit for generating the final output signal of the swish equation $(x/(1 + e^{-x}))$. The output signal obtained is a smooth, non-monotonic function with a one-sided boundedness at zero as illustrated in Fig. 5 which satisfies the Swish property. Table 1 of Sect. 5 presents the swish-RRAM (this work) and sigmoid-ReLU-memristor device results (from [13, 14]).

4 RRAM-Based Deep Inference Architecture Using Self-Gated Activation Function (Swish)

4.1 Deep Neural Network Architecture

A 2-layer artificial neural network with 4 input neurons, 4 hidden layer neurons, and 4 output neurons is considered as shown in Fig. 3 and two 4 × 4 crossbars fit in as synapses (weights) using the 1T-1RRAM structure as shown in Fig. 4. When a neuron receives a signal at the input layer, the respective layer weights get combined and processes the final output as discussed in Sect. 1.

Fig. 3 Two layer artificial
neural network

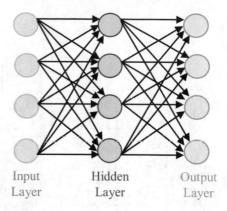

Input   Hidden   Output
Layer   Layer   Layer

4.2 Deep Inference Architecture Using NVM Devices and Self-Gated Activation Functions

The deep neural network has been designed using two 4×4 crossbar array structures comprising of 1T-1RRAM cells acting as switches. The crossbar structure consists of large array of wires and in between each pair of wires there is 1T-1RRAM cell. Initially, all the cells are open (OFF) and no information is passed but if we start closing (ON) some of the cells, we can program the crossbar with the desired information. When a positive/negative voltage is applied, the RRAM device moves the oxygen molecules down/up by switching the RRAM's resistance state from HRS (OFF state) to LRS (ON state) or vice-versa. Depending upon the voltage (V_i) and weights applied, the parallel multiply and accumulate operation draws a current (I) at the end of each column as defined in (3). The dot product works on the principle of Ohm's and Kirchhoff's law [6, 15].

The columnar output current can be expressed as

$$I = \sum (Gij \times Vi) \tag{3}$$

where i and $j = 1,2,3\ldots n$ (depending on size of the network).

The linear current driving at the end of each column is processed by applying the non-linear self-gated activation function as depicted in Fig. 4. and given to the next crossbar layer as the input, the same process continues until a final output at the end of the second layer is obtained. The above process is executed in forward-propagation mode for the deep neural network considered. The proposed architecture has been

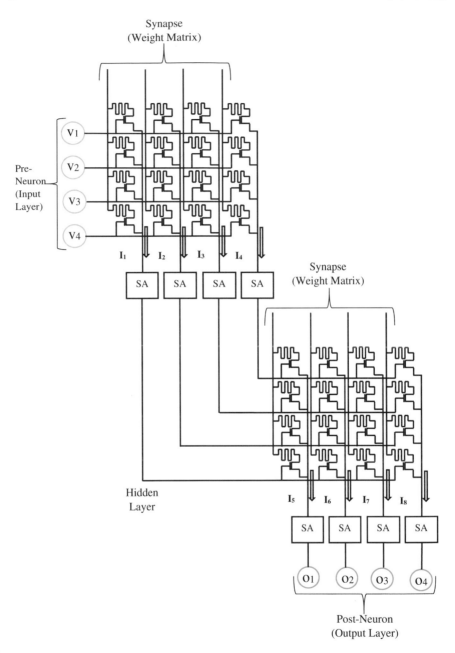

Fig. 4 Design of 2-layer neural networks using 4 × 4 crossbars (SA = swish activation circuit)

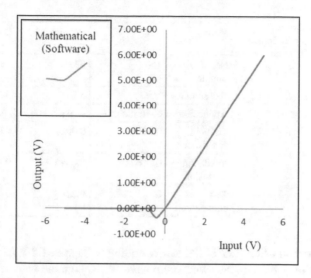

Fig. 5 Analog hardware characteristics of swish activation function

Table 2 Figure of merits: 1T-1RRAM cell

Parameters	1T-1RRAM
Technology node	180 nm
Switching time	2.28 ns
Conductance	17.39 mhos
Ron	267.8 kΩ
Roff	11.4 kΩ
On/Off ratio	23.49

trained 'offline' on Fisher's Iris [16], Balance scale [17], and Bank note authentication [18] datasets to perform the classification task using forward-propagation/inference method on the deep neural network. Table 2 of Sect. 5 presents the device metrics of the proposed architecture. This design can be extended for deeper networks with 'n' number of hidden layers.

5 Results and Discussion

The simulation results of the proposed architecture are presented below along with a comparative analysis of the Self-Gated activation function using RRAM with Sigmoid and ReLU using memristors. The swish activation function with RRAM devices outperforms sigmoid and ReLU with memristors on parameters such as operating voltage, total power, and device resistance states (ON & OFF). The swish

Table 3 Performance metrics of the deep inference architecture on different datasets

Metric	Iris	Balance scale	Bank note authentication
No. of samples	150	625	1372
Test samples	10%	5%	5%
Application	Classification	Classification	Classification
Training confusion	0.0167	0.0924	0.0105
Validation confusion	0.0667	0.0645	0
Test confusion	0	0.129	0

activation function using RRAM has low operating voltage of 1.2 V and low power consumption of 498uW (Peak) when compared to the sigmoid activation function with memristors that used $\pm$ 3 V operating voltage and almost 3mW of total power. The resistance switching characteristic from ON state to OFF state is observed at 2.38 ns with a conductance of 17.39mhos in the 1T-1RRAM cell structure of the deep inference architecture as in Table 2. Further, the performance metrics of the architecture on three datasets have been shown in Table 3. The iris and bank note authentication dataset have a test confusion rate of '0' which signifies that the network has classified correctly from the trained samples and have a 100% classification accuracy, whereas the balance scale dataset has a test confusion rate of 0.129 with a classification accuracy of 99.87% for the deep neural network considered. The outputs obtained for the deep inference architecture using three datasets have been plotted in Fig. 6. depicting the activations for the desired combination of inputs.

6   Conclusion

The role of non-linear activation functions in analog hardware was demonstrated through a comparative analysis of the Swish activation function with RRAM on Sigmoid and ReLU functions with memristors. The simulation results illustrate that the swish function has low operating voltage of 1.2 V, low power consumption of 498uW as opposed to sigmoid with memristors and the resistance switching behavior was observed at 267.8 k (ON state) and 11.4 k (OFF state) as opposed to the ReLU function with memristors. Also, the deep inference architecture with swish activation function using RRAM devices have resistance switching speed at 2.38 ns with 100% classification accuracy on iris and bank note authentication datasets and 99.87% classification accuracy on balance scale dataset.

Fig. 6 Inference outputs of the deep inference architecture

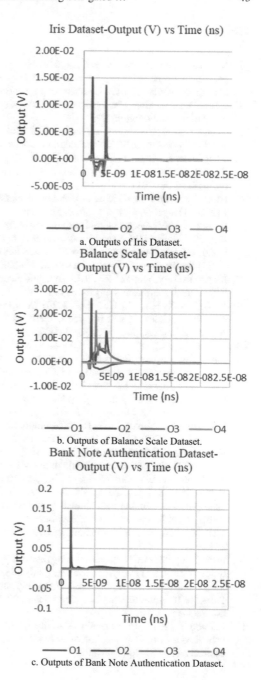

a. Outputs of Iris Dataset.

b. Outputs of Balance Scale Dataset.

c. Outputs of Bank Note Authentication Dataset.

References

1. Bersuker G, Mason M, Jones KL (2018) Neuromorphic computing: the potential for high performance processing in space. Center for space policy and strategy, pp 1–12. https://aerosp ace.org/sites/default/files/2018-12/Bersuker_NeuromorphicComputing_12132018.pdf
2. International Roadmap for Devices and Systems (2020) More Moore. IEEE. https://irds.ieee. org/editions/2020/more-moore
3. Chen PY, Yu S (2015) Compact modeling of RRAM devices and its applications in 1T1R and 1S1R array design. IEEE Trans Electron Devices 62(12):4022–4028
4. Goodfellow I, Bengio Y, Courville A (2016) Deep learning. MIT Press, pp 198–201
5. Ramachandran P, Zoph B, Le QV (2017) Swish: a self-gated activation function. Google brain, pp.1–12, 16 Oct 2017
6. Hu M, Strachan JP, Li Z, Grafals EM, Davila N, Graves C, Lam S, Ge N, Williams RS, Yang J (2016) Dot-product engine for neuromorphic computing: programming 1T1M crossbar to accelerate matrix-vector multiplication. Hewlett packard labs, 3 March 2016
7. Burr GW, Shelby RM, Sebastian A, Kim S, Kim S, Sidler S, Virwani K, Ishii M, Narayanan P, Fumarola A, Sanches LL, Boybat I, Le Gallo M, Moon K, Woo J, Hwang H, Leblebici Y (2017) Neuromorphic computing using non-volatile memory. Adv Phys: X 2(1):89–124
8. Kuzum D, Yu S, Wong H-SP (2013) Synaptic electronics: materials, devices and applications, IOP science. Nanotechnology 24(38)
9. Yu S, Sun X, Peng X, Huang S (2020) Compute-in-memory with emerging non-volatile-memories: challenges and prospects. IEEE custom integrated circuits conference (CICC). Boston, MA, USA, pp 1–4, 23 April 2020
10. Chou C et al (2018) An N40 256K×44 embedded RRAM macro with SL-precharge SA and low-voltage current limiter to improve read and write performance. In: IEEE international solid—state circuits conference—(ISSCC). San Francisco, CA, pp 478–480, 12 March 2018
11. Ye Z, Liu R, Barnaby H, Yu S (2019) Evaluation of single event effects in SRAM and RRAM based neuromorphic computing system for inference. IEEE international reliability physics symposium (IRPS). Monterey, CA, USA, pp 1–4, 23 May 2019.
12. Rajendran B, Alibart F (2016) Neuromorphic computing based on emerging memory technologies. IEEE J Emerg Sel Top Circuit Syst 6(2):198–211
13. Kaiyrbekov N, Krestinskaya O, James AP (2018) Variability analysis of memristor-based sigmoid function. In: International conference on computing and network communications (CoCoNet). Astana, Kazakhstan, pp 206–209, 19 May 2018
14. Bala A, Yang X, Adeyemo A, Jabir A (2019) A memristive activation circuit for deep learning neural networks. In: 8th International symposium on embedded computing and system design (ISED). Cochin, India, pp 1–5, 2 May 2019
15. Yu S (2018) Neuro-inspired computing With emerging nonvolatile memory. IEEE 106(2):260–285
16. Fisher RA (1988) UCI machine learning repository. Irvine. CA: University of California, School of Information and Computer Science, 1 July 1988. https://archive.ics.uci.edu/ml/datasets/iris
17. Siegler RS (1994) UCI machine learning repository. Irvine. CA: University of California, School of Information and Computer Science, 22 April 1994. http://archive.ics.uci.edu/ml/dat asets/balance+scale
18. Lohweg V (2013) UCI machine learning repository. Irvine. CA: University of California, School of Information and Computer Science, 16 April 2013. https://archive.ics.uci.edu/ml/datasets/banknote+authentication

Development of Universal Polynomial Equation for All the Sub-phases of Human Gait

Astha Verma, Vijay Bhaskar Semwal, and Koushlendra Kumar Singh

1 Introduction

To understand problem of the patients who has a walking disability and to provide rehabilitation training, gait training robots have been developed. These robots assist the patient in performing the gait cycle. Robot-based assistance is better than traditional manual artificial lower limbs rehabilitation and medical equipment for rehabilitation which do not meet the requirements of disabled people [1]. For these robots, motion planning is needed to train people. Motion planning is done by generating trajectories through human walking model. So in real-time system, the motion of normal human walking can be simulated by 3-link manipulator. The bipedal robot walk be simulated using the human walking model. So in our work OpenSim is used which is a real-time system having human walking model. Here, trajectories are generated for normal human walk. Trajectories are generated by solving inverse kinematics. This method provides accurate joint angle results in less amount of time [2].

Earlier for gait retraining, researchers have used direct kinematics in real time for calculation of joint angles assuming markers are attached to segments. Joint angles are computed as biofeedback variables, instead of inverse kinematics. Inverse kinematics globally optimizes generalized coordinates of model to minimize marker tracking errors. The joint angles computed by direct kinematics are less accurate, and it takes more time for calculation [3].

The work is supported by SERB, DST of Government of India under Early Career Award to Dr. Vijay Bhaskar Semwal with DST No: ECR/2018/000203 dated 04- June-2019.

A. Verma (✉) · V. B. Semwal
Maulana Azad National Institute of Technology, Bhopal, India

K. Kumar Singh
National Institute of Technology, Jamshedpur, India

© The Author(s), under exclusive license to Springer Nature Singapore Pte Ltd. 2021
M. K. Bajpai et al. (eds.), *Machine Vision and Augmented Intelligence—Theory and Applications*, Lecture Notes in Electrical Engineering 796,
https://doi.org/10.1007/978-981-16-5078-9_5

1.1 Author's Contribution

The first Contribution of our work is that a model-based method for solving inverse kinematics in real time is presented. Joint trajectories of knee, hip, and ankle joint angles for two different models of OpenSim are computed [4].This method provides accurate joint angle results in less amount of time.

The other Contribution is to design the polynomial equations for all sub-phases of human gait by using time series gait data. This data is generated by solving inverse kinematics in OpenSim for Gait 2354 model, which generate human like trajectories. Then generated equation trajectories are compared with both the OpenSim model gait2354 and gait 2392 models. It is observed that the polynomial equations are universal and can act alternative for human walk [5].

1.2 Organization of Paper

This paper is organized as follows. In Second Section, different methods proposed by some earlier researchers for solving inverse kinematics are explained. In Method Section, our method for solving model-based inverse kinematics in real time is explained. In Sect. 4, the algorithm for solving the inverse kinematics in OpenSim is discussed. In Result Section, Comparison of polynomial equation generated trajectories with both OpenSim model trajectories is shown. Next, in the Conclusion Section, summary of our work is presented.

2 Literature Review

Nearchou et al. in 1998 has presented idea on solving the inverse kinematics problem of redundant robots that are operating in complex environments through a modified genetic algorithm [6].

Dutra et al. in 2008 has presented idea on solution of the inverse kinematics problem using Simulated Annealing [7].

Semwal et al. in [8] has presented idea on Generation of Joint Trajectories Using Hybrid Automate-Based Model [9].

3 Method

In OpenSim, for every time frame, we calculate inverse kinematics, using the walking data which is experimentally collected. It computes joint angles for a walking model by reducing weighted sum of marker errors [10].

1. To minimize the marker error, OpenSim solves a weighted least square optimization problem.
2. Marker error is the distance between the location of experimental marker and corresponding model marker location.
3. Each marker has its own weight value, which tells by how much that marker's error term should be reduced in least square problem.

The minimization of weighted sum of marker errors can be expressed by this equation

$$\min_q \left[\sum i \in \text{markers } Wi \left\| X^{i^{exp}} - Xi(q) \right\|^2 \right] \tag{1}$$

where
q = vector of calculated joint angles.
xi^{exp} = cartesian position of the experimental marker i.
$xi(q)$ = cartesian position of the corresponding model marker i (it depends on q).
wi = weight value of marker i.

4 Implementation

Algorithm explaining the procedure to solve inverse kinematics for gait analysis.

Algorithm   1 Solving Inverse Kinematics

Input: subject01_simbody.osim - scaled model
gait2354_ Setup_ IK.xml - This file has pre-configuredsettings for inverse kinematics tool to compute joint angles for time varying coordinates, including marker tracking weights.
subject01_ walk1.trc - Experimental marker trajectory file.
Output: subject01_walk1 ik.mot - Inverse Kinematics Solution will save in motion file(i.e. file contains the joint angles computed by IK).
Begin:
//Load model

load muskuloskeletal model (gait2354 simbody.osim).
//Scale model
provide Scale setup xml file to the model.
(This file will scale the model to the dimensions of a subject whose experimental   data is used here).

We will get scaled model with name subject01 with pink markers.
//Setup inverse kinematics analysis
provide ik tool setup file subject01_ Setup_ IK.xml to the model
//Solve inverse kinematics problem

When model walks for one complete gait cycle, then Inverse Kinematics problem starts to solve for each time frame of experimental data by minimizing root mean square error for each time frame.
EndBegin

Experimental Marker File (Table-I) This is the input dataset which contains markers that are placed on the body segment of the model. These markers describe the cartesian position of different segments of leg during motion [11] (Table 1).

Below table shows Root Mean Square Error for each time frame:

This table shows minimization of root mean square error for each time frame while solving inverse kinematics in OpenSim (Table 2).

5   Result

This is the output dataset which is motion file generated after solving inverse kinematics. This file contains 6 joint angles(left and right ankle,hip,knee) of leg varying with time during motion. This data is for one gait cycle ranges from 0.4 s to 1.6 s at 1 m/s speed (Table 3).

Generating the polynomial equations for each phase

The time series gait data of gait2354 model is divided into different phases of gait. The divided data is then used for generating equations in python [12]. The equations are generated using curve fitting (Tables 4, 5 and 6).

The data is plotted for a certain range of time values and the curve is fitted for that. After curve fitting we get the polynomial equation of different orders which depends on the accuracy of fitting of the curve[13] (Tables 7, 8 and 9).

Here, equations are generated for each phase of gait cycle, so to get less error in each phase and more accuracy, the polynomial equations of degrees which varies from second order to eight order are generated [14].

The polynomial functions for all the joints and for all the seven phases of human gait cycle are given below.

The trajectory of actual gait (OpenSim model gait2354 and gait 2392 model) and polynomial function generated trajectory are compared.

It is observed that joint trajectories by polynomial equations are same as the human like trajectories of both OpenSim models [15]. So these are generalized equations with time as input [16]. So these equations are correct and can be used for finding joint trajectories of any model [17]. Figure 1 shows the comparison between the Gait2392 model, Gait2354 model and our developed polynomial equation trajectories for all the different joints, i.e., right and left hip, knee and ankle.

6   Conclusion and Futuristic Research Directions

This section consists of conclusion of this research article and future research direction.

Table 1 Experimental marker file(subject01_walk1.trc)

Frame number	Time	R.ASIS			V.Sacral			R.Thigh.Upper		
–	–	X1	Y1	Z1	X2	Y2	Z2	X3	Y3	Z3
1	0	617.24762	1055.27502	170.78198	430.86984	1051.26465	29.96675	517.3327	741.09601	212.08337
2	0.017	617.99811	1053.21753	168.51317	432.34061	1050.23743	26.84679	516.61377	740.4259	211.21942
3	0.033	620.29224	1051.77124	165.85938	434.09943	1049.34143	23.81936	517.77893	739.68091	209.92978
4	0.05	621.54041	1050.55212	163.5325	436.27994	1048.70715	20.95202	519.19745	739.32581	208.32521
5	0.067	624.58844	1050.92834	161.24614	438.82794	1048.45105	18.27267	522.16846	738.27905	206.22354
6	0.083	628.15863	1051.42017	158.44899	441.57205	1048.66125	15.77033	526.8028	738.1261	205.65331
7	0.1	630.80774	1051.99683	155.28273	444.30652	1049.38757	13.38743	535.10321	738.08984	203.62639
8	0.117	634.3573	1053.59888	151.48531	446.83075	1050.62231	11.01402	544.72296	738.2121	201.64484
9	0.133	636.58606	1055.25659	148.46054	448.95215	1052.28821	8.53319	554.57361	738.0722	201.58772
10	0.15	637.73926	1057.85437	144.71632	450.49979	1054.27356	5.88769	563.95862	737.61774	199.39542

Table 2 Root mean square error

Time(sec)	Root mean square error
0.4	0.0210096
0.417	0.0210009
0.433	0.0211359
0.45	0.021289
0.467	0.0214533
0.483	0.0214502
0.5	0.0214141
0.517	0.0212732
0.533	0.0212037
0.55	0.0211697

Table 3 A motion file containing the joint trajectories computed by IK

Time	r Hip flexion	r Knee angle	r Ankle angle	l Hip flexion	l Knee angle	l Ankle angle
0.4	20.16323127	−55.18730856	2.73637463	−5.79549243	−7.33535694	5.39710797
0.417	20.63387013	−50.31535853	2.7472313	−7.28440892	−6.33404953	5.62863786
0.433	20.96628697	−44.98985076	2.64343298	−8.72478157	−5.3167808	5.88912383
0.45	20.78903614	−39.2013406	2.37092498	−10.30761725	−4.47841451	6.24166928
0.467	20.7798154	−33.1576252	1.94532109	−11.49059775	−3.84790562	6.64969224
0.483	20.17300853	−26.49001002	1.39318234	−12.96257351	−2.9398077	6.9878691
0.5	19.64774636	−19.896284	0.91078464	−14.38123778	−2.07650312	7.3261432
0.517	19.16114122	−13.68136495	0.62807694	−15.66585779	−1.46152018	7.75051873
0.533	18.6821211	−8.10851422	0.6415855	−16.80471433	−1.13023352	8.31867189

Table 4 Polynomial functions and Values of Coefficients a1, a2, a3, a4, a5, a6, a7 of the trajectory polynomial for all the seven phases for right ankle joint

for loading response phase, terminal stance phase polynomial function is $a1 x^4 + a2 x^3 + a3 x^2 + a4 x + a5$						
for preswing phase, midswing phase polynomial function is $a1 x^5 + a2 x^4 + a3 x^3 + a4 x^2 + a5 x + a6$						
for initial swing polynomial function is $a1 x^5 + a2 x^4 + a3 x^3 + a4 x^2 + a5 x + a6$						
for midstance, terminal swing polynomial function is $a1 x^6 + a2 x^5 + a3 x^4 + a4 x^3 + a5 x^2 + a6x + a7$						
Gait subphases	a1	a2	a3	a4	a5	a6	a7
Loading Response	4.172e+04	-7.374e+04	4.854e+04	-1.412e+04	+1534	0	0
midstance	-1.634e+06	6.096e+06	-9.4e+06	7.667e+06	-3.49e+06	8.408e+05	-8.378e+04
terminal stance	1.051e+04	-3.539e+04	4.443e+04	-2.462e+04	5074	0	0
Pre Swing	3.2e+06	-1.516e+07	2.873e+07	-2.721e+07	1.288e+07	-2.439e+06	0
Initial Swing	-2386	7698	-5002	-7524	1.122e+04	-3999	0
Mid Swing	2.169e+05	-1.406e+06	3.641e+06	-4.705e+06	3.036e+06	-7.824e+05	0
Terminal Swing	-5.32e+06	4.805e+07	-1.807e+08	3.62e+08	-4.076e+08	2.446e+08	-6.108e+07

Table 5 Polynomial functions and Values of Coefficients a1, a2, a3, a4, a5, a6, a7, a8, a9 of the trajectory polynomial for all the seven phases for left ankle joint

for loading response phase polynomial function is
a1 x^5 + a2 x^4 + a3 x^3 + a4 x^2 + a5 x+a6
for midstance polynomial function is
a1 x^8 +a2 x^7 + a3 x^6 + a4 x^5+a5 x^4+ a6x^3+ a7x^2 +a8 x+ a9
for terminal stance polynomial function is
a1 x^7 + a2 x^6 + a3 x^5+a4 x^4+ a5 x^3+ a6 x^2 +a7 x+ a8
for preswing phase polynomial function is
a1 x^5 + a2 x^4 + a3 x^3 + a4 x^2 + a5 x+a6
for initial swing polynomial function is
a1 x^6 +a2 x^5 + a3 x^4 + a4 x^3+a5 x^2+ a6x+a7
for midswing phase polynomial function is
a1 x^7 + a2 x^6 + a3 x^5+a4 x^4+ a5 x^3+ a6 x^2 +a7 x+ a8
for terminal swing polynomial function is
a1 x^6 +a2 x^5 + a3 x^4 + a4 x^3+a5 x^2+ a6x+a7

Gait subphases	a1	a2	a3	a4	a5	a6	a7	a8	a9
Loading Response	5.856e+05	-1.326e+06	1.198e+06	-5.399e+05	1.213e+05	-1.087e+04	0	0	0
Mid Stance	3.102e+08	-1.493e+09	3.139e+09	-3.764e+09	2.814e+09	-1.344e+09	4.001e+08	-6.794e+07	5.036e+06
Terminal Stance	4.402e+07	-2.373e+08	5.46e+08	-6.948e+08	5.281e+08	-2.398e+08	6.018e+07	-6.442e+06	0
Pre Swing	-2.019e+06	9.554e+06	-1.808e+07	1.71e+07	-8.079e+06	1.526e+06	0	0	0
Initial Swing	8.773e+04	-7.254e+05	2.384e+06	-4.042e+06	3.761e+06	-1.831e+06	3.656e+05	0	0
Mid Swing	2.162e+06	-1.64e+07	5.099e+07	-8.195e+07	6.904e+07	-2.436e+07	-2.29e+06	2.816e+06	0
Terminal Swing	-5.115e+05	4.545e+06	-1.682e+07	3.316e+07	-3.676e+07	2.171e+07	-5.341e+06	0	0

Table 6 Polynomial functions and Values of Coefficients a1, a2, a3, a4, a5, a6, a7, a8, a9 of the trajectory polynomial for all the seven phases for left hip joint

for loading response phase polynomial function is
a1 x^6 +a2 x^5 + a3 x^4 + a4 x^3+a5 x^2+ a6x+a7
for midstance,initial swing,midswing phase, polynomial function is
a1 x^8 +a2 x^7 + a3 x^6 + a4 x^5+a5 x^4+ a6x^3+ a7x^2 +a8 x+ a9
for terminal stance polynomial function is
a1 x^5 + a2x^4 + a3 x^3 + a4 x^2 + a5 x+a6
for preswing phase polynomial function is
a1 x^5 + a2 x^4 + a3 x^3 + a4 x^2 + a5 x+a6
for terminal swing polynomial function is
a1 x^8 +a2 x^7 + a3 x^6 + a4 x^5+a5 x^4+ a6x^3+ a7x^2 +a8 x+ a9

Gait subphases	a1	a2	a3	a4	a5	a6	a7	a8	a9
Loading Response	2.694e+08	-7.248e+08	8.113e+08	-4.837e+08	1.62e+08	-2.891e+07	2.146e+06	0	0
Mid Stance	4.545e+08	-2.177e+09	4.55e+09	-5.423e+09	4.031e+09	-1.913e+09	5.661e+08	-9.552e+07	7.035e+06
Terminal Stance	5497	9497	-6.96e+04	1.021e+05	-6.029e+04	1.281e+04	0	0	0
Pre Swing	5.124e+06	-2.429e+07	4.605e+07	-4.362e+07	2.066e+07	-3.91e+06	0	0	0
Initial Swing	1.752e+07	-1.626e+08	6.591e+08	-1.523e+09	2.197e+09	-2.023e+09	1.162e+09	-3.809e+08	5.449e+07
Mid Swing	4.034e+08	-4.194e+09	1.907e+10	-4.951e+10	8.03e+10	-8.331e+10	5.399e+10	-1.998e+10	3.234e+09
Terminal Swing	-3.578e+06	4.166e+07	-2.119e+08	6.15e+08	-1.114e+09	1.288e+09	-9.287e+08	3.817e+08	-6.844e+07

Table 7 Polynomial functions and Values of Coefficients a1, a2, a3, a4, a5, a6, a7, a8, a9 of the trajectory polynomial for all the seven phases for right hip joint

for loading response phase polynomial function is
a1 x^6 +a2 x^5 + a3 x^4 + a4 x^3+a5 x^2+a6x+a7
for midstance phase polynomial function is
a1 x^8 +a2 x^7 + a3 x^6 + a4 x^5+a5 x^4+ a6x^3+ a7x^2 +a8 x+ a9
for terminal stance,terminal swing phase polynomial function is
a1 x^5 + a2 x^4 + a3 x^3 + a4 x^2 + a5 x+a6
for preswing,initial swing phase polynomial function is
a1 x^5 + a2 x^4 + a3 x^3 + a4 x^2 + a5 x+a6
for mid swing polynomial function is
a1 x^6 +a2 x^5 + a3 x^4 + a4 x^3+a5 x^2+ a6x+a7

Gait subphases	a1	a2	a3	a4	a5	a6	a7	a8	a9
Loading Response	3.647e+08	-9.834e+08	1.103e+09	-6.595e+08	2.215e+08	-3.962e+07	2.949e+06	0	0
Mid Stance	-3.493e+08	1.675e+09	-3.51e+09	4.194e+09	-3.127e+09	1.49e+09	-4.427e+08	7.506e+07	-5.559e+06
Terminal Stance	-2.931e+04	1.244e+05	-2.094e+05	1.748e+05	-7.233e+04	1.19e+04	0	0	0
Pre Swing	1.305e+07	-6.192e+07	1.174e+08	-1.113e+08	5.274e+07	-9.99e+06	0	0	0
Initial Swing	1.157e+05	-6.352e+05	1.393e+06	-1.525e+06	8.339e+05	-1.821e+05	0	0	0
Mid Swing	-3.8e+06	2.957e+07	-9.582e+07	1.655e+08	-1.606e+08	8.311e+07	-1.79e+07	0	0
Terminal Swing	-8.842e+04	6.572e+05	-1.953e+06	2.9e+06	-2.152e+06	6.38e+05	0	0	0

Table 8 Polynomial functions and Values of Coefficients a1, a2, a3, a4, a5, a6 of the trajectory polynomial for all the seven phases for left knee joint

for loading response,midstance,preswing,initial swing phase polynomial function is $a1\ x^5 + a2\ x^4 + a3\ x^3 + a4\ x^2 + a5\ x+a6$						
for terminal stance, midswing,terminal swing phase polynomial function is $a1\ x^5 + a2\ x^4 + a3\ x^3 + a4\ x^2 + a5\ x+a6$						
Gait subphases	a1	a2	a3	a4	a5	a6
Loading Response	-4.278e+06	9.66e+06	- 8.708e+06	3.918e+06	- 8.795e+05	7.88e+04
Mid Stance	-1.461e+05	4.342e+05	- 5.151e+05	3.042e+05	- 8.934e+04	1.042e+04
Terminal Stance	9.225e+04	- 4.161e+05	7.465e+05	- 6.647e+05	2.931e+05	- 5.117e+04
Pre Swing	-4.397e+06	2.087e+07	- 3.962e+07	3.76e+07	- 1.783e+07	3.382e+06
Initial Swing	-4.264e+04	2.192e+05	- 4.547e+05	4.764e+05	- 2.521e+05	5.379e+04
Mid Swing	1.44e+04	- 1.199e+05	3.857e+05	- 6.044e+05	4.639e+05	- 1.4e+05
Terminal Swing	9.042e+04	- 6.754e+05	2.016e+06	- 3.005e+06	2.237e+06	- 6.651e+05

Table 9 Polynomial functions and Values of Coefficients a1, a2, a3, a4, a5, a6, a7, a8, a9 of the trajectory polynomial for all the seven phases for right knee joint

for loading response phase polynomial function is $a1\ x^3 +a2\ x^2 + a3\ x +a4$								
for midstance,preswing phase polynomial function is $a1\ x^5 + a2\ x^4 + a3\ x^3 + a4\ x^2 + a5\ x+a6$								
for terminal stance,midswing,terminal swing phase polynomial function is $a1\ x^5 + a2\ x^4 + a3\ x^3 + a4\ x^2 + a5\ x+a6$								
for initial swing phase polynomial function is $a1\ x^8 +a2\ x^7 + a3\ x^6 + a4\ x^5+a5\ x^4+ a6x^3+ a7x^2 +a8\ x+ a9$								
Gait subphases	a1	a2	a3	a4	a5	a6	a7	a8	a9
Loading Response	-2178	3620	- 1576	135.3	0	0	0	0	0
Mid Stance	-4.177e+05	1.308e+06	- 1.623e+06	9.964e+05	- 3.022e+05	3.618e+04	0	0	0
Terminal Stance	8.051e+04	- 3.258e+05	5.242e+05	- 4.186e+05	1.657e+05	- 2.596e+04	0	0	0
Pre Swing	-1.123e+07	5.327e+07	- 1.01e+08	9.574e+07	- 4.535e+07	8.591e+06	0	0	0
Initial Swing	1.4e+09	- 1.233e+10	4.753e+10	- 1.046e+11	1.438e+11	- 1.264e+11	6.941e+10	- 2.177e+10	2.986e+09
Mid Swing	2.861e+05	- 1.836e+06	4.71e+06	- 6.036e+06	3.864e+06	- 9.886e+05	0	0	0
Terminal Swing	7.047e+04	- 5.329e+05	1.611e+06	- 2.433e+06	1.833e+06	- 5.515e+05	0	0	0

Conclusion

For fast and accurate model-based inverse kinematics calculations, an inverse kinematics solution in real time using experimental data is presented to compute the joint angles for a musculoskeletal model during movement [18, 19]. To analyze a movement of model, the hip, knee, and ankle trajectories have been generated from both models of OpenSim [20]. Our other contribution is the generation of polynomial equations using gait data of gait2354 model [21], and then generated joint trajectories of bipedal motion using polynomial equations. These equations are suitable for generating walking trajectories of any bipedal robots [22]. Since these equations are designed using actual normal human gait captured data, so they are stable.

Comparison of trajectories generated by these equations with the OpenSim model gait2354 and gait2392 trajectories shows the equations which we have developed are correct [19].

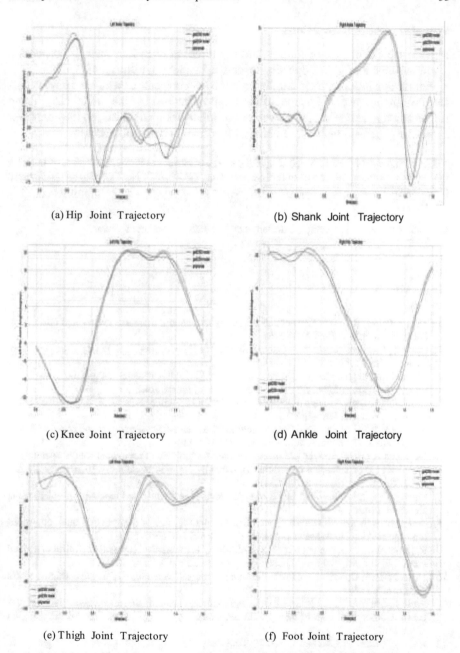

(a) Hip Joint Trajectory

(b) Shank Joint Trajectory

(c) Knee Joint Trajectory

(d) Ankle Joint Trajectory

(e) Thigh Joint Trajectory

(f) Foot Joint Trajectory

Fig. 1 Gait pattern of different joints for Gait 2354 model, polynomial function trajectories and Gait2392 **a** hip joint **b** shank joint **c** knee joint **d** ankle joint **e** thigh joint **f** foot joint

Futuristic research directions

May be the calculation of torques and net forces at each joint, which produces a given movement of joints, by using inverse dynamics algorithm [24].

For the dynamics of the manipulator, these joint trajectories which we have generated by solving inverse kinematics are required as input to the model [25]. These forces and torque control the movement of joints of biped robots, so the controller should be generated which resembles with normal human walk [26].

Acknowledgements The author(s) would like to express thanks to SERB, DST govt. of India for funding project under the schema of Early career award (ECR), DST No: ECR/2018/000203 dated on 04/06/2019.

Conflict of Interest The author(s) declare that they have no conflict of interest.

References

1. Diaz I, Gil JJ, E (2011) Lower-limb robotic rehabilitation: literature review and challenges. https://doi.org/10.1155/2011/759764
2. Jindal D, Randhawa JS, Kant S, Gupta I, Singla S (2017) Conversion of gait data into OpenSim. Int Res J Eng Technol (IRJET) 04(06)
3. Pizzolato C, Reggiani M, Modenese L, Lloyd DG (2017) Biofeedback for gait retraining based on real-time estimation of tibiofemoral joint contact forces. IEEE 25
4. Reinbolt JA, Seth A, Delp SL (2011) Simulation of human movement: applications using OpenSim. Procedia IUTAM 2:186–198
5. Semwal VB (2016) Design of vector field for different subphases of gait and regeneration of gait pattern. IEEE Trans Autom Sci Eng 15(1):104–110
6. Nearchou A (1998) Solving the inverse kinematics problem of redundant robots operating in complex environments via a modified genetic algorithm. https://doi.org/10.1016/S0094-114X(97)00034-7
7. Dutra MS, Salcedo IL, Diaz LP (2008) New technique for inverse kinematics problem using simulated annealing
8. Semwal VB, Nandi GC (2016) Generation of joint trajectories using hybrid automate-based model: a rocking block-based approach. IEEE SensS J 16 5805–5816
9. Raj M, Semwal VB, Nandi GC (2018) Hybrid model for passive locomotion control of a biped humanoid: the artificial neural network approach. IJIMAI 5(1):40–46
10. Hicks J (2016) OpenSim documentations: how inverse kinematics works. https://simtk-conflu ence.stanford.edu
11. Porsa S, Lin YC, Pandy MG (2016) Direct methods for predicting movement biomechanics based upon optimal control theory with implementation in OpenSim. Ann Biomed Eng 44 2542–2557
12. Rai JK, Tewari R, Chandra D (2009) Trajectory planning for all sub phases of gait cycle for human-like walking. Int J Eng Syst Model Simul. https://doi.org/10.1504/IJESMS.2009.031353
13. Wiley (1978) Curve fitting and optimal design for prediction. J R Stat Soc Seri. B (Methodological) 40(1):1–42. https://www.jstor.org/stable/2984861
14. Pourkarimia L, Yaghoobib MA, Mashinchib M (2011) Efficient curve fitting: an application of multiobjective programming. https://doi.org/10.1016/j.apm.2010.06.009

15. Nandi GC (2016) Modeling bipedal locomotion trajectories using hybrid automata. IEEE region 10 conference (TENCON)
16. Semwal VB (2015) Biologically-inspired push recovery capable bipedal locomotion modeling through hybrid automata. Robot Auton Syst 70 181–190
17. Semwal VB, Nandi GC (2015) Toward developing a computational model for bipedal push recovery–a brief. IEEE SensS J 15(4):2021–2022
18. Arnold EM, Ward SR, Lieber RL, Delp SL (2010) A model of the lower limb for analysis of human movement. Ann Biomed Eng. https://doi.org/10.1007/s10439-009-9852-5
19. Seth A, Hicks JL, Uchida TK, Habib A, Dembia CL, DunneJJ, Ong CF, DeMers MS, Rajagopal A, Millard M (2018) Opensim: simulating musculoskeletal dynamics and neuromuscular control to study human and animal movement. PLoS Comput Biol. https://doi.org/10.1371/journal.pcbi.1006223
20. Seth A, Sherman M, Reinbolt JA, Delp SL (2011) OpenSim: a musculoskeletal modeling and simulation framework for in silico investigations and exchange. Procedia IUTAM 2:212–232
21. Semwal VB, Gaud N, Nandi GC (2019) Human gait state prediction using cellular automata and classification using ELM. Machine intelligence and signal analysis. Springer, Singapore, 135–145
22. Gupta A, Semwal VB (2020) Multiple task human gait analysis and identification: ensemble learning approach. Emotion and information processing. Springer, Cham, 185–197
24. Ewing, Katie A (2016) Prophylactic knee bracing alters lower-limb muscle forces during a double-leg drop landing. J Biomech 49(14):3347–3354
25. Barrios JA, Crossley KM, Davis IS (2010) Gait retraining to reduce the knee adduction moment through real-time visual feedback of dynamic knee alignment. J Biomech 43:2208–2213
26. Lee LF, Umberger BR(2016) Generating optimal control simulations of musculoskeletal movement using OpenSim and matlab. https://doi.org/10.7717/peerj.1638
27. Bijalwan V, Semwal VB, & Mandal TK (2021) Fusion of multi-sensor based biomechanical gait analysis using vision and wearable sensor. IEEE Sens J
28. Gupta A, & Semwal VB (2020) Multiple task human gait analysis and identification: ensemble learning approach. Emotion and information processing. Springer, Cham. 185–197
29. Semwal VB et al (2021) Pattern identification of different human joints for different human walking styles using inertial measurement unit (IMU) sensor. Artificial Intelligence Review 1–21
30. Jain R, Semwal VB & Praveen K (2021) Deep ensemble learning approach for lower extremity activities recognition using wearable sensors. Expert Systems e12743
31. Semwal VB, Anjali G & Praveen L (2021) An optimized hybrid deep learning model using ensemble learning approach for human walking activities recognition. The J Supercomputing 1–24
32. Semwal VB et al (2021) Speed, cloth and pose invariant gait recognition-based person identification. Machine Learning: Theoretical Foundations and Practical Applications 39–56
33. Semwal VB, Nandi GC (2014) Study of humanoid push recovery based on experiments. arXivarXiv-1405
34. Semwal VB & Yash G (2021) Performance analysis of data-driven techniques for solving inverse kinematics problems. Proceedings of SAI Intelligent Systems Conference. Springer, Cham

Application of Equipment Utilization Monitoring System for ICU Equipment Using Internet of Things (IoT)

Barath Kumar Babu and Bhoomadevi A

1 Introduction

Medical devices vary in both their intended use and indications to be used. Examples range from straightforward, low-risk devices like tongue depressors; medical thermometers, disposable gloves, and bedpans to complex, high-risk devices that are implanted and help sustain life. The planning of medical devices constitutes a serious segment of the sector of biomedical engineering. Albeit medical devices are indispensable for all aspects of healthcare, many appropriate technologies are inaccessible to the bulk of the people that need them, particularly in low and middle-income countries.

In India, the lack of proper management of medical equipment has limited the capacity of health institutions to deliver adequate health care. It is estimated that only about 61% of medical equipment found in Indian public hospitals and other health facilities are functional at any given time. Medical equipment management defines the organization and coordination of activities that make sure the successful management of kits associated with patient care during a clinic.

This study is meant to spot the reported reasons that contributed to availability also as utilization of medical devices within the respective hospitals. This may help hospital administrators and other stakeholders to make awareness as a way of resolving problems through communication and take informed actions for better healthcare delivery.

B. K. Babu
MBA (Hospital and Health Systems Management) Faculty of Management Sciences, SRIHER (DU), Chennai, Tamil Nadu, India

B. A (✉)
Associate Professor Faculty of Management Sciences, SRIHER (DU), Chennai, Tamil Nadu, India

© The Author(s), under exclusive license to Springer Nature Singapore Pte Ltd. 2021
M. K. Bajpai et al. (eds.), *Machine Vision and Augmented Intelligence—Theory and Applications*, Lecture Notes in Electrical Engineering 796,
https://doi.org/10.1007/978-981-16-5078-9_6

1.1 Need for Monitoring System

Monitoring systems are liable for controlling the technology employed by a hospital to research their operation and performance and to detect and alert the possible errors. An honest monitoring system is in a position to watch devices, infrastructures, applications, services, and even business processes. Monitoring may be a tremendously broad and sophisticated activity; it is not a closed concept, but it depends on the requirements of every company. However, monitoring systems often have a variety of common features, including the following:

a. Analysis in real-time
b. Regular system alerts
c. Graphic visualization
d. Production of reports
e. Record the availabilities
f. Distinction supported user type.

1.2 Traditional Monitoring Versus Real–Time Monitoring

1. Traditional monitoring requires data to be entered manually. For instance, patient wheel-in time and wheel-out time in an ICU is employed to calculate the ICU charges for a patient; whereas in real-time monitoring, the wheel-in, wheel-out times are directly pushed to the HIS of the hospital in order that the billing is often done easily.

2. Traditional monitoring consumes man-hours, whereas real-time monitoring does not involve man-hours because automation is done.

3. Real-time monitoring provides answers in real-time, whereas traditional monitoring post analysis has got to be done to get user-friendly statistics.

1.3 Internet of Things (IoT)

The Internet of things (IoT) is the extension of Internet connectivity into physical devices and everyday objects. Embedded with electronics, Internet connectivity, and other sorts of hardware (such as sensors), these devices can communicate and interact with others over the web and that they are often remotely monitored and controlled.

1.3.1 IoT in Healthcare

The Internet of Medical Things (also called the web of health things) is an application of the IoT for medical and health-related purposes, data collection and analysis for research, and monitoring.

IoT devices are often want to enable remote health monitoring and emergency notification systems. These health monitoring devices can range from vital sign and pulse monitors to advanced devices capable of monitoring specialized implants, like pacemakers, Fit bit electronic wristbands, or advanced hearing aids. Some hospitals have begun implementing "smart beds" which will detect once they are occupied and when a patient is attempting to urge up. It also can adjust itself to make sure appropriate pressure, and support is applied to the patient without the manual interaction of nurses. A 2015 Goldman Sachs report indicated that healthcare IoT devices "can save us quite $300 billion in annual healthcare expenditures by increasing revenue and decreasing cost." Moreover, the utilization of mobile devices to support medical follow-up led to the creation of 'm-health', used "to analyze, capture, transmit and store health statistics from multiple resources, including sensors and other biomedical acquisition systems".

Advances in plastic and fabric electronics fabrication methods have enabled ultra-low-cost, use-and-throw IoMT sensors. These sensors, alongside the specified RFID electronics, are often fabricated on paper or e-textiles for wirelessly powered disposable sensing devices. Applications are established for point-of-care medical diagnostics where portability and low system-complexity are important.

As of 2018 IoMT was not only being applied within the clinical laboratory industry but also being applied within the healthcare and insurance industries. IoMT within the healthcare industry is now permitting doctors, patients, et al. involved (i.e., guardians of patients, nurses, families, etc.) to be a part of a system, where patient records are saved during a database, allowing doctors and therefore, the remainder of the medical staff to possess access to the patient's information. Moreover, IoT- based systems are patient-centered, which involves being flexible to the patient's medical conditions. IoMT within the insurance industry provides access to raise and new sorts of dynamic information. This includes sensor-based solutions like biosensors, wearables, connected health devices, and mobile apps to track customer behavior. This will cause more accurate underwriting and new pricing models.

The application of the IOT in healthcare plays a fundamental role in managing chronic diseases and in disease prevention and control. Remote monitoring is formed possible through the connection of powerful wireless solutions. The connectivity enables health practitioners to capture patient's data and applying complex algorithms in health data analysis.

2   Literature Review

[1] considered that a lot of technologies can reduce overall costs for the prevention or management of chronic diseases. Among these technologies are devices that monitor health indicators, automatic administration therapies, or devices that track health data in real-time when a patient self-administers therapy. Because high-speed Internet access and smartphones have increased, many patients began using mobile applications (applications) to manage various health needs. These mobile devices and

applications are increasingly used and integrated with telemedicine and tales aloud through the medical Internet of Things (mIoT) [2] explained that new operational data sources will cause a replacement design of systems to supply health services and ways to support operational planning and decision-making. Technologies like Real-Time Location Systems (RTLS) provide unique insight and understanding of how healthcare adjustments behave and answer operational design changes. This text uses RTLS data from an outpatient clinical environment to spot the acceptable number of planned providers to enhance clinical space utilization while balancing the negative effects of clinical congestion [3] study show that the important motivation for this research is to develop an efficient system that will monitor the health parameters of multiple patients simultaneously and effectively provide data to patients where it is stored permanently. The present traditional health monitoring is achieved by individual PCs attached to every patient bed. The varied parameters that are monitored are vital signs, temperature, ECG, and EEG. Our research explores the potential of WSN together, send, and process these multiple multi-patient parameters simultaneously and in real-time. This research manages to show the patient's traditional individual monitor and requirements into a tool capable of reliably monitoring the varied parameters of up to six patients at an equivalent time, in real-time [4] described that accurate motion tracking can provide detailed information through qualitative and quantitative chemical analysis of patient movements within the field of rehabilitation and, therefore, it is often an efficient tool for handling motion problems. Patients are usually doing rehabilitation training programs under the guidance of their supervisor just for a couple of small fragments (1–2 h) of the day. Remote motion monitoring can allow qualified medical personnel to closely monitor patient training activities reception throughout the day, so in various parts (morning, afternoon, night) training sessions are often easily included in lifestyle, and in some cases (e.g., stroke rehabilitation) this will significantly improve the healing process and may cause better restoration results. This text focuses mainly on its internal architecture and its usage scenarios within the sector of telerehabilitation.

3   Methodology

There are several ways to measure the utilization of equipment. There are no right or wrong ways but only ways that best fit the need(s).A study on Application of Equipment Utilization Monitoring System for ICU Equipment using Internet of Things (IoT) was conducted in MGM Healthcare Pvt. Ltd, Chennai, with the support of Tenx Health Technologies Pvt. Ltd, Coimbatore, in order to enhance the process of monitoring equipment throughout the hospital. The study was confined to the ICU owing to time constraints.

This study was conducted to enhance the monitoring of vital equipment in the ICU using IoT technology. This enables the equipment to be remotely monitored and used in automated billing when integrated to the HIS of the hospital.

Equipment included in the study are Ventilators, Monitors, Syringe pumps, and Infusion pumps.

The research design of this project is Proof of concept (POC) based Descriptive Research. Proof of Concept is a type of research where a small demonstration of certain ideas in certain disciplines is carried out in order to prove the practical potential of the idea.

This POC based Descriptive Research design focuses on providing an accurate description of the ideas that have practical potential. It involves observing and describing the behavior of a subject without influencing it in any manner.

The primary data was collected through an observational checklist to track the movement of nurses in the ICU.

4 Results

4.1 Real Time Location System (RTLS)

Due to time and cost constraints, Medium Integration was done to ensure that both the patient and staff are present at the same location. By ensuring this, it is assumed that the equipment is utilized as both of them are in the same location hence fulfilling the purpose of the equipment.

Figure 1 depicts the technician that is in the Nursing Station—considered to be a ICU for a period of 9 h 58 min and also shows the patient named Mr. Raman was in the same nursing station for 36 min. Since both the patient and the technician were present in the same location along with the equipment, it is considered that the equipment in the ICU was utilized for 36 min. Thus the utilization for all the equipment can be found in the same way.

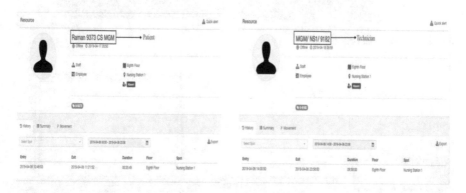

Fig. 1 Screenshot of Patient named Raman and Screenshot of Technician

4.2 Raspberry Pi-Based IoT

The Raspberry Pi is a series of small single-board computers developed in the United Kingdom by the Raspberry Pi Foundation in order to promote basic computer science knowledge in schools and in developing countries. The original model has become far more popular than anticipated. It does not include peripherals like keyboards and cases, but some accessories have been included in several official and unofficial bundles (Fig. 2).

CONFIGURING CoMeT CONNECT™ EDGE DEVICE

1. Connect the CoMeT Connect™ Edge Device to a Computer via a Standard Cross Over Cable (LANCable). Then Set the Ethernet IP of the Computer to **192.168.0.10** (Figs. 3 and 4).

Windows 10

1. Go to Settings > Network and Internet > Ethernet > Change Adapter options
2. Right click on the Ethernet connection

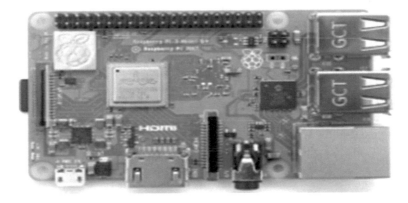

Fig. 2 Raspberry Pi based IoT

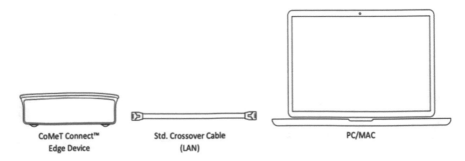

Fig. 3 Comet connect to computer via LAN

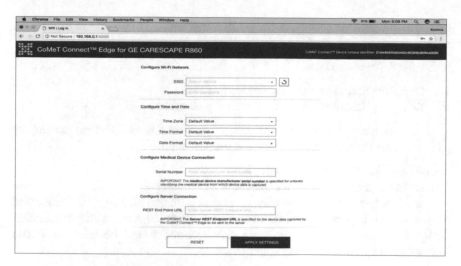

Fig. 4 Comet connect webpage

3. Go to Properties and select

    'Internet Protocol Version 4(TCP/IPV4)'

4. Click on the Properties button
5. Select the radio button, 'Use the following IP address'
6. Change the IP Address to "**192.168.0.10**" and 'Subnet Mask' to "**255.255.255.0**".

Mac OSX

1. Go to System Preferences > Network > Select the LAN
2. Change 'Configure IPv4' to "Manually"
3. Enter 'IP Address' to "**192.168.0.10**" and 'Subnet Mask' to "**255.255.255.0**"
4. Open a web browser (preferably Google Chrome) and enter "192.168.0.1:5000" in the address bar.
5. The following web page opens:

2. Fill the form:

a. Configure Wi-Fi network.

i.   Select the Wi-Fi network SSID from the drop-down list.
ii. Enter password.

Please note: CoMeT Connect™ Edge device only supports 2.4 GHz Wi-Fi networks. If you are unable to find some Wi-Fi Network SSIDs in the list, it could be due to different network types like 5 GHz. It is advised to work with the network administrator and arrange for a 2.4 GHz Wi-Fi network.

b. Configure Time and Date:

i.   Select the time zone from the drop-down list.
ii.   Select the date/time format from the drop-down list.

If you are unable to find the time zone or date time format you are looking for, please contact the Cohere Med Solutions support team.

c. Configure Medical Device Connection:
    i. Enter the medical device manufacturer serial number.

The Manufacturer Serial Number is used as a unique identifier for the medical device. It is an important piece of information which helps to identify the medical device from which the data is being acquired and would be used for further identification by other receiving applications.

d. Configure Server Connection:

i.   Enter the REST end point URL for the Web service which is hosted and managed by any compatible information system for further processing the device data.
3.   Click "Apply Settings" button:

The changes will be applied and the CoMeT Connect™ Edge Device will be restarted. Please do not close the browser window and allow the page to refresh automatically. It may take a few minutes to refresh the page.

4.   Success

The form will be presented with the Wi-Fi Network displaying the status "Connected" and other entered values will be populated (Figs. 5 and 6).

5.   In case of Failure:

The form will be presented with the error message. Please take necessary action (Fig. 7).

Troubleshooting Tips:

1.   Check the Connecting Cable for loose connections.
2.   Check the Medical Device to see whether it is powered on.
3.   Check the CoMeT Connect™ Edge device to see whether it is powered on.
4.   Check the Wi-Fi network for connectivity/change of password etc.
5.   Check the RESTful Web service to see whether it is up and running.

The configuration to be done in each device is listed below:

    1. **Philips IntelllvueMX450**:

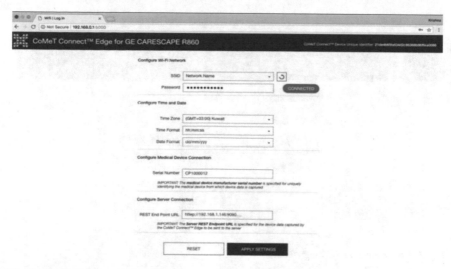

Fig. 5 Comet connect—settings success

Fig. 6 Comet connect—settings success

The initial configuration requires the LAN port of the IoT device must be connected with the monitor through a RJ 45 cable (Fig. 8).

To configure the IP address of the monitor manually switch the monitor into **service mode**.

After that under **Main Menu → Bed Information** change the IP configuration as shown in following figure:

By selecting "IP Config" a new dialog will appear. Please change the setting "BootP" to "Manual". Now you can edit the fields to enter a new IP address and subnet mask (Fig. 9).

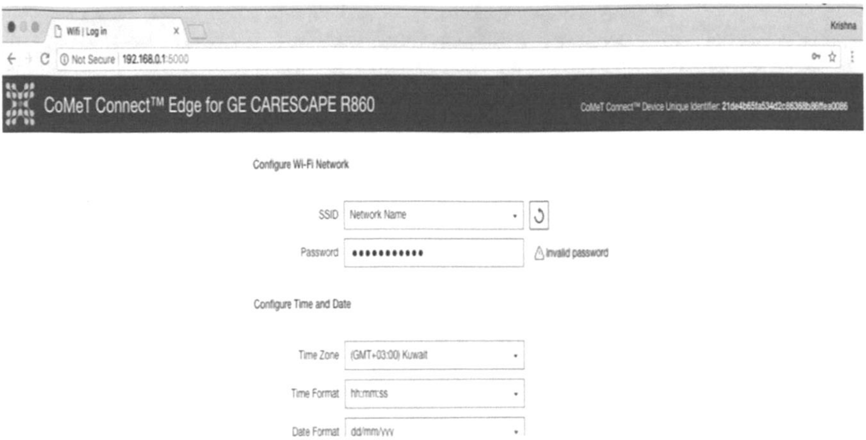

Fig. 7 Comet connect—settings failure

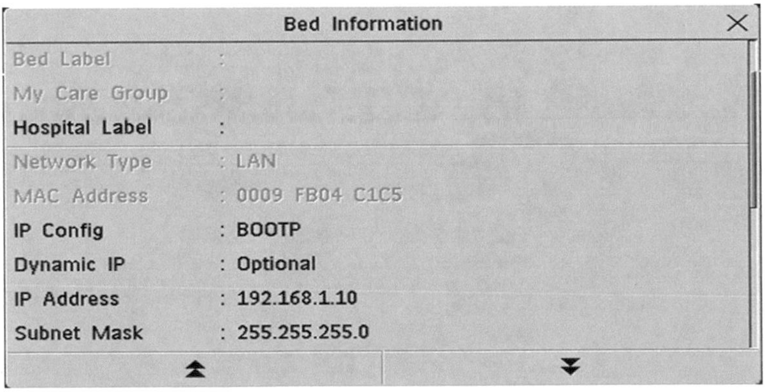

Fig. 8 Philips monitor settings

Finally select "Store" at the bottom menu bar to save the new settings (Fig. 10).

2. **Macquet Ventilator**:

The initial configuration of the Macquet Ventilator just requires an RS 232 to USB cable to be connected. The RS 232 port is connected in the ventilator, and the USB port is connected in the IoT device. There are no other configurations to be done in the device. Troubleshooting: In order to obtain the values from the device in the initial stage (without a patient being connected with the ventilator), a test lung can be connected to the ventilator to check if the vitals are being charted (Fig. 11).

3. **Syringe and Infusion Pump**:

Fig. 9 Philips
monitor—network setup

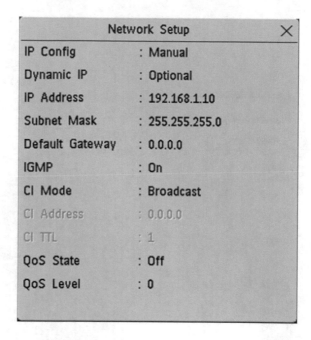

The initial configuration of the Syringe pump (Graseby-2100) and infusion pump (Graseby-1200) requires an RS 232 to USB cable to be connected. The RS 232 port is connected in the pump, and the USB port is connected in the IoT device. There are no other configurations to be done in the device. To check vitals, enter random values in the pumps and select start.

Thus the device is configured with the IoT device. It is then used to extract the data from the equipment using the respective drivers. Two types of data can be extracted from the device.

i. Online/Offline status of the equipment ii. Vitals from the equipment

Every equipment in the hospital is connected to the IoT device. The IoT device gives the Online/Offline status of the equipment throughout (Figs. 12, 13 and 14).

From the above image the following can be obtained:

Device Type: Type of equipment that is connected example, Monitor, Ventilator, etc.

Device Name: Device name can be renamed and can be associated with the model of the equipment used and the bed linked to it.

Serial No: Serial number refers to the device number that is connected.

Status: Status is the ON/OFF status of the equipment.

Total Up Time: It refers to the total working time of the equipment.

Last Location: Location of the device last used.

Last active: Date when the equipment was last active.

From the above information, the following data can be obtained:

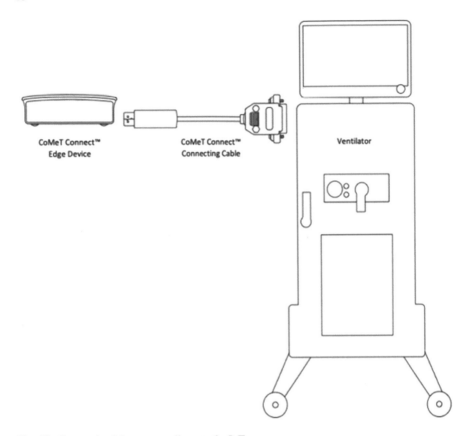

Fig. 10 Connecting Macquet ventilator to the IoT

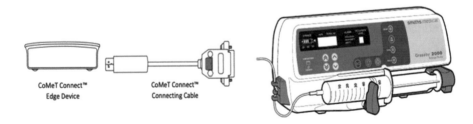

Fig. 11 Connecting infusion and syringe pump to the IoT

i.   The ON/OFF status of the equipment is obtained in JSON format which is then converted into csv file. The csv file is then pushed to the URL where the utilization details are displayed.

ii.   The entire equipment in the hospital can be monitored remotely—Refer figure above.

Device Type	Device Name	Serial No.	Status	Total Up Time	Last Location	Last Active
Patient Monitor	Philips Intellivue MX450	TestMX450	ONLINE	0hr 16min	Dept_01	12-04-2019
Infusion pump	Smiths Graseby-1200	Test1200	OFFLINE	0hr 15min	Dept_01	12-04-2019
Ventilator	Maquet Servo-i	TestMaquet	ONLINE	0hr 13min	Dept_01	12-04-2019
Infusion pump	Smiths Graseby-2100	Test2100	ONLINE	0hr 14min	Dept_01	12-04-2019
Infusion pump	Smiths Graseby-C9	171300101	ONLINE	20hr 4min	Dept_01	12-04-2019
Infusion pump	Smiths Graseby-2100	171200101	ONLINE	20hr 26min	Dept_01	12-04-2019
Infusion pump	Smiths Graseby-1200	171100101	ONLINE	20hr 21min	Dept_01	12-04-2019
Patient Monitor	Nihon Kohden Vismo	NK-00001	OFFLINE	19hr 41min	Dept_01	12-04-2019

Fig. 12 Online/Offline Status of the equipment

2019-03-22 18:24:51,163 [1] INFO ConnectCapture.PublishDeviceData (null) - {"time":"22/03/2019 18:24:50","deviceId":"b62b3ee7eafc4e98955fc95b54fe9b74","status":"off"}
2019-03-22 18:25:52,094 [1] INFO ConnectCapture.Main (null) - Starting
2019-03-22 18:26:12,871 [1] ERROR ConnectCapture.Main (null) - Error opening/writing to UDP port :: Connection timed out
2019-03-22 18:26:13,381 [1] INFO ConnectCapture.PublishDeviceData (null) - {"time":"22/03/2019 18:26:12","deviceId":"b62b3ee7eafc4e98955fc95b54fe9b74","status":"off"}
2019-03-22 18:26:13,680 [1] INFO ConnectCapture.PublishDeviceData (null) - HTTP Resp is OK
2019-03-22 18:26:13,693 [1] INFO ConnectCapture.PublishDeviceData (null) - {"time":"22/03/2019 18:26:12","deviceId":"b62b3ee7eafc4e98955fc95b54fe9b74","status":"off"}
2019-03-22 18:27:14,644 [1] INFO ConnectCapture.Main (null) - Starting
2019-03-22 18:27:15,437 [1] INFO ConnectCapture.PublishDeviceData (null) - {"time":"22/03/2019 18:27:14","deviceId":"b62b3ee7eafc4e98955fc95b54fe9b74","status":"on"}
2019-03-22 18:27:15,908 [1] INFO ConnectCapture.PublishDeviceData (null) - HTTP Resp is OK
2019-03-22 18:27:15,924 [1] INFO ConnectCapture.PublishDeviceData (null) - {"time":"22/03/2019 18:27:14","deviceId":"b62b3ee7eafc4e98955fc95b54fe9b74","status":"on"}

On Fri, Mar 22, 2019 at 5:58 PM   wrote:
2019-03-22 17:40:57,935 [1] INFO ConnectCapture.Main (null) - Starting
2019-03-22 17:41:18,461 [1] ERROR ConnectCapture.Main (null) - Error opening/writing to UDP port :: Connection timed out
2019-03-22 17:41:18,981 [1] INFO ConnectCapture.PublishDeviceData (null) - {"time":"22/03/2019 17:41:18","deviceId":"b62b3ee7eafc4e98955fc95b54fe9b74","status":"off"}
2019-03-22 17:41:19,310 [1] INFO ConnectCapture.PublishDeviceData (null) - HTTP Resp is OK
2019-03-22 17:41:19,323 [1] INFO ConnectCapture.PublishDeviceData (null) - {"time":"22/03/2019 17:41:18","deviceId":"b62b3ee7eafc4e98955fc95b54fe9b74","status":"off"}
2019-03-22 17:42:20,207 [1] INFO ConnectCapture.Main (null) - Starting
2019-03-22 17:42:41,042 [1] ERROR ConnectCapture.Main (null) - Error opening/writing to UDP port :: Connection timed out
2019-03-22 17:42:41,554 [1] INFO ConnectCapture.PublishDeviceData (null) - {"time":"22/03/2019 17:42:41","deviceId":"b62b3ee7eafc4e98955fc95b54fe9b74","status":"off"}
2019-03-22 17:42:41,846 [1] INFO ConnectCapture.PublishDeviceData (null) - HTTP Resp is OK
2019-03-22 17:42:41,859 [1] INFO ConnectCapture.PublishDeviceData (null) - {"time":"22/03/2019 17:42:41","deviceId":"b62b3ee7eafc4e98955fc95b54fe9b74","status":"off"}
...

Fig. 13 ON/OFF status obtained in JSON

iii. The total usage of the device can be found which provides useful insights like total equipment utilization, etc.

iv. The downtime of the equipment is obtained which is used to interpret the effectiveness of the biomedical engineers.

v. The equipment that are not put to use can also be calculated which enhances decision making to downsize the equipment.

vi. The billing can be automated in the ICU for the utilization of equipment based on the actual time used rather than the round off value.

ii. Vitals from the Equipment:

The monitor, ventilator, and the pumps can be connected to the IoT to obtain the vitals of the patient connected to the respective equipment. This can be directly connected

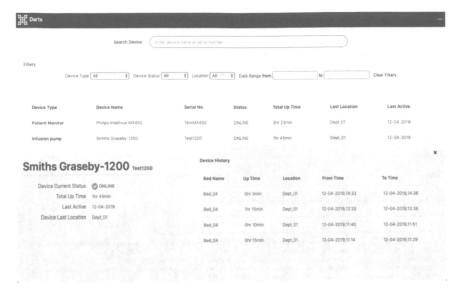

Fig. 14 Device time status

with the Electronic Medical Records of the hospital. Due to this the time taken by the nurses can be reduced to a great extent (Fig. 15).

The above figure indicates the values obtained for every 30 minutes. The values are obtained from all the equipment for a particular patient, and it is displayed. These values are directly imported to the EMR of the hospital (Figs. 16, 17, 18, 19 and 20).

The UI displays the following:

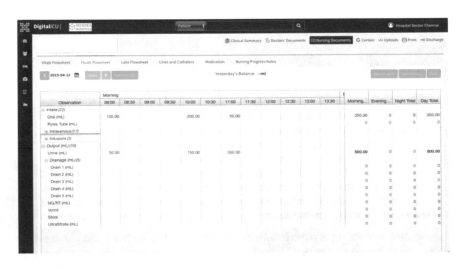

Fig. 15 Vitals from the equipment

Fig.16 IoT dashboard

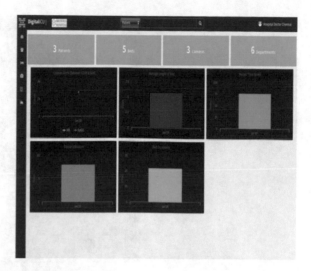

Fig.17 Vitals trend i.e., data from monitor & ventilator of the patients are charted

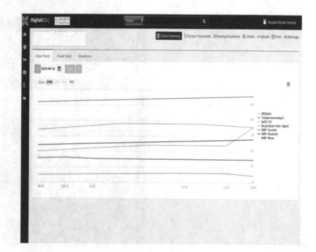

Vitals Flowchart: The vitals from the monitor and ventilator are displayed here

Fluid Flowchart: The vitals from the syringe and infusion pumps are displayed here

The benefits obtained from the data obtained are as follows:

i. The patient vitals are updated automatically to the EMR which reduces the time taken by the nurses to note it down manually (the checklist is attached in the report below).

ii. An alert is provided to the doctors and other staff nurses for the critical patient values (threshold values) that are obtained from the monitor and ventilator. This reduces the compulsion and need for doctors to always be on rounds.

Fig. 18 Fluid trend

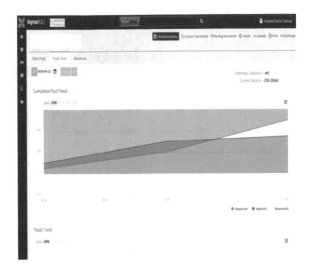

Fig. 19 Doctor's
document–procedure

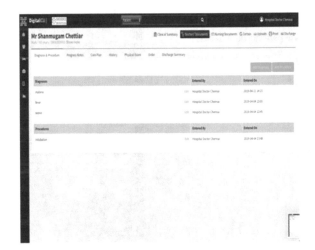

iii. By obtaining these records the discharge process can be made simpler.

Process flow in an ICU:
Process flow after IoT based equipment monitoring:

Fig. 20 Doctor's
document—history

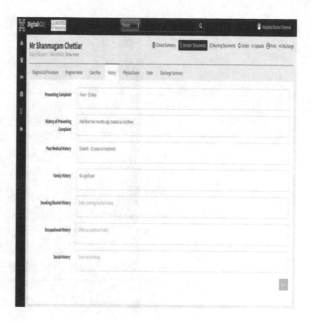

4.3 Observation of Traditional Process Flow Versus Process Flow After IoT Application

a. In the traditional process flow, manual entry of equipment and patient data makes the process slow (Figs. 21, 22, 23, 24 and 25).

b. When the equipment is connected to an IoT, the manual data can be avoided and the patients can be monitored remotely. This avoids the nurses to enter the data manually for every 30 min which is a standard for NABH.

When the data is remotely monitored, alerts can be provided for the doctors and staff nurses which makes it convenient for the doctors to attend the patients at the time of emergency (Figs. 26, 27 and 28).

Checklist for tracking nursing time spent:

Average time taken by the patient = Total time/Number of samples

$$=2581/30$$
$$=86.03 \text{ secs/patient}$$

The nurse on an average takes manual readings for every 30 min.

When the work time of the nurse is considered to be for 8 h, then the nurse takes 16 readings per day.

So the total time taken by one nurse = 16 * Average time taken by the patient.

$$=16 * 86.03$$
$$=1376.48 \text{ secs (or) } 22.94 \text{ mins}$$

When the data are remotely monitored, the nurse time can be saved as much as 22.94 min on an average per day.

So calculating the same per year,

Fig.21 Nursing document

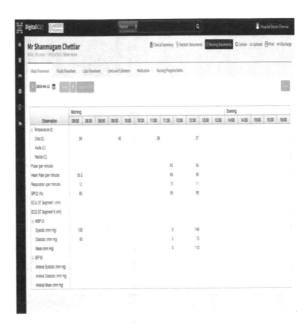

Fig.22 Nursing document

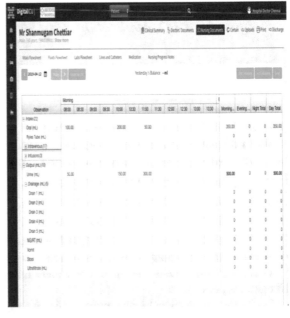

Fig. 23 Discharged patient's reports

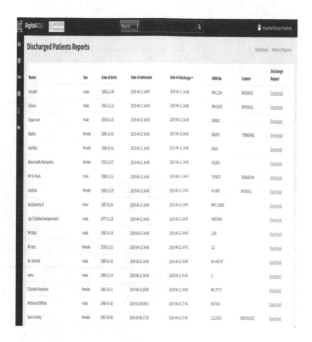

Total time saved per year = 22.94 min/ day * Number of days.

(Considering the average working per year is 262 days) = 22.94 * 262.

=6010.28 mins (or) 100.17 hours

Considering an average of 262 days, a nurse time can be saved up to 100 h.

Traditional discharge process vs IoT based discharge process:

In the traditional discharge process, the following processes take place,

1. Discharge decision taken by the physician and the discharge process is initiated. Here time is consumed for manually checking the case reports of the patients.

2. Preparation of discharge note by the physician and the time is consumed for getting the investigation report to be merged with the discharge note.

3. Further processing of discharge note by ward secretary. Centralized discharge summary preparation process takes place. Time consumed for proof reading.

4. Preparation of rough discharge summary by the editor. Time consumed for getting billing and insurance clearance.

5. Completed discharge summary after proof read and signed by the physician.

6. Handover of discharge summary to the patients.

In the IoT based discharge process, the following steps takes place.

1. Discharge decision taken by the physician, and hence he collects all the records which are captured through the IoT device.

2. Data is proof read by the physician and it is signed.

3. Handing over off discharge summary after being signed by the physician.

Lean Quality tool—Jidoka:

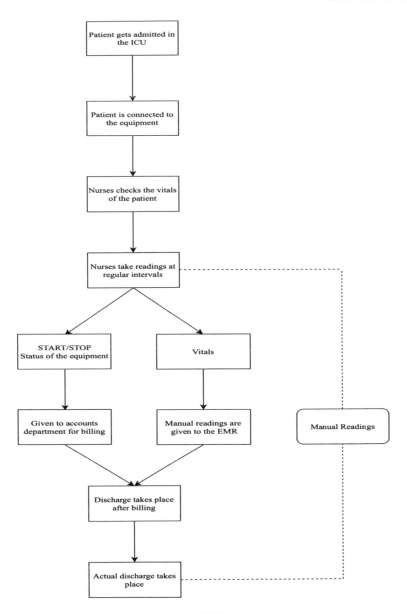

Fig. 24 Normal process flow taking place in an ICU

These are the four basic principles of Jidoka. These principles will be discussed in detail below:

i. To detect a problem: The details required for the discharge is not provided by the staff nurses and doctors on time.

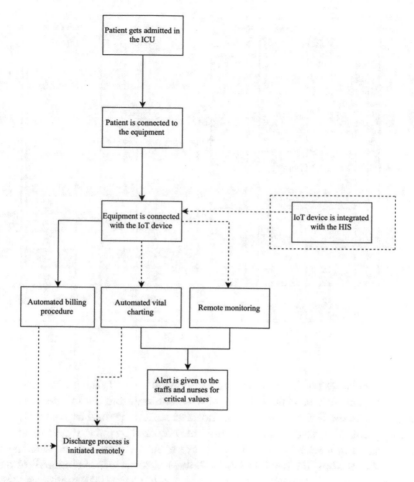

Fig. 25 Process flow after IoT based equipment monitoring

ii. To stop the process: This can be avoided by not obtaining the data from the doctors and nurses.

iii. Fix the problem immediately: The solution to this is by obtaining the data from remote devices i.e., an IoT device.

iv. Investigate the cause of the problem: The cause of the problem is because of the two reasons. One is busy schedule of the doctors and nurses. The other is because of the human error done by the nurses at the time of entering the manual data

It is suggested that doctors and other staff nurses can make use of IoT device to remotely monitor the vitals of the patient and prepare discharge summary (Figs. 29 and 30.

Patient ID	Nurses time taken (secs)	Patient ID	Nurses time taken (secs)
1	57	16	132
2	49	17	71
3	64	18	75
4	72	19	80
5	55	20	95
6	98	21	77
7	78	22	120
8	91	23	94
9	73	24	83
10	107	25	127
11	85	26	100
12	92	27	66
13	80	28	86
14	63	29	99
15	120	30	92
		Total	2581

Fig. 26 Checklist

Alerts can be set for the patient for threshold values so that the doctors can make prior arrangements and do the necessary. The summary from the IoT device can be integrated with the HIS and EMR of the hospital so that the discharge summary can be easily prepared. Based on the utilization rate prepared by the IoT device, decision making can be done. Decisions like purchase of new equipment, downsizing the equipment in the hospital can be taken with the statistical values obtained from the device. Medico-legal cases can be easily handled through the EMR reports generated by the IoT device. Cases like failure of equipment, etc. can be easily proved with the data generated by the device. Third Party Administrators (TPA) before approving the claims can verify if the utilization is based on the actual coverage. Once the equipment utilization monitoring system is introduced throughout the hospital, the standards can be improved and it can be remotely monitored by the NABH and JCI assessors. They do not have the necessity to come and visit the hospital at regular intervals. These are the suggested cases where the IoT can also be utilized.

5   Limitations of the Study

The study is confined only to four critical equipment in the ICU, namely, monitor, ventilator, syringe, and infusion pump. The HIS integration was done only for the Idea Med Hospital Information System, and it is not configured to the other HIS used

Traditional discharge process:

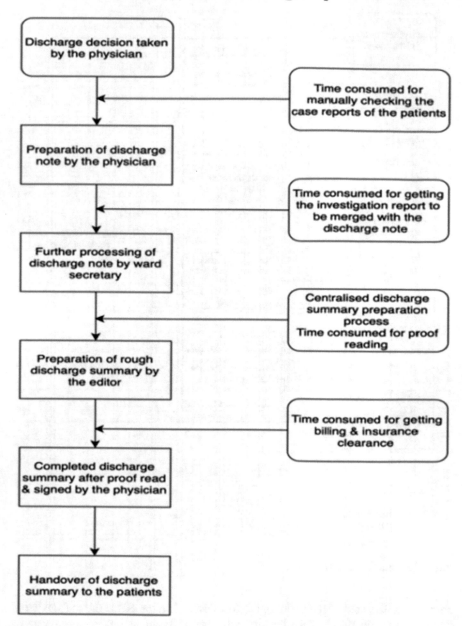

Fig. 27 Normal discharge process

IoT based discharge process:

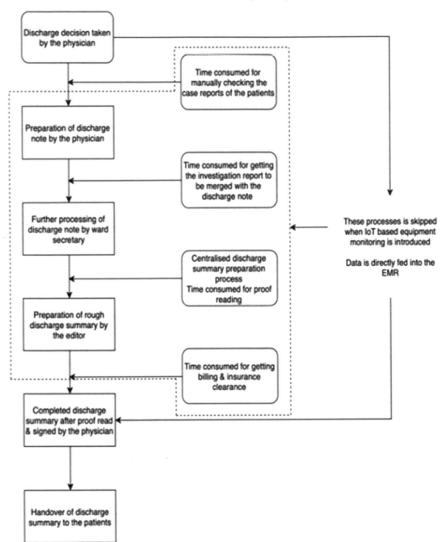

Fig. 28 IoT based discharge process

commonly. The cost of maintaining the IoT device is high. Since the IoT device is configured to the Wi-Fi of the hospital with the TCP enabled, it is more prone to cyber security attacks.

Fig. 29 Equipment
utilization time/duration

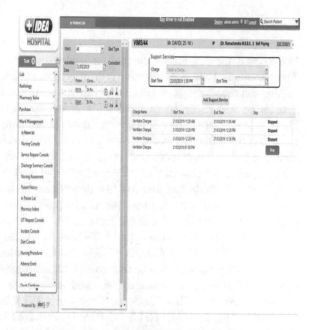

Fig. 30 Equipment
utilization charges

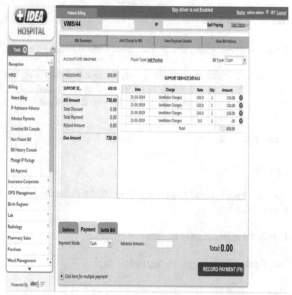

6 Conclusion

In a hospital, the ICU is considered to be generating higher revenue compared to other departments and hence its effective utilization is considered to be of high importance. Traditional monitoring systems consume a lot of time and perform unnecessary data generation which can be avoided through IoT-based equipment monitoring. The Quality department can easily use these data for decision making. Data like Average Length of Stay, Bed Occupancy Rate, etc. are generated by the IoT based on the data gathered (when implementation is done throughout the hospital). Based on these data, upscaling or downscaling of equipment can be done.

It is an inevitable fact that IoT is emerging in the field of medicine, and it may take a longer time to come under practice. Application of IoT in healthcare is quite challenging as the infrastructure of the existing hospitals and the equipment that are used in them do not readily support IoT-based healthcare delivery. In order to apply IoT in healthcare, every process of the department must be understood. Once the process is understood, it can be improved with IoT-based health systems. RTLS is a disruptive IoT technology that can be used vastly in the field of Healthcare. IoT in healthcare has over 100 different used cases, and RTLS is one among them. Different POCs were done based on RTLS in MGM Healthcare Pvt. Ltd as a part of this study. Doctors, staff nurses, equipment, etc. can be tracked using the RTLS device which makes it simpler for the non-clinical department to function smoothly.

Acknowledgements The authors would like to acknowledge all the participants in this study.

Author's Contributions: BKB and ABD conceptualized the study. BKB and ABD collected, analyzed the data and wrote the first draft of the manuscript. BKB and ABD contributed to the essential discussion points in the paper. All the authors have read and approved the final draft of the manuscript.

Funding: Nil.

Declarations

Ethics Approval and Consent to Participate: Institution Ethics approval and informed consent was obtained.

Consent for publication: Yes

Availability of Data and Materials: Yes.

Competing Interests: The authors hereby declare there is no potential competing interest.

References

1. Dimiter V Dimitrov (2016) Medical internet of things and big data in healthcare from the article. Health Care Inf Res 156–163

2. Bjorn Berg, Grant Longley, Jordan Dunitz (2019) Improving clinic operational efficiency and utilization with RTLS. J Med Syst 43
3. Megalingam RK, Kaimal DM, Ramesh MV (2012) Efficient patient monitoring for multiple patients using WSN. In: 2012 International conference on advances in mobile network, communication and its applications. Bangalore, pp. 87–90
4. Kozlovszky M (2013) Enabling patient remote rehabilitation through motion monitoring and analysis. In: IEEE 14th International symposium on computational intelligence and informatics (CINTI), Budapest, pp. 95–98

Suryanamaskar Pose Identification and Estimation Using No Code Computer Vision

Ujjayanta Bhaumik, Siddharth Chatterjee, and Koushlendra Kumar Singh

1 Introduction

Suryanamaskar, or Salute to the Sun, is a sequence of yoga asanas that originated from the old Indian yogic traditions [1]. It is a sequence of twelve asanas: Pranamasana, Hastauttanasana, Hasta Padasana, Ashwa Sanchalanasana, Dandasana, Ashtanga Namaskara, Bhujangasana, Dandasana, Ashwa Sanchalanasana, Hasta Padasana, Hastauttanasana, and Pranamasana. Five pose pairs are identical: first and twelfth, second and eleventh, third and tenth, fourth and ninth, and fifth and eighth. The sequence of asanas is designed in a way that each asana complements its previous one. Suryanamaskar has been known to reduce blood pressure, resting pulse rate, and improve cardio-vascular rates in individuals [2]. The current research examines a Suryanamaskar pose in isolation and aims to identify the pose as one of the seven different poses defined earlier. The developed software has been trained with multiple pose images and can accurately classify poses in real time. Microsoft lobe, a no code machine learning tool, has been used for the classification purpose. 700 images each of the seven poses were used in the training phase, and the accuracy obtained was 98%.

U. Bhaumik
Sustainable Living Labs, Singapore, Singapore
e-mail: ujjayanta.bhaumik.18@ucl.ac.uk

S. Chatterjee (✉)
The Math Company, Bengaluru, Karnataka 560025, India
e-mail: siddharth.chatterjee@themathcompany.com

K. Kumar Singh
NIT, Jamshedpur, Jharkhand, India
e-mail: koushlendra.cse@nitjsr.ac.in

© The Author(s), under exclusive license to Springer Nature Singapore Pte Ltd. 2021
M. K. Bajpai et al. (eds.), *Machine Vision and Augmented Intelligence—Theory and Applications*, Lecture Notes in Electrical Engineering 796,
https://doi.org/10.1007/978-981-16-5078-9_7

2 Literature Review

With the advent of deep learning, human posture recognition has been addressed in a lot of research. Posture recognition has found use in many fields like Human computer interaction, physical training, and awareness of surroundings. Huang et al. developed a posture recognition system based on indoor positioning technology by considering keypoints in the human body [5]. Barros et al. studied natural communication using hand gestures in human beings and their application in robotics [3]. Yan et al. used convolutional neural networks to predict whether particular driving postures are safe or unsafe [4]. Posture recognition can be a real boon in analyzing physical training as wrong postures can cause harm to the body. The recognized postures can be analyzed and compared to correct postures. Thar et al. proposed a method for finding out abnormalities in Yoga poses for self-learning using multipart detection with a PC camera [6]. Islam et al. proposed a technique for yoga posture recognition using Microsoft Kinect to aid the user in performing yoga [7]. They explored the use of Kinect with multiple methods like decision trees, support vector machines, naive bayes, and neural networks. The current work focuses particularly on Suryanamaskar, and Microsoft Lobe is used to detect the poses to aid the user in doing the asana.

Traditionally, machine learning is associated with lots of code. But in the past decade, there has been a rise of "no-code" approach in implementing web technologies, machine learning, app development, and so on [8–10]. No code approach would generally present users with a graphical user interface to guide them in designing elements without any coding requirements. No code gives one the ability to achieve the same things as one can do with code. It is more like programming in the visual domain. The current work uses this approach to tackle a machine learning problem in the form of yoga pose detection. The Microsoft Lobe platform is a graphical user interface that allows both automatic and manual labeling of images, and training is done with no code as well. All the programming abstractions and coding complexities are avoided in no code approach.

3 Data

This research data has been collected from Suryanamaskar videos by participants who decided to take part in the study. Frames were extracted from the videos using Python and labeled manually for each of the seven individual asanas. The images collected were taken in different conditions like different lighting conditions and different angles. Seven different individuals took part of the study. In total, there were 700 images each for each of the different asanas.

4 Methodology

The 700 different Suryanamaskar pose images are passed through the ResNet50V2 model with 50 layers (Fig. 1).

The extracted poses are automatically put into seven groups: Pranamasana, Hastauttanasana, Hasta Padasana, Ashwa Sanchalanasana, Dandasana, Ashtanga Namaskara, and Bhujangasana. Some image preprocessing is done in order to enhance the quality of input images, and also image augmentation is done to increase input points. The ResNet-50V2 architecture is trained in the backend by Microsoft Lobe [12]. Following the training, the inferencing is done in real-time as the users perform Suryanamaskar in front of the camera.

The key frames adopted from videos are then used for keypoint detection and pose estimation. For the pose estimation part, COCO keypoint dataset has been used. This step involves estimating where different body joints are located. Posenet

Fig. 1 Pose detection, identification, and estimation steps

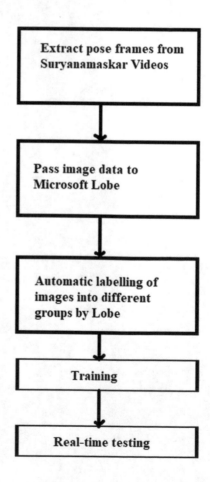

is a computer vision model where human pose estimation can be done in real time, for example, where someone's elbow shows up in an image (Fig. 2).

The reason behind using the COCO keypoint dataset is that it is a multi-person 2D pose estimation dataset that is incredibly robust. The pose estimation steps include removing the image background to focus on the human subject, extracting features from the image to build a confidence map to identify keypoints. The keypoints detected in order from 0 to 18 in the image below correspond to nose, neck, right shoulder, right elbow, right wrist, left shoulder, left elbow, left wrist, right hip, right knee, right ankle, left hip, left knee, left ankle, right eye, left eye, right ear, left ear, and background (Fig. 3).

Fig. 2 Residual learning building block

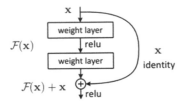

Fig. 3 Detected Keypoints for Pose Estimation

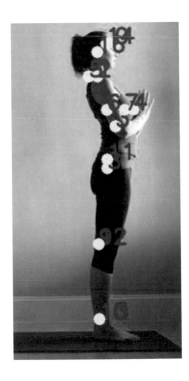

5 Experiments and Results

Microsoft Lobe allows classification by manual labeling of images or automatic labeling of images. In this case, the images were automatically labeled (Fig. 4).

Lobe is a no code app that uses machine learning in the backend to do computer vision tasks. The model was optimized for accuracy and not for speed which meant that the model gave slow but accurate results. The ResNet-50V2 model has been used for classification. ResNet-50V2 has 50 neural network layers where the weight layers are pre-activated. Batch normalization and ReLU activation are applied to the input before being multiplied with the weight matrix [11, 12]. Small variations of data are created during training to include more variations (Fig. 5).

The model predicted 99% of the images correctly. Some of the results are shown here:

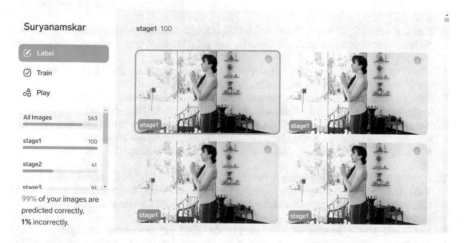

Fig. 4 Training stage

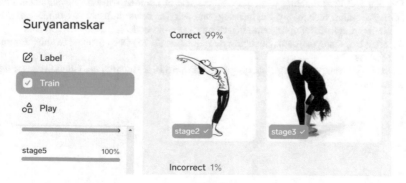

Fig. 5 Prediction results

6 Conclusion and Future Scope

The current work analyzes the utility of computer vision and machine learning in analyzing Suryanamaskar. The designed model achieved an accuracy of 99% in recognizing Suryanamaskar poses. The model also worked in real-time. As an extension, pose estimation done using models like the Coco model can be compared with an expert for further diagnosis.

References

1. Carol Mitchell (2003) Yoga on the ball. inner traditions. 48
2. Pratima M Bhutkar, Milind V Bhutkar, Govind Taware, Vinayak Dojiad, Doddamani BR (2008) Effect of Suryanamaskar practice on cardio-respiratory fitness parameters: a pilot study. 126–129
3. Barros P, Magg S, Weber C, Wermter SA (2014) Multichannel convolutional neural network for hand posture recognition. In: Wermter S, et al. (eds) artificial neural networks and machine learning
4. Chao Yan, Frans Coenen, Bailing Zhang (2016) Driving posture recognition by convolutional neural networks. 103–114. https://doi.org/10.1049/iet-cvi.2015.0175
5. Huang Xiaoping et al (2019) "A Posture Recognition Method Based on Indoor Positioning Technology." Sensors (Basel, Switzerland). https://doi.org/10.3390/s19061464
6. Thar MC, Winn KZN, Funabiki N (2019) A proposal of yoga pose assessment method using pose detection for self-learning. In: 2019 International conference on advanced information technologies (ICAIT), Yangon, Myanmar, 137–142. https://doi.org/10.1109/AITC.2019.8920892
7. Muhammad Islam, Hasan Mahmud, Faisal Ashraf, Iqbal Hossain, Md. Kamrul Hasan (2017) Yoga posture recognition by detecting human joint points in real time using microsoft kinect, IEEE Region 10 humanitarian technology conference (R10-HTC). https://doi.org/10.1109/r10-htc.2017.8289047
8. Data predictions in minutes, without writing code (2020) https://www.obviously.ai/
9. Create no-code predictive models with Azure machine learning (2020) https://Docs.Microsoft.Com/. https://docs.microsoft.com/en-us/learn/paths/create-no-code-predictive-models-azure-machine-learning/
10. Caballar RD Programming without code: the rise of no-code software development (2020) IEEE spectrum: technology, engineering, and science news. https://spectrum.ieee.org/tech-talk/computing/software/programming-without-code-no-code-software-development
11. Kaiming He, Xiangyu Zhang, Shaoqing Ren, Jian Sun (2015) Deep residual learning for image recognition
12. Kaiming He, Xiangyu Zhang, Shaoqing Ren, Jian Sun (2016) Identity mappings in deep residual networks

A Review on Digital Watermarking-Based Image Forensic Technique

Sanjay Kumar⬦ and Binod Kumar Singh⬦

1 Introduction

Advances in digital imaging technology have raised new concerns and problems about verification and integrity regarding digital images [14, 33]. Ensuring the integrity of obtained images and original possession for possible flaws in the security of non-private internet poses a challenge. The analysis of the authenticity of images along with their elements, recognizing source, and detection of forgery is termed digital image forensics [7]. By applying different methods for authenticating digital images, digital forensics has popped up in the past years. Active and passive are the two categories in which the approaches for authentication for images can be classified [1, 4, 13, 20]. Advanced knowledge of components related to the cover image is required in the active methods. Passive techniques do not require any prior knowledge about the original image. Active authentication techniques are classified further into two techniques: digital signatures and digital watermarking [20]. In a watermarking-based image forensics technique, insertion of the watermark within the cover image takes place. Fragile, semi-fragile, and robust are the three classes in which the watermarking scheme can be classified. For authentication fragile and semi-fragile watermarking schemes are used.

Apart from digital forensics watermarking is also used in applications like copyright protection, copy control, data aggregation, etc. [9–12]. In the recent Covid-19 outbreak, there has been a fast growth of telemedicine where medical images are mainly used for diagnosis [2]. This lead to a rise in concern for the privacy and security of medical images. Watermarking-based techniques can be used to protect privacy as well as security of medical data. In the case of the region of interest (ROI)-based watermarking, the information produced from the ROI is embedded

S. Kumar (✉) · B. K. Singh
National Institute of Technology, Jamshedpur, India
e-mail: 2017rscs001@nitjsr.ac.in

© The Author(s), under exclusive license to Springer Nature Singapore Pte Ltd. 2021
M. K. Bajpai et al. (eds.), *Machine Vision and Augmented Intelligence—Theory and Applications*, Lecture Notes in Electrical Engineering 796,
https://doi.org/10.1007/978-981-16-5078-9_8

into the region of non-interest (RONI). Watermark embedding and extraction are the two steps in the process of watermarking. Traditionally, watermarks are embedded in the cover image either in the frequency domain or in the spatial domain [10, 14]. But in the last few decades, several hybrid domain watermarking schemes are proposed [18, 26, 29]. Spatial domain watermarking is suitable for data authentication, whereas frequency domain and hybrid domain watermarking are generally suitable for copyright protection.

The major benefaction of this work is:

1.   A comprehensive literature review of watermarking-based image forensics is carried out.
2.   Comprehensive analysis of active and passive image forensics is disused.
3.   Various issues and challenges of active image forensics are discussed.

The outline of the rest of the paper is as follows: In Sect. 2, an overview of digital image forensics techniques is briefly discussed. Digital watermarking is briefly discussed in Sect. 3. In Sect. 4, some of the recent state-of-the-art watermark-based image forensics are disused. The issues and challenges of active image forensics are discussed in Sect. 5, and in Sect. 6 conclusion is drawn.

2   Digital Image Forensics Technique

Digital image forensics is an investigation sphere that focuses on the ratification of the authenticity of images [22]. To date, several techniques are developed to validate digital images and are broadly classified into two classes: active and passive [1, 4, 20]. Further, active techniques can be subdivided into two sub-classes: digital watermarking and digital signature. Cryptography algorithms like hash functions are used to gain the signature information when techniques based on signature are applied to an image. High security to the key agreement and unchanged cover image during authentication are the advantages of digital signature-based image forensics. However, a disadvantage of digital signature-based techniques is that the detection and localization of the corrupted regions of the changed images are not possible [5, 16]. On the contrary, binary sequence, binary logo, or information data are inserted as a watermark on the unrevealed regions of the image in watermarking-based techniques. In order to detect corrupted or altered areas of the image extracted watermarks are put to use. In addition to image authentication and tamper detection, watermarking is used in several other applications like copyright protection, copy control, fingerprint, etc. The various characteristics that an image authentication technique must have are discussed in the following [32]:

- Invisibility/imperceptibility: The watermark inserted into the cover image must be not visible.
- Sensitivity: The watermarking system must be able to sense malicious manipulations.

- Tolerance: Watermarking system should endure losing some information (lossy compression).
- Payload: The higher size of authentication data may alter the quality of the original image.

On the contrary, the passive techniques can be subdivided into five subclasses: geometry-based, format-based, pixel-based, physical environment-based, and camera-based. Passive techniques are based on the hypothesis that the underlying statistics could change, even if visual evidence is not left by forgery as a result of tampering [20]. Figure 1 depicts various image forgery detection techniques. Table 1 shows the comparison between the digital watermark-based and passive image forensics techniques.

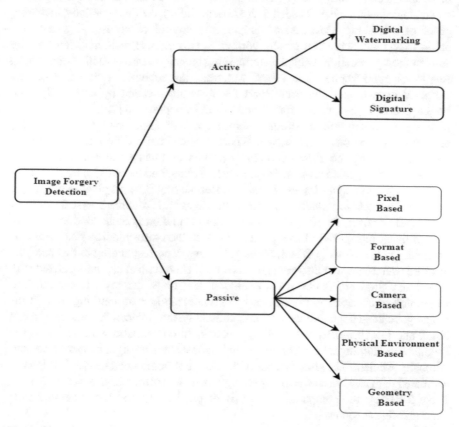

Fig. 1 Classification of image forensics techniques

Table 1 Comparison between digital watermarking and passive techniques

–	Digital watermarking	Passive technique
Accuracy	High	Low as compared to watermark-based technique
Computational complexity	Low	High

3 Digital Watermarking

Digital watermarking can be defined as the method of inserting some information (watermark) into a digital multimedia element (image, video, or audio), probably in an undetectable way such that the quality of the content didn't get degraded. At any later level, such embedded data are detected for various functions, including proof of ownership, detection of tamper, and control of access. A watermark-based image authentication system comprises two phases: watermark embedding and tampering detection. Digital watermarking techniques are classified into robust, fragile, or semi-fragile. In a robust watermarking scheme, watermarks can be extracted even though the watermarked images are violated by commonly used image processing techniques, for example, JPEG compression [23]. In fragile watermarking, the watermark is extremely sensitive to tampering, even though there are only minor alterations in the image. Whereas semi-fragile watermarking methods focus on resisting the allowable content-preserving changes and notice malevolent content changes. Pixel-wise fragile watermarking and block-wise fragile watermarking are two major classes of fragile watermarking [25]. In pixel-based fragile watermarking scheme watermark information is gained from the grayscale value of each pixel of cover. Besides, this watermark information is embedded into the list of significant bits (LSB) of that pixel itself or to the corresponding pixel which is mapped. In case, if any grayscale value got changed, corresponding to that pixel the inserted watermark will also change hence each altered pixel can be localized with ease. Each block created by the small block division of the cover image contains watermark information in the case of block-wise fragile watermarking. Here if the image got changed intentionally or unintentionally, the watermark contained in that block and the corrupted block will not match. In comparison with a pixel-based fragile watermarking scheme, block-based fragile watermarking schemes are computationally efficient. The effectiveness of the fragile watermark technique is primarily estimated with two criteria: security strength and tamper localization accuracy [15]. Table 2 depicts the comparative analysis of pixel-based and block-based fragile watermarking schemes.

Table 2 Comparison between pixel-based and block-based fragile watermarking

–	Pixel-based fragile watermarking scheme	Block-based fragile watermarking scheme
Complexity	High	low
Imperceptivlity	Low	high
Tamper localization accuracy	High	low
Security	Vulnerable to attacks	Can resist various attacks

4 State-of-the-Art

Recently, several works are carried out in the field of digital watermarking-based image forensics techniques. In this section, some of the recent digital watermarking-based image forensic techniques are summarized below.

Tiwari et al. proposed an image watermarking scheme based on vector quantization (VQ) for image authentication [31]. Experimental results exhibit that the average false rate of this scheme is 0.00021, whereas 0.0014 is the average false negative rate achieved. In [28] a semi-fragile watermarking scheme using integer wavelet transform (IWT) and discrete cosine transform (DCT) is proposed. Here two different watermarks, namely authentication watermark and recovery watermark, are used. The use of a tamper detection map and normalized hamming similarity (NHS) increases the performance of this watermarking scheme. Thanki and Borra have presented a hybrid domain non-blind fragile watermarking scheme for the detection of tamper and copyrights of sensitive images [30]. As this scheme uses a non-blind technique so only the authorized person can extract the watermark. For image authentication pixel-based fragile watermarking is proposed by Zhang et al. [33]. Further, Arnold transform is used twice at the time of watermark embedding for the security of the watermark. Kamili et al. proposed a dual watermarking framework for tamper detection and content authentication for industrial images [8]. DCT domain is used for robust watermarking whereas in the spatial domain the fragile watermark is embedded. For protecting the authenticity and integrity of medical images, Liu et al. proposed a reversible watermarking scheme [17]. This scheme consists of a total of four phases, i.e., watermark generation; watermark embedding; watermark extraction; and security verification. Here, without dividing ROI and RONI watermarks are inserted into the entire medical images.

Gul and Ozturk proposed a block-based fragile watermarking scheme using the SHA-256 hash function and LSB substitution [5]. Here, the cover image is divided into blocks of size 32×32 which are non-overlapping. Further, each of these blocks is subdivided into four subblocks of size 16×16. From the first three subblocks, the binary watermark is generated using SHA-256 and is embedded into the fourth subblock. In [6] self-embedded fragile watermarking technique is proposed with triple recovery information embedding method. Here, the MD-5 hash function and

LSB substitution technique are used. In [24] self-embedding fragile watermarking scheme using block truncation coding (BTC) is proposed. Further, LSB substitution is used to embed the watermark. For the efficient localization of corrupted image content, Prasad and Pal proposed a fragile watermarking scheme [21]. This scheme robustly detects forged image content at the block level. Here, a watermark is created by Hamming code from the most significant bit (MSB) of each pixel. Haghighi et al. proposed a semi-fragile watermarking technique for the detection of tamper and recovery with the use of LWT, DCT, and feed-forward neural network (FNN) [3]. Here, one level of LWT is applied over the host image, and DCT is applied to each 2 × 2 block of diagonal details. Further, by correlating DC coefficients a random binary sequence is inserted in every block. For color images to deliver effective image tamper detection and self-recovery, Sinhal et al. proposed a fragile watermarking scheme [27]. Here, for inserting each channel of the RGB image is split up into 2 × 4 size blocks which are non-overlapping. Further, in these blocks watermark is embedded using LSB techniques. The summary of the recent state-of-the-art techniques is depicted in Table 3.

5 Issues and Challenges of Digital Signature and Watermarking-Based Image Forensics Techniques

One of the major limitations of the active image forensic technique is that watermarks or signatures need to be embedded in the image before distribution. However, most cameras in the market nowadays are not equipped with the function of watermark embedding. The digital signature-based technique cannot detect and localize the tampered regions of the altered images. Also in the case of the digital signature, it is very challenging to keep private keys safely [7]. For signature-based authentication, the time complexity is very high for key generation and verification. Further, the storage of all previous keys is another issue. The digital signature approach fails to provide confidentiality to the images. In the field of medical imaging, confidentiality is its prime concern.

One of the major challenges for the watermarking-based approach is that to embed the watermark, specialized hardware or software is needed. In a digital watermarking-based approach there is always a trade-off between its various features [10]. Furthermore, in various watermarking techniques, blocks that are small in size are used for the watermark inserting process. However, the visual quality of images that are watermarked gets reduced when a huge amount of data is inserted into small blocks. However, an area like fine artwork, military image, or medical images requires restoring of original host images. This indicates that irreversible image verifying schemes cannot protect integrity suitably in this area [19]. From the above discussion, it is clear that a lot of work can be done in the area of watermark-based image forensics.

Table 3 Summary of state-of-the-art techniques

References	Technique Used	Result	Remarks
[31]	Vector quantization, modified index key—based method	Average FPR = 0.00024, average FNR = 0.0012, average PSNR = 42 dB, accuracy = 99.8%	Can recognize crop, text addition, and cut attacks as malicious attacks
[28]	IWT, DCT	Average PSNR = 40.84 dB	NHS and tamper detection map improve the performance of this scheme
[30]	CS theory, discrete wavelet transform (DWT), and non-subsampled contourlet transform (NSCT)	For grayscale watermark average PSNR = 42.66 dB, average CC = 0.9971	This method can be used for authentication along with detection of tamper of sensitive color images
[33]	Singular value decomposition (SVD), LSB substitution, Arnold transform	Average PSNR = 51.16 dB	Experimental outcomes reveal that the watermarked images obtained have an acceptable visual effect
[8]	DCT, chaotic, and DNA encryption	Average NCC for signal attack = 0.95, average NCC hybrid attack = 0.90, for a payload of 8192 bits PSNR is more than 41 dB	This scheme can be used for protecting vital and precious industrial images
[17]	Integer wavelet transform, block truncation coding, Slantlet transform, SVD	Average PSNR = 41.29 dB, average SSIM = 0.9607, average BER = 0.0476	To avoid the threats caused due to segmentation of the image in a spatial manner, here watermarks are inserted into complete medical images
[5]	SHA-256, LSB substitution	For 1024 × 1024 size image average PSNR = 57.16 dB, watermark embedding time = 7.328386 s, tamper detection time = 7.480778	The proposed scheme uses the quarter part of non-overlapped blocks for embedding the watermark
[6]	MD-5, LSB substitution	Watermarked image PSNR = 44.14, recovered image PSNR = 30.49	Every block of the image holds recovery information of the other three blocks that offers a triple chance of tampered area recovery

(continued)

Table 3 (continued)

References	Technique Used	Result	Remarks
[24]	Block truncation coding, LSB substitution	Average PSNR = 39.0 dB	The proposed scheme gives high-quality recovery fidelity along with negilagble blocking artifacts
[21]	Block-level pixel adjustment process, pixel-value differencing, Hamming code	Average PSNR = 42.08 dB, average SSIM = 0.9993, average IF = 0.9839	As this scheme offers indirect data hiding process, the watermark embedding technique causes less distortion
[3]	LWT, feed-forward neural network, DCT	Average PSNR = 44.23 dB, average SSIM = 0.9925	It is appropriate for real-time applications because of IALF efficiency and simplicity
[27]	LSB substitution	Accuracy = 99%, PSNR = 49.68	Controlled random watermark as presented in this work makes the technique more strong against block-wise attacks

6 Conclusion and Future Direction

Watermarking is one of the computationally efficient approaches for image authentication. In this paper, an overview of active and passive image forensics techniques is briefly discussed. Further, digital watermarking in image authentication is discussed in this work. We have also presented various issues and challenges of watermark-based image forensics technique. From the extensive discussion in this work, it is noticed that there is always a trade-off between the different features of the watermarking scheme.

A lot of work can be done by the researcher to satisfy these trade-offs. Also, in the field of medical image watermarking, it is challenging for the researcher to develop a watermarking scheme such that along with authentication the confidentiality of the medical image is also ensured. Also for authentication, several works have been carried out for the grayscale images, but it is a burning research issue for color and 3D image authentication. The authors believe that this paper will prove to be an aid for the researcher to further work in the direction of watermark-based image forensics.

References

1. Akhtar Z, Khan E (2018). Revealing the traces of histogram equalisation in digital images. https://doi.org/10.1049/iet-ipr.2017.0992
2. Bokolo Anthony Jnr (2020) Use of telemedicine and virtual care for remote treatment in response to COVID-19 pandemic. J Med Syst 44(7):132. https://doi.org/10.1007/s10916-020-01596-5
3. Bolourian Haghighi B et al (2020) An effective semi-fragile watermarking method for image authentication based on lifting wavelet transform and feed-forward neural network. Cognit Comput 12(4):863–890. https://doi.org/10.1007/s12559-019-09700-9
4. Ferreira WD et al (2020) A review of digital image forensics. Comput Electr Eng 85. https://doi.org/10.1016/j.compeleceng.2020.106685
5. Gul E, Ozturk S (2019) A novel hash function based fragile watermarking method for image integrity. Multimed Tools Appl. https://doi.org/10.1007/s11042-018-7084-0
6. Gul E, Ozturk S (2020) A novel triple recovery information embedding approach for self-embedded digital image watermarking. Multimed Tools Appl. https://doi.org/10.1007/s11042-020-09548-4
7. Jisha TE, Monoth T (2019) Authenticity and integrity enhanced active digital image forensics based on visual cryptography. Springer Singapore. https://doi.org/10.1007/978-981-13-1927-3_19
8. Kamili A et al (2020) DWFCAT: dual watermarking framework for industrial image authentication and tamper localization. IEEE Trans Ind Inform 3203 c, 1–1. https://doi.org/10.1109/tii.2020.3028612.
9. Kumar C et al (2018) A recent survey on image watermarking techniques and its application in e-governance. Multimed Tools Appl 77(3):3597–3622. https://doi.org/10.1007/s11042-017-5222-8
10. Kumar S et al (2020) A recent survey on multimedia and database watermarking. Multimed Tools Appl 79(27–28):20149–20197. https://doi.org/10.1007/s11042-020-08881-y
11. Kumar S et al (2020) Role of digital watermarking in wireless sensor network. Recent Adv Comput Sci Commun 13. https://doi.org/10.2174/2666255813999200730230731
12. Kumar S, Dutta A (2016) A novel spatial domain technique for digital image watermarking using block entropy. In: 2016 International conference on recent trends in information technology. 1–4. https://doi.org/10.1109/ICRTIT.2016.7569530
13. Kumar S, Nagori S (2017) Key-point based copy-move forgery detection in digital images. J Stat Manag Syst 20(4):611–621. https://doi.org/10.1080/09720510.2017.1395181
14. Kumar S, Singh BK (2020) Entropy based spatial domain image watermarking and its performance analysis. Multimed Tools Appl. https://doi.org/10.1007/s11042-020-09943-x
15. Li C et al (2013) Multi-block dependency based fragile watermarking scheme for fingerprint images protection. Multimed Tools Appl 64(3):757–776. https://doi.org/10.1007/s11042-011-0974-z
16. Li X et al (2015) Image integrity authentication scheme based on fixed point theory. IEEE Trans Image Process 24(2):632–645. https://doi.org/10.1109/TIP.2014.2372473
17. Liu X et al (2019) A novel robust reversible watermarking scheme for protecting authenticity and integrity of medical images. IEEE Access 7:76580–76598. https://doi.org/10.1109/ACCESS.2019.2921894
18. Liu XL et al (2018) Blind dual watermarking for color image's authentication and copyright protection. IEEE Trans Circuits Syst Video Technol 28(5):1047–1055. https://doi.org/10.1109/TCSVT.2016.2633878
19. Nguyen TS et al (2016) A reversible image authentication scheme based on fragile watermarking in discrete wavelet transform domain. AEU Int J Electron Commun 70(8):1055–1061. https://doi.org/10.1016/j.aeue.2016.05.003
20. Pandey RC et al (2016) Passive forensics in image and video using noise features: a review. Digit Investig 19(182):1–28. https://doi.org/10.1016/j.diin.2016.08.002

21. Prasad S, Pal AK (2020) A tamper detection suitable fragile watermarking scheme based on novel payload embedding strategy. Multimed Tools Appl 79(3–4):1673–1705. https://doi.org/10.1007/s11042-019-08144-5
22. Redi JA et al (2011) Digital image forensics: a booklet for beginners. Multimed Tools Appl 51(1):133–162. https://doi.org/10.1007/s11042-010-0620-1
23. Shen JJ et al (2020) A self embedding fragile image authentication based on singular value decomposition. Multimed Tools Appl. https://doi.org/10.1007/s11042-020-09254-1
24. Singh D, Singh SK (2019) Block Truncation Coding based effective watermarking scheme for image authentication with recovery capability. Multimed Tools Appl 78(4):4197–4215. https://doi.org/10.1007/s11042-017-5454-7
25. Singh D, Singh SK (2017) DCT based efficient fragile watermarking scheme for image authentication and restoration. Multimed Tools Appl 76(1):953–977. https://doi.org/10.1007/s11042-015-3010-x
26. Singh RK, Shaw DK (2018) A hybrid concept of cryptography and dual watermarking (LSB-DCT) for data security. Int J Inf Secur Priv 12(1):1–12. https://doi.org/10.4018/IJISP.2018010101
27. Sinhal R et al (2020) Blind image watermarking for localization and restoration of color images. IEEE Access:1–1. https://doi.org/10.1109/access.2020.3035428
28. Sivasubramanian N, Konganathan G (2020) A novel semi fragile watermarking technique for tamper detection and recovery using IWT and DCT. Comput 102(6):1365–1384. https://doi.org/10.1007/s00607-020-00797-7
29. Taher F et al (2016) A new hybrid watermarking algorithm for MRI medical images using DWT and hash functions. In: Proceedings of Annual International Conference of the IEEE Engineering in Medicine and Biology Society (EMBS). 2016 Oct, 1212–1215. https://doi.org/10.1109/EMBC.2016.7590923
30. Thanki R, Borra S (2019) Fragile watermarking for copyright authentication and tamper detection of medical images using compressive sensing (CS) based encryption and contourlet domain processing. Multimed Tools Appl 78(10):13905–13924. https://doi.org/10.1007/s11042-018-6746-2
31. Tiwari A et al (2017) Watermarking based image authentication and tamper detection algorithm using vector quantization approach. AEU Int J Electron Commun 78:114–123. https://doi.org/10.1016/j.aeue.2017.05.027
32. Tuncer T (2018) A probabilistic image authentication method based on chaos. Multimed Tools Appl 77(16):21463–21480. https://doi.org/10.1007/s11042-017-5569-x
33. Zhang H et al (2017) Fragile watermarking for image authentication using the characteristic of SVD. Algorithms 10:1. https://doi.org/10.3390/a10010027

An IoT-Enabled Smart Waste Segregation System

Subham Divakar, Abhishek Bhattacharjee, Vikash Kumar Soni,
Rojalina Priyadarshini, Rabindra Kumar Barik, and Diptendu Sinha Roy

1 Introduction

Enormous development in technology in the field of Internet of Things (IoT) has changed how people used to live and work. It is a rising technology and represents the future of the entire world. IoT provides exchange and linkage between low-energy devices and interactions through the Internet [1, 2]. IoT is making machines smarter day by day. But a bit of caution is that IoT consumes energy and produce e-wastes, so this does not seem to be environment-friendly. We should always go for the technology which contributes to reduce emissions, low pollutions and minimize power consumption [3–5]. Waste management becomes a cause of concern these days for the world. In a recent survey, it was recorded that 2.1 billion tons of municipal solid waste generates every year and 35% of the waste materials are not able to manage in an environmentally safe manner. Owing to this in many smart cities, IoT-enabled waste management system service is present, which not only focuses on the collection of waste materials but also transports the waste materials to its given

S. Divakar
Persistent Systems, Pune, India

A. Bhattacharjee
Cognizant Solutions, Bangalore, India

V. K. Soni
Infosys, Bangalore, India

R. Priyadarshini (✉)
C.V.Raman Global University, Bhubaneswar, India

R. K. Barik
KIIT Deemed To Be University, Bhubaneswar, India

D. S. Roy
NIT Meghalaya, Shillong, India

© The Author(s), under exclusive license to Springer Nature Singapore Pte Ltd. 2021   101
M. K. Bajpai et al. (eds.), *Machine Vision and Augmented Intelligence—Theory
and Applications*, Lecture Notes in Electrical Engineering 796,
https://doi.org/10.1007/978-981-16-5078-9_9

locations [6]. IoT-based waste management model performs an important role in improving the way of living and human well-being by increasing energy efficiency, enhancing governance and reducing cost [7, 8]. With the increase in waste in this growing world, we also need a solution to manage, control and understand the waste generated in our day to day life. If done so then waste management and control will go hand in hand with protecting the environment. This paper deals with such waste management which was achieved with IoT and deep learning (DL) technology [9]. It shows how we can separate waste materials into two categories: (1) organic waste (2) and recyclable waste. The use of IoT was such that the waste bins are smart bins that are fitted with IoT components such as Raspberry Pi, infrared sensors and a camera. The DL comes to action with the help of IoT components as infrared sensors detect the waste and trigger the camera and the camera, in turn, takes the images of the waste and the trained DL model helps to separate the waste. The training of the models is explained further in the paper below. This method of separation of waste is unique and can help out in any environment and word-related works. The major contributions of this work are as follows: (1) Automatic segregation of waste by capturing the images of waste. (2) Use of DL-based intelligent solutions to categorize the waste. The rest of the paper is divided into five sections. The first section is the introduction, the second section talks about related works, the third section deals with our proposed work in detail, followed by the fourth section which talks about results and discussion, and the last section discusses the conclusion and future scope.

2   Related Works

The use of sensors in waste management is studied in this section and discussed over here. Misra et al. in their work showed the use of ultrasonic sensors and various gas sensors to detect hazardous gases and the maximum limit of waste. They also used cloud and mobile app-based monitoring systems [10]. Singh et al. used infrared sensors connected to a Raspberry Pi board to collect real-time data from the waste bins to check the level of waste present in the bins and communicated the results to the waste managers [11]. Hong et al. in their proposed work developed an IoT-based smart garbage system for food management. They connected many smart garbage bins together with routers and servers and collected the data and status from each waste bin and the solution focused on reducing the waste and saving cost [12]. Malapur and Pattanshetti in their suggested work discussed an IoT-based approach where they collected the information of waste from the bins to get the details of the volume of waste being generated and developed an efficient trip planning for the collection of the waste according to their density. This optimal trip planning helped to reduce cost and time for waste collection [13]. Kumar et al. in their paper checked the waste level of garbage bins using sensor systems [14]. Once the limit of the garbage in the bin exceeds the limit, then the concerned authorized garbage collection agency is informed using a GPRS/GSM system placed in the waste bin itself. Bharadwaj et al. showed how by making use of sensors they collected data from the garbage bins and sent them to a gateway using LoRa technology [15]. They sent the data from various garbage bins to the cloud over the internet using the MQTT (Message Queue Telemetry Transport) protocol. The main advantage of their proposed system is the use of LoRa technology for data communication which enables long-distance data transmission along with low-power consumption as compared to Wi-Fi, Bluetooth or Zigbee.

The majority of the cited work tries to find the level of waste to generate a notification that can be used to plan an effective way for the management of the waste. Some of the work focused on developing an efficient as well as economical solution. Our proposed work combines the power of IoT and DL to come up with an automatic waste segregation system that also alerts the government/user when the bin is full. It is no longer only IoT or only DL that is working, but both working together and that too in real time. Automatic segregation of waste enabled by machine learning algorithm is a useful idea and seems to be effective also. In this case the images of waste could be captured by the camera and then these real images are passed through a trained machine learning model that can classify waste into different types. This classification process further helps to monitor the waste and to better plan the strategy to manage this. But the real challenge while developing an automatic segregation unit is the constrained computing power of IoT devices. In this work we tried to develop a DL model that could work in this constrained environment. Thus this becomes the key contribution to the project.

3 Proposed Work

In this work a synergy of DL and IoT is employed which could be used to develop a solution for waste disbursal and management. This work is around a waste collection and segregation technique. The designed system is a centralized one and can be easily installed by the government authorities for proper waste collection and segregation. The proposed system is composed of three main components as depicted in Fig. 1.

- **Cloud:** The cloud is the most important aspect of any IoT system because it is the cloud through which the data is sent or received. Also in our proposed system we have not only used the cloud for communication but also for storing the saved deep learning model.
- **Smart bin:** The smart bin contains Raspberry Pi, an ultrasonic sensor to find a full dustbin and a camera module for taking live snapshots of the waste put on

Fig. 1 Workflow diagram of proposed work showing the three entities and the data communicated between them

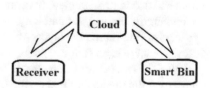

the tray of the bin. The camera module picks up snapshots and the deep learning model classifies the waste, and accordingly, the tray tilts to the R or O side.

– **Receiver:** The core implementation of the project lies in the receiver end for it can be used at home and also by the government authorities who are the receivers who will receive the signal from the bin when it is full.

Inside the dustbin, the person puts the waste on the tray in the dustbin. Owing to real-time running camera, it takes the snapshots in real time and the deep learning model immediately classifies the image as R or O (R—recyclable or O—organic) and the tray tilts either to the right side or left side depending upon R or O category. The tilting of the tray is managed by the motors connected with the Raspberry Pi. Thus the automatic waste segregation happens and also the ultrasonic sensors tell whether the bin is full or not and if it is full, it sends an alert.

3.1 Hardware Implementation

The hardware consists of one Raspberry Pi module, one motor, one camera module and one ultrasonic sensor. The camera is connected to Raspberry Pi with the internet via Wi-Fi.

3.2 Deep Learning-Based Waste Segregation

DL has been used extensively nowadays with the evolvement of computing power; however, as far as IoT is considered, DL falls a little behind because of the low computational power available with the IoT devices as compared to modern computers. However, with the recent developments by NVIDIA, they have developed DL-based IoT boards like Jetson Nano, yet the price seems to be an issue. In our proposed work we have taken a public available dataset from Kaggle [10], which contains two categories of data belonging to O—organic waste and R—recyclable waste. It contains data already divided into train and test categories. The train part contains 9999 images belonging to the O category and 12,565 images belonging to the R category. The test part contains 1401 images belonging to the O category and 1112 images belonging to the R category. Thus we have used train set for training and test set for testing, upon which the accuracy of the classifier is evaluated. We have used the process of transfer learning for training the models because it not only saves time but also is very efficient in terms of accuracy when the dataset contains images belonging to the general category of images. In this paper we have also used the process of fine-tuning the layers of the pre-trained models for achieving better accuracy. We have used four pre-trained models, which are (1) Inception, (2) VGG16, (3) VGG19 and (4) MobileNetsV2. These are pre-trained models. For our paper we have used the models trained on the Imagenets dataset. The full code is available on Kaggle and can be accessed from the link [16]. The results obtained from each model are discussed below along with their comparison. Also we have shown two states of each model and the accuracy after fine-tuning. Figure 2 shows the plots of training accuracy versus validation accuracy and training loss versus validation loss for the Inception model. Similarly, Figs. 3, 4 and 5 present the accuracy and loss functions for VGG16 model, VGG19 model and MobileNetsV2 model, respectively.

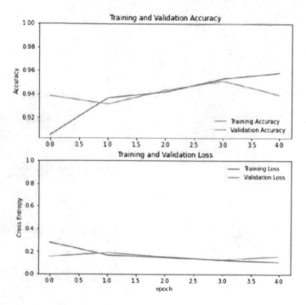

Fig. 2 Plots of accuracy and cross-entropy for inception model

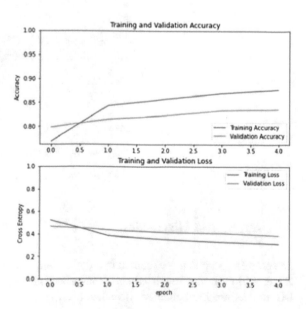

Fig. 3 Plots of accuracy and cross-entropy for VGG16 model

Fig. 4 Plots of accuracy and cross-entropy for VGG19 model

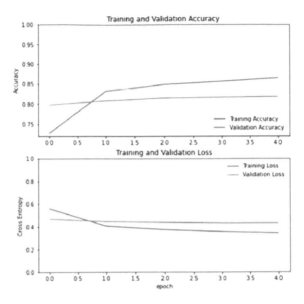

Fig. 5 Plots of accuracy and cross-entropy for MobileNetsV2 model

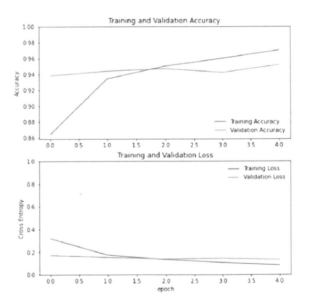

4 Results and Discussion

The entire experiment is executed in a Python environment. All the used DL models are tested in the same environment. Tensorflow and Keras are the backend in which DL models are implemented. It makes use of several libraries present in OpenCv

Table 1 Accuracy, precision and F1 score for inception, VGG16 and VGG19 model

Used model types	Accuracy in percentage	Precision	F1 score
MobileNetsV2 model	0.8993	0.9077	0.8977
Inception model	0.8917	0.8976	0.8903
VGG16 model	0.8730	0.8784	0.8713
VGG19 model	0.8746	0.8802	0.8729

and Sklearn as well. The comparison of all four models along with their accuracy, F1 score and precision are shown in Table 1 and sorted in decreasing order of their accuracy. From Table 1, it is evident that MobileNetsV2 is the best model as it has the highest accuracy among all the models. This result has been obtained on a separate test dataset as mentioned in Sect. 3.1. Also, we cannot rule out that this high accuracy is almost similar for the top-two models, thus both could perform well in real scenarios. However, for the purpose of implementation, we used MobileNetsV2 since it had the best accuracy.

5 Conclusion and Future Scope

Thus in this work, we have presented a deep learning and IoT-based waste segregation system which can be implemented by the government authorities or at home for proper waste segregation. The use of IoT and deep learning together open up a whole new way of achieving new milestones, and the purpose of this paper is to show that when deep learning is combined with IoT the whole IoT system becomes more intelligent and it gives digital brains to the system. Energy efficiency is an issue in the present system, which needs to be addressed. The future scope of this project lies in the ability to make models lighter than the MobileNetsV2 so that less use of API calls is done which will make the system faster and more reliable than the present ones.

References

1. Pradhan B, Vijayakumar V, Pratihar S, Kumar D, Reddy KHK, Roy DS (2020) A genetic algorithm based energy efficient group paging approach for iot over 5g. J Syst Arch 101878
2. Roy DS, Behera RK, Reddy KHK, Buyya R (2018) A context-aware fog enabled scheme for real-time cross-vertical iot applications. IEEE Internet Things J 6(2):2400–2412
3. Pardini K, Rodrigues JJ, Kozlov SA, Kumar N, Furtado V (2019) Iot-based solid waste management solutions: a survey. J Sens Actuator Netw 8(1):5
4. Reddy KHK, Behera RK, Chakrabarty A, Roy DS (2020) A service delay minimization scheme for qos-constrained, context-aware unified iot applications. IEEE Internet Things J 7(10):10527–10534

5. Roy DS (2019) A study on drx mechanism for wireless powered lte-enabled iot devices. In: 2019 IEEE international conference on consumer electronics-Taiwan (ICCE- TW). IEEE, pp. 1–2
6. Fan YJ, Yin YH, Da Xu L, Zeng Y, Wu F (2014) Iot-based smart rehabilitation system. IEEE Trans Industr Inf 10(2):1568–1577
7. Marques P, Manfroi D, Deitos E, Cegoni J, Castilhos R, Rochol J, Pignaton E, Kunst R (2019) An iot-based smart cities infrastructure architecture applied to a waste management scenario. Ad Hoc Netw 87:200–208
8. Xu B, Da Xu L, Cai H, Xie C, Hu J, Bu F (2014) Ubiquitous data accessing method in iot-based information system for emergency medical services. IEEE Trans Industr Inf 10(2):1578–1586
9. Priyadarshini R, Barik RK, Panigrahi C, Dubey H, Mishra BK (2020) An investigation into the efficacy of deep learning tools for big data analysis in health care. In: Deep learning and neural networks: concepts, methodologies, tools, and applications. IGI Global, 654–666
10. Misra D, Das G, Chakrabortty T, Das D (2018) An iot-based waste management system monitored by cloud. J Mater Cycles Waste Manage 20(3):1574–1582
11. Singh A, Aggarwal P, Arora R (2016) Iot based waste collection system using infrared sensors. In: 2016 5th international conference on reliability, infocom technologies and optimization (Trends and Future Directions) (ICRITO). IEEE, pp. 505–509
12. Hong I, Park S, Lee B, Lee J, Jeong D, Park S (2014) Iot-based smart garbage system for efficient food waste management. Sci World J 2014
13. Malapur B, Pattanshetti VR (2017) Iot based waste management: an application to smart city. In: 2017 international conference on energy, communication, data analytics and soft computing (ICECDS). IEEE, pp 2476–2486
14. Kumar SV, Kumaran TS, Kumar AK, Mathapati M (2017) Smart garbage monitoring and clearance system using internet of things. In: 2017 IEEE international conference on smart technologies and management for computing, communication, controls, energy and materials (ICSTM). IEEE, pp 184–189
15. Bharadwaj AS, Rego R, Chowdhury A (2016) Iot based solid waste management system: a conceptual approach with an architectural solution as a smart city application. In: 2016 IEEE annual india conference (INDICON). IEEE, pp. 1–6
16. Diwakar S, Bhattacharya A, Priyadarshini R (2020) DataSet and code link. https://www.kaggle.com/shubhamdivakar/ai-and-iot-based-system-conference-paperAccessed 28 Oct 2020

Ear Localization and Validation Using Ear Candidate Set

**Ayushi Rastogi, Ujjayanta Bhoumik, Chhavi Choudhary,
Akbar Sheikh Akbari, and Koushlendra Kumar Singh**

1 Introduction

Human traits cannot be stolen or forgotten because of which it is extremely beneficial to use these traits for recognition and verification in all security spheres [1].
Behavioral and physiological characteristics are utilized by theses systems in order
to perform human recognition. Structural and shape-related information of a human
body fall under the category of physiological characteristics. These include ear, face,
palm print or hand geometry, iris, fingerprint, retina, veins, etc. Human behavior
and habitual traits fall under behavioral characteristics [2, 3]. These include voice,
signature, gait, keystroke dynamics, etc. Human identification and verification have
seen ear to be a very promising candidate among all the other physiological characteristics because of its reliability and scalability [4]. There are various reasons behind
the growing popularity of ear biometrics. It falls under passive biometrics, meaning,
it seeks very little human intervention for getting the accuracy right. The fact that the
shape of ear changes from 4 to 8 months and then after 70 years gives it credibility for
being a stable means. Ear biometrics is consistent to a great extent as it is expression-
invariant and has a relatively good size, smaller than the face but larger than the thum
or iris [5]. Automated ear recognition has seen several approaches in the literature.
Burge and Burger gave a technique using formable colors for ear detection [6]. They
also came up with the approach of vernoi diagrams. 2D and 3D images were used
for ear recognition in various systems. Nanni and Lumini, came up with fusion of
color spaces for authentication of ear [2]. Force field feature extraction was used by
Hurley, Nixon, and Carter for ear biometrics [7]. Alvarez et al. used a void model for

A. Rastogi · U. Bhoumik · C. Choudhary · K. Kumar Singh (✉)
National Institute of Technology Jamshedpur, Jharkhand 831014, India
e-mail: koushlendra.cse@nitjsr.ac.in

A. S. Akbari
Leeds Beckett University, Room 207, Caedmon Hall, Headingely Campus, Leeds LS6 3QR, UK

© The Author(s), under exclusive license to Springer Nature Singapore Pte Ltd. 2021   109
M. K. Bajpai et al. (eds.), *Machine Vision and Augmented Intelligence—Theory
and Applications*, Lecture Notes in Electrical Engineering 796,
https://doi.org/10.1007/978-981-16-5078-9_10

developing a fitting ear contour [8]. Two line landmarks were used for ear recognition by Yan and Bowyer [9]. A technique based on skin color and contour was proposed by Yuan and Mu [10]. The proposed technique is able to detect subject's ear across its similar ear image instances. Identification of individual become challenging if the systems database consist of subject's ear without variations, and the verification check is done after certain variations in pose and angle is observed [11]. The implemented method proves that individual verification is being achieved, despite of slight changes that occurs in subject's ear due to variations in pose and angle [12]. Subject's ear is captured and feeded into the computer after taking a photo of it [13, 14]. Various preprocessing steps are applied on this captured image [15]. After this, edge detection and approximation of these edges are carried out on the picture. The processed ear is then used to extract features like mean, standard deviation, skewness, and pixel counts [16, 17]. Matching is being conducted between subject's captured ear images with all the images previously stored in the database. To decide the identity of the person, this match is compared against predefined ranges and threshold values.

2 Proposed Methodology

The ear localization and validation technique comes across various challenges. This is because, the ear may vary in terms of pose, out-plane rotation, in-plane rotation, scale, and piercing. An efficient design and development of an ear biometric system for ear localization from a side face image and validation using ear candidate set is done through a technique which will be shape-, rotation-, and scale-invariant. The technique involves a combination of several steps like

2.1 Color-Based Skin Segmentation

An image falling under RGB color space gives information about color as well as luminance which differs according to lighting conditions of different areas of the face. So, utilization of RGB color space in order to determine skin and non-skin region becomes undependable and unreliable. We have thus chosen a method where we can separate chrominance and luminance information. This can be achieved through YCbCr color space, where Cb and Cr components provide only the information related to color and separates any luminance information attached. The image segmentation is performed in this color space, and a proper thresholding is done after which skin regions are denoted as white and non-skin regions are denoted by black pixels. All the detected skin regions will not contain the ear, and hence, ear localization technique will have to be used to some extent in order to locate ear in all the skin-like segments.

2.2 Skins-Region Edge Computation

Edge computation is the next step following the color-based skin segmentation. For this purpose, a canny edge operator is used. Edge points are connected together into a pixel coordinate pair sequence for computing the edges and populating the edge list. In this process, we need to be careful whenever an edge junction is encountered. If an edge junction comes across, for each branch, a separate sequence of edge points is generated after terminating the edge. It is then added to the list. The edge list, thus, consists of a set of edges containing two end points.

2.3 Approximation of Edges

The edges obtained after performing the edge-detected algorithm may contain some edges, which may be a part of ear or may not be a part of it. There would be certain number of junctions, which are needed to be removed. For doing so, thinning is performed on the binary image of edges to get thinned edges. If a point at the end is connected to the edge with only one point, then that point belongs to a thinned edge. If we take a thinned edge and pick any point on it, we can observe that every point is connected to one neighborhood pixel. If a case arises where two neighborhood pixels are found to be connected to any point on the edge, then there exists a junction. In the process of thinning, the junction with that point is then removed from that edge.

2.4 Feature Extraction

We considered five features for matching the captured and stored images which are as follows:

A.. **Count of white pixel**: This gives us the count of pixels which fall in the edge region.
B. **Difference of Black and White Pixels**: This gives us the measure of how many pixels are not belonging to edge regions relative to those pixels which fall in the edge region.
C. **Mean:** This feature helps in mean value calculation of the image.
D. **Standard deviation:** It gives us the average distance from the mean of the data set to a point. For calculating this, we can compute the squares of the distance from each data point to the mean of the set.
E. **Skewness**: This feature gives us the measure of symmetry of an image. If a dataset or a distribution looks the same to the left and right of the center point, it is said to be symmetric.

2.5 *Matching*

Matching is performed after all the required features are extracted from the ear image. Subject's ear image is taken to be as the source image. Its features are compared with the features of all the images stored in the database, and depending upon the threshold range computed, its match is found and accuracy rate of matching is determined. This is done for all the images in the dataset, and overall accuracy of matching is determined for the system.

3 Algorithms

/*This algorithm is used for skin segmentation in YcbCr color space and for thresholding.*/

i. ALGORITHM 1:
Skin Segmentation=[Input: I, cb, cr, w, h, Output: Segmented image]

Input: I, cb, cr, w, h
    I: Original image
   cb: blue difference
   cr: red difference
   w: width
   h: height
Output: Segmented image

begin
    Read the original input file
    Convert it into a double format
    Convert rgb color space to hsv color space
    Calculate cb = 0.148*I(:,:,1) - 0.291*I(:,:,2)+0.439*I(:,:,3)+128
    Calculate cr = 0.439*I(:,:,1) -0.368*I(:,:,2)-0.071*I(:,:,3)+128

for i=1 to w
    for j=1 to h
       if 140<=cr(i,j) && cr(i,j)<=165 && 140<=cb(i,j) && cb(i,j)<=195 &&
0.01<=hue(i ,j) && hue(i,j)<=0.1
         Segment(I,j)=1
      else
         Segment(I,j)=0
      end if
    end for
  end for
end

This algorithm is used for obtaining an edge detected image from a segmented image/

ii. ALGORITHM 2:
Edge Detection = [Segmented image, edge detected image]
Input: Segmented image
   segment: *Skin segmented image*
     EI: *Edge detected image*
Output: *Edge detected image*
begin
  EI = edge(segment, 'canny')
end

/*This algorithm is used for approximation edges in an edge detected image*/

iii. *ALGORITHM 3:*

Thinning = [EI, EMorph]
Input: Edge Detected Image
   EI :   *Edge Detected Image*
   EMorph: *Thinned Image*
Output: *Image After Thinning*
begin
     EMorph = bwmorph(EI, 'thin')
end

/*This algorithm is used for calculation of major features of an image after the edge approximation is complete*/

iv. ALGORITHM 4:
Features = [EMorph, mean, standard_deviation, skewness, whitePixels, DiffBlackWhite]
Input: Thinned Image
  EMorph: *Thinned Image*
  mean: *Table of mean difference*
  standard_deviation: *Table of standard deviation*
                    difference
  skewness: *Table of skewness difference*
  whitePixels: *Table of white pixels difference*
  DiffBlackWhite: *Table of black and white pixels difference*
Output: *mean, standard_deviation, skewness, whitePixels, DiffBlackWhite*

begin
   for *each image in the directory*
     find all the features and store in an array
     for *all images in the directory*
       calculate the difference of all the
       features considered and store in respective tables
end

/*This algorithm is used for calculating the accuracy of each class of image based on the difference tables of mean, standard deviation, skewness, white pixels and difference of black and white pixels*/

v. *ALGORITHM 5:*

AccuracyCalculation=[Input: mean, standard_deviation, skewness, whitePixels, DiffBlackWhite Output: AccuracyPercentage]
Input: mean, standard_deviation, skewness, whitePixels,
     DiffBlackWhite
  mean: *Table of mean difference*
  standard_deviation: *Table of standard deviation difference*
  skewness: *Table of skewness difference*
  whitePixels: *Table of white pixels difference*
  DiffBlackWhite: *Table of black and white pixels difference*
Output: *AccuracyPercentage*

begin
          set the ranges for each class for respective feature categories

for *all the images in the directory*
              set the class each time
              for *all the images in the directory*
                       calculate the count of images falling in the ranges
                       determined for the class but don't belong to that class
                       calculate the accuracy based on the count for that class
                   end for
      end for
    end

/*This algorithim is used for matching an input image against the ranges of each class calculated and stored previously. The class and accuracy of matched image is returned afterwards*/

          vi. *ALGORITHM 6:*

Matching=[Input: I Output: class, accuracy]
Input: I
  I: *input image*
  class: *class of matched image*
  accuracy: *accuracy of matched image*
Output: *class, accuracy*

begin
         calculate features of input image
         calculate the feature difference array of input image with respect to
         all the images in the dataset

     for *all the images in the directory*
             compare the feature difference with computed ranges of
             respective classes and return the matched class and accuracy
             percentage
         end for
     end

4 Experiments and Results

The proposed algorithm has been tested on data base of AMI which contains the total 60 images of different peoples of different color. The both left and right ears of the same person are also in the data base (Figs. 1, 2, 3, 4, 5, 6, 7 and 8).

Figures 1 and 5 show the raw RGB images directly taken from the dataset. These images undergo various preprocessing steps. After the color-based skin segmentation is performed, they turn out to be like the Figs. 2 and 6. Canny edge operator is then used on these images in order to obtain edge-detected images like in Figs. 3 and 7. Final step of preprocessing is applied to carry out approximation of theses edge segments by thinning, and this results in Figs. 4 and 8.

Fig. 1 For a left ear sample original RGB image

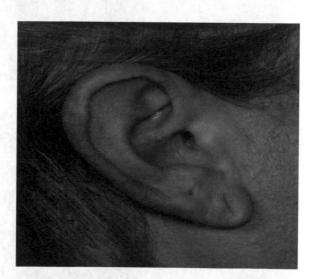

Fig. 2 For a left ear sample skin segmented image

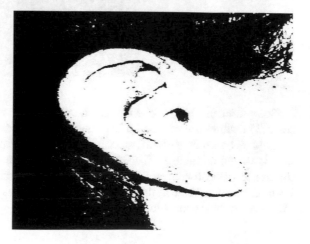

Fig. 3 For a left ear sample edge detected image

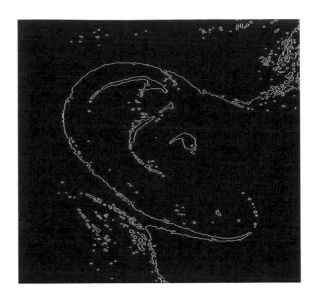

Fig. 4 For a left ear sample thinned image

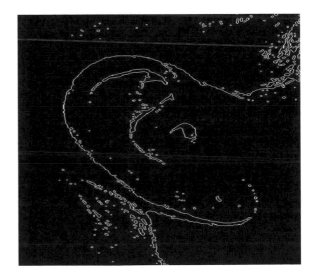

   Soon after the image is obtained as an output from the preprocessing steps, required features are calculated like mean, standard deviation, skewness, count of white pixels, and count of difference of black and white pixels for all the images. This data is shown in Table 1. These features are then used to calculate corresponding difference tables for mean (Table 2), standard deviation in Table 3, skewness has been tabulated in Table 4, the value of white pixels has been shown in Table 5, and difference of black and white pixels in Table 6.

Fig. 5 For a right ear sample original RGB image

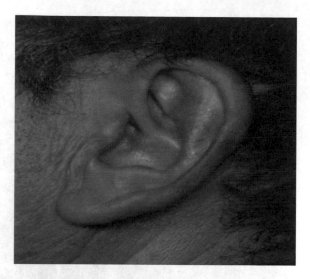

Fig. 6 For a right ear sample skin segmented image

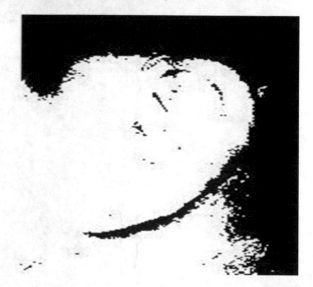

5 Conclusions

The results of the experiments performed clearly show that the colored image is segmented into skin and non-skin regions. All detected skin regions do not necessarily contain ear, but since ear is rich in edges and is the only part which shows much variations in pixel intensities in a side face image, we have thus tried to exploit this fact in our further steps. We took a dataset of 60 images from AMI (Applied Market Information Limited) and performed color-based skin segmentation, edge detection, and thinning as preprocessing steps on it. Then, we calculated various features like

Fig. 7 For a right ear
sample edge detected image

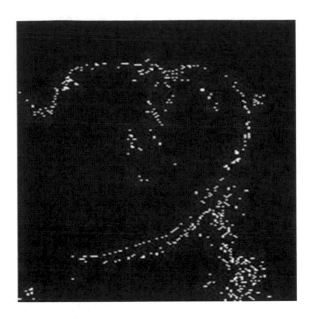

Fig. 8 For a right ear
sample thinned image

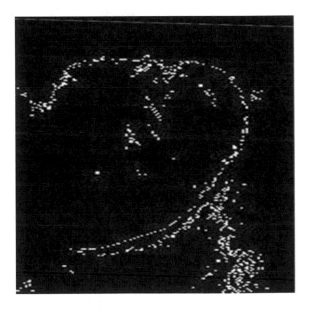

the count of white pixels, mean, standard deviation, skewness, and the count of difference of black and white pixels. We exploited these features to determine the extent to which they help in matching images which are similar to each other with an overall system accuracy of 80 percent.

Table 1 Feature calculation

	Mean	Standard deviation	Skewness	White pixels	Difference of black and white pixels
Image 1	2.3240	30.4216	7.9626	1927	341,530
Image 2	3.2681	26.8294	9.0953	1505	342,374
Image 3	2.3774	22.9809	10.698	1118	343,148
Image 4	2.6169	24.0877	10.183	1243	342,898
Image 5	2.2667	22.3989	10.9815	1079	343,226

Table 2 Mean difference

	Image 1	Image 2	Image 3	Image 4	Image 5
Image 1	0	0.9441	0.0534	0.2929	0.0573
Image 2	0.9441	0	0.8907	0.6512	1.0014
Image 3	0.0534	0.8907	0	0.2395	0.1107
Image 4	0.2929	0.6512	0.2395	0	0.3502
Image 5	0.0573	1.0014	0.1107	0.3502	0

Table 3 Standard deviation difference

	Image 1	Image 2	Image 3	Image 4	Image 5
Image 1	0	3.5921	7.4407	6.3339	8.0226
Image 2	3.5921	0	3.8486	2.7418	4.4305
Image 3	7.4407	3.8486	0	1.1068	0.5819
Image 4	6.3339	2.7418	1.1068	0	1.6887
Image 5	8.0226	4.44305	0.5819	1.6887	0

Table 4 Skewness difference

	Image 1	Image 2	Image 3	Image 4	Image 5
Image 1	0	1.1327	2.7354	2.2204	3.0189
Image 2	1.1327	0	1.6026	1.0877	1.8862
Image 3	2.7354	1.6026	0	0.515	0.2835
Image 4	2.2204	1.0877	0.515	0	0.7985
Image 5	3.0189	1.8862	0.2835	0.7985	0

Table 5 White pixels difference

	Image 1	Image 2	Image 3	Image 4	Image 5
Image 1	0	422	809	684	848
Image 2	422	0	387	262	426
Image 3	809	387	0	125	39
Image 4	684	262	125	0	164
Image 5	848	426	39	164	0

Table 6 Difference of black and white pixels

	Image 1	Image 2	Image 3	Image 4	Image 5
Image 1	0	844	1618	1368	1696
Image 2	844	0	774	524	852
Image 3	1618	774	0	250	78
Image 4	1368	524	250	0	328
Image 5	1696	852	78	328	0

References

1. Nanni L, Lumini A (2007) A multi-matcher for ear authentication. Pattern Recogn Lett 28(16):2219–2226
2. Nanni L, Lumini A (2009) Fusion of color spaces for ear authentication. Pattern Recogn 42(9):1906–1913
3. De Marsico M, Michele N, Riccio D (2010) Hero: human ear recognition against occlusions. In: Proceedings of computer vision and pattern recognition workshops (CVPRW). pp 178–183
4. Prakash S, Gupta P (2011) An efficient ear recognition technique invariant to illumination and pose
5. Prakash S, Gupta P (2012) An efficient ear localization technique
6. Burge M, Burger W (2000) Ear biometrics in computer vision. In: Proceedings of international conference on pattern recognition (ICPR' 00), vol 02. pp 822–826
7. Hurley J, Nixon MS, Carter JN (2005) Force field feature extraction for ear biometrics. Comput Vis Image Understand 98(3):491–512
8. Alvarez L, Gonzalez E, Mazorra L (2005) Fitting ear contour using an ovoid model. In: Proceedings of IEEE international carnahan conference on security technology (ICCST' 05). pp 145–148
9. Chen H, Bhanu B (2004) Human ear detection from side face range images. In: Proceedings of international conference on pattern recognition (ICPR'04), vol 3. pp 574–577
10. Yuan L, Mu Z-C (2007) Ear detection based on skin-color and contour information. In: Proceedings of international conference on machine learning and cybernetics (ICMLC' 07), vol 4. Hong Kong, pp 2213–2217
11. Yan P, Bowyer K (2005) Empirical evaluation of advanced ear biometrics. In: Proceedings of international conference on computer vision and pattern recognition-workshops, vol 3. pp 41–48
12. Bandyopadhyay S, Narayan D (2013) Detection of an individual after piercing using ear biometric. IJCSMC 2(6):369 375
13. Sana A, Gupta P (2009) Ear biometrics: a new approach. In: Proceedings of the 7th International conference on Advances in pattern recognition. ICAPR
14. Singh KK, Bjapi MK, Pandey RK, Munshi P (2017) A novel non-invasive method for extraction of geometrical and texture features of wood. Res Nondestr Eval 28(3):150–167
15. Malathy C, Annapurani K (2013) Analysis of fusion methods for ear biometrics. IJARCSSE
16. Singh KK, Bajpai MK, Pandey RK (2018) A novel approach for enhancement of geometric and contrast resolution properties of low contrast images. IEEE/CAA J Automat Sin 5(2): 628–638
17. Suman S, Jha RK (2017) A new technique for image enhancement using digital fractional-order Savitzky- Golay differentiator. Multidimension Syst Signal Process 28(2):709–733

Study of Communication Pattern for Perfect Difference Network

Sunil Tiwari, Manish Bhardwaj, and Rakesh Kumar Katare

1 Introduction

This paper presents communication patterns of Perfect Difference Network (PDN) and explores topological properties [1]. This communication pattern is a class of connectivity of nodes. The algorithm helps in the distribution and exchange of information between processing elements of the interconnection network [2]. The study of communication pattern is useful in various forms based on the application of interconnection patterns, such as Fast Fourier transform (FFT) might cause the shuffle permutation like sorting applicant and fluid dynamics simulation exhibit neighbour pattern [3]. The current study approach is to find an augmenting communication pattern in the interconnection network. The thought of the study is based on the reachability from the source node to the sink node covering all the links in the interconnection network, a message packet is sent on one of the paths. All the possible paths of the network are covered from source to sink node. It is assumed that at any moment, each node can transmit on at most 2δ incident links, where δ is prime or power of a prime.

James Singer had represented point and line in form of a perfect difference set (PDS). Further, Parahmi and Rakov contributed to developing the topological properties and graphical model for the analysis of perfect difference set. Data transfer and message communication play an important role in the usefulness of an interconnection network. Other research groups have made Perfect Difference Network popular by evaluating this model through various metrics: degree, diameter, average distance, bisection width, blocking and non-blocking network and static and dynamic. The communication aspect of the interconnection network is also discussed in a paper, which is used to measure the cost and performance of the interconnection network

S. Tiwari (✉) · M. Bhardwaj · R. K. Katare
Department of Computer Science, A.P.S. University Rewa, Madhya Pradesh, India

© The Author(s), under exclusive license to Springer Nature Singapore Pte Ltd. 2021
M. K. Bajpai et al. (eds.), *Machine Vision and Augmented Intelligence—Theory and Applications*, Lecture Notes in Electrical Engineering 796,
https://doi.org/10.1007/978-981-16-5078-9_11

Fig. 1 PDN with
communication pattern

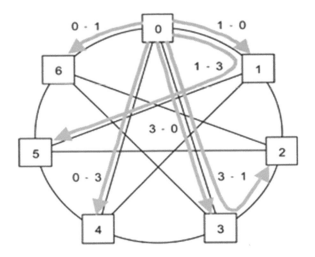

to solve the problem. We critically examine and analyse the structure of PDN. The
following isomorphic structures have been contemplated:

Graphical, Functional, Ordering, Equivalence, Algebraic and Discrete Mathematical Perfect Difference Network constitutes a class of robust, high-performance
interconnection network for parallel processing. The rich connectivity of PDN
makes it possible to circumvent faulty nodes and links with negligible increase in
communication distance and performance of the network.

2 Communication Pattern

Communication has a very wide range of applications in real-world problems such as
engineering, science, linguistics and in numerous other areas. The study of communication patterns can be used to represent almost any communication situation
involving broadcasting, multiplexing and discrete relationship among objects. We
consider a PDN [4, 5] where $n = (\delta^2 + \delta + 1)$, $\delta = 2$ and PDS = {0, 1, 3} Fig. 1.
PDN with the shortest path from node 0 to all other nodes is highlighted and labelled
with corresponding differences.

Perfect difference networks constitute a class of robust, high-performance interconnection networks for parallel and distributed computation [6, 7]. PDNs may not
be desirable for large networks with wired connectivity, but they offer attractive
alternatives for wireless and optical smaller interconnection networks in hierarchical
architectures. So, network flow in PDN is possible in numerous ways as discussed
below:

Node '0'.

Ring Link (clockwise network flow)　　　　　Ring Link (anti-clockwise network flow)

$n_0 + 1 \longrightarrow n_1$	$n_0 - 1 \longrightarrow n_6$
$n_1 + 1 \longrightarrow n_2$	$n_6 - 1 \longrightarrow n_5$
$n_2 + 1 \longrightarrow n_3$	$n_5 - 1 \longrightarrow n_4$
$n_3 + 1 \longrightarrow n_4$	$n_4 - 1 \longrightarrow n_3$
$n_4 + 1 \longrightarrow n_5$	$n_3 - 1 \longrightarrow n_2$
$n_5 + 1 \longrightarrow n_6$	$n_2 - 1 \longrightarrow n_1$
$n_6 + 1 \longrightarrow n_0$	$n_1 - 1 \longrightarrow n_0$

Chordal Ring network flow:

$n_0 + s_j \,(\text{mod } n) \longrightarrow$	n_3
$n_0 - s_j \,(\text{mod } n) \longrightarrow$	n_4
$n_0 + s_j \,(\text{mod } n) - 1 \longrightarrow$	n_2
$n_0 - s_j \,(\text{mod } n) + 1 \longrightarrow$	n_5
$n_0 - s_j \,(\text{mod } n) + 2 \longrightarrow$	n_6
$n_0 + s_j \,(\text{mod } n) - 2 \longrightarrow$	n_1

The chordal link or circular links [8], 9 are capable to broadcast any message in a perfect difference network individually. In PDN, if any node fails, then there is an alternate link to complete communication. But it is critical for large δ to tolerate more faulty (mix of circular and chord) of links. Now, we convert connectivity in PDN into a matrix through formulation ni $\pm$ 1 and ni $\pm$ sj (mod n).

1 represents a communication link, and

0 represents a path with no direct communication link.

Remainder theorem N = D*Q + R where N: numerator, D: divisor, Q: quotient and R: remainder, and modular arithmetic has explored the connectivity of PDN. The node number in PDN is labelled as $0,1,2,\ldots, \delta^2 + \delta$, and the rules for operation are the same as arithmetical operation with modular arithmetic. According to modular arithmetic, if a number Q (output) equals or greater than $N(\delta^2 + \delta + 1)$, it is divided by $\delta^2 + \delta + 1$, the Q is discarded and the remainder is used in place of Q. The modulo $(\delta^2 + \delta + 1)$ is shown below:

+	0	1	2	3	4	5	6
0	0	1	2	3	4	5	6
1	1	2	3	4	5	6	0
2	2	3	4	5	6	0	1
3	3	4	5	6	0	1	2
4	4	5	6	0	1	2	3
5	5	6	0	1	2	3	4
6	6	0	1	2	3	4	5

$n_i + S_j \bmod (\delta^2 + \delta + 1)$	3	3	3	3	3	3	3
0	3						
1		4					
2			5				
3				6			
4					7 = 0		
5						8 = 1	
6							9 = 2

From the above table, we verified that the set 0, 1, 2, ..., $\delta^2 + \delta$ with the addition or modulo arithmetic $\delta^2 + \delta + 1$ is a field because $\delta^2 + \delta + 1$ is a prime number. Such a field is also called a Galois field GF(2). The above table is also explored as follows:

Let $i = 1$

$n_1 + 1 = n_2$, $n_1 - 1 = n_0$ and $n_1 + 3 (\bmod \delta^2 + \delta + 1) = n_4$.

$n_1 - 3 (\bmod \delta^2 + \delta + 1) = 1 - 3 \bmod 7 = -2 \bmod 7 = 5 = n_5$

1		1		1	1	

Let $i = 2$

$n_2 + 1 = n_3$, $n_2 - 1 = n_1$ and $n_2 + 3 (\bmod \delta^2 + \delta + 1) = n_5$.

$n_2 - 3 (\bmod \delta^2 + \delta + 1) = 2 - 3 \bmod 7 = -1 \bmod 7 = 6 = n_6$

	1		1		1	1

Let $i = 3$

$n_3 + 1 = n_4$, $n_3 - 1 = n_2$ and $n_3 + 3 (\bmod \delta^2 + \delta + 1) = n_6$.

$n_3 - 3 (\bmod \delta^2 + \delta + 1) = 3 - 3 \bmod 7 = 0 = n_0$

1		1		1		1

Let $i = 4$

$n_4 + 1 = n_5$, $n_3 - 1 = n_3$ and $n_4 + 3 (\bmod \delta^2 + \delta + 1) = n_7 = n_0$.

$n_4 - 3 (\bmod \delta^2 + \delta + 1) = n_1$

1	1		1		1	

Let $i = 5$

$n_5 + 1 = n_6$, $n_5 - 1 = n_4$ and $n_5 + 3 (\bmod \delta^2 + \delta + 1) = n_8 = n_1$.

$n_5 - 3 (\bmod \delta^2 + \delta + 1) = n_2$

1		1		1		1	

Let $i = 6$

$n_6 + 1 = n_{7=}n_0$, $n_6 - 1 = n_5$ and $n_6 + 3 \pmod{\delta^2 + \delta + 1} = n_9 = n_2$.

$n_6 - 3 \pmod{\delta^2 + \delta + 1} = n_3$

1		1	1		1	

Hence, 9 mod 7 = 2 is the connective node for node 6.

Similarly, we can find all connectivity of corresponding node number in the Perfect Difference Network. Therefore, it is possible to make communication either circular or chord link with these network flow patterns. It helps to balance the load and fault tolerance in PDN. Now, we discuss PDN with GF(2), then every number has seven bits can only be either 0 or 1. If PDN is considered a complete graph, 27 vectors are possible. The following representation shows a vector in a $(\delta^2 + \delta + 1)$ dimensional vector space over the field GF(2).

N_0						
(0	1	0	1	1	0	1)
N_1						
(1	0	1	0	1	1	0)
N_2						
(0	1	0	1	0	1	1)
N_3						
(1	0	1	0	1	0	1)
N_4						
(1	1	0	1	0	1	0)
N^5						
(0	1	1	0	1	0	1)
N_6						
(1	0	1	1	0	1	0)

Lemma 1: The degree of each node of the perfect difference network is even.

Proof: A PDN has $\delta^2 + \delta + 1$ node [10] where δ is a prime or power of prime. The corresponding value of δ and PDS [11, 12] is shown below:

Table1 shows that the value of δ can be even or odd.

The multiplication of odd or even number is:

Table 2 also shows that multiplication is associative and commutative. If we regroup terms, the result will never change, 4*5 = 5*4 = 20. The result of.

Table 1 PDS of order δ in normal form and n = δ² + δ + 1

δ	N	PDS of order δ in normal form
2	7	0, 1, 3
3	13	0, 1, 3, 9
4	21	0,1,4,14,16
5	31	0,1,3,8,12,18
7	57	0,1,3,13,32,36,43,52
8	73	0,1,3,7,15,31,36,54,63
9	91	0,1,3,9,27,49,56,61,77,81
11	133	0,1,3,12,20,34,38,81,88,94,104,109
13	183	0,1,3,16,23,28,42,76,82,86,119,137,154,175
16	273	0,1,3,7,15,31,63,90,116,127,136,181,194, 204,233,238,255

Table 2 Nature of operation

	Operation		Result	Example
Even	*	Even	Even	4*4 = 16
Even	*	Odd	Even	4*5 = 20
Odd	*	Even	Even	5*4 = 20
Odd	*	Odd	Odd	5*5 = 25

$2 * δ = δ * 2$.

From the definition of PDN, the degree of a node is $2δ$. For the multiplication of even number with even or odd number, the result will be even.

δ	Degree (2*δ)	
2	2*2 = 4	even*even = even
3	2*3 = 6	even*odd = even
4	2*4 = 8	even*even = even
5	2*5 = 10	even*odd = even
7	2*7 = 14	even*odd = even
8	2*8 = 16	even*even = even
9	2*9 = 18	even*odd = even
11	2*11 = 22	even*odd = even
13	2*13 = 26	even*odd = even
16	2*16 = 32	even*even = even

Therefore, the product of any δ value with 2 is always even. The degree of each node is also even. Hence, it is proved that the degree of each node of PDN is always even.

3 Study of Connectivity Between Nodes in PDN

Set theory and algebraic structure are powerful tools in connectivity as well as in the network flow. They assist in a thorough understanding of communication pattern and to do analysis or manipulating it algebraically, if we wish to enlist the aid of an interconnection network in reducing the connectivity and complexity of PDN. Subsets $N_0, N_1, N_2, N_3, N_4, N_5, N_6$ are collection of some of the nodes of PDN. The two most common combinations between vectors, the union($\cup$) and intersection ($\cap$), are contemplated. PDN has closure with respect to union.

N_0	0	1	0	1	1	0	1
N_1	1	0	1	0	1	1	0
$N_0 \cup N_1$	1	1	1	1	1	1	1

Union with any two vector of PDN shows perfect difference network is connected. PDN is associated with respect to union.

$(N_0 \cup N_1) \cup N_2 = N_0 \cup (N_1 \cup N_2)$.

$N_0 \cup N_1$	1	1	1	1	1	1	1
N_2	0	1	0	1	0	1	1
$(N_0 \cup N_1) \cup N_2$	1	1	1	1	1	1	1

N_0	0	1	0	1	1	0	1
$N_1 \cup N_2$	1	1	1	1	1	1	1
$N_0 \cup (N_1 \cup N_2)$	1	1	1	1	1	1	1

Intersection between two vectors of PDN represents those vectors that are alternate PE to complete the communication between processors.

4 Conclusion

A comprehensive study of communication patterns of the interconnection network has been performed. The topological properties of PDN were also highlighted with their importance. Efforts have been made to find the inter-relationship between the communication patterns of the PDN and FFT. This helps the distribution of information between nodes of the interconnection networks. The study of communication patterns is useful in various forms based on application and interconnection patterns, such as fast Fourier Transform. It may cause the shuffle permutation and neighbour simulation pattern in fluid dynamics. This study helps in finding augmenting communication patterns in interconnection networks for parallel and distributed systems.

References

1. Katare RK, Chaudhari NS (2007) A comparative study of hypercube and perfect difference network for parallel and distributed system and its application to sparse linear system, vol. 2. Sandipani Academic, Ujjain, pp 13–30
2. Katare RK, Chaudhari, NS (2008) Study of parallel algorithms for sparse linear systems and different interconnection networks. J Comp Math Sci Appl Ser Publ New Delhi
3. Deo N (2000) Graph theory, with application to engineering and computer science. Prentice Hall of India pvt. Ltd., New Delhi. ISBN 81–203–0145–5
4. Parhami B, Rakov MA (2005) Performance, algorithmic and robustness attributes of perfect difference network. IEEE Trans Parallel Distrib Syst 16(8)
5. Parhami B, Rakov MA (2005) Perfect difference networks and related interconnection structures for parallel and distributed systems. IEEE Trans Parallel Distrib Syst 16(8)
6. Tiwari S, Katare RK (2015) Alliance study of perfect difference network & hex-cell architecture. Int J Emerg Technol Adv Eng 5(3):25
7. Tiwari S, Katare RK (2015) A study of fabric of architecture using structural pattern and relation. Int J Latest Technol Eng Manag Appl Sci 4(9), ISSN 2278–2540
8. Tiwari S, Katare RK, Singh N Computing and comprehending parameters for structural analysis of PDN ad hex-cell architecture. Res J A.P.S. University, Rewa 6(12), ISSN 0976–9986
9. Tiwari S, Katare RK, Sharma V, Tiwari CM (2016) Study of geometrical structure of perfect difference network(PDN). Int J Adv Res Comp Commun Eng 5(3) ISSN(online) 2278–1021,(print) 2319–5940
10. Tiwari S, Katare RK, Sharma V, Tiwari CM, (2016) Study of geometrical structure of perfect difference network (PDN). Int J Adv Res Comp Commun Eng 5(3), ISSN(online) 2278–1021,(print) 2319–5940
11. Tiwari S, Katare RK (2017) A study of interconnection network for parallel and distributed system. BEST Int J Manag Inform Technol Eng 5(6): 69–74. ISSN (P): 2348–0513, ISSN (E): 2454–471X
12. Tiwari S, Katare RK, Sharma V (2017) A study of parallel programming techniques for inter-connection network. Int J Emerg Technol Adv Eng 7(9) E-ISSN 2250–2459 (UGC Approved List Journal No-63196)
13. Tiwari S, Katare RK, Sharma V (2017) Study of structural representation of perfect difference network. IJRSET 5(11)
14. Tiwari S, et.al (2019) Vector operation on nodes of PDN using logical operators. Int J Adv Res Comp Sci 10 ISSN 0976–5697
15. Tiwari S, Singh GP, Katare RK (2020) A study of structural analysis of PDN. Int Res J Sci Eng Technol 10(2) ISSN 2454–3195

An Approach for Denoising of Contaminated Signal Using Fractional Order Differentiator

Koushlendra Kumar Singh, Ujjayanta Bhaumik, Anand Sai, Kornala Arun, and Akbar Sheikh Akbari

1 Introduction

Calculus is an integral part of our life, and from everything imaginable, from artificial intelligence to social networks, every minute visualization can afford a shadow of calculus [1]. From taking baby steps to finding the derivative of a linear function to realizing the verisimilar graphics in movies and games, calculus is intermingled in every detail. But there is a more subtle side to the story, and an even more beautiful side expands when the fractional side is considered. Fractional calculus is something that has gained immense popularity in recent years. Riemann–Liouville, Caputo, Grunwald–Letnikov, and several others defined fractional derivatives in their own ways which proved breakthroughs in the calculation of fractional derivatives [2, 3]. Robotics, algorithms in genetics, basic sciences, telecommunication, diffusion, and different image processing applications are just some of the areas upon which fractional derivative has bestowed its grace and this is just a sneak peak of the list [2]. Fractional order SavitzkyGolay differentiator has been also used for image enhancement [4, 5]. Singh et al. designed a new fractional order differentiator based on Chebyshev polynomial and successfully detected the internal structure of wood with this differentiator [6]. Chen et al. designed a new method based on fractional order differentiator for finite impulse response [7]. Chen et al. also discretized a fractional order differentiator and integrator for signal reconstruction [8]. Especially with regards to signal processing, fractional differentiation has helped make scalar

K. Kumar Singh (✉) · U. Bhaumik · A. Sai · K. Arun
Department of Computer Science and Engineering, National Institute of Technology Jamshedpur, Jamshedpur, Jharkhand 83014, India
e-mail: koushlendra.cse@nitjsr.ac.in

A. S. Akbari
Leeds Beckett University, Caedmon, 207, Headingley Campus Leeds, UK

© The Author(s), under exclusive license to Springer Nature Singapore Pte Ltd. 2021
M. K. Bajpai et al. (eds.), *Machine Vision and Augmented Intelligence—Theory and Applications*, Lecture Notes in Electrical Engineering 796,
https://doi.org/10.1007/978-981-16-5078-9_12

129

advances [9]. The SavitzkyGolay differentiator based on fractional order differentiation helps in approximating a signal using regression technique on polynomials [10, 11]. Digital Fractional Order differentiator, in fact, can be utilized as a model for studying how digital signals behave under differentiation, and both continuous and discrete time-based modes are available. There are various methods available for the continuous domain, like methods of Roy, Chareff, Carlson, and Matsuda, whereas the discrete domain is supported by Taylor and Newton series, expansion using continued fraction. But the methods in popular use are not that effective when a contaminated signal is used as an input [12–16].

Recently, there has been a lot of interest in fractional calculus, and different applications have been proposed, like those in control systems by Podlunby, processing of signals in bio-medical systems by Margin, noise processing by Ninness, processing splines and wavelets by Usher and Blu [17–19]. Many different techniques were proposed by Baba et al. to use Savitzky Golay filter to enhance geophysical signals, Bai et al. to devise anisotropic diffusion using fractional order derivative, and Magin et al. to use fractional differentiation in bioengineering [20–22]. Pu et al. created masks by utilizing the concepts of Grunwald–Letnikov and Riemann–Liouville fractional derivative definitions [23]. There has been remarkable progress in the field of signal processing and denoising too.

The authors have proposed a noble method of signal denoising that involves breaking a signal into parts and treating them, so that the irrelevant or the redundant noise components could be removed, and high frequency and low frequency noises both could be removed with relevant techniques. Signal denoising helps in reconstruction of the original signal and also helps in estimating the nature and source of noise. Fractional order SavitzkyGolay differentiator is a manifestation of the SavitzkyGolay differentiator, so that the order is changed from integer to fraction according to the Riemann–Liouville definition. The authors propose an alternative approach by which fractional order SavitzkyGolay differentiator can be used with smaller differentiator lengths to approximate the derivative of the original signal with a large number of sample points. The proposed Digital Fractional Order SavitzkyGolay Differentiator (DFOSGD), in this work, is used to approximate known signals like sinusoidal, exponential, and trigonometric functions. The proposed method calculates the fractional derivative of a signal by breaking into small piecewise signals and then applies the differentiator on the individual signals. The novel approach, here, experiments on the size of the sliding window, and calculates the accuracy of the differentiator for different window sizes, unlike the other differentiators described in the literature. Efforts have been made to experimentally determine the effect of changing differentiator length on standard signals.

The structure of the paper is as follows: Sect. 2 portrays the proposed methodology. Section 3 documents the experimental results and analysis. Section 4 gives conclusion of the work done and is followed by the references.

2 Methodology

Often unwanted additions are there to the signals because of factors which can be represented as:

$$x_e(t) = x(t) + e(t) \tag{1}$$

where $x(t)$ is the clean signal, $e(t)$ the unwanted addition, and $x_e(t)$ the resultant. Given a signal that is sampled at uniform intervals, the aim is to estimate its xth order derivative using a differentiating window with L points and to examine the effect that variation of L has on derivative. The signal is approximated using a least-square polynomial of degree n, where n is less than L. The approximated signal can be represented as:

$$A_x = \sum_{i=0}^{n} a_i x_L^i \tag{2}$$

Here, $A(x)$ approximates the given signal, and x represents the L sample points of the signal on which the differentiator window is applied (i.e., $j = 1, 2, ..., L$). a_i is ith coefficient of the least-square polynomial function [24]. To estimate a_i, a form of regression analysis called least squares method is applied.

Let M be the measured signal points for the sample points in the differentiating window such that $M = [m_1, m_2, ..., m_L]$. Let A be a vector representing the coefficients of the least-square polynomial such that $A = [a_1, a_2, ..., a_L]$. Let δ denote the error made during estimating the least-square polynomial and V be an $L \times (n + 1)$ Vandermonde Matrix. The Vandermonde matrix is shown below.

$$V = \begin{bmatrix} 1^0 \ 1^1 \ 1^2 \ \cdots \ 1^n \\ 2^0 \ 2^1 \ 2^2 \ \cdots \ 2^n \\ \cdots \cdots \cdots \cdots \cdots \\ L^0 \ L^1 \ L^2 \ \cdots \ L^3 \end{bmatrix} \tag{3}$$

For ease of understanding, the problem can be represented using matrices as follows:

$$M = V A + \delta \tag{4}$$

The coefficients of the polynomial are chosen such that they minimize the total squared error between the data points and the approximated polynomial. Thus:

$$A = (V'V)^{-1} V'M \tag{5}$$

Here, V' is transpose of the Vandermonde matrix defined in (3). Using Eq. (5) to replace A in (4) and ignoring delta, we get:

$$M_{approx} = V A \qquad (6)$$

$$\Rightarrow Mapprox = V\left((V'V)^{-1}V'M\right) \qquad (7)$$

$$\Rightarrow M_{approx} = U M \qquad (8)$$

Here, U acts as a differentiator window that approximates and smooths the given signal. Given U, we can calculate the smoothed signal from the original signal.

The Riemann–Liouville definition is used to determine fractional order derivative in the proposed approach. The Riemann–Liouville definition for fractional order derivatives is shown below:

$$_0D_x^\alpha f(x) = \frac{1}{\Gamma(1-\alpha)} \frac{d^L}{(dx^L)} \int_0^x (x-t)^{(L-\alpha-1)} f(t)dt \qquad (9)$$

Here, $0 \le (l-1) < \alpha < l$ [25]. The signal is approximated to least-square polynomials which are in the form of $f(i) = \sum_{i=0}^n a_i j^i$, thus knowing the Riemann–Liouville definition for αth derivative of j^i can help determine the derivative of the signal:

$$_0D_x^\alpha j^i = \frac{\Gamma(i+1)}{\Gamma(i-\alpha+1)} j^{(i-\alpha)} \qquad (10)$$

Here, Γ operator is defined as $\Gamma n = (n-1)!$. Using linearity of Riemann–Liouville definition, the following can be inferred:

$$_0D_x^\alpha f(i) \qquad (11)$$

$$\Rightarrow {}_0D_x^\alpha \sum_{i=0}^n a_i j^i \qquad (12)$$

$$\Rightarrow \sum_{i=0}^n a_{i0} D_x^\alpha j^i \qquad (13)$$

Using Eq. (10) and Eq. (13) can be written as:

$$\Rightarrow \sum_{i=0}^n a_i \frac{\Gamma(i+1)}{\Gamma(i-\alpha+1)} j^{(i-\alpha)} \qquad (14)$$

The above logic can be generalized using matrices. The αth order derivative of the ith point is given as:

$$_lM^\alpha_{approx} = V^\alpha_l A = U^\alpha_l M \tag{15}$$

Using the results in Eq. (14) in Eq. (15), the following can be inferred:

$$_lM^\alpha_{approx} = a(V'V)^{-1}V'M \tag{16}$$

As evident from Eq. (14), a is

$$a = [\frac{\Gamma(1)}{\Gamma(1-\alpha)}i^{-\alpha}, \frac{\Gamma(2)}{\Gamma(2-\alpha)}i^{1-\alpha}, \cdots, \frac{\Gamma(n+1)}{\Gamma(n+1-\alpha)}i^{n-\alpha}] \tag{17}$$

Thus, U^α_l is obtained using:

$$U^\alpha_l = a(V'V)^{-1}V' \tag{18}$$

Using this U^α_l, the αth derivative at any point i of the signal can be approximated, provided the original signal is given. The sampling interval (θ) is taken as one. A generalized expression for non-unitary theta can be obtained in a similar fashion. The proposed algorithm is demonstrated as follows:

```
ALGORITHM
    Initialize: L, n, α
Input: M(i) where i = 1,2,3,...,l
Output: N(i) where i = 1,2,3,...,l
temp_signal=M(1 to L)
derivative_of_temp = DIFFERENTIATOR(L, n,  temp_signal,
α)
final_signal(1 to L) = derivative_of_temp
fori : L+1 to l
temp_signal=M(i-L+1 to i)
derivative_of_temp = DIFFERENTIATOR(L, n, temp_signal, α)
final_signal(i) = derivative_of_temp(L)
endfor


    BEGIN DIFFERENTIATOR (L, n, temp_Signal, α)
    J=temp_Signal.length()
    fori : 1 to J
    for j : 0 to n
    a[j + 1] = j^(j-α)/Γ(j + 1 - α)
    endfor

    U^α_1 = aV^(-1)
        output_Signal[i] = U_l^α * temp_Signal
    endfor
    returnoutput_S
    signal
    END DIFFERENT
```

3   Results and Analysis

The proposed method has been examined using four different experiments. The proposed method has also been compared with existing methods in literature. The different signals chosen in the experiments arc parabola with axis as the y axis and a sinusoidal curve, with the fractional derivatives being calculated at several points. The sinusoidal and parabolic signals are chosen to represent a variety of signals and also because of ease of comparison with other results. The signals to noise ratios show that the proposed differentiator calculates the fractional derivatives with a high degree of accuracy. The results of the derivatives calculated by the proposed differentiator are compared with the methods of Euler, Oustaloup, Tustin, Al-Alaoui, Simpson, New IIR, and DFOSGD differentiator. The experiments are as follows:

A. Experiment 1

The aim of this experiment is to test the accuracy of the proposed method by using the moving window coefficients to obtain the derivatives and by comparing these derivative values against standard values. The moving window's weight U_i^{α} at the ith point x_i is computed for different values of α, which represents the order of the derivative, with values in the set 0.0, 0.1, 0.2, 0.3, 0.4, 0.5, 0.6, 0.7, 0.8, 0.9, 1.0. In this experiment, the order of the polynomial is taken as 2 ($n = 2$) and the length of the differentiator is taken as 10 ($L = 10$). The assumption is that the given signal is a parabolic function having equation $y = x^2$. It is assumed that the given signal is sampled at first 10 integers, i.e., $I = 1,2,3, \ldots,10$. The results of the experiment are listed in Table 1 which gives the values of the derivative of the function at various sample points for various values of α. For instance, at the sample point 5, the derivative of the function at $\alpha = 0.5$ has a value of 16.8209.

The graph for the original derivative of the signal and the derivative calculated using the proposed method is shown in Fig. 1. The green line shows the original derivative of the function at $\alpha = 1$ and the blue line shows the derivative calculated through proposed method at $\alpha = 1$. It is clear from Fig. 1 that the proposed method calculates the derivative accurately, and by comparing the values of the derivatives obtained via the experiment with the standard values of the derivative for the above parabolic function at $\alpha = 1$, we obtain a mean-square error of 7.8676×10^{-9}.

In addition, the proposed method has been tested using the signal $h(t) = t^{0.5}$. It is assumed that the given signal is sampled at first 10 integers, i.e., $I = 1,2,3, \ldots,10$. The result is shown in Fig. 2. In Fig. 2, the blue line indicates the original signal $h(t)$, the curve colored green indicates the original derivative of $h(t)$ at $\alpha = 1$, and the curve colored red indicates the derivative of $h(t)$ calculated using the proposed method at $\alpha = 1$. By comparing the values of the derivatives obtained via the experiment with the standard values of the derivative for the above parabolic function at $\alpha = 1$, we obtain a mean-square error of 0.0343.

It can be deduced that the proposed method works as a differentiator accurately, and the errors obtained can be accounted for the estimation error.

Table 1 Values of the derivatives of the function at various values of alpha

Points	0.0	0.1	0.2	0.3	0.4	0.5	0.6	0.7	0.8	0.9	1.0
1	1.000	1.0945	1.1930	1.2948	1.3990	1.5045	1.6101	1.7142	1.8152	1.9112	2.0000
2	4.00	4.0847	4.1542	4.2067	4.2409	4.2554	4.2490	4.2209	4.1703	4.0967	4.0000
3	9.00	8.8255	8.6188	8.3810	8.1134	7.8177	7.4958	7.1503	6.7838	6.3993	6.0000
4	16.0	15.244	14.4656	13.6676	12.8560	12.0361	11.2133	10.3931	9.58073	8.7814	8.0000
5	25.0	23.294	21.6160	2 19.972	18.3722	16.8209	15.3253	13.8909	12.5225	11.2245	10.0000
6	36.0	32.9379	30.0125	27.2301	24.5953	22.1117	19.7817	17.6062	15.5851	13.7172	12.0001
8	64.0	56.8958	50.3724	44.4063	38.9721	34.0433	29.5922	25.2909	22.0109	1,808,234	16.0001
9	81.0	71.1656	62.2684	54.2506	47.0542	40.6219	34.8973	29.8253	25.3525	21.4273	18.0001
10	100	686.94	75.2717	64.8922	55.6943	47.5770	40.4438	34.2034	28.7693	24.0603	20.0002

Fig. 1 Original and proposed derivative of $y = x^2$ at $\alpha = 1$

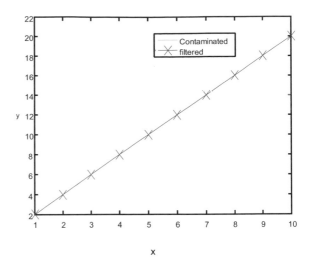

Fig. 2 Original and proposed derivative of $y = x^2$ at $\alpha = 1$

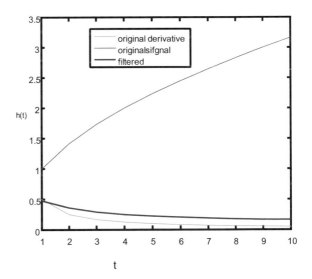

B. Experiment 2.1

This experiment is carried out using a sine curve. The signal used in this experiment is $h(t) = sin(t)$. The parameters are set as follows: the order of the polynomial is taken as 5 ($n = 5$) and the length of the differentiator window is taken as 10 ($L = 10$). The effect on the curve is visualized using the variable parameter α which denotes the order of derivative, and the orders are taken as 0.0, 0.1, 0.2, 0.3, 0.4, 0.5, 0.6, 0.7, 0.8, and 0.9. The curve is sampled a 1000 times between $t = 0$ and $t = 4$. The value of the sine curve is examined at angles varying with increments of 15 degrees starting with 0 degree and going up-to 90 degrees. The variation in these values is

Table 2 Values of derivative of $sin(t)$ at various α and t

t,α	0.0	0.1	0.2	0.3	0.4	0.5	0.6	0.7	0.8	0.9
0°	0.00004	50.0013	0.0028	0.0056	0.0105	0.0199	0.0388	0.0834	0.2281	1
15°	0.2639	0.2683	0.2741	0.2817	0.2923	0.3082	0.3344	0.3856	0.5266	0.9657
30°	0.5059	0.5098	0.5149	0.5217	0.5312	0.5452	0.5682	0.6124	0.7297	0.8649
45°	0.7130	0.7162	0.7203	0.7252	0.7334	0.7446	0.7628	0.7971	0.8826	0.7044
60°	0.8709	0.8732	0.8761	0.8799	0.8851	0.8927	0.9048	0.9268	0.9745	0.4953
75°	0.9688	0.9699	0.9713	0.9732	0.9757	0.9792	0.9845	0.9926	0.9993	0.2521
90°	0.9999	0.9998	0.9997	0.9995	0.9991	0.9983	0.9962	0.9900	0.9552	0.0085

examined as α is varied. The observations are recorded in Table 2 which gives the derivative of the function at various standard points for various values of α. For an instance, the value of derivative of the function at sample point 75 degrees and $\alpha = 0.5$ is 0.9792.

In Fig. 3, the blue-colored curve represents original derivative and the red-colored curve represents proposed derivative at $\alpha = 0.1$.

Similarly, Fig. 4 represents the plot between original derivative and proposed derivative at $\alpha = 1$. As evident from the figures, the proposed method estimates the derivative of the sinusoidal signal accurately (with some error due to an estimation error of least-square polynomial). As evident from the data, the values of the derivatives obtained through the proposed method are very close to the real value. The mean-square error between the first order derivative ($\alpha = 1$) and the curve $h(t) = \cos t$ comes to 2.6194×10^{-7}. This is a clear indicative that the proposed method works as a differentiator very well.

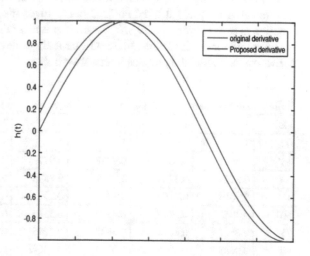

Fig. 3 Original and proposed derivative of $h(t) = sin(t)$ at $\alpha = 0.1$

Fig. 4 Original and
proposed derivative of $h(t) =$
$sin(t)$ at $\alpha = 1$

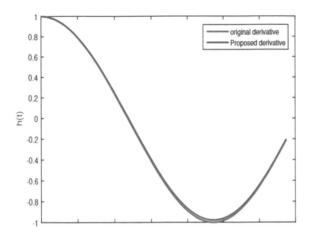

C. Experiment 2.2

This experiment is fabricated using a sine curve and the signal used is $h(t) = sin(t)$.
The order of the polynomial is taken as 5 ($n = 5$) and the order of the derivative is
taken as 1 ($\alpha = 1$). The length of the differentiator (L) is varied and the values are
recorded in a similar way as done in experiment 2.1. Mean-square error is calculated
between the derivative obtained using proposed differentiator and standard derivative
of $h(t)$ which is equal to $cos(t)$ for every value of L. The values of L considered are 10,
15, 20, 25, 30, 50, and 100. The results are shown in Table 3 which gives a derivative
of the function at various values of L keeping $\alpha = 1$. For an instance, the value of
the derivative of the function at $L = 20$ at the point 75 degrees is 0.2835.

In Figs. 5, 6, and 7, the blue-colored curve gives the original derivative of the
function at $\alpha = 1$ and the red-colored curve gives the proposed derivative of the
function at $\alpha = 1$. From the Figs. 5, 6, and 7, it is clear that as the value of the length
of differentiator (L) increases, there will be a slight deviation between the original
derivative curve and the proposed derivative curve.

Table 3 Values of derivative of $sin(t)$ at various values of L and t

t,L	10	15	20	25	30	50	100
0°	1	1	1	1	1.000	1	1
15°	0.9657	0.9697	0.9737	0.9773	0.9807	0.9916	0.9685
30°	0.8649	0.8728	0.8807	0.8885	0.8961	0.9236	0.9744
45°	0.7044	0.7156	0.7271	0.7385	0.7496	0.7920	0.8823
60°	0.4953	0.5091	0.5233	0.5375	0.5515	0.6058	0.7294
75°	0.2521	0.2675	0.2835	0.2995	0.3153	0.3778	0.5262
90°	0.0085	0.0075	0.0241	0.04048	0.0574	0.1238	0.2867
MSE	2.6194×10^{-7}	1.3686×10^{-4}	5.4383×10^{-4}	0.0012	0.0022	0.0087	0.0437

Fig. 5 Original and proposed derivative of $h(t) = sin(t)$ at $L = 10$

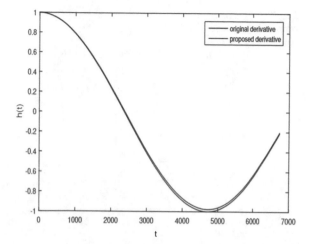

Fig. 6 Original and proposed derivative of h(t) = sin(t) at L = 50

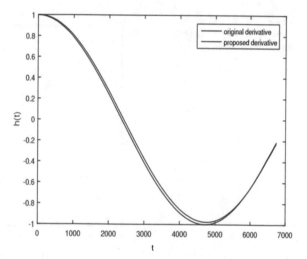

Figure 8 gives the plot between Mean Square Error (MSE) and Length of differentiator L, which shows that MSE increases with increase in value of L and decreases at $L = 25$, and then increases with increase in L. The effect of differentiator length on the mean-square error can be seen in Table 3 and the Figs. 5, 6, and 7. As the length of the differentiator increases, the mean-square error also increases. Higher differentiator lengths imply larger Vandermonde Matrices. Large Vandermonde matrices have poor conditioning. This leads to errors in inverse calculations, and thus increasing mean-square error.

Fig. 7 Original and
proposed derivative of h(t) =
sin(t) at L = 100

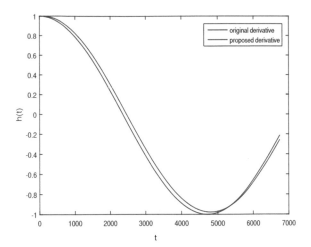

Fig. 8 Variance of mean
square error with respect to
length of diffrentiator

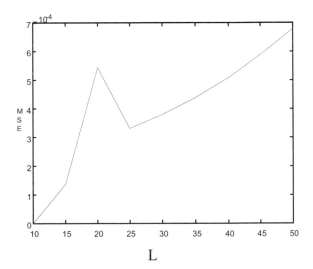

D. Experiment 3

The third experiment is dedicated to the comparison of the proposed method with
established methods like those of Euler, Tustin, Oustaloup, and others. The curve
which is used to show the robustness of the proposed method is $h(t) = e^{-t}.sin(3t +$
1). In this experiment, the length of differentiator is taken as 10 ($L = 10$) and the
order of the polynomial is taken as 5 ($n = 5$). A uniformly distributed random noise
with amplitude ranging from -0.1 to 0.1 and having Signal to Noise Ratio (SNR)
of 24 dB is added to the signal $h(t)$ to contaminate it. This contaminated signal
is passed through the proposed differentiator to get the differentiatored signal. To
compare the efficiency of this method with other methods, Root Mean Square value

for the contaminated signal and the differentiatored signal is compared for different methods mentioned above. The results are listed in Table 4 which gives comparison of Root Mean Square (RMS) values for different methods with the proposed methods for $\alpha = 0.1, 0.3, 0.5, 0.7, 0.9$.

In Fig. 9, the curve colored green depicts the signal contaminated with noise and the red-colored curve depicts the filtered signal after passing through the proposed differentiator at $\alpha = 0.1$. Similarly, in Fig. 10, the curve colored green depicts the signal contaminated with noise and the red-colored curve depicts the filtered signal after passing through the proposed differentiator at $\alpha = 0.1$.

Furthermore, Fig. 11 gives us the plot between the RMS Error and different values of $\alpha = 0.1, 0.3, 0.5, 0.7, 0.9$, and it can be derived that the method gives the least RMS Error for $\alpha = 0.3$. From the error comparison from Table 4, it can be seen that

Table 4 Comparison of RMS error for $\alpha = 0.1, 0.3, 0.5, 0.7, 0.9$

Method	$\alpha = 0.1$	$\alpha = 0.3$	$\alpha = 0.5$	$\alpha = 0.7$	$\alpha = 0.9$
Oustaloup	0.0304	0.0677	0.1486	0.3308	0.7295
Tustin	0.0364	0.0997	0.3189	1.3448	13.6736
Euler	0.0333	0.0741	0.1589	0.3605	0.8474
Al-Alaoui	0.0342	0.0782	0.1728	0.4084	1.0064
Simpson	0.0359	0.0799	0.1563	0.3298	0.7437
New IIR	0.0351	0.0801	0.1712	0.3907	0.9387
DFOSGD	0.0056	0.0087	0.0137	0.0217	0.0343
Proposed Method	0.0026	0.0013	0.0042	0.0046	0.0048

Fig. 9 Original and proposed derivative of $h(t) = e^{-t}.sin(3t + 1)$ at $\alpha = 0.1$

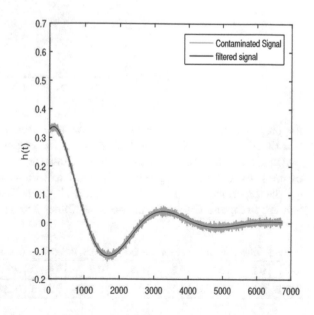

Fig. 10 Original and
proposed derivative of h(t) =
e − t.sin(3t + 1) at α = 0.3

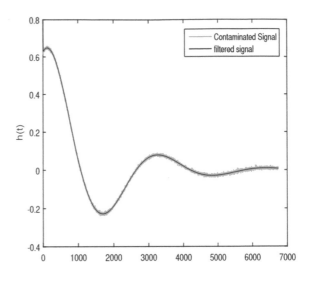

Fig. 11 Plot for root mean
square error and α

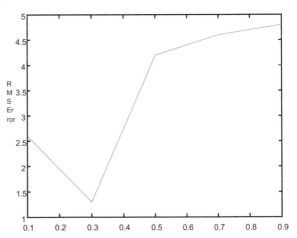

the proposed method is better than the existing methods such as Oustloup, Tustin, and Euleretc. It is evident from the Table and the graphs that the proposed method which acts as a diffrentiator also can act as a tool for denoising of the signal and can be used as a method to reduce noise in many real-life applications.

The experiment is repeated with Additive White Gaussian Noise (AWGN) of varying strengths. The results are noted in Tables 5 and 6.

Table 5 Mean Square error for $\alpha = 0.1, 0.3, 0.5, 0.7, 0.9, 1$ in order of 10^{-2}

α	0.1	0.2	0.3	0.4	0.5	0.6	0.7	0.8	0.9	1.0
MSE	0.1501	0.1703	0.1906	0.2173	0.2434	0.2718	0.2996	0.3248	0.3620	0.3895

Table 6 Mean Square error for different Signal to Noise Ratio (SNR) in order of 10^{-2}

SNR	10	20	30	40	50
MSE	2.189	0.8208	0.2599	0.0817	0.0256

Table 5 shows the variation of mean-square error with the change in order of derivative (α) keeping the signal to noise ratio (SNR) of the signal fixed at 35 dB. Table 6 shows the variation of mean-square error of the denoised signal at different values of SNR. Order of derivative (α) is kept fixed at 0.1.

4 Conclusions

Fractional order derivative is very important in the field of signal denoising. The proposed method works well as differentiator. For polynomial functions, the order of mean-square error is 10^{-9}, and for sinusoidal functions, the order of mean-square error is 10^{-7}. This is because polynomial functions can be exactly represented using least square method, whereas other functions are only approximated using least square methods. The outcome of this study clearly defines relation between length of differentiator and derivative obtained through the differentiator. The effects of varying length of differentiator are tested by comparing against standard derivatives of first order and its mean-square error. The order of mean-square error varies from 10^{-7} for smaller values of L to 10^{-2} for larger values of L. It is clear that the length of differentiator has a significant impact on determining the derivatives, and large lengths of differentiator perform badly due to conditioning issues with the matrix. The proposed method is successfully able to minimize the noise of contaminated signal. The denoised signal has a minimum root mean-square error of 0.0013 at $\alpha = 0.3$.

References

1. Vinagre et.al (2000) Some approximations of fractional order operators used in control theory and applications. Fract Calc Appl Analalysis 4
2. Liu D-Y et al (2015) Fractional order differentiation by integration and error analysis in noisy environment. IEEE Trans Automatic Control 60:2945–2960
3. Podlunby (1999) Fractional differential equations: an introduction to fractional derivatives, fractional differential equations, to methods of their solution and some of their applications, p 198
4. Suraj S, Jha RK (2017) A new technique for image enhancement using digital fractional-order Savitzky–Golay differentiator. Multidim Syst Sign Process 28:709–733
5. Chen D et al (2012) 1-D and 2-D digital fractional order Savitzky Golay differentiator. Signal Video Image Process SIViP 6:503–511
6. Singh et al (2017) A novel non-invasive method for extraction of geometrical and texture features of wood. Res Non Destr Eval 28(3):150–167

7. Chen YQ et al (2003) A new IIR-type digital fractional order differentiator. Signal Process 83(11):2359–2365
8. Chen YQ et al (2002) Discretization schemes for fractional-order differentiators and integrators. IEEE Trans Circuits Syst Fundamental Them 49:363–367
9. Roy S (1967) On the realization of a constant-argument immittance or fractional operator. IEEE Trans Circuit Theory 3:264–274
10. Luo J et al (2005) Properties of Savitzky—Golay digital differentiators. Digital Signal Process 15:122–136
11. Savitzky A, Golay ME (1964) Smoothing and differentiation of data by simplified least squares procedures, Anal Chem 36:1627–1639
12. Ninness (1998) Estimation of 1/f noise
13. Tseng CC (2001) Design of fractional order digital fractional differentiator. IEEE Signal Process 8:77–56
14. Tseng et al (2000) Computation of fractional derivatives using fourier transform and digital FIR differentiator. Signal Process 80:151–159
15. Engheta N (1996) On fractional calculus and fractional multipoles in electro magnetism. IEEE Trans Antennas Propagat 44:554–566
16. Quan Q et al (2012) Time domain analysis of the Savitzky-Golayfilters. Digit Signal Process 2:238–245
17. Podlubny I (1999) Fractional-order systems and PID. Controllers 44:208–214
18. Usher et al (2000) Fractional splines and wavelets. SIAM Rev
19. Ferdi Y (2011) Fractional order calculus based filters for biomedical signal processing. In: Middle east conference on biomedical engineering, pp 73–76
20. Baba et al (2014) Enhancing geophysical signals through the use of Savitzky-Golay filtering method. Geoficia Int 53:399–409
21. Bai et al (2007) Fractional-order anisotropic diffusion for image denoising. IEEE Trans Image Process 2492–5202
22. Magin et al (2004) Fractional calculus in bioengineering. Crit Rev Biomed Eng 1–104
23. Pu et al (2010) Fractional differential mask: a fractional differential-based approach for multiscale texture enhancement. IEEE 19:491–511
24. Rajesh KP et al (2014) An approximate method for abel inversion using chebyshev polynomials. Appl Math Comput 237:120–132
25. Singh KK, Bajpai MK, Pandey RK(2018) A novel approach for enhancement of geometric and contrast resolution properties of low contrast images. IEEE/CAA J Autom Sin 5(2):628–638

Performance Analysis of Machine Learning-Based Breast Cancer Detection Algorithms

Sanjay Kumar, Akshita, Shivangi Thapliyal, Shiva Bhatt, and Naina Negi

1 Introduction

Breast Cancer is a serious health hazard for women in many countries. It is well known that the best way to cure breast cancer is early detection. Around 2.1 million women are affected by breast cancer each year. American Cancer Society estimated that new cases in 2020 will be 2,76,480 which is 15.3% of all new cancer cases. Mammography, Ultrasound, MRI are some common methods to detect breast cancer [1]. Breast cancer does not display any symptoms in its initial stage, and this is why women above 40 years of age are advised to take mammograms (X-Ray of the breast) once a year [2]. It is possible to miss a small tumor when reviewing a mammogram with naked eyes. Accurate prediction of cancer has become one of the most challenging tasks for physicians, which is why an accurate, rapid, and automatic diagnosis system is required for breast cancer. This is where machine learning has outsmarted human intelligence, as it can detect even a small tumor in mammograms by scanning through the image thoroughly. Machine learning techniques help us to extract information and knowledge from this experience and detect hard-to-perceive patterns from large and noisy datasets [3]. In the medical field, ML techniques are used to increase the prediction rate of breast cancer. Also, Wisconsin (Diagnostic) Data Set is mostly used to train the model. Many research papers concluded that the Support Vector Machine and Random Forest are giving the best accuracy [4, 5].

In this work, we made several calculative contributions which are as follows:

- In this work, we studied and implemented different supervised machine learning algorithms such as SVM, CNN, and RF for breast cancer detection.

S. Kumar (✉)
National Institute of Technology Jamshedpur, Jamshedpur, India
e-mail: 2017rscs001@nitjsr.ac.in

Akshita · S. Thapliyal · S. Bhatt · N. Negi
Women Institute of Technology Dehradun, Dehradun, India

- Performance analysis is carried out over two datasets, i.e., Breast Cancer Wisconsin (Diagnostic) Data Set and the Breast Histopathology Images Dataset.
- K-fold cross-validation technique is used to check the effectiveness of the machine learning model.

The rest of the paper is organized as follows: Related work has been discussed in Sect. 2. Methodology and Material is discussed in Sect. 3. Implementation and result analysis is presented in Sect. 4. Finally, the conclusion has been drawn in Sect. 5.

2 Related Work

Breast cancer detection has evolved thoroughly in the past years. In this section, some of the breast cancer detection techniques are discussed.

Abdel et al. [6] presented different models to classify among pre-segmented breast cancer masses and trained multiple CNN models to improve classification results by obtaining average of predictions. Yamlome et al. [7] presented an efficient training strategy involving transfer learning data augmentation along with high-resolution complete image training. This approach yielded 95.27% classification accuracy and 96.35% patient score accuracy. The main goal of Chaurasia et al. [8] work is improvement of accuracy of prediction using a new statistical method of feature selection. Here, six integrated models are applied in the reduced attribute data subset (12 features). Ragab et al. [9] proposed a new CAD system with two segmentation techniques. Extraction was performed by DCNN and this was further connected to an SVM model. This model yielded an accuracy of 80.5% and can also be used for other anomalies in breasts along with a classification of amiable and vicious breast cancer. Nagendra et al. [10] designed and developed dual-layered CNN (DL-CNN) parted into two sections to score a TPR of 0.9726 and the lowest value of FPI 0.3976. Rohan et al. [11] proposed a model that outperformed all the existing ones. This model used 11 features and 10 attributes and enhanced the performance of the classifiers. Kumar et al. [12] have applied CNN combined with changing the parameter and testing it on Break His dataset image of breast cancer using deep learning framework TensorFlow. It is observed in this research that the classification accuracy majorly depends on how CNN brings out and learns the characteristics in different layers with the variation in parameters. Alkhaleefah et al. [13] provided a possible solution to the classification of amiable or vicious breast cancer by using a hybrid approach which uses a combination of CNN and RBF-based SVM. Sharma et al. [5] proposed a model for comparative study of different ML algorithms for detection and classification of breast cancer. This study revealed that supervised ML algorithms work better and give an accuracy of above 94%. Khourdifi et al. [4] researched the algorithms that help predict breast cancer. They concluded that the SVM classifier gave the best possible results. Gupta et al. [14] researched on multilayered perception which proved to be better than all of the other classifiers. Al-masni et al. [15] presented a

YOLO-based CAD system for classification and detection of breast cancer, considered different methods, and experimentally determined that SVM classifier was best in detecting microcalcifications in mammography images. Islam et al. [16] proposed an SVM-based model for detection of breast cancer. This model displayed accuracy of 99.68%. Alyami et al. [17] built models with ANN and SVM along with tenfold cross-validation. In this research, ANN achieved an accuracy of 96.7096% and SVM reached 97.1388%. Wang et al. [18] proposed a breast CAD method based on deep learning. The research focused on the application of features extracted by CNN in two stages, namely, mass detection and mass diagnosis. Table 1 depicts the summary of the related work.

3 Methodology and Material

This section is a brief description of the methodology we have used in our models and also the material used to construct them:

3.1 Methodology

Different machine learning algorithms, both supervised and unsupervised, were tested on the two datasets we have used in our work. The three algorithms that made their way into the most suitable ones have been detailed below.

3.1.1 Support Vector Machine

SVM is a supervised machine learning algorithm which is a classifier of discriminative nature which is designed using a hyperplane to classify the data in different classes based on class membership. Two parallel lines that are maximum distance apart and have no data points between them are termed as hyperplane, and the data points closest to a hyperplane are support vectors [19]. Our objective is to find the best, which one is the farthest from the data point. The SVM algorithm is used when the data comprises two classes where the classification is done [2, 16].

3.1.2 Convolutional Neural Network

CNN is a class of neural networks in deep learning. This class is also termed as space (or shift) invariant artificial neural networks (SIANN). CNN is a regular version of multilevel perceptions [7, 13]. This classifier is majorly used when working with images, as it helps to extract features from the images. A benefit of using CNN with images is that it uses fewer data preprocessing in comparison to other algorithms used

Table 1 Summary of the related work

Authors	Related work		
	Techniques and algorithms	Accuracy	Remark
Abdel et al.[6]	Convolutional Neural Networks Transfer Learning	Inception V3-like Model: 79.6% ResNet50-like Model: 85.71%	This model presented different models to classify among pre-segmented breast cancer masses and trained multiple CNN models to improve classification results by obtaining average of predictions
Yamlome et al. [7]	Convolutional Neural Networks (CNN)	Image level: 91% Patient Scores: 95%	A reliable step towards authentic automation of medical diagnostics
Chaurasia et al. [8]	CART, SVM, Naïve Bayes, KNN, Linear Regression, and MLP	99%	The features of dataset will be reduced using statistical method mode
Ragab et al. [9]	CNN, SVM, DDSM, CBIS-DDSM	80.5%	The model is efficient enough to detect and classify benign or malignant breast cancer. It can also identify other anomalies in breasts
Nagendra et al. [10]	Dual Layered Convolutional Neural Networks (DL-CNN)	97.26%	Rate of false positive has been minimized using this model
Rohan et al. [11]	Random Forest ensemble learning	98.5714%	This proposed approach plays a major role in the research related to the diagnosis of breast cancer. The use of ADABOOST structure is a plus point
Kumar et al. [12]	CNN	90%	The room for improvement in this technique is high
Alkhaleefah et al. [13]	CNN, SVM classifier based on Radial Basis Function	92%	The hybrid approach is giving best results

(continued)

Table 1 (continued)

Authors	Related work		
	Techniques and algorithms	Accuracy	Remark
Sharma et al. [5]	Random Forest, KNN, and Naïve Bayes	94%	Supervised machine learning techniques are reported to give better results
Khourdifi et al. [4]	Random Forest, Naïve Bayes, SVM, and KNN	SVM highest, i.e., 97.9%	The findings help to decide the most appropriate ML algorithm for breast cancer detection
Gupta et al. [14]	Decision Tree, SVM, KNN	SVM highest, i.e., 93.09%	The result shows that multilayer perceptron performs better than other techniques
Al-masni et al. [15]	You Only Look Once (YOLO)	85.52%	The proposed model overcomes many problems that existed in classification systems
Islam et al. [16]	SVM and KNN	99.68%	To get an accurate outcome, system uses tenfold cross-validation
Alyami et al. [17]	Support Vector Machine (SVM), Artificial Neural Network (ANN)	SVM: 97.1388% ANN: 96.7096%	Different data partitioning is an important feature developed by this research
Wang et al. [18]	Convolutional Neural Networks (CNN) fused with Unsupervised Extreme Learning Machine (US-ELM)	ELM > CNN	This method outperforms others of its kind with a large dataset

in image classification. CNN was useful in working with the Breast Histopathology Image Dataset [12]. It played a major role in extracting features from the images in the dataset. Along with this, the fact remains that the dataset did not have pixel-rich images, and the proficiency of CNN was helpful in this field a lot.

CNN is the type of ML algorithm that requires an image input. Since the Breast Cancer Wisconsin (Diagnostic) dataset has a non-image kind of data, therefore, it has not been trained using CNN.

3.1.3   Random Forest Algorithm

The Random forest classifier is the supervised learning Algorithm that consists of the maximum number of ensemble decision trees. This technique is based on recursion; basically, it is used for classification problems [19]. The rules of the random forest mechanism are, first, we have to create a decision tree based on given samples; after that, predict from each, collect the votes for prediction, and in the end for result, select a higher voted prediction sample. For applying in our dataset, firstly, we divided the dataset into train and test, then used a simple random forest algorithm in each feature individually (mean, standard error, and worst). The Random forest algorithm has the property for identifying the most important features from all given features; so, we used this property and trained our model by using important features from all three parts: mean, standard error, and worst [2].

3.2   Material

The materials required for this model were the two datasets that have been explained below.

3.2.1   Breast Cancer Wisconsin (Diagnostic) Dataset

The Dataset "Breast cancer Wisconsin (Diagnostic)" is retrieved from UC Irvine machine learning repository named as Breast Cancer Wisconsin (Diagnostic) Data Set, and this dataset also can be found through the UW CS File transfer protocol server [3, 4]. The Features are calculated from digitized images of a Fine Needle Aspirate of a Breast mass, and these features describe the characteristics of the cell nuclei present in the Image. Dataset has 569 instances and 33 data columns; one data column has null values so it is removed, after that there are 32 data columns which are used for data analysis. All have 0 non-null values. Here, instances are divided into three features, first is mean, second is standard error, and last one is worst. Each feature contains ten parameters: Radius, texture, area, perimeter, smoothness, compactness, concavity, concave points, symmetry, and fractal dimension. By using these features, we have to predict the stage of cancer, Malignant (M) and Benign (B) [3–5].

3.2.2   Breast Histopathology Images Dataset

The dataset named "Breast Histopathology Images" has been retrieved from CCO which is a public Machine Learning repository. Originally, there were 162 complete slide images of BC specimens scanned at 40x. From these 162 images, 277,524 patches were extracted of size 50 × 50 of which 198,738 were IDC negative and

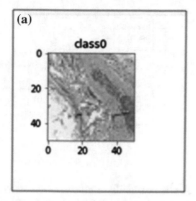 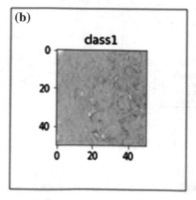

Fig. 1 Two Mammogram samples: **a** labeled as 0 (non-IDC), **b** labeled as 1 (IDC)

78,786 were IDC positive. Each patch's file name is of the format: uxXyYclassC.png —> example 10253idx5 × 1351y1101class0.png. Where u represents the patient ID (10253idx5), X and Y are the x-coordinate and y-coordinate of where the patch was cropped from respectively, and C will be the class where: 0 means non-IDC (Fig. 1a) and 1 means IDC (Fig. 1b). We can also see that image patches are closeups of the actual mammograms, and therefore it becomes harder for the human eye to read them.

The dataset has the following features: area, bounding box, centroid, convex area, convex hull, convex image, eccentricity, Equiv diameter, Euler number, extent, extrema, filled image, filled area, image, major axis length, minor axis length, orientation, perimeter, pixel index list, pixel list, solidity, weighted centroid, sub-array index, thinness ratio, elongation (EN), circularity1, circularity2, compactness, distortion and disorientation (DP), and shape index (SI). The area computes the actual number of pixels in the region and hence is the scalar value, while the centroid computes the center of the tumor region, therefore, is the vector. On data visualization, we can conclude that the brighter region is more than the dark region in our image.

4 Implementation and Result Analysis

Figure 2 shows the whole process of the proposed work. In this paper, we will use two datasets. We first import libraries like matplotlib used for plotting the graph, seaborn used to plot interactive graph, sklearn, etc. After that we explore the data, here we remove those columns which have null values and not needed. In the next phase, we do data analysis and feature selection process. In this phase, data is split into training data and testing data. In the next phase, we apply classification algorithms like SVM, CNN, and RF in our training data and compute the accuracy of

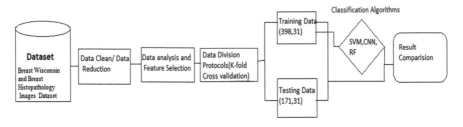

Fig. 2 Process of proposed work

datasets. Then, we compare all the accuracy. However, this method is not very reliable, because the accuracy we got with one test set can be different if we use a different training set on the same model. Here K-fold cross-validation comes into Fig. 2, which divides the data into k-folds and each fold uses a different test set. In K-fold cross-validation, train and test data will change in every iteration. This will help to validate the model properly. Here are the steps which are followed in our model for k-fold cross-validation. In the first step, we split the data into k-fold and the value of k is 5. In the second step, recording the error of each prediction, it will repeat 5 times because of the value of k. The recorded value of error is called cross-validation error and it will serve as the performance of our model.

In Feature Selection, the best features from a dataset are extracted to improve the accuracy of the model and to reduce the complexity of a model. Feature Selection is categorized into three parts, i.e., Wrapper Method, Filter Method, and Embedded Method. The Wrapper Method is used to select the subset of features, and then with every subset, we used to analyze the model's accuracy. The wrapper method is best for smaller datasets. In the Filter Method, we used to select the beast subset of features among all features, and then apply the learning algorithm and analyze the performance of the model. This model can be used for larger datasets. Embedded method combines the features of filter and wrapper methods.

In Breast Histopathology Images datasets, we are using ten features, i.e., area, centroid, major axis length, axis length, eccentricity, orientation, filled area, extrema, solidity, and equiv diameter, after performing wrapper feature selection. Parameter values are taken for SVM, CNN, RF is described in Tables 2, 3 and 4 respectively for both the datasets. And the result of the breast histopathology images dataset in terms of accuracy is depicted in Table 5.

From Table 5, it is clear that CNN for selected features gives the higher accuracy. Experimental results show that for CNN accuracy is 92.4%, whereas for SVM accuracy is 89.01%.

In the Breast Cancer Wisconsin (Diagnostic) dataset, instances are divided into three features: mean, standard error, and worst. In this dataset, we have used the Univariate Feature selection method to select the best feature. We had 33 features in the beginning and we reduced it to ten using wrapper feature selection technique. These ten selected features are radius, texture, area, perimeter, smoothness,

Table 2 Parameter value taken for SVM (for both datasets)

Breast cancer wisconsin (Diagnostic) dataset		Breast histopathology images dataset	
Parameters	Values	Parameter	Values
Kernel Function	Gaussian Kernel Radial Basis Function	Kernel Function	Gaussian Kernel Radial Basis Function
Gamma	Auto	Gamma	Auto
Cache size	200		
C (The penalty Parameter)	1.0		
Decision function shape	Ovr		

Table 3 Parameter value taken for CNN (Breast histopathology Images dataset)

Operation layer	Number of output features	Size of output features
Input layer	1	15×15
Convolutional layer C1	5	8×8
Maximum pooling layer C1	5	4×4
Convolutional layer C2	10	5×5
Maximum pooling layer C2	10	2×2

Table 4 Parameter value taken for RF (for both datasets)

Breast cancer wisconsin (Diagnostic) dataset		Breast histopathology images dataset	
Parameters	Values	Parameter	Values
N_estimators	100	N_estimators	10
Random_state	1	Random_state	0
Criterion	Gini	Criterion	Entropy

Table 5 Performance analysis of breast histopathology Images dataset in terms of accuracy

	SVM	CNN	RF
Precision (%)	70.087	88.01	77.66
Recall (%)	82.608	88.00	67.49
F1-score (%)	75.834	88.00	72.22
Accuracy (%)	87	90	74.17
Accuracy after fivefold cross-validation (%)	89.01	92.4	87.8

compactness, concavity, concave points, symmetry, and fractal dimension. By using these features, we have to predict the stage of cancer, Malignant (M) and Benign (B).

Table 6 Performance analysis of breast cancer wisconsin dataset in terms of accuracy

	SVM		RF	
	For all features	Important features	For all features	Important features
Mean (%)	90	89	92	86
Standard error (%)	91	87	89	89
Worst (%)	88	85	95	93
Overall accuracy after fivefold cross-validation (%)	95.27		98.91	

From Table 6, it is clear that RF gives higher accuracy. Experimental results show that for RF accuracy is 98.91%, whereas for SVM accuracy is 95.27%.

5 Conclusion

This paper presents a performance analysis of breast cancer detection techniques based on machine learning. In this work, two datasets: Breast cancer Wisconsin (Diagnostic) and Breast Histopathology Images Dataset are used. It considers three machine learning algorithms that are Support Vector Machines (SVM), Random Forest (RF), and Convolutional Neural Network (CNN). Based on the results achieved, both SVM and RF are used for Breast cancer Wisconsin (Diagnostic) dataset, and SVM and CNN are used for Breast Histopathology Images Dataset. Experimental results show that the highest accuracy is achieved for RF on Wisconsin dataset. Whereas for Breast Histopathology Images Dataset, CNN gives the highest accuracy. Further, k-fold cross-validation is carried out to validate the performance. In the future, performance analysis of the other ML techniques for the detection of breast cancer can be performed. Also, the performance analysis of existing ML techniques can be performed over the other datasets.

References

1. Aaqib M, Muhammad T, Shahzad A (2019) A novel deep learning based approach for breast cancer detection. In: 2019 13th International conference on mathematics, actuarial science, computer science and statistics (MACS). IEEE
2. Kajala A, Jain VK (2020) Diagnosis of breast cancer using machine learning algorithms-a review. In: 2020 International conference on emerging trends in communication, control and computing (ICONC3). IEEE
3. Shahnaz C, et al (2017) Efficient approaches for accuracy improvement of breast cancer classification using wisconsin database. In: 2017 IEEE region 10 humanitarian technology conference (R10-HTC). IEEE

4. Khourdifi Y, Mohamed B (2018) Applying best machine learning algorithms for breast cancer prediction and classification. In: 2018 International conference on electronics, control, optimization and computer science (ICECOCS). IEEE
5. Sharma S, Archit A, Tanupriya C (2018) Breast cancer detection using machine learning algorithms. In: 2018 International conference on computational techniques, electronics and mechanical systems (CTEMS). IEEE
6. Rahman ASA, et al (2020) Breast mass tumor classification using deep learning. In: 2020 IEEE international conference on informatics, IoT, and enabling technologies (ICIoT). IEEE
7. Yamlome P, et al (2020) Convolutional neural network based breast cancer histopathology image classification. In: 2020 42nd Annual international conference of the IEEE engineering in medicine & biology society (EMBC). IEEE
8. Chaurasia V, Pal S (2020) Applications of machine learning techniques to predict diagnostic breast cancer. SN Comput Sci 1(5):1–11
9. Ragab DA, et al (2019) Breast cancer detection using deep convolutional neural networks and support vector machines. Peer J 7:e6201
10. Kumar MN, Anand J, Narayanappa CK (2019) Probable region identification and segmentation in breast cancer using the DL-CNN. In: 2019 International conference on smart systems and inventive technology (ICSSIT). IEEE
11. Rohan TI, et al (2019) A precise breast cancer detection approach using ensemble of random forest with AdaBoost. In: 2019 International conference on computer, communication, chemical, materials and electronic engineering (IC4ME2). IEEE
12. Kumar K, Rao ACS (2018) Breast cancer classification of image using convolutional neural network. In: 2018 4th International conference on recent advances in information technology (RAIT). IEEE
13. Alkhaleefah M, Wu C-C (2018) A hybrid CNN and RBF-based SVM approach for breast cancer classification in mammograms. In: 2018 IEEE international conference on systems, man, and cybernetics (SMC). IEEE
14. Gupta, M, Bharat G (2018) A comparative study of breast cancer diagnosis using supervised machine learning techniques. In: 2018 Second international conference on computing methodologies and communication (ICCMC). IEEE
15. Al-masni MA, et al (2017) Detection and classification of the breast abnormalities in digital mammograms via regional convolutional neural network. In: 2017 39th Annual international conference of the IEEE engineering in medicine and biology society (EMBC). IEEE
16. Islam MM, et al (2017) Prediction of breast cancer using support vector machine and K-nearest neighbors. In: 2017 IEEE region 10 humanitarian technology conference (R10-HTC). IEEE
17. Alyami R, et al (2017) Investigating the effect of correlation based feature selection on breast cancer diagnosis using artificial neural networks and support vector machines. In: 2017 International conference on informatics, health & technology (ICIHT). IEEE
18. Wang, Z, et al (2019) Breast cancer detection using an extreme learning machine based on feature fusion with CNN deep features. IEEE Access 7:105146–105158
19. Kumar, G (2019) Breast cancer detection using decision tree, naïve bayes, KNN and SVM classifiers: a comparative study. In: 2019 International conference on smart systems and inventive technology (ICSSIT). IEEE

Static Gesture Classification and Recognition Using HOG Feature Parameters and k-NN and SVM-Based Machine Learning Algorithms

C. V. Sheena and N. K. Narayanan

1 Introduction

For the last two decades, gesture recognition has been an active area of research. Unresolved problems such as reliable identification of gesturing phase, size sensitivity, variations in shape and speed, and problems due to occlusion maintain the recognition of hand gestures in a research area that is still very active [1]. Recognition of gestures has so many applications. They are an interpretation of sign language, interactive smart home control, software interface control and virtual environment control, the interaction between humans and robots, and robot hand control [2, 3]. Among the possible applications, this paper performed an interpretation of static hand gestures for HCI. The present study analyzes the effectiveness of histogram-oriented gradient (HOG) features in static hand gesture recognition (SHGR) using k-nearest neighbor (k-NN) and support vector machine (SVM) classifier. In computer vision (CV), HOG descriptors provided excellent performance. Our study evaluates the efficiency of HOG features in static hand gesture recognition (SHGR) using the two well-known machine learning (ML) algorithms: k-nearest neighborhood (k-NN) and support vector machine (SVM).

In this paper recognition of a subset of static hand gestures is done using HOG features. The objective of the study is to interpret a hand gesture for human–computer interaction. As part of the study, we created a database of 10 classes of hand gestures. Each class contains 60 static hand gestures, images of numbers 0, 1, 2, 3, 4, 5, 6, 7, 8, and 9. The images are static hand gestures of a single individual captured using a Nokia digital camera. The remaining part of this paper is organized as follows:

C. V. Sheena (✉)
Department of Information Technology, Kannur University, Kannur, Kerala, India

N. K. Narayanan
Indian Institute of Information Technology, Kottayam, Kerala, India
e-mail: nknarayanan@iiitkottayam.ac.in

© The Author(s), under exclusive license to Springer Nature Singapore Pte Ltd. 2021
M. K. Bajpai et al. (eds.), *Machine Vision and Augmented Intelligence—Theory and Applications*, Lecture Notes in Electrical Engineering 796,
https://doi.org/10.1007/978-981-16-5078-9_14

In Sect. 2, related studies are described briefly. Section 3 describes the proposed hand gesture recognition system and the different steps involved in the classification. Section 4 presents the recognition of static hand gesture using k-NN and SVM. Section 5 presents a discussion of the results presented in Sect. 4. Finally, Sect. 5 summarizes the above sections and their results.

2 Related Works

Before the evolution of verbal languages, gesture is one of the earliest modes of communication. It is a form of non-verbal communication made with a part of a body. Natural interaction that does not use any mechanical instruments is possible between a human and a machine through gesture recognition [4]. In human–human interaction, gestures are widely used and play a significant role in communication when participants are unable to speak/hear, or the condition does not enable participants to speak/hear, etc. The gestures also play as an off-set-input to the other mode of communication; for example, gesture and speech are co-expressive and they organize a portion of rich human conversational features.

Gestures can be categorized with respect to different criteria. Based on the type of information which one should like to express it is classified into three. They are symbolic gestures, deictic gestures, and iconic gestures. Based on the movement of objects and those taking part in gesture production, the gestures are classified into two: static and dynamic gestures [5]. For a natural interaction to become true, computers want to automatically recognize gestures that may be static or dynamic. Initially, researchers used hardware-based devices for automatic gesture recognition. In such contact-based gesture recognition, cyber gloves and magnetic trackers are used for motion detection and trajectory modeling of gestures. It may be wired or wireless. A wired glove is an input device for HCI worn like a glove. In wired gloves, various sensor technologies are used to capture physical data such as bending of the fingers. Often, a motion tracker such as a magnetic tracking device or inertial tracking device is attached to capture the global position/rotation of the glove. These movements are then interpreted by the software that accompanies the glove [6, 7]. Gestures can then be categorized into useful information such as recognizing sign language or other symbolic functions. These kinds of technologies are very expensive also, so they prevent natural interaction because of the devices that we want to wear. Computer vision-based (CV) technologies are a solution to these kinds of inconveniences.

Computer vision-based analysis of gestures is the most natural way of constructing a human–computer gestural interface. In CV-based gesture recognition, one or more cameras are used to capture input. Using different image processing techniques, these input videos are analyzed to get motion information of gestures and are converted into data for the recognition process. Different types of sensors that are used for CV-based gesture recognition are infrared cameras, monocular cameras, stereo cameras, pan-tilt-zoom (PTZ) cameras, and body markers [7]. From the literature, it is found that CV-based gesture recognition techniques can be further classified into two approaches: the body model-based approach and the appearance-based approach. The first approach uses geometrical primitives, such as cylindrical models [8]. These approaches are not suitable for virtual reality applications, in which recognition results are required within acceptable time intervals. On the other hand, appearance-based approaches estimate the gesture class by applying machine learning (ML) algorithms. Although these methods require the target gestures to be learned beforehand, there is no need for the user to wear special markers or devices and the recognition task is not affected by frequent occlusions. The work done by Gupta et al. reports a color and contour-based classification of hand gesture recognition [9]. The studies of Mohandes et al. report a CV-based approach combined with a sensor-based technique for recognizing Arabic sign language [10]. P. K. Pisharady et al. used shape, texture, and color with the SVM classifier for image recognition against complex background [11]. Dalal et al. proposed [12] HOG method for human detection, which we applied in our database. In this method, a gradient image is used for detecting the orientation of the object in the image so that it can uniquely represent the posture of the object. Jaya Prakash et al. proposed vision-based static hand gesture principle component analysis-based (PCA) reduced deep neural network features and SVM classifier [13]. They used pre-trained Alex Net feature parameters. The dimensionality of the feature set was reduced using PCA. The feature parameters are classified using the SVM classifier. From the literature survey, it is clear that the result of gesture recognition is affected by the data set used for the experiment, problems such as lighting, hand segmentation, and similarity in gesture posture. We aim to investigate the effectiveness of HOG features to classify similar static hand gestures using ML algorithms.

3 Gesture Recognition System

The structure of the proposed gesture recognition system is given in Fig. 1. Different steps involved in the proposed gesture recognition system are image acquisition, preprocessing, feature extraction, and classification. As part of image acquisition, a database containing 600 static gesture images is constructed using a digital camera with a simple background. The database consists of 10 classes of static hand gesture that represent sign language digits 0–9. Other major steps involved are: hand localization using skin color segmentation, HOG feature extraction, and classification of extracting features using SVM and k-NN machine learning techniques.

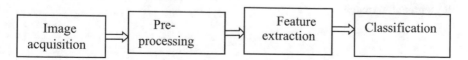

Fig. 1 Gesture recognition system

3.1   Hand Segmentation Using Skin Color Detection

The experiment used the RGB-based skin color segmentation technique for the segmentation of hand gestures from the background. There are many color space models for skin color detection. The most popular models are RGB model, normalized RGB, HSI, and YCrCb. RGB-based methods have gained a lot of popularity among these color space models due to the computational complexity over other methods and are the commonly used color spaces for digital image data storage. One of the widely used sources of information is skin color in human–computer interaction (HCI). It is used to segment the human face and gesture from the complex background of the image. We have to come up with the selection of RGB values in the RGB color space model, where human skin lies. It is important to identify each pixel as either a skin pixel or a non-skin pixel. There are various skin color types that must be all classified as one class, i.e., skin color. The study adopted the algorithm proposed by Xiang [14]. The decision rule for classifying a given pixel as skin or non-skin is done using the following algorithm:

Pseudo Code for Skin Color Segmentation Algorithm

```
function skin_seg(I)
   for no_row_image
      for no_col_image
         R = I(no_row,no_col,1);
         G = I(no_row,no_col,2);
         B = I(no_row,no_col,3);
         if(R > 95 && G > 40 && B > 20)
         v = [R,G,B];
         if((max(v) - min(v)) > 15)
         if(abs(R-G) > 15 && R > G && R > B)
           seg_image=I;
           return seg_image
          end if
      end for
 end function
```

The pixels that fall in the region of the above decision rule in the pseudo-code are segmented to localize the hand region and are used for feature extraction. The original image and the segmented image obtained for gesture digit 5 is shown in Fig. 2. The following section discusses how a feature vector can be generated from the segmented image.

Fig. 2 Original image and its corresponding segmented image obtained using a skin color segmentation algorithm for digit 5

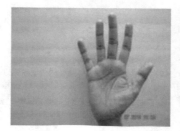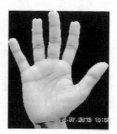

3.2   Feature Extraction

In any typical gesture recognition system feature extraction is a crucial part. The classification experiment of human gesture data is a challenging problem because of the difficulty in modeling human gestures for the extraction of appropriate feature parameters due to significant intra-class variations, viewpoint change, partial occlusion, and background dynamic variations. In the past one decade, a great deal of research has been directed toward finding human gesture characteristics that are effective for action recognition using HOG features [15]. The method is based on evaluating well-normalized local histograms and image gradient orientation in a dense grid. The appearance and shape of an object in an image can be characterized by the distribution of local intensity gradients or edge direction. It is not necessary to have the correct gradient or edge position information. This provides the underlying basic concept of HOG features. Practically, this is implemented by dividing the image into smaller spatial regions. For each spatial region, a local 1-D histogram of gradient direction over the pixels of the spatial region is computed. These regions are grouped into overlapping blocks. The block-level histogram is computed and normalized to evaluate changes in illumination and contrast. All block histograms are combined to represent a feature vector of the image.

3.2.1   Computation of Gradient Image

The first process involved in the extraction of HOG feature parameters is the computation of gradient image. The horizontal and vertical gradients I_x and I_y for the segmented grayscale image I are obtained by a convolution operation with a one-dimensional filter using Eqs. 1 and 2, respectively.

$$I_x = I * F_x \tag{1}$$

$$I_y = I * F_y \tag{2}$$

where F_x and F_y are one-dimensional filter kernels

$$F_x = [-1 \quad 0 \quad 1] \tag{3}$$

$$F_y = [1 \quad 0 \quad -1]^T \tag{4}$$

We computed the magnitude of gradient G and gradient 0 for all pixels in the 8 × 8 spatial regions of the segmented grayscale using Eqs. 5 and 6, respectively.

$$|G| = \sqrt{I_x^2 + I_y^2} \tag{5}$$

$$\theta = \tan^{-1}\left(I_x / I_y\right) \tag{6}$$

3.2.2 Computation of Gradient Histogram

The next step is the computation of the histogram of the oriented gradient of the spatial region. Each pixel in the spatial region casts a weighted vote for orientation-based histogram bins corresponding to the value in the gradient computation. The histogram bins are evenly divided over 0° to 180°. The spatial regions are then grouped into overlapping blocks to evaluate changes in the lightning and contrast.

3.2.3 Block Normalization

The blocks composed of 8 × 8 pixel regions are normalized to avoid changes in the illumination and contrast. The equation used for normalization is as follows:

$$V_{diff} = \frac{v}{\sqrt{\|v\|_2^2 + \varepsilon^2}} \tag{7}$$

where v is the feature vector of a spatial region before normalization and ϵ is a small constant introduced to avoid the division by zero. The normalized block histograms are combined to form an entire HOG feature vector.

3.3 Gesture Recognition

After computing HOG features from the segmented gesture images, classification is performed using two different supervised machine learning techniques: the k-nearest neighbor classification (k-NN) algorithm and support vector machine (SVM) classification algorithm. The k-NN algorithm is a simpler and more stable pattern recognition technique and has a good classification performance on a wide range of real-world data sets [16, 17]. It has been studied extensively and applied success-fully in many pattern recognition applications. The simulation experiment and result obtained using the k-NN classification algorithm is computed and discussed below. An average recognition accuracy of 96 is obtained by applying the k-NN algorithm on HOG features. A simulation experiment is conducted on a different number of neighbors and it is found that maximum recognition accuracy is obtained when the number of neighbors is equal to 3.

As part of this study, we also evaluated the efficiency of a multiclass SVM clas-sification algorithm for static gesture recognition. Experiments are conducted for different kernel functions, such as linear kernel, RBF kernel, and polynomial kernel. It is found that the polynomial kernel is the most suitable kernel function of the SVM model based on static gesture interpretation of the extracted features. Comparative accuracy analyses for the two classifiers are given in the following section.

4 Accuracy Analyses

The static hand gesture recognition system was tested on a data database of 10 gestures by constructing a database of 600 images. We tried to interpret the different gestures using SVM and k-NN with the HOG feature descriptor. From the normalized feature parameter set, 80% of the data were used for training and the remaining 20% of the data are used for testing. A simulation experiment was performed for a different number of neighbors of the k-NN classifier. A graphical representation of the error rate obtained for a different number of neighbors during a simulation experiment for the k-NN with HOG descriptor is shown in Fig. 3. It is found that the error is

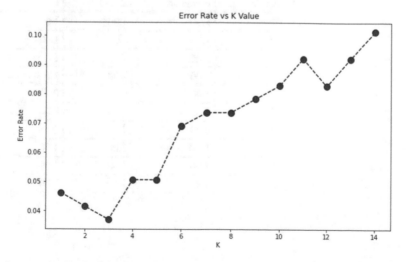

Fig. 3 Error rate obtained for different number of neighbors in k-NN

minimized by fixing a value threefor "k" number of neighbors. Using this value classification is performed and an average recognition accuracy of 96% is obtained. A classification report obtained using k-NN and HOG feature parameters is shown in Table 1.

Support vector machine is a supervised machine learning technique. The basic SVM only supports binary classification, but extensions have been proposed to handle multiclass classification problems [18]. In this study SVM with polynomial kernel function is used for static gesture recognition using the HOG feature parameter and an average recognition accuracy of 98% is obtained. A classification report obtained using the SVM and HOG feature parameter is shown in Table 2.

Table 1 Classification report of k-NN

Class	Precision	Recall	F1 score
1	1.00	1.00	1.00
2	1.00	1.00	1.00
3	1.00	1.00	1.00
4	1.00	0.67	0.80
5	1.00	1.00	1.00
6	1.00	1.00	1.00
7	0.88	1.00	0.93
8	0.80	1.00	0.89
9	1.00	0.86	0.92
10	1.00	1.00	1.00

Table 2 Classification report of SVM

Class	Precision	Recall	F1 score
1	1.00	1.00	1.00
2	1.00	1.00	1.00
3	1.00	1.00	1.00
4	1.00	1.00	1.00
5	1.00	0.88	0.93
6	1.00	1.00	1.00
7	0.75	1.00	0.86
8	1.00	1.00	1.00
9	1.00	1.00	1.00
10	1.00	1.00	1.00

5 Conclusions

In this study, two well-known machine learning algorithms: SVM and k-NN are performed for static gesture interpretation using HOG feature vector parameters. Experimental results show that among these two classifiers SVM got 98% of average accuracy with a polynomial kernel function. The average performance of k-NN was only 96%. It is found that the performance of the SVM classifier is better than the k-NN classifier for static gesture prediction using HOG feature parameters. However, recognition accuracy can be improved by using more than one feature extraction techniques. The study can be further extended to interpret dynamic gestures which have got a wide range of applications in human–computer interaction.

References

1. Pramod K et al (2015) Recent methods and database in vision-based hand gesture recognition: a review. Comput Vis Image Underst
2. Rautaray SS, Agrawal A (2015) Vision based hand gesture recognition for human computer interaction: a survey. Artif Intell Rev. https://doi.org/10.1007/s10462-012-9356-9
3. Francis Q et al (2002) Gesture and speech multimodal conversational interaction. ACM Trans Comput Hum Interact 9(3):171–193
4. Mithra S, Acharya T (2007) Gesture recognition—a survey. IEEE Trans Syst Man Cybern Part C Appl Rev 37(3):311–324
5. Keith M (2003) Building meaning in interaction: rethinking gesture classification. Cross Roads Lang Interact Cult 5:29–47
6. Harshith et.al (2010) Survey on various gesture recognition techniques for interfacing machines based on ambient intelligence. IJCSES 1(2)
7. Pragathi G et al (2009) Vision based hand gesture recognition. World Acad Sci Eng Technol 49:972–977
8. Pavlovic et al (2002) Visual interpretation of hand gesture for human computer interaction: a review. IEEE Trans Pattern Anal Mach Intell 19(7):677–695
9. Gupta L, Ma S (2001) Gesture-based interaction and communication: automated classification of hand gesture contours. IEEE Trans Syst Man Cybern Part C Appl Rev 31(1)
10. Mohandes et al (2014) Image-based and sensor-based approaches to arabic sign language recognition. IEEE Trans Hum Mach Syst 44(4):551–557
11. Pisharady PK et al (2013) Attention based detection and recognition of hand posters against complex background. Int J Comput Vision 101(03):403–419
12. Dalal N, Triggs B (2005) Histograms of oriented gradients for human detection. In: 2005 IEEE computer society conference on computer vision and pattern recognition (CVPR'2005). ISBN: 0-7695-2372-2
13. Sahoo JP et al (2019) Hand gesture recogntion using PCA based deep CNN educed features and SVM classifier. In: 2019 IEEE international symposium on smart systems. https://doi.org/10.1109/iSES47678.2019.00056
14. Xiang FH et al (2013) Fusion of multi color space for human skin region segmentation. Int J Inf Electron Eng 3(2):172–174
15. Freeman WT, Roth M (1995) Orientation histograms for hand gesture recognition. In: Proceedings of the International workshop on automatic face and gesture recognition. IEEE, pp 296–301
16. Dardas et al (2011) Real time hand gesture detection and recognition using bag of features and support vector machine techniques. IEEE Trans Instrum Meas 60(11):3592–3607

17. Ghosh AK, Murthy CA (2005) On visualization and aggregation of nearest neighbor classifiers. IEEE Trans Pattern Anal Mach Intell. https://doi.org/10.1109/TPAMI.2005.204
18. Vapnik V (1998) Statistical learning theory. Wiley, NY

Multiagent-Based GA for Limited View Tomography

Raghavendra Mishra and Manish Kumar Bajpai

1 Introduction

Computed tomography (CT) plays a critical role in engineering and medical application. It is a non-destructive testing method widely used to know the internal structure of objects. The CT methods are used in engineering and medical applications. However, in practical engineering applications, complete access of the object under scan is impossible. In medical imaging, the CT methods reconstruct internal organs with unmatched precision for medical diagnosis and treatments. However, the use of too much ionizing radiation in CT methods may induce cancer and other diseases in patients. The promising reconstruction methods reduce radiation dose or X-ray projections across the human body. Hence, we need a limited view of reconstruction methods or sparse reconstruction.

Image reconstruction has been done with mainly three types of methods, namely transformation-based method, iterative methods (algebraic methods), and optimization methods. Transform-based method reconstructs the images with high accuracy if a complete set of projection data is given, i.e., back-projection (BP) and filter back-projection (FBP). Transform-based methods provide poor-quality images with limited projection data, due to the "soft-field" effect and the nonlinearity. Hence, transform-based methods are not suitable for limited data reconstruction. The iterative methods are suitable for limited data reconstruction. These methods are used to overcome this limitation. However, iterative methods can reconstruct images in fewer projections data, but these methods are computationally expensive. Gorden et al. have

R. Mishra (✉) · M. K. Bajpai
Department of Computer Science and Engineering, Design and Manufacturing Jabalpur, Indian Institute of Information Technology, Jabalpur, India
e-mail: raghavendra@iiitdmj.ac.in

M. K. Bajpai
e-mail: mkbajpai@iiitdmj.ac.in

© The Author(s), under exclusive license to Springer Nature Singapore Pte Ltd. 2021
M. K. Bajpai et al. (eds.), *Machine Vision and Augmented Intelligence—Theory and Applications*, Lecture Notes in Electrical Engineering 796,
https://doi.org/10.1007/978-981-16-5078-9_15

published the first algebraic method. This method works completely on asymmetric objects [1]. The sparse reconstruction method improves image quality and reduces the artifacts for limited view tomography [1–4]. It has been observed that compared to the transformation-based method, iterative algorithms provide improved image quality but demand intensive computations [5–7].

Reference [8] has performed a comparative study between GA and multiplicative algebraic reconstruction techniques (MART). Its results show that GA provides much better results than MART.

The optimization methods are suitable for limited data reconstruction. The optimization methods divide into two categories: machine learning (CNN, DNN) and evolutionary algorithm. The machine learning-based methods and DNN-based methods provide excellent results with limited projection data [9]. Although machine learning-based models continue to dominant medical image reconstruction fields in terms of accuracy, these methods have plenty of remaining challenges. The image reconstruction is an inverse problem. Hence, the DNN methods require a huge number of epochs for network training, and each epoch increases computational overhead. Reference [10] addresses these challenges of machine learning methods in computed tomography. There are very few labeled data available to develop a new DNN model in medical applications. Owing to privacy concerns, it is difficult to get a large amount of medical data. However, the significant computational load required to train the neural networks result in reduced image resolution. The DNN-based methods require a complete set of projection data for training and testing purposes. Hence, DNN-based methods are not suitable for limited data reconstruction.

The reconstruction problem can formalize as an optimization problem. Genetic algorithm is the most popular optimization method based on genetic evolution. Kodali et al. have proposed a GA-based methodology for image reconstruction [11]. This method uses simulated data for reconstruction. Yan et al. have proposed an adaptive GA for two-phase flow. This study uses adaptive crossover and mutation rates, which significantly improve the performance of the algorithm. Seyedali et al. have proposed a GA-based methodology for image reconstruction. References [12–14] have proposed evolutionary algorithm-based image/signal reconstruction methods with limited projection data, or sparse data, or noisy data. It has been observed during the exhaustive literature survey that the evolutionary algorithm (EA) shows great potential to solve global optimization problems. The image reconstruction is an optimization problem. However, the EA phase is challenged in large-scale optimization problems, i.e., local optima problem, slower convergence, and selection of crossover and mutation rates. On the basis of a comprehensive literature survey, we identified the following objectives:

1. Reduce the radiation dose
2. Reduce the cost per scan
3. Reduce computation overhead
4. Reconstruct using limited projection data or noisy data
5. Improve the convergence speed and reduce the chance of local stagnation.

As shown in the literature, the GA phase has slow convergence and is stuck in local optima. This article proposes a multiagent-based GA (MAGA) for image reconstruction. This method uses dynamic crossover and mutation rates, which increase the convergence rate and reduce the chance of local stagnation.

This method significantly improves the perforce and reduces the loss of diversity of the population. The method uses two different types of crossover and mutation rates: dynamic decreasing of high mutation rate/dynamic increasing of crossover rate (DHM/ILC) and dynamic increasing of low mutation rate/dynamic decreasing of high crossover rate (ILM/DHC). The proposed algorithm is suitable for limited data reconstruction. The contribution of the paper is as follows:

1. The proposed algorithm efficiently reconstructs the image with limited data. Here, we take 26 numbers of projection.
2. The proposed algorithm uses dynamic crossover and mutation rates, which efficiently improve the performance of the algorithm.
3. The proposed algorithm provides a higher convergence rate and reduces the chance of local optima.
4. The proposed algorithm produces satisfactory results when compared with the other state of reconstruction methods. Our method produces higher accuracy compared to other reconstruction methods.

The organization of the paper is as follows: Sect. 2 explains the methodology of MAGA. Section 3 discusses the proposed algorithm, and Sect. 4 presents the results and discussion.

2 Methodology

CT methods reconstruct the internal structure of the objects using its projection data. The projection data can be formulated as a linear equation:

$$P = AX \tag{1}$$

If we consider noise during the collection of projection data (1) is reformulated as:

$$P = AX + \Psi \tag{2}$$

Here, $P \in R^M$ is the projection data; $A \in R^{M \times N}$ is a matrix. Here, M is the number of rays and N is the total number of pixels in the image. The proposed multiagent-based GA refined the initial solution until it finds an optimal solution or a maximum number of generations is completed. The fitness function Θ defines here the difference between the given projection data and simulated projection data.

$$\Theta = \frac{1}{\Theta_A \times P} \sum_{j}^{\Theta_A} \sum_{k}^{P} \left\{ \left| MD_{(j,k)} - SD_{(j,k)} \right|^2 \right\} \tag{3}$$

Here, Θ is the fitness function to calculate the difference between simulated projection data (MD) and measured projection data (SD). P indicates projection data and θ indicates angles. The fitness values calculate all the population members in each generation.

In the proposed multiagent model, each individual identifies as an agent, and a set of agents are recognized as an agent society. These agents are computational systems, and several agents interact or work together in order to achieve goals. The interaction between agents is performed using the crossover and mutation operations [11, 15–17]. Here, we adjust the crossover and mutation rates dynamically [17]. The dynamic crossover and mutation rates improve the performance of the proposed algorithm.

2.1 Crossover

This crossover operation generates new population members. In this study, we perform a crossover operation between two parents. Figure 1 shows a crossover operation, parent 1 and parent 2 interchanging grid between us and generates two new offspring. Here, we perform a single-point crossover operation; the interchanging point selects randomly, then swap grids between two parents.

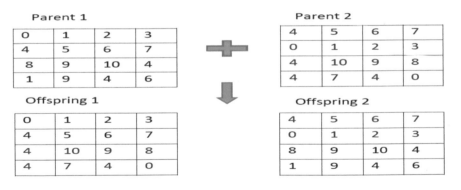

Fig. 1 Crossover operation (single-point crossover)

Parent

O	1	2	3
4	5	6	7
8	9	10	4
1	9	4	6

Offspring

O	1	2	3
6	5	5	7
8	9	10	4
1	8	4	7

Fig. 2 Mutation operation

2.2 Mutation

The mutation operation performs after the crossover operation. This operation introduces a new random solution in the population and improves the exploration capacity of the algorithm. Figure 2 shows the mutation operation.

2.3 Termination

The stopping criterion of the proposed algorithm is an average error if the difference between the reconstructed image and the original image (ground truth image) is less than 0.01 or maximum generation.

2.4 Crossover and Mutation Rates

The standard GA method uses fixed crossover and mutation rates. Finding the optimal values of the crossover (P_c) and mutation rate (P_m) is still an optimization problem. The optimal values of crossover and mutation rates considerably improve the performance of the algorithm. Reference [17, 18] explains the new dynamic adjustable methods for crossover and mutation rates. This study uses two methods for crossover and mutation rates, namely dynamic decreasing of high mutation rate/ dynamic increasing of crossover rate (DHM/ILC) and dynamic increasing of low mutation rate/ dynamic decreasing of high crossover rate (ILM/DHC).

2.4.1 DHM/ILC

This method's initial crossover rate is 0 and mutation rate 1. The crossover and mutation rates calculated in every generation are as follows:

$$P_c = C_G / \text{MaxGen}$$
$$P_m = 1 - (C_G / \text{MaxGen})$$

(4)

Here, C_G is the current generation, MaxGen indicates the maximum generation of the MAGA.

2.4.2 ILM/DHC

This method's initial crossover rate is 1 and mutation rate 0. The crossover and mutation rates calculated in every generation are as follows:

$$P_c = 1 - (C_G / \text{MaxGen})$$
$$P_m = (C_G / \text{MaxGen})$$

(5)

Here, C_G is the current generation, MaxGen indicates the maximum generation of the MAGA. The dynamic P_c and P_m are calculated in every generation. The crossover and mutation rates change in parameters values linearly based on the mathematical Eqs. 4 and 5.

3 MAGA Model

The proposed MAGA model initially generates a random population using prior information, and afterward calculates the fitness of the population. If the stopping criterion is satisfied then stop MAGA; otherwise, perform selection, crossover, and mutation operation and generate new population until the desired solution is found or maximum generation is completed.

Algorithm: Multiagent Based GA for Limited View Tomography
INPUT:
   M – Population size
   P_c- Crossover rate
   P_m- Mutation rate
   P_e - Elitism rate
Fitness Function $\Theta(i) = \dfrac{1}{\Theta_A \times P}\sum_j^{\Theta_A}\sum_k^P\{|MD_{(j,k)} - SD_{(j,k)}|^2\}$

Here, $\Theta(i)$ – Difference between computed projection data and simulated projection data, Θ-indicate angles, P - projection data
OUTPUT:
   I_r- Reconstructed image
Begin
   Initialize M population members,
   Initialize P_c
   Initialize P_m
   Initialize P_e
   $G \leftarrow 0$
   Calculate the fitness $\Theta(i)$; $i \in \{1, 2, 3, ..., M\}$;
   While $\Theta(i) > 0.01$ **do**
      Select two parent randomly based on the fitness values
      $P_c = G/MaxGen$
      $P_m = 1-(G/MaxGen)$
      Crossover operation,
      If $U(0, 1) < P_c$ **then**
          $[X'_1, X'_2] = crossover(X_1, X_2, P_c)$
      End if
      Mutation operation,
      If $U(0, 1) < P_m$ **then**
          $[X''_1] = mutation(X'_1, P_m)$
          $[X''_1] = mutation(X'_1, P_m)$
      End if
      Calculate fitness $\Theta(i)'$; $i \in \{1, 2, 3, ..., M'\}$;
      Perform Elitism $ne = Pe*M$;
      $M' = M'+ ne$;
      New population $M \leftarrow M'$;
      If $MaxGen > G$ **then**
            Exit
      End if
      $G = G+1$;
   End while
   Reconstructed image Ir
End Begin

4   Experimental Results and Discussion

The simulation has been performed on CPU: i7-4790, 3.6 GHz; with RAM 4 GB and we used Matlab-17. The other experimental settings are given in Tables 1 and 2.

We have performed the simulation on a numerical head phantom. The numerical head phantom is used for the numerical accuracy of the proposed algorithm. The performance of the proposed algorithm is calculated in terms of average error (AE) and structural similarity index (SSIM). The average error is calculated as:

$$AE = \frac{1}{m.n} \sum_i^m \sum_j^n \left(|GroundImage_{(i,j)} - RecImage_{(i,j)}| \right) \tag{6}$$

Here, AE indicates the average error, and m, n are grid sizes of ground truth images or reconstructed images.

4.1   Analysis

This study presents a multiagent-based GA with dynamic crossover and mutation rates. The performance of the proposed algorithm is analyzed in a qualitative and quantitative manner. Figure 3 shows the qualitative results, proposed algorithm, and other reconstruction methods. The proposed algorithm produces good results with dynamic crossover and mutation rates. Here, we show both dynamic approach results with constant parameters, population size (50), generation (1000), and Elite rate (0.2). It is observed that both approaches, DHM/ILC or ILM/DHC, produce identical results. Table 3 shows that the quantitative results of the proposed algorithm produce satisfactory results in terms of average error and SSIM.

Table 1 Experimental settings for DHM/INC

Population size M	50
Crossover rate P_c	0
Mutation rate P_m	1
Elites rate P_e	0.3
Maximum generation	1000

Table 2 Experimental settings for ILM/DHC

Population size M	50
Crossover rate P_c	1
Mutation rate P_m	0
Elites rate P_e	0.3
Maximum generation	1000

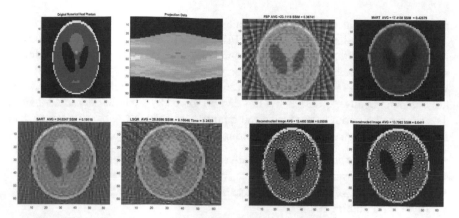

Fig. 3 Reconstruction results, ground truth image (Head phantom), Projection data, FBP (AE = 23.1118 and SSIM = 0.36741) [19], MART (AE = 17.4138 and SSIM = 0.42679) [8], SART (AE = 24.0247 and SSIM = 0.19118) [20], LSQR (AE = 28.8556 and SSIM = 0.16646) [21], proposed DHM/ILC (AE = 13.4495 and SSIM = 65.086), proposed ILM/DHC (AE = 12.6392 and SSIM = 0.63207)

Table 3 Quantitative results of the proposed algorithm

Methods	FBP [19]	MART [8]	SART [20]	LSQR [21]	MAGA (DHM/ILC)	MAGA (ILM/DHC)
AE	23.118	17.4138	24.0247	28.08556	13.4495	12.6392
SSIM	0.36741	0.42679	0.19118	0.16646	0.65086	0.63207

The proposed algorithm is compared with other reconstruction methods. These reconstruction methods belong to transform-based methods and iterative methods. A comparative study has been performed on a numerical head phantom with limited projection data. Here, we reconstruct an image with 26 views limited in [0, Π]. The projection data are collected uniformly in [0, Π]. The proposed algorithm produces satisfactory results with very few projection data. The proposed algorithm initially explores the search space and after that exploits the search space. It is observed that initial convergence is high; after 500 generations convergence rates reduce; and after 600 generations the algorithm is stuck in local optima.

5 Conclusion

The proposed algorithm is tested on numerical head phantom and yields a satisfactory result. As we know, the optimal value of crossover and mutation probability significantly improves the performance of the MAGA. The proposed algorithm uses two types of dynamic crossover and mutation rates methods, and these methods produce good results compared to the traditional fixed crossover and mutation rates. The proposed algorithm compares with FBP, MART, SART, and LSQR methods. It has been observed that the proposed algorithm produces excellent results in terms of average error and SSIM. The execution time of the proposed algorithm increases with the resolution of the image. However, we know that the optimization methods are computationally expensive, but this can be solved by a parallel implementation. The proposed algorithm provides good quality results with limited projection data or noisy data or sparse data. The key finding of the proposed algorithm is as follows:

- There is no prior information required regarding the object under scan.
- Dynamic crossover and mutation rates produce satisfactory results.
- If the resolution of the image increase then execution time also increases.
- There is no training required.
- The proposed algorithm is suitable for sparse reconstruction if projection data is unorganized or noisy algorithm does not require any modification.

References

1. Sun Y, Chen H, Tao J, Lei L (2019) Computed tomography image reconstruction from few views via log-norm total variation minimization. Digit Signal Process 88:172–181
2. Tovey R, Benning M, Brune C, Lagerwerf MJ, Collins SM, Leary RK, Midgley PA, Schonlieb CB (2019) Directional sinogram inpainting for limited angle tomography. Inverse Probl 35(2):024004
3. Wei W, Zhou B, Połap D, Woźniak M (2019) A regional adaptive variational pde model for computed tomography image reconstruction. Pattern Recognit 92:64–81
4. Xu J, Zhao Y, Li H, Zhang P (2019) An image reconstruction model regularized by edge-preserving difusion and smoothing for limited-angle computed tomography. Inverse Probl 35(8):085004
5. Bajpai M, Gupta P, Munshi P, Titarenko V, Withers PJ (2013) A graphical processing unit-based parallel implementation of multiplicative algebraic reconstructiontechnique algorithm for limited view tomography. Res Nondestruct Eval 24(4):211–222
6. Bajpai M, Gupta P, Munshi P (2015) Fast multi-processor multi-gpu based algorithm of tomographic inversion for 3d image reconstruction. Int J High Perform Comput Appl 29(1):64–72
7. Bajpai M, Schorr C, Maisl M, Gupta P, Munshi P (2013) High resolution 3d image reconstruction using the algebraic method for cone-beam geometry over circular and helical trajectories. NDT & E Int 60:62–69
8. Kodali SP, Deb K, Munshi P, Kishore N (2009) Comparing ga with mart to tomographic reconstruction of ultrasound images with and without noisy input data. In: 2009 IEEE congress on evolutionary computation. IEEE, pp 2963–2970
9. Kalare KW, Bajpai MK (2020) Recdnn: deep neural network for image reconstruction from limited view projection data. Soft Comput 24
10. Zhang HM, Dong B (2020) A review on deep learning in medical image reconstruction. J Oper Res Soc China 1–30
11. Kodali SP, Bandaru S, Deb K, Munshi P, Kishore N (2008) Applicability of genetic algorithms to reconstruction of projected data from ultrasonic tomography In: Proceedings of the 10th annual conference on Genetic and evolutionary computation. IEEE, pp 1705–1706

12. Li L, Yao X, Stolkin R, Gong M, He S (2013) An evolutionary multi objective approach to sparse reconstruction. IEEE Trans Evol Comput 18(6), 827{845 (2013)
13. Yan, B., Zhao, Q., Wang, Z., Zhang, J.A.: Adaptive decomposition-based evolutionary approach for multi objective sparse reconstruction. Inf Sci 462, 141{159 (2018)
14. Yan B, Zhao Q, Wang Z, Zhao X (2017) A hybrid evolutionary algorithm for multiobjective sparse reconstruction. Signal, Image Video Process 11(6):993–1000
15. Yan M, Hu H, Otake Y, Taketani A, Wakabayashi Y, Yanagimachi S, Wang S, Pan Z, Hu G (2018) Improved adaptive genetic algorithm with sparsity constraint applied to thermal neutron ct reconstruction of two-phase ow. Meas Sci Technol 29(5):055404
16. Mirjalili S, Dong JS, Sadiq AS, Faris H (2020) Genetic algorithm: theory, literature review, and application in image reconstruction. In: Nature-inspired optimizers. Springer, pp 69–85
17. Hassanat A, Almohammadi K, Alkafaween E, Abunawas E, Hammouri A, Prasath V (2019) Choosing mutation and crossover ratios for genetic algorithms- a review with a new dynamic approach. Information 10(12):390
18. Dong X, Deng C, Tan Y (2017) Dynamic differential evolution with oppositional orthogonal crossover for large scale optimisation problems. Int J Comput Sci Math 8(5):414–424
19. Chetih N, Messali Z (2015) Tomographic image reconstruction using _ltered back projection (fbp) and algebraic reconstruction technique (art). In: 2015 3rd International conference on control, engineering & information technology (CEIT). IEEE, pp 1–6
20. Andersen AH, Kak AC (1984) Simultaneous algebraic reconstruction technique (sart): a superior implementation of the art algorithm. Ultrason Imaging 6(1):81–94
21. Chillarón M, Vidal V, Verd G (2020) Evaluation of imagelters for their integration with lsqr computerized tomography reconstruction method. PloS One 15(3):e0229113

A Transfer Learning-Based Multi-cues Multi-scale Spatial–Temporal Modeling for Effective Video-Based Crowd Counting and Density Estimation Using a Single-Column 2D-Atrous Net

Santosh Kumar Tripathy and Rajeev Srivastava

1 Introduction

The crowd analysis using crowd count and density estimation (CCDE) is one of the emerging research areas in computer vision application. The CCDE is an interdisciplinary research area that spans video-based applications (crowd counting and vehicle counting), biological applications (cell counting) and agricultural applications (crop counting), and so forth. Tasks such as, but not limited to CCDE, crowd commotion detection [1], crowd behavior analysis [2], crowd flow analysis, crowd congestion-level analysis [3], and all together accomplish the crowd analysis task. The importance of CCDE can be understood as handy to provide the density of crowd in a particular area that can be used further to deduce inferences for crowd analysis like crowd congestion and crowd behavior. The following Fig. 1 shows a general workflow diagram for CCDE.

Broadly, the CCDE approaches are of three types such as:

- Detection-based [4]
- Regression-based [5] and
- Density map-based regression (DMR) [6–20].

The detection-based approaches use the face, shoulder, or body part attributes. The major drawback of the approaches is a deficient performance in the dense crowd. On the other hand, the regression-based approaches utilize the regression mapping function that maps the spatial and/or temporal features onto a single count

S. K. Tripathy (✉) · R. Srivastava
Computing and Vision Lab, Department of Computer Science and Engineering,
Indian Institute of Technology (BHU), Varanasi, UP 221005, India
e-mail: santoshktripathy.rs.cse.18@iitbhu.ac.in

R. Srivastava
e-mail: rajeev.cse@iitbhu.ac.in

© The Author(s), under exclusive license to Springer Nature Singapore Pte Ltd. 2021   179
M. K. Bajpai et al. (eds.), *Machine Vision and Augmented Intelligence—Theory and Applications*, Lecture Notes in Electrical Engineering 796,
https://doi.org/10.1007/978-981-16-5078-9_16

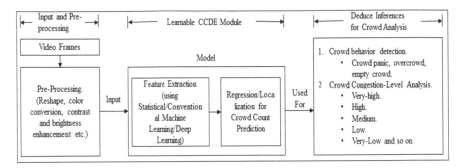

Fig. 1 General workflow diagram for the CCDE

value. The drawback of such approaches is that the mapping function ignores the crowd's spatial distribution in the scene and just maps on to a single count as a global value. The density map-based regression (DMR) approaches overcome these drawbacks by defining a mapping function that maps the learned features on the frame's density map, thereby considering the frame's spatial distribution. The density maps are obtained by using the given annotated head notations.

The proposed approach is a DMR-based CCDE approach. Basically, the existing approaches for DMR-based CCDE can be broadly divided into two different ways, such as static-based and video-based. Conventional and deep-learning approaches have been developed for both approaches. One of the major drawbacks of the static-image-based CCDE approaches is that they do not consider the temporal relation between frames for video datasets. A few works have been developed for video-based CCDE. These approaches extract spatial and/or temporal features for CCDE and lack to address the following major issues:

- Scale variation because of perspective distortion in the frame (multi-scale spatial features).
- Scale variation due to perspective distortion across the volume of frames (multi-scale temporal features).
- Multi-scale spatial features concerning to foreground of the frame by minimizing the background influence.
- Multi-scale temporal features concerning to volume of the foreground of the frames by minimizing the background influence.

So, to fulfill these issues, we developed an 'A Transfer Learning-based Multi-Cues Multi-Scale Spatial–Temporal Modelling for Effective Video-based Crowd Counting and Density Estimation using a Single-Column 2D-Atrous Net'. The contributions are as follows:

- The proposed model extracts multi-scale features for four different frame(s) cues from video using a transfer learning technique. The four different frame(s) cues are frame (RGB), the volume of frames, frame foreground map, and volume of frame foreground maps.

- The transfer learning approach utilizes an Inception-V3 model to extract multi-scale spatial–temporal (from frame and volume of frames) and multi-scale foreground spatial–temporal features from four different image types cues.
- The extracted multi-scale features are fused and inputted into a single column 2D-Atrous-Net for crowd density estimation.
- The proposed model has experimented on two publicly available datasets, i.e., the Mall and the Venice dataset.

The paper's organization is as follows: Sect. 1 discussed the introduction, Sect. 2 describes the literature review, Sect. 3 discusses the proposed model, Sect. 4 discusses the datasets, performance metrics, and the result analysis, followed by the conclusion in Sect. 5.

2 Related Works

Most of the recent DMR-based CCDE approaches try to overcome challenging issues like scale variation due to the distortion of the crowd scene. Models like convolution neural networks (CNN), sequential networks, and encoder–decoders have been explored to fulfill such challenging issues. CNN-based approaches like multi-column CNN, hydra-CNN, switch-CNN, and multi-density map fusion for crowd counting (MDMF-CC) extract multi-scale features of CCDE. Unlike handling the scale variation issues, Zhang et al. [7] focused on developing a cross-scene model that minimizes the domain gap across different datasets for CCDE. Likewise, Wei et al. [21] extract spatial–temporal features from the super-pixel blocks of extracted crowd regions by developing a deep accumulated learning-based support vector regression (DAL-SVR). Xu et al. [22] developed a hybrid model for CCDE. The model extracts near-view and far-view from the crowd scene by using depth information. The YOLO is used to count people from the near-view, and a CNN-based model counts the crowd from the far-view. The total count is based on the sum of the results obtained from two views.

Apart from the CNN-based approaches, generative models are also developed to fulfill the scale variation issue by extracting multi-scale features. Zhou et al. [19] focused on generating high-quality density maps by developing a multi-scale generative adversarial network (MS-GAN). The authors utilized two models like a multi-scale CNN (MS-CNN) and another CNN model as a generator and a discriminator, respectively. The MS-CNN encodes the multi-scale features and generates crowd density maps from the input frame, whereas the discriminator focuses on obtaining high-quality density maps by discriminating the ground-truth and predicted density maps. Although the above discussed are benchmark models, these models treat the video dataset frames as static and do not consider the temporal relationship. A few video-based CCDE models can be found in the literature in which we can find the different ways of spatial–temporal modeling of frames for the CCDE. Models like fully convolution neural network (FCN) and residual long short-term memory

(FCN-rLSTM) [11], a bidirectional Conv-LSTM [10], and spatial–temporal CNN (ST-CNN) [6] utilized spatial–temporal modeling for the CCDE from crowd videos. Saqib et al. [12] proposed a region-based deep-CNN (RDCNN) for CCDE in low-resolution crowd datasets. The RDCNN is composed of two models. The first one is a region-based CNN to identify pedestrians from localized regions, and the second one performs spatial–temporal modeling using motion-guided filters from the extracted crowd regions to count crowds.

Although the video-based CCDE approaches [6, 10, 12] utilize spatial–temporal modeling for the CCDE, they have noticeable drawbacks:

- Scale variation due to perspective distortion in the frame (multi-scale spatial features).
- Scale variation due to perspective distortion across the volume of frames (multi-scale temporal features).
- Multi-scale spatial features concerning to foreground of the frame by minimizing the background influence.
- Multi-scale temporal features concerning to volume of the foreground of the frames by minimizing the background influence.
- They neglect the background influence from the frame.
- The use of 2D CNN [6] for spatial feature extraction from the RGB frame ignores the depth information and treats them as 2D.
- The models that possess a high difference between MAE and RMSE indicate that these models are not robust.

Hence, to satisfy these gaps, we are motivated to design and extract multi-cue multi-scale spatial–temporal features using transfer learning and designed a single-column 2D-Atrous-Net for CCDE. The proposed model utilizes Inception-V3 for transfer learning. The details of the proposed model are described in the following subsection.

3 Proposed Model

Figure 2 presents the detailed architecture of the proposed model. The proposed work comprises two tasks such as:

- Extraction of multi-cues multi-scale spatial–temporal features.
- CCDE using a 2D-Atrous-Net.

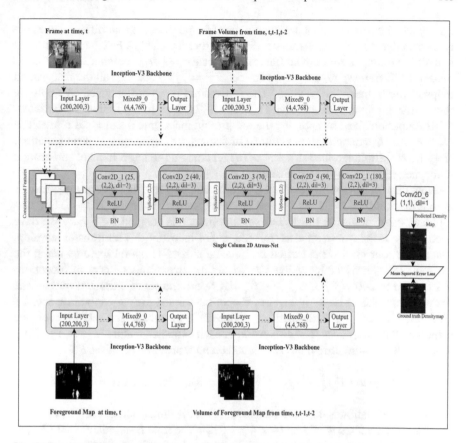

Fig. 2 Detail architecture of the proposed model

3.1 Extraction of Multi-cues Multi-scale Spatial–Temporal Features

We have used a transfer learning technique using a pre-trained Inception-V3 to extract multi-scale features. The Inception-V3 is known for its multi-scale feature extraction capabilities. So, we have used its knowledge in our application. Instead of extracting multi-scale features for single RGB frames, we have used four different cues for a video. These multi-cues represent the frame (RGB), the volume of frames, foreground maps of the frame, and the volume of foreground maps. Frames (RGB) and foreground maps (RGB) are used to extract multi-scale spatial features, whereas the volume of frames and volume of foreground maps are used to extract multi-scale temporal features.

The volume of frames or volume of foreground maps are obtained by stacking three consecutive grayscale frames or grayscale foreground maps for frames at timestamp t, t −1, t −2. The resolution of all the four video cues are set to [200 × 200 ×

3]. Let the video dataset contains N number of frames. Let the four different cues are represented as sets like Fr (frame), FF (foreground frame), VF (volume of frame) and VFF (volume of foreground frame). The set $Fr = \{fr_i\}$ contains a collection of resized RGB frames, $fr_i|_{i=1,2,...,N}$. The set $FF = \{ff_i\}$ contains all the foreground maps of the frames, $ff_i|_{i=1,2,...,N}$. The foreground maps are obtained by applying the Gaussian mixture model (GMM) [23, 24]. The foreground frames are basically RGB frames obtained by applying the foreground mask onto the original frame. The set $VF = \{vf_i\}$ contains all the volume of frames, i.e., $vf_i|_{i=1,2,...,N}$ at time-stamp t ($t = 1 to N$). Similarly, the set $VFF = \{vff_i\}$ contains all the volume of foreground maps, i.e., $vff_i|_{i=1,2,...,N}$ at time-stamp t ($t = 1 to N$).

Note that for time-stamp t $= 1$, the volume contains a replication of three frames at that time and for t $= 2$ the volume contains frames containing at t $= 2$ and two replications of frames at t $= 1$. The same approach is adopted for VFF. We have used a very deep layer (named as 'mixed9_0') of Inception-V3 for transfer learning. For all the four cues we extracted multi-scale spatial–temporal features using the 'mixed9_0' layer of the Inception-V3. We set the size of input tensor of Inception-V3 to [200 × 200 × 3]. Let $f_1, f_2, f_3,$ and f_4 are the set of extracted multi-scale features from the 'mixed9_0' layer of Inception-V3 and the corresponding sets are $Fr, FF, VF,$ and VFF respectively, where N is the size of the sets which is the same for all the four cues. The dimension of each extracted feature is [4 × 4 × 768]. The extracted features are then concatenated and represented as a set FS

$$FS = Concate\left(\left[f_1^i, f_2^i, f_3^i, f_4^i\right], axis = 3\right), \quad for \ each \ i = 1 \ to \ N \quad (1)$$

The concatenation is done elementwise. Now, the dimension of each entry of the concatenated features would be [4 × 4 × 3072]. The final fused feature set (FS) is then used as input to a single column 2D-Atrous-Net for CCDE which is discussed in the following subsection.

3.2 CCDE Using a Single-Column 2D-Atrous-Net

We have designed a single-column 2D-Atrous-Net for the CCDE. The Atrous-Net is also known as dilated CNN. We have chosen Atrous-Net because of the following reasons:

- The receptive field of the convolution kernel will increase with the increase of the dilation rate.
- It can cover a large area by keeping the filter elements the same.

A detail architecture of the proposed 2D-Atrous-Net is shown in Fig. 2. Table 1 shows the details of the layers used in the proposed model.

The model constitutes of six dilated convolutions among which the sixth dilated convolution is used for CCDE using density map-based regression. The details of the layer are shown in Table 1. The model has three upscale layers to increase the

Table 1 Details of the layers of 2D-Atrous-Net

Layer name	Kernel size	Number of kernels	Dilation rate
Conv2D_1	(2, 2)	25	(2, 2)
Conv2D_2	(2, 2)	40	(3, 3)
Conv2D_3	(2, 2)	70	(3, 3)
Conv2D_4	(2, 2)	90	(3, 3)
Conv2D_5	(2, 2)	180	(3, 3)
Conv2D_6	(1, 1)	1	(1, 1)
UpScale_1	(2, 2)	NA	NA
UpScale_2	(2, 2)	NA	NA
UpScale_3	(2, 2)	NA	NA

scale of its input features. We have used ReLU as an activation function for all the layers except the final atrous layer. The linear activation function is used in the final layer. Every convolution layer is followed by an activation layer, which is again followed by a batch normalization (BN) layer except the final layer. Three upscale layers are used each after the first three batch normalization layers. We have included bias to every layer of the proposed Atrous-Net and set the padding to the same. Let $\emptyset_{Net} = [W_{Net}, b_{Net}]$ represents the set of weights and biases of the proposed single-column atrous net. The output of the sixth dilation convolution layer is used to predict the density maps. For this, we need to have the ground-truth density maps which are discussed in Sect. 4. The total crowd count is obtained by summing the obtained density map of that frame. Now, for training, we need to obtain the loss function. In our case, we have used the mean squared error (MSE) as a loss function. Let the sets $P = \{p_i\}, i = 1\,to\,N$ and $GT = \{gt_i\}, i = 1\,to\,N$ represent the set of predicted density maps and the ground-truth density maps, respectively. Let the loss function for the proposed model is defined as

$$Loss(\emptyset_{Net}) = \frac{1}{N} \sum_{i=1}^{N} (p_i - gt_i)^2, i = 1\,to\,N \tag{2}$$

Now, the problem statement can be treated as an optimization problem for which we have to minimize the loss function as described in Eq. 3. The problem statement can be represented as in Eq. 3, which is optimized by using a backpropagation algorithm [25] with Adam optimizer [26]

$$\underset{\emptyset_{Net}}{argmin}\, Loss(\emptyset_{Net}) \tag{3}$$

4 Datasets and Ground-Truth Density Maps, Performance Metrics Training Details, and Result Analysis

4.1 *Datasets and Ground-Truth Density Maps Generation*

4.1.1 Datasets

We have demonstrated experiments on two publicly available datasets like the Mall [27] dataset and the Venice [28] dataset. The datasets comprise varying densities. The crowd densities of the Mall dataset vary from 11 to 53. The modality of both datasets is RGB. The resolution of the Mall dataset is [$480 \times 640 \times 3$] and contains a total number of 2000 sequences among which the first 800 are taken for training and the rest 1200 samples for testing. The Venice is high-definition crowd videos where the density varies from 86 to 421. It contains a total number of 167 sequences of which 80 sequences are used for training and 87 sequences for testing. The resolution of these sequences is [$1280 \times 720 \times 3$].

4.1.2 Ground-Truth Density Maps Generation

We use the geometric adaptive kernel [13] to generate ground-truth density maps. Let an image I has L number of annotated head points. We can represent the image, I with L number of head points as a function $H(I)$ which can be represented as

$$H(I) = \sum_{i=1}^{L} \delta(I - I_i) \tag{4}$$

Now according to [13], we will find the K nearest distance for every head points of the image. Let us obtain m different distances $\left(\{d_1^i, d_2^i, \ldots\ldots .d_m^i\} \right)$ for a given head pixel i. Next, we will obtain the average of these distances which can be represented as

$$d^i = \frac{1}{m} \sum_{k=1}^{m} d_k^i \tag{5}$$

Finally, the density maps (DM) can be obtained by convolving the $H(I)$ with a Gaussian kernel with variance δ_i, i.e., $G_{\delta_j}(I)$ for an image, I and it is represented as

$$DM(I) = \sum_{i=1}^{L} \delta(I - I_i) * G_{\delta_i}(I), \tag{6}$$

Fig. 3 Frame of Mall dataset

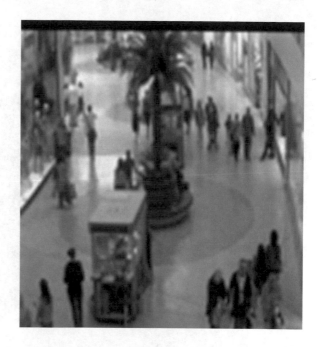

where $\delta_i = \beta d^i$. We fixed the value of $\beta = 0.3$ and K $= 4$. Figures 3, 4, 5 and 6 show some of the examples of frames and their ground-truth density maps of the Mall and Venice datasets.

Fig. 4 Density map of the frame of Mall dataset

Fig. 5 Frame of Venice
dataset

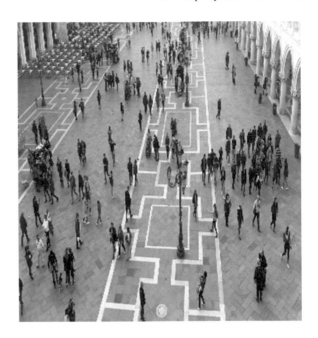

Fig. 6 Density map of the
frame of the Venice dataset

The resolution of the output layer of the proposed single-column Atrous-Net is [32 × 32], so we have to rescale the ground-truth density maps to [32 × 32] by preserving the total count of the frame.

4.2 Performance Metrics

We used mean absolute error (MAE) and root mean square error (RMSE) to measure the performance of the model. The MAE defines the accuracy whereas the RMSE defines the robustness of the model. The MAE and RMSE are defined as

$$MAE = \frac{1}{N} \times \sum_{I=1}^{N} |gt_i - p_i| \qquad (7)$$

$$RMSE = \sqrt{\frac{1}{N} \times \sum_{I=1}^{N} |gt_i - p_i|^2} \qquad (8)$$

Here N is the total number of frames.

4.3 Training Details

The model is trained by setting the maximum number of epochs to 500 and the learning rate to 0.001. We used Adam optimizer [26] to optimize the model. We employed two regularization techniques to avoid overfitting. These are L_2 norm and callbacks. We set the L_2 regularization parameter for kernel as well as biases to 0.01 and the patience parameter of callback to 5. The momentum of the batch normalization layer is set to 0.95. We set the batch sizes of Mall and Venice datasets to 64 and 8, respectively. The proposed model is trained using an inteli7 8th generation processor with 4 GB GPU and 16 GB RAM).

4.4 Results Analysis

4.4.1 The Mall Dataset [27]

The comparative analysis of the results on the Mall dataset is shown in Table 2. It can be observed from Table 2 that the results of 13 state-of-the-art approaches are compared with the proposed model. The proposed model obtains MAE = 3.72 and RMSE = 4.74. Figure 7 presents the predicted crowd count on the Mall dataset [27] using a bar graph.

From Table 2, we can notice that the performance of the conventional approaches [27, 29] is very poor as compared with the deep learning approaches. Among the single-image-based techniques [13, 21, 22, 30–32] DAL-SVR [21] possesses better performance with MAE and RMSE of 2.4 and 9.57, respectively. Among the video-based CCDE approaches [6, 10, 12] and the proposed model, R-DCNN has the better

Table 2 Comparative analysis of results on the Mall dataset [27]

Model name	MAE	RMSE
LBP + ridge regression [27]	6.73	19.18
Count forest [29]	5.75	10.88
CNN-MRF [30]	4.66	9.01
Faster R-CNN [31]	4.65	7.26
MCNN [13]	4.74	8.64
CCNN [32]	5.36	9.34
ConvLSTM-nt [10]	2.53	11.2
ConvLSTM [10]	2.24	8.5
Bidirectional ConvLSTM [10]	2.10	7.6
DAL-SVR [21]	2.40	9.57
DIGCrowd [22]	3.21	16.4
R-DCNN [12]	1.27	5.62
ST-CNN [6]	4.03	5.87
Proposed model	3.72	4.74

Fig. 7 Predicted crowd counts of the proposed model on the Mall dataset [27]

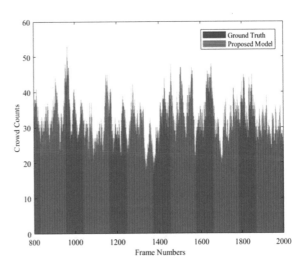

MAE but the proposed approach achieves better RMSE (=4.74). As we know that for a model the value of MAE and RMSE should be minimum as well as the difference between them should be minimum. But in the case of R-DCNN the difference between MAE and RMSE is very high and comparing it with the proposed model the difference is minimum. Hence, we can conclude that the proposed model performs better.

Table 3 Comparative analysis of results on the Venice dataset [28]

Model name	MAE	RMSE
MCNN [13]	145.4	147.3
Switch-CNN [16]	52.8	59.5
CSR-Net [33]	35.8	50.00
ECAN [28]	20.5	29.9
Proposed model	49.17	58.22

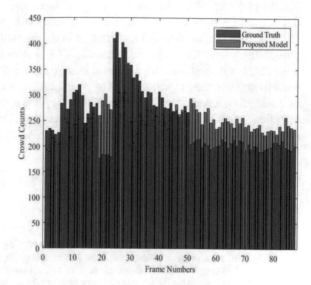

Fig. 8 Predicted crowd counts of the proposed model on the Venice dataset [28]

4.4.2 The Venice Dataset [28]

The result analysis of several approaches on the Venice dataset [28] is shown in Table 3. It can be observed that ECAN [28] obtain better MAE and RMSE. The proposed model results are MAE = 49.17 and RMSE = 58.22. Figure 8 presents the plotting of predicted count versus ground-truth count on the Venice dataset [28]. The proposed model exhibits better than MCNN [13] and switch-CNN [16] and places third position in the list. We can conclude that the proposed model gives moderate results on the Venice dataset [28] but is still very effective.

5 Conclusion

We have proposed a multi-cue multi-scale spatial–temporal modeling for video-based CCDE. The proposed model utilizes a pre-trained Inception-V3 to extract multi-scale spatial–temporal features from four image cues—the image cues like

RGB frames, foreground maps, the volume of frames, and the volume of foreground maps. The main aim behind extracting the multi-scale features is to handle the scale-variation issue due to perspective distortion. The extracted multi-scale features are concatenated and fed into a single-column 2D-Atrous-Net. The model's effectiveness is obtained by experimenting on two datasets like the Mall dataset [27] and the Venice dataset [28]. The proposed model obtains better results on the Mall dataset compared with the existing video-based CCDE [6, 10, 12] by obtaining MAE = 3.72 and RMSE = 4.74. For the Venice dataset, the model achieves an MAE of 49.17 and RMSE of 58.22. Nevertheless, the model obtains moderate results on the Venice dataset, but the obtained result is still better than the benchmark CCDE approaches [13, 16]. The proposed model's advantage is that it exploits multi-scale multi-cues spatial–temporal features for video-based CCDE, performs better in moderate crowd densities, but its performance decreases in high crowd densities. In our future work, we will improve the proposed model by developing more sophisticated deep models and analyzing models' performance in other applied areas like cell counting, wheat counting, and vehicle counting. Overall, we can conclude that the model performs quite better in varying datasets by utilizing multi-scale multi-cue spatial–temporal features.

References

1. Yang DS, Liu CY, Liao WH, Ruan SJ (2020) Crowd gathering and commotion detection based on the stillness and motion model, Multimed. Tools Appl 79(27–28):19435–19449
2. Chen DY, Huang PC (2013) Visual-based human crowds behavior analysis based on graph modeling and matching. IEEE Sens J 13:2129–2138. https://doi.org/10.1109/JSEN.2013.2245889
3. Tripathy SK, Srivastava R (2020) A real-time two-input stream multi-column multi-stage convolution neural network (TIS-MCMS-CNN) for efficient crowd congestion-level analysis. Multimedia Syst 26(5):585–605
4. Liu Y, Shi M, Zhao Q, Wang X (2019) Point in, box out: beyond counting persons in crowds. Proc IEEE Comput Soc Conf Comput Vis Pattern Recognit 2019-June:6462–6471. https://doi.org/10.1109/CVPR.2019.00663
5. Hu Y, Chang H, Nian F et al (2016) Dense crowd counting from still images with convolutional neural networks. J Vis Commun Image Represent 38:530–539. https://doi.org/10.1016/j.jvcir.2016.03.021
6. Miao Y, Han J, Gao Y, Zhang B (2019) ST-CNN: spatial-temporal convolutional neural network for crowd counting in videos. Pattern Recogn Lett 125:113–118. https://doi.org/10.1016/j.patrec.2019.04.012
7. Zhang C, Li H, Wang X, Yang X (2015) Cross-scene crowd counting via deep convolutional neural networks. In: Proceedings of the IEEE computer social conference computer vision pattern recognit. pp 833–841. https://doi.org/10.1109/CVPR.2015.7298684
8. Shi X, Li X, Wu C, et al (2020) A real-time deep network for crowd counting
9. Liu Z, Chen Y, Chen B et al (2019) Crowd counting method based on convolutional neural network with global density feature. IEEE Access 7:88789–88798. https://doi.org/10.1109/ACCESS.2019.2926881
10. Xiong F, Shi X, Yeung DY (2017) Spatiotemporal modeling for crowd counting in videos. In: Proceedings of the IEEE International Conference on Computer Vision 2017-October. pp 5161–5169. https://doi.org/10.1109/ICCV.2017.551

11. Zhang S, Wu G (2017) FCN-rLSTM : deep spatio-temporal neural networks for. Iccv 3687–3696
12. Saqib M, Khan SD, Sharma N, Blumenstein M (2019) Crowd counting in low-resolution crowded scenes using region-based deep convolutional neural networks. IEEE Access 7:35317–35329. https://doi.org/10.1109/ACCESS.2019.2904712
13. Zhang Y, Zhou D, Chen S, et al (2016) Single-image crowd counting via multi-column convolutional neural network. In: Proceedings of the IEEE conference on computer vision pattern recognition. pp 589–597. https://doi.org/10.1002/slct.201701956
14. Boominathan L CrowdNet : a deep convolutional network for dense crowd counting
15. Zeng L, Xu X, Cai B, Qiu S, Zhang T (2017) Multi-scale convolutional neural networks for crowd counting. School of Electronic and Information Engineering South China University of Technology, Guangzhou, China, pp 465–469
16. Sam DB, Surya S, Babu RV (2017) Switching convolutional neural network for crowd counting. In: Proceedings–30th IEEE Conference on Computer Vision Pattern Recognition, CVPR 2017 2017-Janua. pp 4031–4039. https://doi.org/10.1109/CVPR.2017.429
17. Zhang L, Shi M, Chen Q (2018) Crowd counting via scale-adaptive convolutional neural network. in Proceedings–2018 IEEE winter conference appl comput vision, WACV 2018 2018-Janua. pp 1113–1121. https://doi.org/10.1109/WACV.2018.00127
18. Wang Y, Hu S, Wang G et al (2020) Multi-scale dilated convolution of convolutional neural network for crowd counting. Multimed Tools Appl 79:1057–1073. https://doi.org/10.1007/s11042-019-08208-6
19. Zhou Y, Yang J, Li H, et al (2020) Adversarial learning for multiscale crowd counting under complex scenes. IEEE Trans Cybern 1–10. https://doi.org/10.1109/TCYB.2019.2956091
20. Wang Y, Zhang W, Liu Y, Zhu J (2020) Multi-density map fusion network for crowd counting. Neurocomputing. https://doi.org/10.1016/j.neucom.2020.02.010
21. Wei X, Du J, Liang M, Ye L (2019) Boosting deep attribute learning via support vector regression for fast moving crowd counting. Pattern Recogn Lett 119:12–23. https://doi.org/10.1016/j.patrec.2017.12.002
22. Xu M, Ge Z, Jiang X et al (2019) Depth information guided crowd counting for complex crowd scenes. Pattern Recognit Lett 125:563–569. https://doi.org/10.1016/j.patrec.2019.02.026
23. Kaewtrakulpong P, Bowden R (2002) An improved adaptive background mixture model for realtime tracking with shadow detection. In: Proceedings of the 2nd eur work adv video based surveill syst AVBS01, video based surveill syst comput vis distrib process
24. Stauffer C, Grimson WEL (1999) Adaptive background mixture models for real-time tracking. IEEE Comput Soc Conf Comput Vis Pattern Recognit 2:2246–2252
25. Rumelhart DE, Hinton GE Williams RJ (1986) Learning representations by back-propagating errors. 533–536
26. Kingma DP, Ba J (2014) Adam: a method for stochastic optimization. 1–15
27. Chen K, Loy CC, Gong S, Xiang T (2012) Feature mining for localised crowd counting. BMVC 1:1–11
28. Liu W, Salzmann M, Fua P (2019) Context-aware crowd counting. In: Proceedings of the IEEE comput soc conf comput vis pattern recognit 2019-June. pp 5094–5103. https://doi.org/10.1109/CVPR.2019.00524
29. Pham VQ, Kozakaya T, Yamaguchi O, Okada R (2015) COUNT forest: co-voting uncertain number of targets using random forest for crowd density estimation. In: Proceedings of the IEEE International Conference on Computer Vision 2015 Inter. pp 3253–3261. https://doi.org/10.1109/ICCV.2015.372
30. Han K, Wan W, Yao H, Hou L Image crowd counting using convolutional neural network and markov random field. 1–6
31. Zhang L, Lin L, Liang X, He K (2016) Is faster R-CNN doing well for pedestrian detection? Lect Notes Comput Sci 9906 LNCS:443–457. https://doi.org/10.1007/978-3-319-46475-6_28

32. Onoro-Rubio D, López-Sastre, RJ (2016) Towards perspective-free object counting with deep learning. In: European Conference on Computer Vision. Springer, Cham, pp 615–629. https://doi.org/10.1007/978-3-319-46478-7_38
33. Li Y, Zhang X, Chen D (2018) CSRNet: dilated convolutional neural networks for understanding the highly congested scenes. In: Proceedings of the IEEE computer social conference computer vision pattern recognition. pp 1091–1100. https://doi.org/10.1109/CVPR.2018.00120

Modeling and Predictions of COVID-19 Spread in India

Saurav Karmakar, Dibyanshu Gautam, and Purnendu Karmakar

1 Introduction

The current global coronavirus disease occurrence caused by severe acute respiratory syndrome coronavirus 2 (SARS-CoV-2) is the COVID-19 pandemic, also referred to as the coronavirus pandemic [1]. On 30 January 2020, the first case of COVID-19 in India, originating from China, was identified. As of 27 October 2020, 79,46,429 cases have been recorded and 1,19,502 deaths, while 72,01,070 have recovered [2]. India currently has the most confirmed cases in Asia and the second-highest number of cases after the United States [3]. India is striving hard through various strategies to alleviate the transmission of COVID-19: imposing nationwide lockdown, encouraging social distancing, closing educational institutes, government offices, and private offices, closing transport, imposing curfews, and sealing most affected locations by dividing them into zones, and is still not able to contain it effectively.

To gain insights into the possible spread and implications of COVID-19, accessibility to accurate outbreak prediction models is essential. In order to determine the efficacy of applied policies, governments and other administrative bodies depend on forecast models to recommend new policies to meet the increasingly growing demand for health facilities.

S. Karmakar
Birla Institute of Technology, Ranchi, India
e-mail: thesauravkarmakar@gmail.com

D. Gautam
Vellore Institute of Technology, Chennai, India

P. Karmakar (✉)
The LNM Institute of Information Technology, Jaipur, India
e-mail: purnendu.karmakar@lnmiit.ac.in

© The Author(s), under exclusive license to Springer Nature Singapore Pte Ltd. 2021
M. K. Bajpai et al. (eds.), *Machine Vision and Augmented Intelligence—Theory and Applications*, Lecture Notes in Electrical Engineering 796,
https://doi.org/10.1007/978-981-16-5078-9_17

Consequently, to produce a more accurate outcome, epidemiological models face new challenges. To overcome this challenge, many models have emerged that incorporate several assumptions for modeling (e.g., SIR, SEIR, SEIRD, etc.).

To tackle this, herein, we propose the use of machine learning methods for time series and deep learning models to predict the number of cases. More specifically, five different types of approaches are used, Facebook's Prophet forecasting model [4], multi-layer perceptron (MLP) [5], long short-term memory (LSTM) [6], a mathematical model, and lastly, we proposed a metric based on Levitt's metrics.

In terms of evaluation metrics, the root mean square error (RMSE) was employed to assess each model's performance. Although there is no one-size-fits-all approach for predicting cases, the results indicate that the mathematical model demonstrates superior performance.

2 Literature Survey

Owing to a sudden outbreak of COVID-19, there was a dire need for predicting and analyzing the pandemic to take necessary actions. Many researchers used the epidemiological model to analyze the situation [7], but due to COVID-19's uncertainty, standard models do not prove useful. Forecasting such a pandemic can be a challenging task due to various parameters that can be looked into, and even after that, the uncertainty of the results is always looming on us. The work on modeling the spread using a network-based approach was new, but due to not getting access and accurately maintaining the data of inter-state movements, it is not a viable option to use that [8].

Time-series classical models have been popular for quite a time for forecasting, and they were used to predict the same [9]. One such approach [10] included an exponential smoothing family [11, 12], which was derived and improved to create state-space models that helped in automated forecasting. Many limitations have occurred, like missing values affected the model. Also, they do not work well in the long-term forecast, and we have used Facebook Prophet out of all the time-series models to prove this.

Since the data was more like a time-series model, some papers tried to implement ANNs to predict the curve accurately. Some of them included the use of LSTMs [13] to create models to provide some insights [14]. We have tried to implement LSTM as well to compare and evaluate it.

Many different types of research were aimed to predict the end of the pandemic, and many of these used a popular metric developed by Michael Levitt in his data analysis in March 2020 [15] by using data from Hubei, China which showed a linear decrease over some time. Many other papers tried to modify and create an even better metric to understand the curve better.

3 Materials

3.1 Contribution

Our vision was to get the best possible prediction to arrive at various conclusions about India's preventive measures on spread and effect. For that, we used different models to predict and compare to get the most accurate results. Recent research has already used MLPs and other neural network architectures like LSTMs to get precise predictions over the time-series data. However, we tried to do mathematical modeling with the help of MATLAB to obtain the necessary details and compare all the available solutions out there. Transmission interactions in a population are convoluted. It is not easy to assimilate the dynamics of disease spread without a mathematical model's formal structure, which leads us to experiment with that. The paper also includes a modified version of the Levitt metric based on the recovery rate to analyze the current situation and predict the future scenario.

3.2 Dataset

A publicly accessible dataset available on Kaggle was used for model creation and analysis purposes in this research: the "COVID-19 in India" [16]. Additionally, we used the primary dataset available at Coronavirus Outbreak in India [17] from which the Kaggle dataset was made.

The dataset has information from India's states and its districts and union territories at a daily level. Additionally, the number of tests conducted daily in each state is also present. The distribution as of 27 October 2020 of the total cases is shown in (Fig. 1).

Few conclusions we drew from the dataset. The most distressed states are displayed in Figs. 2 and 3, which show us the top ten districts with more than 50,000 confirmed cases, and we can infer that the southern part of India is hugely impacted. It may be due to the high population density in the states. Also, the main reason might be due to the high number of tests being conducted.

4 Methods

Many researchers used the existing compartmental models for forecasting COVID-19 spread, but due to its uncertainty, it is quite challenging to modify parameters like the SIR model got converted into SEIR, then SEIRD and various others. It is not feasible to modify the parameters or change the equation every time, so we used various forecasting techniques. A great deal of effort and research has been generated

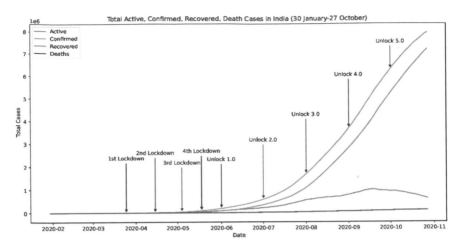

Fig. 1 Total active, confirmed, recovered, and death cases in India from 30 January till 27 October

over the past several decades to build and enhance time-series forecasting models and deep learning models.

In this section, five methods are presented.

4.1 Facebook Prophet

Prophet, a Facebook-developed time-series forecasting model, is focused on decomposable models. It was originally planned to tackle problems in the business time series. It offers easy-to-tune intuitive parameters. This can be used by even someone who lacks the experience to make meaningful predictions about a number of problems.

$$y(t) = g(t) + s(t) + h(t) + \varepsilon_t \tag{1}$$

where

- $g(t)$: for modeling non-periodic shifts in time series, the piecewise linear or logistic growth curve
- $s(t)$: periodic adjustments (e.g. weekly/annual seasonality)
- $h(t)$: impact of holidays (user-provided) with irregular schedules
- ε_t: the error term accounts for any unusual adjustments that the model does not handle (Fig. 4)

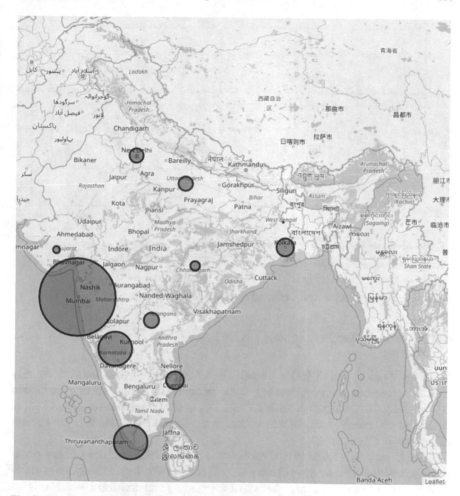

Fig. 2 Top ten most affected states with the highest COVID-19 caseload in India

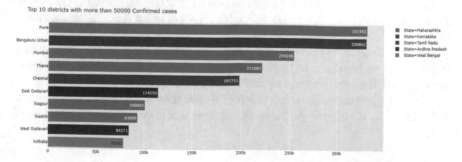

Fig. 3 India's top ten most affected districts with more than 50,000 reported COVID-19 cases

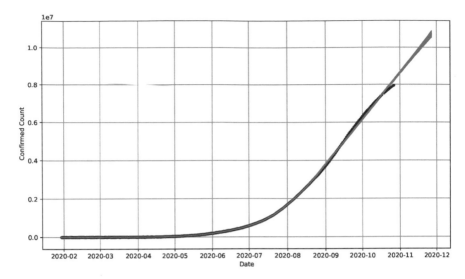

Fig. 4 Forecasting the number of confirmed cases using facebook's prophet

4.2 Multi-Layer Perceptron (MLP)

Multi-layer perceptron (MLP) is an artificial neural feed-forward network entirely linked to at least three layers. An input layer, an output layer, and one or more hidden layers are used in the architecture. MLP usually consists of input neurons equal to the data input and consists only of one neuron in the output layer, which is the number of patients in this situation.

MLP is easy to implement and takes less time on training than its heavy counterparts, making it an obvious choice in predicting the outbreak using ANN architectures. MLP working mainly consists of forwarding and backward propagation. It is based on calculating the current layer neurons' values as an activated summation of previous layer neurons with initial weights as random. The weights are eventually adjusted with backward propagation, but its explanation is not in our discussion scope.

Using MLP regressor, we had many different options for hyperparameter tuning and different architectures to improve our results and help predict as close to the actual spread. For easy iterations among all these combinations, we used a grid search algorithm. Hyperparameter tuning using grid search makes it more comfortable as it checks for all the other hyperparameter options that have been set (Tables 1 and 2 and Fig. 5).

Table 1 MLP model parameters

Hyperparameter	Possible values	Count
Solver	Adam, LBFGS	2
Initial learning rate	0.1, 0.01, 0.5, 0.00001	4
Learning rate adjustment	Adaptive, constant, invscaling	3
Hidden layer sizes	(4,4,4,4), (4,4), (4,4,3,3), (4,3,4), (10,10,10,10,10), (3,), (6,6,6,6), (4,4), (10,5,5,10), (6,), (12,12,12), (3,3,3), (6,6,6), (3,3,3,3,3), (12, 12, 6, 6, 3, 3)	15
Activation functions	ReLU, Identity, Logistic, tanh	4
Regularization parameter	0.01, 0.1, 0.001, 0.0001	4

Table 2 MLP model summary

Layer (type)	Output shape	No. of parameters
Dense	(None,12)	48
Dense	(None,8)	104
Dense	(None,1)	9

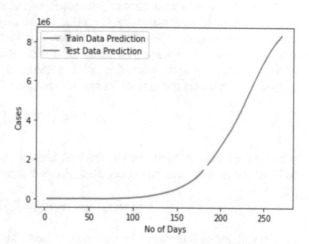

Fig. 5 Forecasting the number of confirmed cases using MLP

4.3 Long Short-Term Memory (LSTM)

Recurrent neural networks (RNNs) are a dominant form of neural network intended to deal with sequence dependency. Conventional RNNs suffer from short-term memory loss. Over time, input from earlier time steps becomes less significant.

Hence, RNNs can fail to retain the context from those earlier steps of the data. Back-propagation through time is the cause of RNNs failing to retain information. Over time gradients become too small to the point, and they become insignificant for updating the weights.

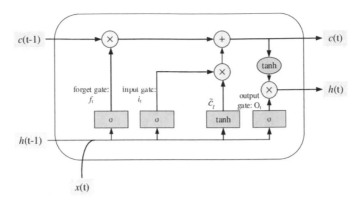

Fig. 6 In an LSTM cell, the repeating module comprises four interacting layers [18]

A special form of RNN, capable of learning long-term dependencies, is the long short-term memory network or LSTM. By using gates that can control the flow of the data going through, they are used to reduce short-term memory.

The LSTM structure consists of four gates, i.e., input gate, forget gate, control gate, and output gate, shown in Fig. 6; each row carries a whole vector from one node output to another node inputs. The pink circles, like vector addition, represent pointwise operations, while the yellow boxes are neural network layers that are taught. Merging lines indicate concatenation, while a forking line denotes the content being copied and the copies going to different locations [19]. The input gate is defined as

$$i_t = \sigma(x_t * U_i + h_{t-1} * W_i) \tag{2}$$

which is responsible for updating the cell state. Forget Gate determines which information is allowed to be kept or discarded and is defined as:

$$f_t = \sigma(x_t * U_f + h_{t-1} * W_f) \tag{3}$$

The cell update is regulated by the control gate as it is multiplied and added by all the other components, so the cell state value fluctuates, and the following equations are given:

$$C_t^{\sim} = tanh(x_t * U_c + h_{t-1} * W_c) \tag{4}$$

$$C_t = f_t * x_t * U_c + h_{t-1} * W_c \tag{5}$$

The hidden layer (h_{t-1}) is changed by the output layer, which is also responsible for determining the value of the next hidden state as given by the output layer:

Table 3 LSTM model summary

Layer (type)	Output shape	No. of parameters
LSTM	(None, 3, 50)	10,400
LSTM	(None, 50)	20,200
Dense	(None, 1)	51

Fig. 7 Forecasting the number of confirmed cases using LSTM

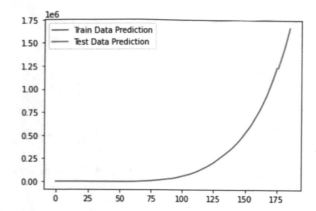

$$O_t = \sigma (x_t * U_o + h_{t-1} * W_o) \qquad (6)$$

$$h_t = o_t * tanh(C_t) \qquad (7)$$

In the above equations,

x_t: Input vector
h_{t-1}: Previous cell output
h_t: Current cell output
C_t: Current cell memory
W, U: Weight vectors

We used the LSTM for regression using the time-window approach, segregated the dataset into a subset of three days, and then calculated the next day (Table 3 and Fig. 7).

4.4 Mathematical Model

It is possible to describe mathematical models as a means of reproducing real-life scenarios with predictive mathematical equations. Mathematical models play a role in epidemiology as a method for studying the spread and control of infectious diseases by changing parameters [20].

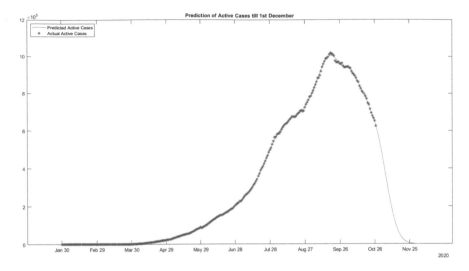

Fig. 8 Forecasting the number of active cases using a mathematical model

In the case of COVID-19 trying to choose parameters is challenging. There are many epidemiological models like in the SIR model it has suspected, infected, and recovered as parameters, and then there is another model, SEIR, which adds exposed as a parameter.

In India, each day, there is a different situation to tackle, so there are many different policies, which is why it is quite challenging to use SIR models, and it is derivatives. We used MATLAB (ver.2020b)'s curve fitting tool, and after tuning the parameters, it is noticed that the data follows a Gaussian distribution, as shown in Fig. 8.

$$f(x) = a_1 e^{-(x-b_1)/c_1^2} + a_2 e^{-(x-b_2)/c_2^2} + a_3 e^{-(x-b_3)/c_3^2} + a_4 e^{-(x-b_4)/c_4^2} \tag{8}$$

4.5 Recovery Metric

The most significant task is to predict when the pandemic rate drops and the effects subside to permissible values. One possible way to predict when the pandemic rate starts declining is to use the Levitt metric on the number of cases/deaths to get a robust prediction of the time taken to get it back to an acceptable state. The advantage of using Levitt's is that it is simple to understand and is independent of the population size.

$$H(t) = \frac{X(t)}{X(t-1)} \tag{9}$$

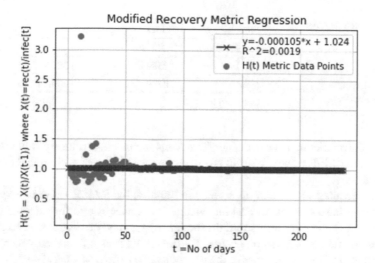

Fig. 9 Forecasting using recovery metrics

where $X(t)$ is the cumulative count until day t.

Although Levitt is quite useful in its way, it still applies to one parameter: either infection rate or the death rate, but it would not be correct to depend on any one of them to conclude that the pandemic has ended. Another way to implement this was to use the same formula by tweaking the parameter as

$$H(t) = \frac{X(t)}{X(t-1)} \tag{10}$$

where $X(t)$ is the cumulative recovered count divided by infected count at day t.

In this way, we can predict the increase or decrease in the rate at which recoveries per infection are happening. This parameter helps us infer how many patients are recovering as compared to the daily infection rate. If it is slowly increasing, then that means the preventive measures show results and a decline in the pandemic effect. Figure 9 shows that gradually we are improving but at a prolonged rate.

5 Results

Our research looked at five critical ways to predict the distribution of COVID-19 cases. Each of the models generated results that were unique in their aspect. Facebook's Prophet, MLP, and LSTM models used confirmed cases as a parameter while our proposed mathematical model used active cases as a parameter and recovery metric used recovery and confirmed cases as a parameter. The performance of each of these methods is shown in Table 4, and as observed, the Gaussian fit proved to be

Table 4 Accuracy metrics

Model	Train set (RMSE)	Test set (RMSE)
Prophet	23,421.46	316,022.46
LSTM	2589.88	301,243.37
MLP	2779.46	206,342.15
Gaussian fit	–	7088.2

the best for predicting over new data. The ANN architectures closely followed it in terms of the RMSE values. We will be discussing the results of each model in a little bit of detail.

Using Prophet, as we can observe from Table 4, the RMSE value is very high, indicating it is less effective. Past knowledge is not adequate to forecast the future, and missing values have influenced the model. To get good predictions, several extra features should be taken into account. By default, it uses a linear model, but it is complicated to forecast because of the unpredictable pattern of COVID-19. We have to find the best parameters that will show the lowest error in forecasting.

Owing to the time-series nature of data, MLP was one of the apparent choices when taking confirmed cases as the base parameter. The findings show that MLP was adequately precise and more comfortable to implement than its counterpart. MLP being easy to use was an obvious choice but it still was prone to discrepancies in the data.

We switched to LSTM, an alternative to the time-series model but an ANN variant that compensates Prophet's drawbacks. They are good at identifying relationships between continuous data points, often in less time over various lengths of timeframes. They can very well recognize trends arising from seasonality. However, the critical problem with deep learning algorithms is that they require a considerable amount of data. Since the RMSE is immense when we split into a test–train dataset allocating fewer data to train data, we needed some alternatives when COVID-19 data was added daily, and it steadily increased.

So, we focused on the mathematical model that predicts nonlinear data very well and requires less data than deep learning algorithms. On the other hand, our modified Levitt metric was formulated, as shown in Fig. 9 in a regression equation. When recoveries are observed per infection, Fig. 9 shows a very constant curve. This means that we recover almost equal to the rate of new infections, giving us a deeper understanding of the present situation and how to improve it in the future.

6   Conclusion

We have shown the various models that we used, and mostly all of these different ways were accurate to some extent. All of these models come with their own set of uncertainties and scope of improvements as well. Many different approaches can differ from these, but we tried to include the maximum of them. Our machine learning approach was primarily based on Prophet, whereas for deep learning, we used multilayer perceptron and LSTM architectures in search of better predictions. These show that AI methods can still generate and predict data for the spread of diseases. The modified Levitt metric that we used helped us understand the rate of recoveries per infection, which makes understanding the whole scenario better by using simple mathematical models.

Future work may include a better architecture or maybe a better parameter grid. Many other models like SIR models take in other parameters to predict the data but come with their challenges. Some different approaches also include hybrid machine learning models of MLP-ICA and ANFIS used in Hungary. The changes in the outbreak and its spread make the modeling strategy very challenging, yet some of these models prove that they can devise a reliable prediction analysis.

References

1. World Health Organization Homepage https://www.who.int/emergencies/diseases/novel-cor onavirus-2019/technical-guidance/naming-the-coronavirus-disease-(covid-2019)-and-the-virus-that-causes-it. Accessed 27 Oct 2020
2. MyGov COVID19 STATEWISE STATUS https://www.mygov.in/corona-data/covid19-statew ise-status/ Accessed 27 Oct 2020
3. WHO Coronavirus Disease (COVID-19) Dashboard https://covid19.who.int/ Accessed 27 Oct 2020
4. Taylor SJ, Letham B (2018) Forecasting at scale. Am Stat 72(1):37–45
5. Car Z, Baressi Šegota S, Anđelić N, Lorencin I, Mrzljak V (2020) Modeling the spread of COVID-19 infection using a multilayer perceptron. Comput Math Methods Med 2020:5714714. https://doi.org/10.1155/2020/5714714
6. Gers FA, Eck D, Schmidhuber J (2002) Applying LSTM to time series predictable through time-window approaches. In: Tagliaferri R, Marinaro M, (eds) Neural nets WIRN Vietri-01. Perspectives in neural computing 2002, vol. 9999. Springer, London, pp. 193–200. https://doi. org/10.1007/978-1-4471-0219-9_20.
7. Banerjee B, Pandey PK, & Adhikari B (2020) A model for the spread of an epidemic from local to global: a case study of COVID-19in India. arXiv preprint arXiv:2006.06404
8. Kumar A (2020) Modeling geographical spread of COVID-19 in India using network-based approach. medRxiv
9. Papastefanopoulos V, Linardatos P, Kotsiantis S (2020) COVID-19: a comparison of time series methods to forecast percentage of active cases per population. Appl Sci 10(11):3880
10. Petropoulos F, Makridakis S (2020) Forecasting the novel coronavirus COVID-19. PLoS One 15(3):e0231236
11. Hyndman RJ, Koehler AB, Snyder RD, Grose S (2002) A state space framework for automatic forecasting using exponential smoothing methods. Int J Forecast 18(3):439–454
12. Taylor JW (2003) Exponential smoothing with a damped multiplicative trend. Int J Forecast 19(4):715–725
13. Schmidhuber J, Hochreiter S (1997) Long short-term memory. Neural Comput 9(8):1735–1780
14. Tomar A, Gupta N (2020) Prediction for the spread of COVID-19in India and effectiveness of preventive measures. Sci Total Environ 138762
15. Levitt M, Scaiewicz A, Zonta F (2020) Predicting the trajectory of any COVID19 epidemic from the best straight line. medRxiv https://doi.org/10.1101/2020.06.26.20140814
16. Rajkumar S, KP D (2020) COVID-19 in India. Kaggle. https://www.kaggle.com/sudalairajku mar/covid19-in-india

17. Coronavirus Outbreak in India-covid19india.org (2020) https://api.covid19india.org/docume ntation/csv/ Accessed 27 Oct 2020
18. Olah C (2015) Understanding LSTM networks. Colah'sBlog. https://colah.github.io/posts/ 2015-08-Understanding-LSTMs/
19. Yuan X, Li L, Wang Y (2020) Nonlinear dynamic soft sensor modeling with supervised long short-term memory net-work. IEEE Trans Ind Inform 16(5):3168–3176. https://doi.org/10. 1109/tii.2019.2902129
20. Naji RK, Hussien RM (2016) The dynamics of epidemic model with two types of infectious diseases and vertical transmission. J Appl Math

A Machine Learning Model for Automated Classification of Sleep Stages Using Polysomnography Signals

Santosh Kumar Satapathy, Hari Kishan Kondaveeti, D. Loganathan, and S. Sharathkumar

1 Introduction

Sleep is one of the important physiological activities for the human body, which directly controls memory consolidation and it also decides the performance of the daily activities. Sleep plays an important role in the human body because it represents the primary functions of the human brain. One human individual is spending one-third of its duration as sleep. Proper quality of sleep maintains the physical and mental fitness of the human body, which alternatively is helpful to perform well in workplaces, control emotions, and able to take proper decisions [1, 2]. Nowadays, it is seen that Sleep diseases (SD) are becoming one of the major causes of death across the world. The main reason for this serious health issue is an imbalance of sleep patterns, and it has occurred due to job pressure and rapid changes in lifestyles across the globe. It has been observed that the prevalence of sleep diseases has significantly increased over the past years. According to the report of the Center for Control of Disease and Prevention (CDC) of the US Government, around 9 million populations have difficulty maintaining good quality sleep [3]. According to a survey of the National Highway Traffic Safety Administration in the USA, it has found that due to the drowsiness factor, around 56,000–100,000 car accidents have happened, which directly reported that more than 1500 have died and 71,000 are affected with injuries annually [4]. It has been found that sleep diseases are considered to be the most predominant death cause with the different age groups of populations across the globe. In general, different types of sleep disorders are categorized, such as

S. K. Satapathy (✉) · D. Loganathan · S. Sharathkumar
Pondicherry Engineering College, Puducherry, India
e-mail: santosh.satapathy@pec.edu

H. K. Kondaveeti
VIT-AP University, Vijayawada, Andhra Pradesh, India

© The Author(s), under exclusive license to Springer Nature Singapore Pte Ltd. 2021
M. K. Bajpai et al. (eds.), *Machine Vision and Augmented Intelligence—Theory and Applications*, Lecture Notes in Electrical Engineering 796,
https://doi.org/10.1007/978-981-16-5078-9_18

obstructive sleep apnea, insomnia, hypersomnia, narcolepsy, breathing-related disorders, stroke, stress, and cardiovascular diseases [5]. All these diseases progressively increased with age. So, early diagnosis is helpful for the human being to prevent the severity of these diseases and it helps to improve the subject's quality of life. The first most important step for sleep diseases is sleep scoring. The most popular test for analyzing sleep quality is the polysomnography (PSG) test. PSG tests include the signals such as electroencephalogram (EEG), electrocardiogram (ECG), electromyogram (EMG), and electrooculogram (EOG). The entire sleep staging procedures are analyzed according to two available sleep standards such as the Rechtschaffen and Kales (R&K) [6] and the American Academy of Sleep Medicine (AASM) [7]. According to R&K sleep guidelines, the whole sleep cycle is categorized into six sleep stages such as wake stage (W), non-rapid eye movement (NREM stage 1 (N1), NREM stage 2 (N2), NREM stage 3 (N3), and NREM stage 4 (N4)), and rapid eye movement (REM) stage. The only changes reflected with the AASM manual incomparable to R&K standards is NREM sleep stages. According to the AASM guidelines, the total sleep stages are five, the NREM stage 3 (N3) and the NREM stage 4 (N4) are combined into one sleep stage called the NREM stage 3. Traditionally, the sleep scoring procedure was conducted through the visual inspection method, where one clinician was monitoring the sleep behavior of the subject for 6–8 h. of sleep. This traditional sleep analysis method requires more human resources for monitoring the whole sleep recordings, and also it consumes more time for analysis, due to more human interpretation, sometimes the results are erroneous [6]. Sometimes, it is also one of the major causes of not achieving higher classification accuracy in the classification of sleep stages. With consideration of all these above-mentioned facts, the automated sleep scoring approach has gained a lot of attention in recent researches [7, 8]. Automated sleep scoring not only causes accuracy improvements but also provides quick diagnosis [9]. It has been observed that the PSG test is one of the costly experiments, and it also gives so many unpleasant scenarios for the subjects, because of its so much connectivity of wires in the different parts of the body [10, 11]. Henceforth, instead of PSG signals, most of the researchers preferred EEG signal, because it directly provides the brain activities during sleep hours. This helps a lot for analyzing the sleep abnormality and it is also more popular for its easier recording facility. In general, EEG signals are combinations of different waveforms, which help to characterize the different sleep stages with different frequency bands such as delta band (0–4 Hz), theta (4–8 Hz), alpha (8–13 Hz), beta (13–30 Hz), spindle (12–14 Hz), sawtooth (2–6 Hz), and k-complex (0.5–1.5 Hz). Finally, the scoring and decisions are taken by the sleep experts through proper interpretation of the quantitative and visual analysis of collected sleep recordings. In some cases, the sleep experts use an algorithm for pre-scoring the entire sleep recordings, and these successive representations of the sleep stages information called hypnograms, which is highly required during the diagnosis of the different types of sleep disorders. Sleep staging is generally a tedious job, which requires highly experienced technicians and experts. This other limitation with subject to sleep staging is variations on sleep scoring from experts to experts, which is also one of the major causes for diagnosing sleep diseases [12, 13].

In this paper, we have obtained a single-channel EEG signal for sleep staging analysis; this approach makes it more interesting because of its ease of operational deployments on mobile devices. It also makes more comfortable situations for the patients due to less cabling used during recordings. It has been observed that most of the contributions with single-channel EEG signals were executed in two-step methodology. In the first step, the different hand-engineered features are extracted from the different waveforms, and in the second step, the extracted features are forwarded to a classifier for classifying the sleep stages based on the feature characteristics. In general, it has been seen that most of the authors obtained one of the three following domains of the features [14] (a) time-domain features, (b) frequency-domain features, (c) non-linear features. Similarly, it has been seen that for classification models, the most common models used by the researchers were support vector machine (SVM) [15], decision trees [16], k-nearest neighbor (KNN) [17], k-means clustering [18], bootstrap aggregating [19], random forest (RF) [20], naïvebayes [21], Gaussian mixture model (GMM) [22], AdaBoost [23], sparse auto encoders (SAE) [24], and artificial neural networks (ANNs) [25]. In [26], the authors obtain the multiscale entropy and autoregressive features and used linear discriminate analysis for classifying the sleep stages.

Zhu et al. [27] proposed automated sleep scoring based on the EEG signal. The author used the features from the visibility graph and uses the SVM classification model for the classification of the sleep stages.

In [28], the authors obtained time–frequency features from the raw EEG signal. The extracted features are fed into the random forest classification model.

Hassan et al. [29] extracted features from an empirical mode decomposition of the signal and use bootstrap-aggregating techniques for multi-class sleep staging classifications.

In [30], the authors extracted spectral features through the tunable Q-factor wavelet transform techniques and use a random forest classifier for the classification of the sleep stages.

In [31], the author considered multiple signals such as EEG, EOG, and EMG for the automated sleep scoring through the extraction of features like skewness, kurtosis, variance, entropy, and used a dendrogram-based SVM (DSVM) classifier for classifying the sleep stages and reported accuracy for the model as 88%.

Hassan et al. [32] applied the EEMD algorithm for signal enhancement from single-channel EEG signal, and extracted statistical features are forwarded into boosting techniques, and the accuracy for two–six sleep stages is reported as 98.15%, 94.23%, 92.66%, 83.49%, and 88.07%, respectively.

Silveria et al. [33] presented a six-state sleep staging approach using a discrete wavelet concept and obtained a random forest classifier, the model achieved 90% accuracy.

Rahman et al. [34] introduced a single-channel EOG sleep scoring approach and extracted statistical features by applying discrete wavelet transform techniques. The average accuracy reported for six-state classifications through RUSBoost, RF, and SVM is 90, 91, and 91.7%.

Memar et al. [35] proposed two-state sleep staging and the acquired signal is decomposed into eight sub-bands, finally, 13 features are extracted from each sub-band epoch. The suitable features are identified through the mRMR feature selection algorithm. The model achieved an overall accuracy of 95.31% through a random forest classifier.

Imtiaz et al. [36] presented automated sleep staging through home-based polysomnography signal, and the model reported accuracy for training and testing dataset as 89% and 72%, respectively, through decision tree classification algorithm.

Dimitriadis et al. [37] proposed one-channel EEG sensor ASSC techniques and estimated cross-coupling frequency (CFC) from each epoch and the system achieved an overall accuracy of 94% through multi-class Naïve Bayes classification techniques.

It has been found that most of the existing state-of-the-art works were based on EEG signals. But sometimes, it has also been seen that other behavior of the human body may also affect the sleep irregularities such as muscle movements and rapid movements of the eye. So, it is also necessary to consider the behavior of the muscle movements and eye blinks during the sleep scoring system. In this research work, we propose an automated sleep staging system based on polysomnography signals. In this study, we retrieved the sleep behavior using the single-channel of EEG, EOG, and EMG signals. The entire research work is carried through the four individual experiments; the first three experiments of sleep staging are executed using single-channel EEG, EOG, and EMG. The final and fourth experiment is conducted with the combinations of the EEG, EOG, and EMG signals. In this study, we have obtained the ISRUC-Sleep subgroup-I (SG-I) data. The entire experiment of the proposed model followed AASM scoring rules. Further, the research work is organized as follows: Sect. 2 explains on the dataset used in this work. Section 3 contains brief descriptions of the experimental results of the proposed model. Section 4 conecludes our proposed research work.

2   Methodology

In this paper, we propose an efficient and reliable automatic sleep staging classification system based on polysomnography signals using machine learning techniques. Figure 1 presents the steps of the proposed sleep staging system and the following sub-stages have described the detail on each step. The proposed sleep staging followed four basic phases. In the first phase, preprocessing the recorded signals, and in the second phase, we extracted the signal properties from the preprocessed signals concerning the time- and frequency-domain. After that, we obtained the feature selection techniques to analyze the relevance of the features of the proposed classification model during the third phase. Finally, in the fourth phase, the screened features are forwarded to the obtained classification model. The entire experimental work was coded and executed through MAT LAB software.

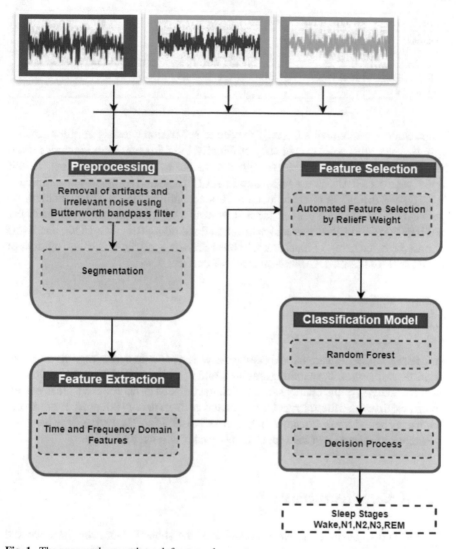

Fig. 1 The proposed research work framework

2.1 Experimental Data

In this study, we use data of subjects who are completely healthy or have different medical conditions. The recorded data was collected from an open-access comprehensive sleep dataset, called ISRUC-Sleep. This dataset includes information from human adults and contains data on both healthy subjects and those with suspected sleep disorders. Data collection was done at the Sleep Medicine Centre of the Hospital of Coimbra University (CHUC) [38]. The first subsection includes 100 subjects, with

Table 1 Description of distribution of sleep stages

Database	Sleep stages					Total samples
	Wake (W)	N1	N2	N3	REM (R)	
ISRUC-Sleep subgroup-I	1001	518	1214	588	429	3750

one recording session per subject. The second subsection consists of eight subjects with two recording sessions per subject. Finally, the third subsection includes information from ten healthy subjects with one recording session per subject. In this study, we used ISRUC-Sleep Subgroup-I (SG-I) dataset. The signals are sampled at 200 Hz, and the length of each epoch is 30 s according to the AASM standard. As per AASM, the sleep stages are labeled as awake (W), NREM (N1, N2, and N3), and REM (R). This dataset contains bio-signal recordings of EEG, EOG, and EMG signals collected using 11 electrodes. Table 1 show the distribution of the number of sleep stages of the ISRUC-Sleep subgroup-I dataset.

2.2 Preprocessing

Since the recorded signals from the subjects were contaminated with different types of artifacts like muscle twitching, motion, and eye blinks, which could potentially limit the analysis of the changes in sleep characteristics of the different sleep stages. So that we discarded these irregular noises and artifacts using 10th order Butterworth bandpass filter with a frequency range from 0.5 to 49.5 Hz. The entire sleep behavior recordings are segmented into epochs, and each epoch length is 30 s.

2.3 Features Extraction

It is difficult to analyze the sleep behavior of the subjects from the preprocessed signals because recorded signals are highly random, and also the behavior of signals continuously changes concerning time and frequency ranges. So, it is highly necessary for proper analysis of the sleep characteristics during sleep scoring. In this study, we have obtained both time- and frequency-domain features for discriminating the sleep characteristics of the subjects. Though human sleep highly changes in nature, so sometimes it is important to study the signal in a non-linearity manner. As a whole, we extracted 29 features, out of that 12 features are time-domain related, 15 features are in frequency-domain-oriented, and 2 features are in the non-linear features, respectively. The 12 time-domain features are mean, median, mode, minimum, maximum, standard deviation, variance skewness, kurtosis, percentile, and Hjorth parameters.

The 15 frequency-domain features are relative spectral power, band power for δ, θ, α, and β frequency sub-bands, seven power ratios, and the non-linear features are zero-crossing rate and spectral entropy.

2.4 Feature Selection

It has been seen that each extracted feature may not be suitable for every subject. Sometimes, it may create a biased performance from the models. So, it is highly important for the proper screening of the features before forwarding them into the classification model. Here, we consider the feature selection algorithm as ReliefF weight, which helps to find out the weightage of the individual features with the help of the generated weight value with regards to the individual features [39].

2.5 Classification

To distinguish the different characteristics of sleep stages, we employ one machine learning classification algorithm, random forest (RF).

Random Forest (RF): This algorithm is proposed by Breimant, and this algorithm is one of the popular classification techniques that uses multiple tree structures for training the data and predict the samples [40]. Each tree requires randomly sampled data values and separate classifiers. The major difference between RF and other classification techniques is that the input is selected in a random manner using bootstrap selection methods. This whole method continues till the noisy and outlier samples are not to desensitize, and at last, the output is computed by voting approaches.

2.6 Model Performance Evaluation

In this proposed study, we have considered performance metrics to validate the proposed system performance with subject to accuracy [41], sensitivity [42], specificity [43], precision [44], and F1score [45].

3 Results and Discussion

The whole research work is conducted with the two different categories of the subjects (SG-I and SG-III) of the ISRUC-Sleep dataset. SG-I category data contains the sleep behavior of the subjects who were affected with the different sleep syndromes, and in opposite, the SG-III data contains the healthy controlled subject's sleep behavior.

The entire sleep recordings annotation was done according to the AASM sleep standards and each epoch length is 30 s. The entire research work is executed in the four individual experiments, the first three experiments are conducted with the individual channel of the EEG (C3-A2), EOG (ROC-A1), and EMG (X1) signals, and the final experiment is executed with the combinations of the EEG, EOG, and EMG signals. Initially, we obtained the preprocessing techniques for eliminating the irrelevant noises, muscle movements, and eye blinks information from the acquired channels using the 10th order Butterworth bandpass filter. Though the brain behavior is highly complicated in nature and to properly analyze the sleep behavior, we have extracted the signal characteristics in both the time and frequency ranges, which directly helps to recognize the disturbances during sleep period time. As a whole, 29 features are extracted from all the input signals. Another advantage of this study is the inclusion of the feature screening algorithm, which decides the most suitable features from the pool of the features which supports to discriminate the sleep characteristics concerning the individual sleep stages. Here, we obtained the selection algorithm as ReliefF feature selection algorithm which decides the importance of the feature by generating the weight value against the individual features, which ultimately decides the more optimal features for a classification task. Finally, the selected features are fed into the classifier for classifying the multi-class sleep stages. In this study, we have considered the classification of the five-sleep state. The whole recordings are segmented into the training and testing portions. The dataset ratio for all the experiments of this proposed research work is training dataset is 70% and the rest of the 30% are considered as testing data. The entire code and execution to be done through the MATLAB software (2017a version) with the system properties of i7-7700HQ 2.81 GHz CPU, 8-GB RAM. At last, the proposed model is tested using certain performance metrics such as accuracy, sensitivity, specificity, and F1score.

3.1 Results with Input of ISRUC-Sleep Subgroup-I Dataset

Experiment-1 (Single-channel EEG signal)

The first experiment is based on EEG signals. The reported confusion matrix with testing data is shown in Table 2 and the results of the performance metrics are presented in Table 3.

It has been observed from Table 3, the highest accuracy, precision, sensitivity, specificity, and F1Score reported from wake stage (99.09%), N2 stage (98.88%), N2 stage (98.19%), REM stage (99.70%), and N1 stage (96.98%), respectively.

Experiment-2 (Single-channel EMG signal)

In this experiment, we obtained the input channel as X1(Chin) of the EMG signal. The reported confusion matrix for this experiment is shown in Table 4 and the performance metrics results are described in Table 5.

Table 2 Confusion matrix obtained using single-channel EEG

Automatic classification	Expert classification					
		W	N1	N2	N3	R
	W	122	1	2	1	1
	N1	1	193	5	0	0
	N2	1	4	489	3	1
	N3	1	1	4	191	1
	R	2	0	2	1	98

Table 3 Classification results of the sleep stages with C3-A2 channel of EEG signal

Performance metrics	W (%)	N1 (%)	N2 (%)	N3 (%)	R (%)	Overall performances (%)
Accuracy	99.09	98.91	98.74	98.91	99.27	98.99
Precision	96.06	96.98	98.99	97.45	97.03	97.30
Sensitivity	96.06	96.98	98.19	96.46	95.15	96.57
Specificity	99.49	99.34	99.18	99.45	99.70	99.43
F1Score	96.06	96.98	98.59	96.95	96.08	96.93

Table 4 Performance values obtained using input of single-channel EMG

Automatic classification	Expert classification					
		W	N1	N2	N3	R
	W	121	1	2	1	2
	N1	3	191	3	2	0
	N2	3	2	489	1	4
	N3	1	1	2	192	2
	R	2	1	3	1	95

Table 5 Performance metrics results using single-channel EMG signal

Performance metrics	W (%)	N1 (%)	N2 (%)	N3 (%)	R (%)	Overall performances (%)
Accuracy	98.64	98.82	98.64	99.00	98.64	98.75
Precision	93.08	97.45	98.99	97.46	92.23	95.84
Sensitivity	95.28	95.98	98.00	96.97	93.14	95.87
Specificity	99.08	99.45	99.17	99.45	99.20	99.27
F1Score	94.16	96.71	98.49	97.22	92.68	95.85

Table 6 Performance values obtained using input of single-channel EOG

Automatic classification	Expert classification					
		Wake	N1	N2	N3	REM
	Wake	120	1	3	1	2
	N1	1	191	2	3	2
	N2	1	1	492	3	1
	N3	3	0	5	189	2
	REM	1	1	2	2	97

Table 7 Performance evaluation results using single-channel EOG channel

Performance metrics	W (%)	N1 (%)	N2 (%)	N3 (%)	R (%)	Overall performances (%)
Accuracy	98.82	99.00	98.64	98.29	98.82	98.71
Precision	95.24	98.45	98.20	95.45	93.27	96.12
Sensitivity	94.49	95.98	98.80	94.97	94.17	95.68
Specificity	99.38	99.67	98.51	99.01	99.30	99.18
F1Score	94.86	97.20	98.50	95.21	93.72	95.90

From Table 5, the highest performance reported in terms of accuracy, precision, sensitivity, specificity, and F1Score is 99% (W stage), 98.99% (N1 stage), 98% (N2 stage), 99.45% (N1 stage), and 98.49% (N2 stage), respectively.

Experiment-3 (Single-channel EOG signal)

The third experiment is conducted with ROC-A1 input channel of EOG signal. The confusion matrix result of this experiment is presented in Table 6 and the performance of the model with different evaluation metrics is presented in Table 7.

From Table 7, it has been seen that accuracy, precision, and specificity are reported highest for the N1 sleep stage, similarly, the highest performance results reported for sensitivity and F1Score is N2 sleep stage, respectively.

Experiment-4 (using EEG+EMG+EOG signals)

In the fourth and final experiment, the input for the model is combinations of the channel of the EEG, EMG, and EOG signal. The confusion matrix result for this experiment is presented in Table 8 and the performance metrics results are presented in Table 9.

It has been noticed from Table 9 that the performance of the model using combinations of the input channel provides better improvements in comparison to the other three individual input channel experiments. The highest accuracy results achieved from N1 stage (99.40%), precision from N2 stage (99.34%), sensitivity from N2 stage (99.26%), specificity from N3 stage (99.71%), and F1score from N2 stage (99.30%).

Table 8 Performance values obtained using input of single-channel EEG+EMG+EOG

Automatic classification	Expert classification					
		Wake	N1	N2	N3	REM
	Wake	652	3	7	4	2
	N1	3	461	5	1	2
	N2	4	2	1206	2	1
	N3	1	2	14	513	21
	REM	3	2	2	1	480

Table 9 Performance values obtained using input of single-channel EEG+EMG+EOG

Performance metrics	W (%)	N1 (%)	N2 (%)	N3 (%)	R (%)	Overall performances (%)
Accuracy	99.19	99.40	99.49	98.63	98.98	99.14
Precision	98.34	98.09	99.34	98.46	94.86	97.82
Sensitivity	97.60	97.67	99.26	93.10	98.36	97.20
Specificity	99.59	99.69	99.62	99.71	99.09	99.54
F1Score	97.97	97.88	99.30	95.71	96.58	97.49

From Table 10, it has been seen that the proposed sleep staging study using PSG signals give the best classification performance of 99.14%. To validate the classification performance results, here, we made the comparisons of the results of the proposed model with the existing state-of-the-art works in Table 11.

Table 10 Overall accuracy results for Experiment-1 to Experiment-4

Experiment number	Five-Sleep states classification task (CT-5)	Accuracy performances of model (%)
		ISRUC-Sleep subgroup-I
	Random forest classifier	Testing data
Experiment-1	Single-channel EEG	98.99
Experiment-2	Single-channel EMG	98.75
Experiment-3	Single-channel EOG	98.17
Experiment-4	Single-channel EEG+EMG+EOG	99.14

Table 11 Performance comparison of state-of-the-art works results with the proposed model performance results

Study	Input signal	Classifier used	Accuracy (%)
Reference [46] 2018	EEG+EMG+EOG EEG+EMG+EOG EEG+EMG+EOG	Decision Tree	80.07
Reference [47] 2018		Hybrid self-attentive model	73.28
Reference [48] 2018		Support vector Machine	92.09
Reference [49] 2019		Convolutional Neural Network	91.22
Proposed study		**Random forest**	**99.14**

4 Conclusion

In this research work, we proposed an automated sleep staging system by using PSG signals, the ReliefF feature selection algorithm, and the RF classification model. To analyze the sleep behavior of the subject, a set of linear and non-linear features was extracted from the PSG signal segments. The proposed methodologies are incorporated to analyze the changes in the sleep behavior during different sleep stages. The proposed research work reported higher sleep staging performance comparable to the existing studies. The proposed model can be used for the diagnosis of any type of sleep-related disorders in a real-time application manner. Further, we will plan to extend our work in the directions of using different epoch lengths as input and apply the deep learning concept.

References

1. Stickgold R (2005) Sleep-dependent memory consolidation, Nature 437(7063):1272
2. Carskadon MA, Dement WC (2005) Normal human sleep: an overview. Principles Pract Sleep Med 4:13–23
3. Ford ES, Wheaton AG, Cunningham TJ (2014) Trends in outpatient visits for insomnia, sleep apnea, and prescriptions for sleep medications among US adults: findings from the National Ambulatory Medical Care survey 1999–2010. Sleep 37:1283–1293
4. Garces Correa A, Orosco L, Laciar E (2014) Automatic detection of drowsiness in EEG records based on multimodal analysis. Med Eng Phys 36:244–249
5. Reynolds CF, O'Hara R (2013) DSM-5 sleep-wake disorders classification: overview for use in clinical practice. Am J Psychiatry 170:1099–1101
6. Boashash B, Ouelha S (2016) Automatic signal abnormality detection using time-frequency features and machine learning: a newborn EEG seizure case study. Knowl Based Syst 106:38–50
7. Hassan AR, Bhuiyan MIH (2017) Automated identification of sleep stages from EEG signals by means of ensemble empirical mode decomposition and random under sampling boosting. Comput Methods Progr Biomed 140:201–210
8. Hassan AR, Bhuiyan MIH (2016) Automatic sleep scoring using statistical features in the EMD domain and ensemble methods. Biocybern Biomed Eng 36(1):248–255

9. Li Y, Luo ML, Li K (2016) A multiwavelet-based time-varying model identification approach for time frequency analysis of EEG signals. Neurocomputing 193:106–114
10. Subasi A (2015) A decision support system for diagnosis of neuromuscular disorders using dwt and evolutionary support vector machines. Signal Image Video Process 9(2):399–408
11. Akben SB, Alkan A (2016) Visual interpretation of biomedical time series using parzen window based density-amplitude domain transformation. PLoS One 11(9):1–13
12. Stepnowsky C, Levendowski D, Popovic D, Ayappa I, Rapoport DM (2013) Scoring accuracy of automated sleep staging from a bipolar electro ocular recording compared to manual scoring by multiple raters. Sleep Med 14(11):1199–1207
13. Wang Y, Loparo KA, Kelly MR, Kaplan RF (2015) Evaluation of an automated single-channel sleep staging algorithm. Nat Sci Sleep 7:101
14. Radha M, Garcia-Molina G, Poel M, Tononi G (2014) Comparison of feature and classifier algorithms for online automatic sleep staging based on a single EEG signal. In: Annual international conference of the IEEE engineering in medicine and biology society, pp 1876–1880
15. Koley B, Dey D (2012) An ensemble system for automatic sleep stage classification using single channel EEG signal. Comput Biol Med 42(12):1186–1195
16. Fraiwan L, Lweesy K, Khasawneh N, Wenz H, Dickhaus H (2012) Automated sleep stage identification system based on time-frequency analysis of a single EEG channel and random forest classifier. Comput Methods Progr Biomed 108(1):10–19
17. Zhang S, Li X, Zong M (2017) Learning k, for kNN classification. ACM Trans Intell Syst Technol 8(3):1–19
18. Shuyuan X, Bei W, Jian Z, Qunfeng Z, Junzhong Z, Nakamura M (2015) An improved K-means clustering algorithm for sleep stages classification. In: 2015 54th Annual Conference of the Society of Instrument and Control Engineers of Japan, pp 1222–1227
19. Awujoola Olalekan J, Francisca O, Odion PO (2020) Effective and accurate bootstrap aggregating (Bagging) ensemble algorithm model for prediction and classification of hypothyroid disease. Int J Comput Appl 176(39):41–49
20. Fraiwan L, Lweesy K., Khasawneh N, Wenz H, Dickhaus H (2012) Automated sleep stage identification system based on time–frequency analysis of a single EEG channel and random forest classifier. Comput Methods Progr Biomed 108:10–19
21. Acharya UR, Chua EC-P, Chua KC, Min LC, Tamura T (2010) Analysis and automatic identification of sleep stages using higher order spectra. Int J Neural Syst 20(06):509–521
22. Wan H, Wang H, Scotney B, Liu J (2019) A novel gaussian mixture model for classification. In: 2019 IEEE international conference on systems, man and cybernetics (SMC), Bari, Italy, pp 3298–3303
23. Tharwat A (2018) AdaBoost classifier: an overview
24. Mienye ID, Sun Y, Wang Z (2020) Improved sparse auto encoder based artificial neural network approach for prediction of heart disease. Informatics in Medicine Unlocked
25. Tagluk ME, Sezgin N, Akin M (2010) Estimation of sleep stages by an artificial neural network employing EEG, EMG and EOG. J Med Syst 34:717–725
26. Liang S-F, Kuo C-E, Hu Y-H, Pan Y-H, Wang Y-H (2012) Automatic stage scoring of single-channel sleep EEG by using multiscale entropy and autoregressive models. IEEE Trans Instrum Meas 61(6):1649–1657
27. Zhu G, Li Y, Wen PP (2014) Analysis and classification of sleep stages based on difference visibility graphs from a single-channel EEG signal,. IEEE J Biomed Health Inf 18(6):1813–1821
28. Hassan AR, Bhuiyan MIH (2016) Computer-aided sleep staging using complete ensemble empirical mode decomposition with adaptive noise and bootstrap aggregating. Biomed Signal Process Control 24:1–10
29. Hassan AR, Bhuiyan MIH (2016) A decision support system for automatic sleep staging from EEG signals using tunable Q-factor wavelet transform and spectral features. J Neurosci Methods 271:107–118
30. Lajnef T, Chaibi S, Ruby P (2015) Learning machines and sleeping brains: automatic sleep stage classification using decision-tree multi-class support vector machines. J Neurosci Methods 250:94–105

31. Zhu G, Li Y, Wen P (2014) Analysis and classification of sleep stages based on difference visibility graphs from a single-channel EEG signal. IEEE J Biomed Health Inform 18(6):1813–1821

32. Hassan AR, Hassan Bhuiyan MI (2016) Automatic sleep scoring using statistical features in the EMD domain and ensemble methods. Bio Cybern Biomed Eng 36(1):248–255

33. Silveiral T, Kozakevıcius J, Rodrıgucs R (2016) Single-channel EEG sleep stage classification based on a streamlined set of statistical features in wavelet domain. Int Fed For Med Biol Eng

34. Rahman MM, Bhuiyan MIH, Hassan AR (2018) Sleep stage classification using single-channel EOG. Comput Biol Med 102:211–220

35. Memar P, Faradji F (2018) A novel multi-class EEG-based sleep stage classification system. IEEE Trans Neural Syst Rehabil Eng 26(1):84–95

36. Imtiaz SA, Rodriguez-Villegas E (2015) Automatic sleep staging using state machine-controlled decision trees. In: Conference of the IEEE Engineering in Medicine and Biology Society, pp 378–81

37. Dimitriadis SI, Salis C, Linden D (2018) A novel, fast and efficient single-sensor automatic sleep-stage classification based on complementary cross-frequency coupling estimates. Clin Neurophysiol 129(4):815–828

38. Khalighi S, Sousa T, Santos JM, Nunes U (2016) ISRUC-Sleep: a comprehensive public dataset for sleep researchers. Comput Methods Programs Biomed 124:180–192

39. Robnik-Šikonja M, Kononenko I (2003) Theoretical and empirical analysis of ReliefF and RReliefF. Mach Learn 53:23–69

40. Shabani F, Kumar L, Solhjouy-Fard S (2017) Variances in the projections, resulting from CLIMEX, boosted regression trees and random forests techniques, Theor Appl Climatol, 1–14

41. Sanders TH, McCurry M, Clements MA (2014) Sleep stage classification with cross frequency coupling. In: Proceedings of 36th annual international conference of the IEEE engineering in medicine and biology (EMBC), pp 4579–4582

42. Bajaj V, Pachori RB (2013) Automatic classification of sleep stages based on the time-frequency image of EEG signals. Comput Methods Progr Biomed 112(3):320–328

43. Hsu Y-L, Yang Y-T, Wang J-S, Hsu C-Y (2013) Automatic sleep stage recurrent neural classifier using energy features of EEG signals. Neurocomputing 104:105–114

44. Yildiz A, Akin M, Poyraz M, Kirbas G (2009) Application of adaptive neuro-fuzzy inference system for vigilance level estimation by using wavelet-entropy feature extraction. Expert Syst Appl 36(4):7390–7399

45. Powers DM (2011) Evaluation: from precision, recall and f-measure to roc, informedness, markedness and correlation

46. Gunnarsdottir KM, Gamaldo CE, Salas RME, Ewen JB, Allen RP, Sarma SV (2018) A novel sleep stage scoring system: combining expert-based rules with a decision tree classifier. In: 2018 40th annual international conference of the IEEE engineering in medicine and biology society (EMBC)

47. Yuan Y, Jia K, Ma F (2018) Multivariate sleep stage classification using hybrid self-attentive deep learning networks. In: IEEE international conference on bioinformatics and biomedicine (BIBM)

48. Huang W, Guo B, Shen Y, Tang X, Zhang T, Li D, Jiang Z (2019) Sleep staging algorithm based on multichannel data adding and multifeature screening. Comput Methods Progr Biomed

49. Yildirim O, Baloglu U, Acharya U (2019) A deep learning model for automated sleep stages classification using PSG signals. Int J Environ Res Public Health 16(4):599

Improved Performance Guarantees for Orthogonal Matching Pursuit and Application to Dimensionality Reduction

Munnu Sonkar, Latika Tiwari, and C. S. Sastry

1 Introduction

Compressed sensing (CS) [1] is an effective technique that provides a sparse signal representation for an undetermined linear system of equations. There exist several greedy as well as convex optimization methods for finding such sparse solutions. Among the sparse signal recovery solvers, Orthogonal Matching Pursuit (OMP) is very popular. The performance guarantee of OMP has been studied in terms of restricted isometry constant (RIC), null-space property, and mutual coherence of the associated sensing matrix. However, in general, computing the RIC of the sensing matrix and establishing the null-space property are hard problems. On the other hand, besides being easily computable, the coherence of the sensing matrix provides a bound on the sparsity (number of nonzero components in the solution to be recovered) towards guaranteeing the success of the greedy OMP. But this bound (detailed in the next section) is known to be pessimistic. In view of this, the present work aims at providing an improved theoretical bound for the success of OMP. We realize our objective via preconditioning. The systems $y = Ax$ and $Gy = GAx$ admit the same set of solutions for an invertible and well-conditioned matrix G. But the coherences of A and GA can be different, implying thereby different coherence-based recovery bounds of OMP for both the systems. Due to the stated equality between the solution sets of both the systems, the improved OMP-recovery bound of new system automatically

M. Sonkar (✉) · L. Tiwari · C. S. Sastry
Department of Mathematics, Indian Institute of Technology Hyderabad, Sangareddy,
Telangana, India
e-mail: ma17resch01001@iith.ac.in

C. S. Sastry
e-mail: csastry@iith.ac.in

© The Author(s), under exclusive license to Springer Nature Singapore Pte Ltd. 2021
M. K. Bajpai et al. (eds.), *Machine Vision and Augmented Intelligence—Theory
and Applications*, Lecture Notes in Electrical Engineering 796,
https://doi.org/10.1007/978-981-16-5078-9_19

holds true for the old system $y = Ax$ as well. In this work, we determine the well-behaved G via a convex optimization in such a way that the sparse recovery guarantees for OMP get improved. The major contributions of this paper may be summarized as follows:

1. Improving recovery guarantees for OMP via preconditioning and providing the conditions on the preconditioner that result in improved bound.
2. Proposing and then solving a convex optimization problem for determining the preconditioner.
3. Demonstrating the efficacy of analytical guarantees empirically towards dimensionality reduction.

The rest of the paper is organized as follows. Sections 2 and 3, respectively, present the basics of Compressed Sensing and a summary of contribution of this paper. While the next two sections, respectively, discuss the proof of improved recovery bound and an optimization problem that finds the preconditioner. Finally, the paper ends with the numerical results and concluding remarks in the last two sections.

2 Compressed Sensing

The undetermined linear system of equations

$$y = Ax, \tag{1}$$

in general, possesses infinitely many solutions, where $A \in \mathbf{R}^{m \times n}$ is a full-rank matrix. Several criteria on solutions give rise to solutions possessing several properties. For instance, imposing minimum norm criterion results in the pseudo inverse solution, which is in general dense. For various applications, one might be interested in obtaining a solution that contains a very few number components. The problem of obtaining such a solution is posed as the following optimization problem:

$$(P_0) \min \|x\|_0 \text{ subject to } y = Ax, \tag{2}$$

which is often referred to as a 0-norm problem. Here, $\|x\|_0$ stands for the number of nonzero components in x. Due to its combinatorial nature, the P_0 problem becomes intractable in high dimensions. A convex relaxation of P_0 problem has been formulated as

$$(P_1) \min \|x\|_1 \text{ subject to } y = Ax, \tag{3}$$

which is referred to as the 1-norm minimization problem. The coherence $\mu(A)$ of a matrix A is the largest absolute normalized inner-product between two different columns of it, that is,

$$\mu(A) = \max_{1 \le i,j \le n, i \ne j} \frac{|a_i^T a_j|}{\|a_i\|_2 \|a_j\|_2},$$

where a_i denotes the i-th column in A. For a k sparse vector x, it is known [2] that the following inequality holds:

$$(1 - (k-1)\mu)\|x\|_2^2 \le \|Ax\|_2^2 \le (1 + (k-1)\mu)\|x\|_2^2. \tag{4}$$

Suppose δ_k is such that $\delta_k \le 1 + (k-1)\mu$. Then, one obtains the following inequality, referred to as the Restricted Isometry Property (RIP)

$$(1 - \delta_k)\|x\|_2^2 \le \|Ax\|_2^2 \le (1 + \delta_k)\|x\|_2^2 \forall \|x\|_0 \le k \tag{5}$$

The sufficient conditions implying the equivalence between the P_0 and P_1 problems have been established through null-space property, restricted isometry property [2]. Two classes of algorithms, viz convex optimization and greedy methods, exist for obtaining the sparse solution of an underdetermined system. Among all solvers, despite being heuristic, Orthogonal Matching Pursuit is very simple and popular. The pseudo-code of OMP is shown in a table below.

Algorithm 1: The pseduo-code of OMP
Data: A, y
Result: x such that $y \approx Ax$ and $\|x\|_0 \le k$
1   initialization: $r_0 = y$, $\Lambda_0 = \emptyset$, $l = 1$;
2   normalize columns of A: $A = [\frac{a_1}{\|a_1\|_2}, \dots, \frac{a_n}{\|a_n\|_2}]$;
3   **while** $l \le k$ **do**
4        $z = |A^T r_{l-1}|$;
5        $\Lambda_l = \Lambda_{l-1} \cup z(k)$;
6        $xl =_{z: supp(z) \subseteq \Lambda l} \| y - Az\|$;
7        $r_l = y - Ax_l$;
8        $l = l + 1$;
9   **end**

The following Theorem 1, however, establishes the performance guarantee of OMP:

Theorem 1 *For a system of linear equations $A x = b$ ($A \in \mathbf{R}^{m \times n}$ full-rank with $m < n$), if a solution x exists obeying.*

$$\|x\|_0 < \frac{1}{2}\left(1 + \frac{1}{\mu}\right), \tag{6}$$

OMP run with threshold parameter $\epsilon = 0$ is guaranteed to find it exactly.

3 Contribution of Present Work

It has been established empirically that the bound in (6) being sufficient is, in general, very pessimistic [3, 4], and that well beyond it, the recovery performance of OMP can be good. An RIP-based improvement has been proposed in [3]. The present work, however, aims at improving the bound on k in (6) by considering an equivalent system $Gy = GA\,x$, where G is an invertible and well-conditioned matrix. We determine G such that

$$\frac{1+\mu}{\mu} < \frac{\lambda_2 + \lambda_1\mu(GA)}{\lambda_2 - \lambda_1 + \lambda_1\mu(GA)} \tag{7}$$

follows. Here λ_2 and λ_1 are the maximum and minimum eigen values of $(GG^T)^{-1}$, respectively. In view of the equivalence of $Ax = y$ and $GAx = Gy$, if at all G exists and satisfies (7), Theorem 1 may be restated as follows:

Theorem 2 *For a system of linear equations $Ax = b$ ($A \in \mathbf{R}^{m \times n}$ full-rank with $m <$ n), if a solution x exists obeying.*

$$\|x\|_0 < \frac{1}{2}\left(\frac{\lambda_2 + \lambda_1\mu(GA)}{\lambda_2 - \lambda_1 + \lambda_1\mu(GA)}\right), \tag{8}$$

OMP run with threshold parameter $\epsilon = 0$ is guaranteed to find it exactly for a suitable preconditioner G such that $\|Ga_i\|_2 = 1 \ \forall \ i \in \{1,2,...,n\}$ and $\frac{\lambda_2}{\lambda_1} \in (1,2)$, where λ_1 and λ_2 stand for the minimum and maximum eigen values of $(GG^T)^{-1}$, respectively.

In [5–7], a projection matrix G has been obtained such that the Gram matrix of the projected matrix GA is close to the identity matrix, which has resulted in a new system with small coherence. In [8], the authors have transformed a given sensing system into a new equivalent sensing system by multiplying a non-singular matrix G, which is suitable for finding a sparse solution numerically. These works have remained focused on reducing the coherence of the given sensing matrix. The present work, nevertheless, aims at improving the bound in (6) while carefully reducing the coherence of the sensing matrix. In particular, we realize our objective by proposing a convex optimization problem (stated in (19)) that results in G satisfying (7), implying thus that (8) is an improved bound.

4 Improved Recovery Bound

In this section, we prove Theorem 2. To begin with, we deduce the following relations for using in the proof of our main result. Since

$$x^T X y = \frac{1}{2}\{x^T X x + y^T X y - (x - y)^T X(x - y)\},$$

we have

$$\frac{1}{2}\{\lambda_1 \|x\|^2 + \lambda_1 \|y\|^2 - \lambda_2 \|x - y\|^2\} \leq x^T X y$$

$$\leq \frac{1}{2}\{\lambda_2 \|x\|^2 + \lambda_2 \|y\|^2 - \lambda_1 \|x - y\|^2\},$$

which implies that

$$\frac{1}{2}\{\lambda_1 \|b_i\|^2 + \lambda_1 \|b_t\|^2 - \lambda_2 \|b_i - b_t\|^2\} \leq b_i^T X b_t$$

$$\leq \frac{1}{2}\{\lambda_2 \|b_i\|^2 + \lambda_2 \|b_t\|^2 - \lambda_1 \|b_i - b_t\|^2\},$$

where, $b_i = G a_i = x$, $b_t = G a_t = y$.

Suppose, without loss of generality, the sparsest solution of the linear system, $Ax = b$ is such that all the nonzero entries occur at first k_0 positions in decreasing order of the values of $|x_j|$. Consequently,

$$b = Ax = \sum_{t=1}^{k_0} x_t(a_t). \tag{9}$$

In view of the stated consideration, for all $i > k_0$, we have

$$|a_1 b| > |a_i b|$$
$$|(G a_1)^T (G^T)^{-1}(G^{-1})(Gb)| > |(G a_i)^T (G^T)^{-1}(G^{-1})(Gb)|. \tag{10}$$

From (9), we obtain

$$Gb = \sum_{t=1}^{k_0} x_t(G a_t). \tag{11}$$

By substituting (11) in (10), we deduce

$$\left| \sum_{t=1}^{k_0} x_t (G a_1)^T (G^{-1})^T G^{-1}(G a_t) \right| > \left| \sum_{t=1}^{k_0} x_t (G a_i)^T (G^{-1})^T G^{-1}(G a_t) \right|.$$

Setting $(GG^T)^{-1}$ to X and $G a_i$ to b_i $\forall i \in \{1,2,...,n\}$, we rewrite the above inequality as

$$\left| \sum_{t=1}^{k_0} x_t b_1^T X b_t \right| > \left| \sum_{t=1}^{k_0} b_i^T X b_t \right|. \tag{12}$$

Now, we obtain the lower bound for the left hand side of the above inequality as

$$\left| \sum_{t=1}^{k_0} x_t b_1^T X b_t \right| \geq |x|_1 |b_1^T X b_1| - \sum_{t=2}^{k_0} |x_t b_1^T X b_t|$$

$$\geq \left| x|_1 \lambda_1 \|b_1\|^2 - \sum_{t=2}^{k_0} |x_t| \cdot |b_1^T X b_t| \right|$$

$$= |x_1| \lambda_1 - \sum_{t=2}^{k_0} |x_t| \cdot |b_1^T X b_t|$$

$$\geq |x_1| \lambda_1 - \sum_{t=2}^{k_0} |x_t| \cdot \left[\frac{1}{2} \left\{ \lambda_2 \|b_i\|^2 + \lambda_2 \|b_t\|^2 - \lambda_1 \|b_i - b_t\|^2 \right\} \right]$$

$$= |x_1| \lambda_1 - \sum_{t=2}^{k_0} |x_t| \cdot \left[\frac{1}{2} \left\{ 2\lambda_2 - 2\lambda_1 \left(1 - b_i^T b_t \right) \right\} \right]$$

$$\geq |x_1| \lambda_1 - \sum_{t=2}^{k_0} |x_t| \cdot (\lambda_2 - \lambda_1 + \lambda_1 \mu(GA))$$

$$= |x_1| \{ \lambda_1 - (k_0 - 1)(\lambda_2 - \lambda_1 + \lambda_1 \cdot \mu(GA)) \}.$$

Similarly, an upper bound for the left hand side of (12) may be obtained as follows:

$$\left| \sum_{t=1}^{k_0} x_t b_i^T X b_t \right| \leq \sum_{t=1}^{k_0} |x_t| \cdot |b_i^T X b_t|$$

$$\leq \sum_{t=1}^{k_0} |x_t| \cdot \left\{ \frac{1}{2} \left(\lambda_2 \|b_i\|^2 + \lambda_2 \|b_t\|^2 - \lambda_1 \|b_i - b_t\|^2 \right) \right\}$$

$$= \sum_{t=1}^{k_0} |x_t| \cdot \left\{ \frac{1}{2} \left(2\lambda_2 - \lambda_1 \left(2 - 2b_i^T b_t \right) \right) \right\}$$

$$\leq \sum_{t=1}^{k_0} |x_t| \cdot (\lambda_2 - \lambda_1 + \lambda_1 \mu(GA))$$

$$\leq |x_1| \cdot k_0 \cdot (\lambda_2 - \lambda_1 + \lambda_1 \cdot \mu(GA)).$$

Suppose G is such that

$$|x_1| \{ \lambda_1 - (k_0 - 1)(\lambda_2 - \lambda_1 + \lambda_1 \cdot \mu(GA)) \} > |x_1| \cdot k_0 \cdot (\lambda_2 - \lambda_1 + \lambda_1 \cdot \mu(GA)),$$

which is same as the following inequality:

$$k_0 < \frac{1}{2}\left(\frac{\lambda_2 + \lambda_1 \mu(GA)}{\lambda_2 - \lambda_1 + \lambda_1 \mu(GA)}\right). \tag{13}$$

This is the desired bound.

As λ_2 and λ_1 are, respectively, the maximum and minimum eigen values of

$$(GG^T)^{-1}, [\kappa(G)]^2 = \kappa(GG^T)^{-1} = \frac{\lambda_2}{\lambda_1}.$$

It may be noted that (7) implies and is implied by

$$\mu(A) - \mu(GA) > \tfrac{\lambda_2}{\lambda_1} - 1, \tag{14}$$

which concludes that (7) holds whenever $\kappa(G) \in (1, \sqrt{2})$. This completes the proof of Theorem 2.

Remark 1 If G exists with desired properties, then (7) and (14), respectively, provide improvements in bound on k and a lower bound on the fall in coherence after preconditioning.

Remark 2 The bound in (13) may be restated in terms of $\kappa(G)$ as follows:

$$k_0 < \frac{1}{2}\left(\frac{[\kappa(G)]^2 + \mu(GA)}{[\kappa(G)]^2 - 1 + \mu(GA)}\right). \tag{15}$$

Consequently, if G happens to be unitary, the above bound coincides with the one in (6).

Remark 3 In this paper, we consider noiseless measurements. As G is very well behaved and invertible matrix, even in the noisy setting (that is, $y = Ax + e$ with $\|e\|$ bounded above by a small quantity), the core result of this work holds true.

5   Construction of Preconditioner G

In the previous section, we have singled out the conditions on G that imply improvement in the recovery bounds of OMP. In this section, we present an optimization problem for obtaining G. Motivated by the result in previous section, we propose to obtain G by solving the following optimization problem:

$$D_0 : \quad \min_{G \neq 0} \max_{i \neq j} \frac{|\langle Ga_i, Ga_j \rangle|}{\|Ga_i\|_2 \|Ga_j\|_2}$$

subject to

$$\kappa\left(\left(GG^T\right)^{-1}\right) \in (1, 2). \tag{16}$$

Since D_0 is non-convex due to the denominator, and in order to meet the requirement of our main result, we consider

$$||Ga_i||_2 = 1, \text{ for all } i = 1, 2, \ldots, n. \tag{17}$$

A convex relaxation problem of D_0 over a closed feasible region may be taken as follows:

$$D_1 : \quad \min_{G \neq 0} \max_{i \neq j} |\langle Ga_i, Ga_j \rangle|$$

subject to

$$1 + \varepsilon <= \kappa((GG^T)^{-1} \leq 2 - \epsilon, \tag{18}$$

for some small $\epsilon > 0$. In view of (17), the above optimization problem may be recast as follows:

$$D_2: \quad \min_Y |a_i^T Y a_j|$$
$$\text{subject to} \quad a_i^T Y a_j = 1, \forall k = 1, \ldots, n$$
$$(1 + \epsilon)I_m \leq Y \leq (2 - \epsilon)I_m, \tag{19}$$

where $Y = G^T G$. As D_2 is in standard convex optimization form, it can be solved using the CVX software. By applying Cholesky decomposition on the solution Y of D_2, one may determine G satisfying $Y = G^T G$.

6 Numerical Results

Since (7) and (14) are equivalent when $\kappa(G) \in (1, \sqrt{2})$, improvement in bound on sparsity is equivalent to the fall in coherence after preconditioning. In view of this, in this section, we demonstrate the efficacy of preconditioning in terms of reduction in coherence that preconditioning brings in.

As an example, we have generated a random matrix of column size 40 with row sizes varying from 2 to 39. For each row size, we have computed G (and hence $\mu(GA)$ along with $\mu(A)$) by solving (19). The averages of values of coherences of A and GA over 100 iterations have been reported in Fig. 1a, b. In generating these

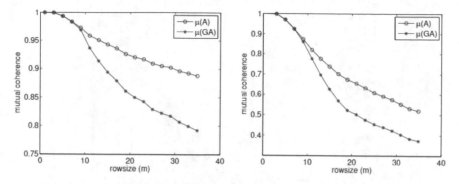

Fig. 1 A comparison of the coherences of A and GA for different row sizes, where the elements of A obey (**a**). Gaussian distribution and (**b**). Uniform distribution. These plots indicate that for certain row sizes, the fall in coherence is significant, implying thereby the improved recovery bound for OMP

plots, we have taken Gaussian and Uniform distributions for the entries of A. The x and y axes in both the plots represent row size and coherence value, respectively. It may be concluded from the plots that preconditioning brings in fall in coherence, implying thereby that (7) holds. With a view to demonstrating the implication of the improved bound, obtained via preconditioning, we have generated y as $y = Ax$, where A is a matrix of size 50×60 with its entries being drawn from Gaussian distribution. Then, we have computed the relative reconstruction errors as $\frac{\|x - x_r\|_2}{\|x\|_2}$, where x_r is the recovered solution from the pair (y, A) or (Gy, GA) via OMP, and x is the original vector. The reconstruction errors obtained from both (y, A) and (Gy, GA) via OMP, reported in Fig. 2, indicate that the improved theoretical bound translates to reduction in reconstruction error.

We now turn to the applicability of proposed theoretical development to dimensionality reduction, which deals with projecting data to a lower dimensional space for applications such as image classification and content-based image retrieval [9]. To this end, we have projected the images in Figs. 3a and 4a, which are of size 128 $\times$ 128, to the space of dimension equal to half of its original size through Gaussian matrix. That is, for a vectorized-image x and the projection matrix A with entries being drawn from a Gaussian distribution, we have generated y as $y = Ax$, where the size of y, as an example, is half of that of x. From the pairs (y, A) and (Gy, GA), the images so recovered via OMP are shown in Figs. 3b, c and 4b, c. For the test image in Fig. 3a, preconditioner improves the PSNR to 14.7415 from 11.2346. While for the one in Fig. 4a, corresponding improvement is 13.9261 from 11.1263. We have computed the PSNR error as $20 \log\left(\frac{\|x\|_\infty}{\|x - x_r\|_2}\right)$. For other reduced sizes, the improvement in reconstruction quality is shown in Table 1. The results in Figs. 3 and 4 and Table 1 vindicate that the preconditioned-OMP improves reconstruction quality, which translates to higher dimensionality reduction via preconditioning for a given error tolerance.

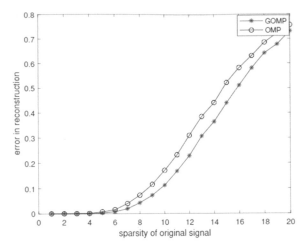

Fig. 2 The reconstruction error (average over 2500 iterations) obtained with OMP and preconditioned-OMP (abbreviated GOMP) solvers. This plot and Table 1 conclude that the OMP with preconditioned sensing matrix provides smaller reconstruction error

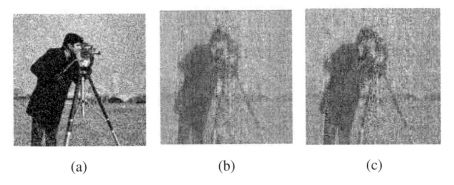

(a)   (b)   (c)

Fig. 3 For the test image in (**a**), the images in (**b**) and (**c**) have been obtained by applying OMP on (y, A) and (Gy, GA), respectively. As an example, size of y has been considered as half of that of x. That is, x has been reconstructed from half of its linearly projected samples. From (b) and (c), it can be concluded that the preconditioned-OMP provides improvement in reconstruction. Needless to say, an increase in size of y leads to an improvement in reconstruction quality

7 Conclusion

Aiming at improving the recovery guarantees of OMP, the present work has posed an optimization problem and derived conditions that imply better recovery conditions. Alongside the proof of concept, we have demonstrated the implications of proposed improved bound towards dimensionality reduction, by considering the reconstruction of a signal or an image from a small set of its linearly projected samples.

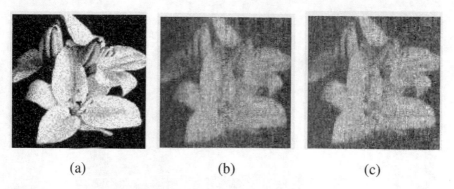

$$(a) \qquad\qquad (b) \qquad\qquad (c)$$

Fig. 4 For the test image in (**a**), the images in (**b**) and (**c**) have been obtained by applying OMP on (y, A) and (Gy, GA), respectively. As an example, size of y has been considered as half of that of x. The results shown on a different test image too vindicate the improvement that preconditioned-OMP brings in

Table 1 Improvement in PSNR with preconditioner for different values of column-to-row ratio. The test image used is Fig. 3a. This table vindicates the improvement in reconstruction quality via preconditioning

n/m	PSNR with (y,A)	PSNR with (Gy,GA)
4	10.2965	13.0610
3.04	10.5652	13.1768
2	11.2346	14.7415

Acknowledgements The first author is thankful to the MHRD, Govt. of India, for its financial support. The third author is grateful to the CSIR, Govt. of India (25(0309)/20/EMR-II) for its support.

References

1. Elad M (2010) Sparse and redundant representations: from theory to applications in signal and image processing. Springer Science & Business Media
2. Foucart S, Rauhut H (2017) A mathematical introduction to compressive sensing. Bull Am Math 54:151–165
3. Chang L-H, Wu J-Y (2014) An improved RIP-based performance guarantee for sparse signal recovery via orthogonal matching pursuit, vol 60. IEEE, pp 5702–5715
4. Schnass K (2018) Average performance of orthogonal matching pursuit (OMP) for sparse approximation. IEEE Signal Process Lett 25:1865–1869
5. Duarte-Carvajalino JM, Sapiro G (2009) Learning to sense sparse signals: simultaneous sensing matrix and scarifying dictionary optimization. IEEE Trans Image Process 18(7):1395–1408
6. Li G, Zhu Z, Yang D, Chang L, Bai H (2013) On projection matrix optimization for compressive sensing systems. IEEE Trans Signal Process 61(11):2887–2898
7. Oey E (2014) Projection matrix design for compressive sensing. In: Proceeding of Makassar international conference on electrical engineering and informatics (MICEEI), pp 124–129

8. Tsiligianni E, Kondi LP, Katsaggelos AK (2015) Preconditioning for underdetermined linear systems with sparse solutions. IEEE Signal Process Lett 22(9):1239–1243
9. Srinivas M, Naidu RR, Sastry CS, Mohan CK (2015) Content based medical image retrieval using dictionary learning. Neurocomputing 168:880–895

Epileptic Seizure Prediction from Raw EEG Signal Using Convolutional Neural Network

Ranjan Jana and Imon Mukherjee

1 Introduction

Epilepsy is a most common neurological disorder of the brain. A seizure is an unpredicted event due to abnormal electrical activity in the brain of an epilepsy patient. Seizure causes loss of awareness and disturbances of movement and sensation [1]. Hence, seizure reduces the quality of living of epilepsy patients. According to World Health Organization, 50 million people have epilepsy around the world [2]. Seizure can be controlled using anti-seizure medicine. However, anti-seizure medicines do not work effectively for one-third of epilepsy patients [3]. The medical practitioners have been predicting seizure by analyzing the EEG signals for more than 25 years [4]. EEG is the recording of the electrical activities of the brain. EEG is recorded by placing metal electrodes on the scalp. The states of the epilepsy patient can be divided into four states: ictal, preictal, interictal, and postictal [5]. Ictal state is the state during the seizure event, whereas preictal state and postictal state are the states before and after the seizure event, respectively. The normal situation of epilepsy patient is called interictal state. Hence, the identification of preictal state is the most important task for seizure prediction in advance. The patterns of the EEG signal are different for each state of epilepsy patient as shown in Fig. 1. The classification of preictal and interictal states is our crucial task for seizure prediction by analyzing the patterns of EEG signal.

In the literature, researchers have proposed different seizure prediction methods to achieve high prediction rate. Most of the researchers have applied different handcrafted features extraction techniques with some machine learning algorithms for

R. Jana · I. Mukherjee
Department of CSE, Indian Institute of Information Technology, Kalyani, India
e-mail: imon@iiitkalyani.ac.in

R. Jana (✉)
Department of IT, RCC Institute of Information Technology, Kolkata, India

© The Author(s), under exclusive license to Springer Nature Singapore Pte Ltd. 2021
M. K. Bajpai et al. (eds.), *Machine Vision and Augmented Intelligence—Theory and Applications*, Lecture Notes in Electrical Engineering 796,
https://doi.org/10.1007/978-981-16-5078-9_20

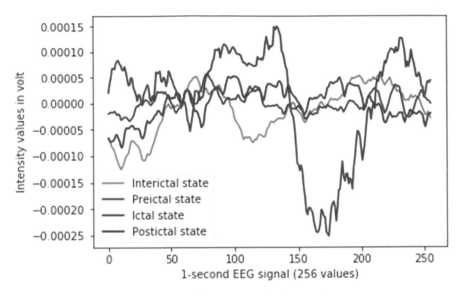

Fig. 1 Sample EEG signal patterns of different states of epilepsy patient

the classification of preictal and interictal states. The handcrafted features extraction techniques are dependent on a particular application and may be unsuitable for other applications. The invention of deep learning was a great achievement in machine learning. Deep learning techniques do not use handcrafted features. They extract most important features automatically from raw input data, which are independent of any application [6]. However, most of the researchers have used some transformation of raw EEG signal to feed the data into deep learning system. The names of some transformations are Short-Term Fourier Transform (STFT) [7], Discrete Wavelet Transform (DWT) [8], and Continuous Wavelet Transform (CWT) [9]. In this work, a patient-specific seizure prediction method is proposed using raw EEG signal without any transformation of EEG signal. A Convolutional Neural Network (CNN) is used for automatic features extraction from raw EEG signal, and it also classifies the preictal and interact states for seizure prediction. The proposed method is capable to inform epilepsy patients about the forthcoming seizure to reduce the life risk of the patients. This work is organized as follows. Section 2 provides the implementation details. The experimental results are shown in Sect. 3. Section 4 summarizes the proposed work and provides the future directions of the research work.

2 Implementation

The proposed method presents a patient-specific seizure prediction method using raw EEG signal. The following steps are applied to implement our proposed method.

2.1 Database Used

In this work, the standard CHB-MIT database [10] is used for training and testing the proposed seizure prediction model. This database is a collection of EEG recordings collected from epilepsy patients of Children's Hospital, Boston. The International 10–20 system was used for placement of electrodes on scalp. All the recordings have 23–38 channels. Most of the recordings contain 23 channels. The duration of each recording is different. The durations of all the recordings are within 1–4 h. There are 256 values for each 1-s EEG signal of each channel. The values are represented in volt. The database consists of 535 non-seizure recordings and 129 seizure recordings.

2.2 Preprocessing of Raw EEG Signal

The classification of preictal and interictal states is our main aim to predict the seizure in advance. The duration of 1-s EEG signal with 22 channels is considered as one sample. A 1-s EEG signal represents 256 values for each channel. Hence, each sample is represented by a 2-D matrix of size 22×256 as shown in Fig. 2. The element D_{ij} of the matrix is represented by jth signal intensity value of ith channel. The normal range of the intensity values of EEG signal is -10^{-4} to $+10^{-4}$, which is extremely

$$
\begin{pmatrix}
D_{1,1} & D_{1,2} & D_{1,3} & \cdots & D_{1,255} & D_{1,256} \\
D_{2,1} & D_{2,2} & D_{2,3} & \cdots & D_{2,255} & D_{2,256} \\
D_{3,1} & D_{3,2} & D_{3,3} & \cdots & D_{3,255} & D_{3,256} \\
\cdot & \cdot & \cdot & \cdots & \cdot & \cdot \\
\cdot & \cdot & \cdot & \cdots & \cdot & \cdot \\
\cdot & \cdot & \cdot & \cdots & \cdot & \cdot \\
D_{21,1} & D_{21,2} & D_{21,3} & \cdots & D_{21,255} & D_{21,256} \\
D_{22,1} & D_{22,2} & D_{22,3} & \cdots & D_{22,255} & D_{22,256}
\end{pmatrix}
$$

Fig. 2. 2-D representation of 1-s EEG signal with 22 channels

narrow. Hence, each intensity value is multiplied with 10^4 to get the range from -1 to $+1$ for faster convergence of the proposed seizure prediction network.

2.3   Features Extraction and Classification

The CNN is a powerful deep learning technique that is competent to extract the most important features from the input data [11, 12]. Here, a CNN is used for important features extraction from raw EEG signal to classify preictal and interictal states for seizure prediction in advance. In this proposed CNN architecture, five convolutional layers and five maxpool layers are used for features extraction, and two fully connected layers are used for features classification as shown in Fig. 3. In the first fully connected layer, the ReLU activation function is used, while the softmax activation function is used in the second fully connected layer, to get the two class probabilities of interictal and preictal state.

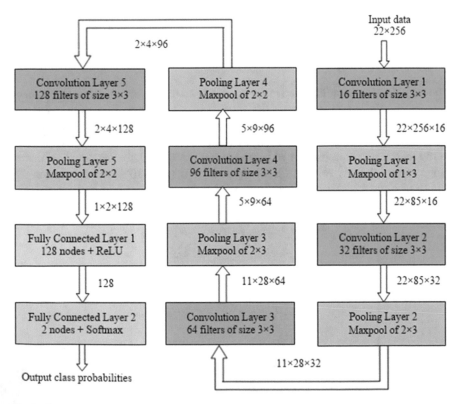

Fig. 3 Proposed CNN architecture

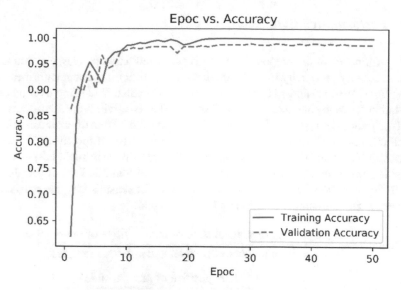

Fig. 4 Training and validation accuracy versus number of epochs

2.4 Training and Testing Method

For simplicity, only 11 patients are considered based on fixed 22 channels of EEG recordings. EEG data before 10 min (600 s) of the seizure event is taken from each seizure recording as preictal samples. Hence, total 1200 preictal samples of 1-s EEG signal are taken for training and validation checking by considering two seizure recordings from each patient. For equal consideration of preictal and interictal states, total 1200 interictal samples of 1-s EEG signal are taken randomly from two non-seizure recordings of each patient. Hence, total number of preictal and interictal samples is 2400. Only 80% of total samples are used for training, and the remaining 20% are used for validation checking. The proposed CNN gets stability after 30 epochs in most of cases as shown in Fig. 4. Hence, only 50 epochs are considered for training the network. Total 49 seizure recordings are considered to calculate the average sensitivity for performance evaluation of the proposed CNN. The average specificity is calculated by considering 40 non-seizure recordings of 81.7 h.

3 Experimental Results

In this section, initially the performance of the proposed method is measured using the sample duration of 1-s EEG signal. Then, the majority voting technique is applied to increase the performance of the proposed method. Finally, a comparative study is done with some previous works.

3.1 Performance Evaluation

The performance of the proposed method is evaluated based on classification accuracy, sensitivity, specificity, and false prediction rate (FPR). The accuracy is measured using Eq. (1). The average classification accuracy is calculated using fivefold cross validation for each patient as shown in Table 1. The sensitivities are measured using Eq. (2) by considering the EEG signal before 10 min and 20 min of seizure event. The specificity and FPR are measured using Eq. (3) and Eq. (4), respectively. The sensitivity, specificity, and FPR of our proposed method are shown in Table 1. The average classification accuracy is 93.80% with a specificity of 86.92%, FPR of 0.1308, and sensitivity of 90.04% before 10 min of seizure event. The results are quite satisfactory by considering the sample duration of 1-s EEG signal.

$$\text{Accuracy} = \frac{\text{True positive of preictal state} + \text{True positive of interictal state}}{\text{Total number of preictal and interictal samples}} \tag{1}$$

$$\text{Sensitivity} = \frac{\text{True positive of preictal state}}{\text{True positive of preictal state} + \text{False positive of interical state}} \tag{2}$$

$$\text{Specificity} = \frac{\text{True positive of interictal state}}{\text{True positive of interictal state} + \text{False positive of preictal state}} \tag{3}$$

$$\text{FPR} = \frac{\text{False positive of preictal state}}{\text{True positive of interictal state} + \text{False positive of preictal state}} \tag{4}$$

Table 1 Accuracy, Sensitivity, Specificity, and FPR using 1-s's sample

Patient ID	Accuracy	Sensitivity before		Specificity	FPR
		10 min	20 min		
Chb01	0.9929	0.9500	0.7767	0.9729	0.0271
Chb02	0.9238	0.9667	0.9458	0.8141	0.1859
Chb03	0.9961	0.9667	0.9458	0.9628	0.0372
Chb04	0.9646	0.9438	0.9688	0.9080	0.0920
Chb05	0.8733	0.8708	0.8833	0.8044	0.1956
Chb06	0.9004	0.8302	0.7125	0.8627	0.1373
Chb07	0.9604	0.9583	0.9958	0.8472	0.1528
Chb08	0.9929	0.9800	0.9817	0.9233	0.0767
Chb09	0.9684	0.8896	0.8750	0.8653	0.1347
Chb10	0.8333	0.7736	0.7958	0.6692	0.3308
Chb23	0.9121	0.7750	0.6383	0.9312	0.0688
Mean	**0.9380**	**0.9004**	**0.8654**	**0.8692**	**0.1308**

Table 2 Sensitivity using majority voting technique

Patient ID	Sensitivity before 10 min			Sensitivity before 20 min		
	30 samples	60 samples	120 samples	30 samples	60 samples	120 samples
Chb01	1.0000	1.0000	1.0000	0.8500	0.8000	0.8000
Chb02	1.0000	1.0000	1.0000	1.0000	1.0000	1.0000
Chb03	1.0000	1.0000	1.0000	1.0000	1.0000	1.0000
Chb04	1.0000	1.0000	1.0000	1.0000	1.0000	1.0000
Chb05	1.0000	1.0000	1.0000	1.0000	1.0000	1.0000
Chb06	0.9063	0.8750	0.8750	0.7500	0.7500	0.7500
Chb07	1.0000	1.0000	1.0000	1.0000	1.0000	1.0000
Chb08	1.0000	1.0000	1.0000	1.0000	1.0000	1.0000
Chb09	1.0000	1.0000	1.0000	0.8750	0.8750	1.0000
Chb10	0.9167	0.9167	0.8333	1.0000	1.0000	1.0000
Chb23	0.9000	1.0000	1.0000	0.8000	0.8000	0.8000
Mean	**0.9748**	**0.9811**	**0.9735**	**0.9341**	**0.9295**	**0.9409**

3.2 Majority Voting Technique

As suggested by medical experts, a 1-s EEG signal is not sufficient to identify the correct state of the epilepsy patient. Hence, majority voting of consecutive n samples is considered to take better decision for identification of correct state. This majority voting technique is applied to get better sensitivity, specificity, and FPR by using consecutive 30 samples, 60 samples, and 120 samples. Two sensitivities are calculated, one for the EEG data before 10 min and another for the EEG data before 20 min of the seizure event. The average sensitivity for the EEG data before 10 min of the seizure event using consecutive 120 samples is 97.35%, as shown in Table 2. The average specificity and FPR using consecutive 120 samples are 93.49% and 0.0651, respectively, as shown in Table 3. It is found that the majority voting technique provides better sensitivity, specificity, and FPR compared with the consideration of one sample to identify the correct state of epilepsy patient.

3.3 Comparison with Other Research Works

The experimental results of the proposed method are compared with some recent previous works for performance evaluation as shown in Table 4. All the previous works mentioned in the comparison table have also used the standard CHB-MIT database. Most of the researchers have applied some transformations of EEG signal to feed the data into the seizure prediction system. The transformations are DWT [8], STFT [7, 14], Wavelet packet decomposition (WPD) [15], spectral band power (SBP), and statistical moment (SM) [13]. Whereas Jana et al. have used only images of EEG

Table 3 Specificity and FPR using majority voting technique

Patient ID	Specificity			FPR/hour		
	30 samples	60 samples	120 samples	30 samples	60 samples	120 samples
Chb01	0.9933	1.0000	1.0000	0.0067	0.0000	0.0000
Chb02	0.9183	0.9600	0.9867	0.0817	0.0400	0.0133
Chb03	0.9792	0.9792	0.9917	0.0208	0.0208	0.0083
Chb04	0.9826	0.9917	0.9944	0.0174	0.0083	0.0056
Chb05	0.9313	0.9542	0.9833	0.0687	0.0458	0.0167
Chb06	0.8542	0.8528	0.8500	0.1458	0.1472	0.1500
Chb07	0.8472	0.8444	0.8472	0.1528	0.1556	0.1528
Chb08	0.9283	0.9267	0.9267	0.0717	0.0733	0.0733
Chb09	0.8923	0.8985	0.8969	0.1077	0.1015	0.1031
Chb10	0.7931	0.8333	0.8500	0.2069	0.1667	0.1500
Chb23	0.9451	0.9504	0.9574	0.0549	0.0496	0.0426
Mean	**0.9150**	**0.9265**	**0.9349**	**0.0850**	**0.0735**	**0.0651**

Table 4 Comparison with other Seizure Prediction Methods

Reference	Feature extraction	Learning technique	Accuracy	Sensitivity	Specificity
Kitano et al. [8]	DWT	SOM	0.911	0.9809	0.8799
Ozcan et al. [13]	SBP and SM	3DCNN	–	0.857	FPR = 0.096
Usman et al. [14]	STFT	SVM	–	0.927	0.908
Zhang et al. [15]	WPD	CNN	0.9	0.922	FPR = 0.12
Jana et al. [16]	Image of EEG signal	DenseNet	0.9066	0.97	0.9587 FPR = 0.0413
Qin et al. [17]	STFT	CNN with extreme learning machine	–	0.9585	FPR = 0.045
Proposed method	Raw EEG data	CNN	**0.938**	**0.9735**	**0.9349** **FPR = 0.0651**

signal without using any transformation of EEG signal [16]. The most commonly used learning techniques are SOM [8], CNN [7, 9, 15], DenseNet [16], and SVM [14]. In this work, only raw EEG data are used to feed the data into CNN for automatic features extraction and classification of preictal and ictal states for seizure prediction. The proposed method provides the average classification accuracy of 93.8%, and the specificity of 93.49% with FPR of 0.0651. It provides the sensitivity of 97.35% before

10 min of seizure event which is one of the most efficient among others as shown in Table 4.

4 Conclusion and Future Research Directions

The proposed method presents a patient-specific seizure prediction technique using raw EEG signal. The CNN is used for automatic features extraction from raw EEG signal for the classification of preictal and interictal states to predict seizure in advance. This method provides a sensitivity of 97.35%, a specificity of 93.49%, and a FPR of 0.0651. It predicts seizure 10 min in advance to avoid life threats of epilepsy patients. Developing a patient-independent seizure prediction will be a challenging task due to unique patterns of EEG signal for each individual. In future, we will try to develop a patient-independent seizure prediction system in spite of unique EEG signal patterns. In this proposed method, 22 channels have been used for seizure prediction. However, implementation of a transportable seizure prediction device using 22 channels will not be suitable. The seizure prediction device using more channels will also consume more power which will not be run for a long time for each power recharge. In future, our research direction will be implementation of a seizure prediction device using minimum number of channels of EEG signal which will be transportable and power efficient.

References

1. Mohseni HR, Maghsoudi A, Shamsollahi MB (2006) Seizure detection in EEG signals: a comparison of different approaches. In: 2006 international conference of the ieee engineering in medicine and biology society, New York, pp 6724–6727
2. World Health Organization (2020) https://www.who.int/. Accessed 15 January, 2020
3. Epilepsy Foundation (2020) https://www.epilepsy.com/. Accessed 21 March, 2020
4. Gadhoumi K, Lina J, Mormann F, Gotman J (2016) Seizure prediction for therapeutic devices: a review. J Neurosci Methods 260:270–282
5. Elgohary S, Eldawlatly S, Khalil . (2016) Epileptic seizure prediction using zero-crossings analysis of EEG wavelet detail coefficients. In: IEEE conference on computational intelligence in bioinformatics and computational biology, Thailand, pp 1–6
6. Bengio Y, Courville A, Vincent P (2013) Representation learning: a review and new perspectives. IEEE Trans Pattern Anal Mach Intell 35(8):1798–1828
7. Truong ND, Nguyen AD, Kuhlmann L, Bonyadi MR, Yang J, Ippolito S, Kavehei O (2018) Convolutional neural networks for seizure prediction using intracranial and scalp electroencephalogram. Neural Netw 105:104–111
8. Kitano LAS, Sousa MAA, Santos SD, Pires R, Thome-Souza S, Campo AB (2018) Epileptic seizure prediction from EEG signals using unsupervised learning and a polling-based decision process. In: International conference on artificial neural networks, Rhodes, Greece, pp 117–126
9. Khan H, Marcuse L, Fields M, Swann K, Yener B (2018) Focal onset seizure prediction using convolutional networks. IEEE Trans Biomed Eng 65(9):2109–2118

10. Goldberger AL, Amaral LAN, Glass L, Hausdorff JM, Ivanov P, Mark RG, Mietus JE, Moody GB, Peng C, Stanley HE (2020) PhysioBank, PhysioToolkit, and PhysioNet: components of a new research resource for complex physiologic signals. Circulation 101(23):e215–e220
11. Lecun Y, Bengio Y (1995) Convolutional networks for images, speech, and time-series
12. Jana R, Bhattacharyya S, Das S (2020) Patient-specific seizure prediction using the convolutional neural networks. In: Advances in intelligent systems and computing, vol 1109. Springer, Singapore, pp 51–60
13. Ozcan AR, Erturk S (2019) Seizure prediction in scalp EEG using 3D convolutional neural networks with an image-based approach. IEEE Trans Neural Syst Rehabil Eng 27(11):2284–2293
14. Usman SM, Khalid S, Aslam MH (2020) Epileptic seizures prediction using deep learning techniques. IEEE Access 8:39998–40007
15. Zhang Y, Guo Y, Yang P, Chen W, Lo B (2020) Epilepsy seizure prediction on EEG using common spatial pattern and convolutional neural network. IEEE J Biomed Health Inform 24(2):465–474
16. Jana R, Bhattacharyya S, Das S (2019) Epileptic seizure prediction from EEG signals using DenseNet. In: IEEE symposium series on computational intelligence (SSCI), Xiamen, China, pp 604–609
17. Qin Y, Zheng H, Chen W, Qin Q, Han C, Che Y (2020) Patient-specific seizure prediction with scalp EEG using convolutional neural network and extreme learning machine. In: 39th Chinese control conference (CCC), Shenyang, China, pp 7622–7625

Social Media Big Data Analytics: Security Vulnerabilities and Defenses

Sonam Srivastava and Yogendra Narain Singh

1 Introduction

Defining trend of today's world is the global connectivity to the Internet. Mobile technologies, including social networks, Internet-of-Things (IoT), and customized services suffer from heavy user utilization. Enormous datasets are created from numerous websites, repositories of multimedia, social networks, and IoT linking a range of devices and sensors. Thus, vast volumes of data are constantly gathered, processed, analyzed, and used by individuals and organizations on multiple channels, including the cloud [1]. The influence of social networking is that the number of globally active social media users would be raised to 3.43 billion monthly by 2023 [2]. The social networking platforms include Facebook, YouTube, WhatsApp, Instagram, etc. [3]. Facebook is the most widespread social network worldwide, with an active user count of 2.7 billion [4].

Social media big data has recently become a budding concept with a substantial influence which transforms businesses worldwide. It is a term used for such a vast array of datasets, possessing specific features such as incredibly enormous, fast-moving, multi-source origin, unstructured, and useful. These features describe the four prominent characteristics of big data, i.e., volume, velocity, variety, veracity, and value [5]. Social media big data analytics is regarded as a contemporary and useful tool for analyzing complicated data to uncover trends that could aid in their successful decision-making [6]. The process of social media analytics employs the following stages, i.e., data acquisition, preprocessing, data representation, analysis, and presentation [6]. It plays a vital role in future data processing and operations in diverse sectors such as healthcare, manufacturing, traffic management, education, and transportation.

S. Srivastava (✉) · Y. N. Singh
Institute of Engineering and Technology, Dr. APJ Abdul, Kalam Technical University, Lucknow, Uttar Pradesh 226 021, India

© The Author(s), under exclusive license to Springer Nature Singapore Pte Ltd. 2021   245
M. K. Bajpai et al. (eds.), *Machine Vision and Augmented Intelligence—Theory and Applications*, Lecture Notes in Electrical Engineering 796,
https://doi.org/10.1007/978-981-16-5078-9_21

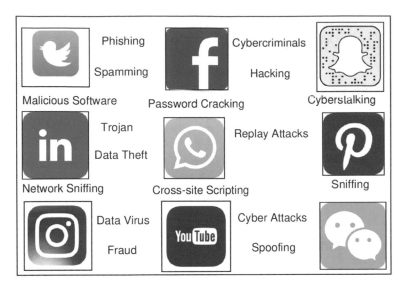

Fig.1 Social media big data security vulnerabilities

Users employ social media platforms to communicate with friends, peers, employers, colleagues, or folks with same interests. Social media serves users with disparate purposes, i.e., entertainment, profit generation, professional networking, career searches, marketing of products, etc. Nowadays, organizations embrace social media big data like never before and employ robust analytical techniques to improve decision-making, find prospects, and maximize efficiency. Being an integral part of people's daily lives, it gives rise to numerous social media big data security concerns. With the enormous growth of data generation, social networking sites face various security vulnerabilities as shown in Fig. 1. For example, theft of user accounts or passwords, spoofing, malware, phishing, fiscal fraud, and spamming are some of the threats to social networks [7]. Social media big data security is the method of safeguarding data and analytics processes against the variety of causes that could threaten the confidentiality [8].

This paper presents an evaluation of security vulnerabilities of social media big data analytics framework and their defenses. Data security is a systematic, ongoing obligation that needs to become an integral part of analytics process of social media big data. This paper presents various risks that are encountered in the distinct stages of social media analytics, i.e., data acquisition, preprocessing, data representation, analysis, and presentation. Securing data requires a comprehensive approach across disparate structures to defend enterprises from a complex threat environment. Securing social media data has several problems that can threaten its privacy. Challenges to secure social media big data are in no way only confined to social media platforms but also to the cloud. Latest technologies for active developments include advanced computational tools for non-relational databases handling unstructured data. Mature authenticating solutions efficiently secure data access and storage. Since, most big data platforms are cluster-based, spanning many nodes and servers, creates numerous vulnerabilities. There are chances of data loss and disclosure in social media big data if the owner does not periodically upgrade security for the environment. These challenges stimulate new technologies and testing initiatives to recognize open questions that pave the way for future research and practice. In accordance with this objective, this paper proposes the defensive strategies to counteract the vulnerabilities of social media analytics framework.

Rest of the paper is organized as follows. The literature review of security issues of social media big data analytics is given in Sect. 2. The security vulnerabilities in social media analytics framework are presented in Sect. 3. Subsequently, their defense and countermeasures are outlined in Sect. 4. Finally, the conclusion is drawn in Sect. 5.

2 Literature Review

Social media big data that refers to a vast array of very large and complicated datasets is facing significant security and privacy concerns. Its typical characteristics are huge size, high velocity, multiple forms, and unstructured nature. Thus, conventional protection and privacy systems are insufficient to cope up with the accelerated data growth in such a dynamic distributed computing environment. Venkatraman et al., have established the existing trends in big data by recognizing the 11 Vs as big data characteristics having an impact on the imminent security problem [9]. They have mapped the identified Vs to the three stages of big data life cycle to excavate the big data security aspects.

Social media platforms have enhanced personal information transparency by making more information accessible online. Irrespective of the security monitoring measures, cyber criminals still find ways to conduct malicious activities. These involve attacking computer servers, data stealing, engaging in phishing activities, cyberbullying, etc. Normally, the threats over the social networking sites spread comparatively faster than other forms of attacks due to trust among the network users. In this context, Deliri et al., have reviewed the most common attacks to online social networks [7]. They have addressed certain countermeasures that can be used against these attacks. Fire et al., have presented an overview of various security and privacy threats which risk the safety of users, especially children [10]. The authors have also listed the existing solutions that could render better protection and security to social media users. Various social media platforms have also challenged ethical aspects regarding security and privacy of user information. The authors Hajli and Lin have examined the security of social networks by considering the users' control over their information exchange behavior [11].

Evidently, the increasing cyber-attacks are posing serious risk to the digital world. The use of social media by people and corporations is skyrocketing. So, the authors Das and Patel have focused on cyber security issues for social networking sites [12]. Their work also proposes some appropriate strategies for a cyber-safe digital environment that can be implemented by individual consumers and government in partnership with the private sector. Rathore et al., have studied threats that arise due to sharing of multimedia content on social networking sites [13]. Their work also explores responsive approaches to accomplish the goal of a trustworthy and stable community of social networks.

3 Security Vulnerabilities in Social Media Analytics

An incident that simultaneously affects the data from multiple sources may be considered a threat to a big data asset. Depending upon different scenarios, different types of vulnerabilities occur in a general digital data analytics frame- work. The likelihood of system vulnerabilities, their nature, and consequences that violate the security of the analytics process have been analyzed for an automated recognition system [14]. In particular, the integrity can be compromised at one or more stages of the analytics framework, i.e., data acquisition, storage, data preprocessing, representation, analysis, and presentation. Generally, the risks that can impact a system during its lifespan can also cause certain steps in a system to fail. Threats such as faults, failures, or attacks on the supporting networks may have a huge effect on social media big data. ENISA 2016 report identified two distinct categories of threats, i.e., big data breach and big data leak [15]. Breach is when the data is stolen by breaking the information and communication technology systems. Whereas, data leak is referred as the complete or partial disclosure of big data asset at a certain point of its lifecycle. Briefly, we present a practical scenario of security threats and their mapping to different stages of social media big data analytics framework as shown in Fig. 2.

The enormous amount of data is generated from online sources. A fraction of the acquired data is structured, whereas most of it is either unstructured or semistructured that need real-time analysis. Due to huge size, high velocity, and variability, the acquired data is vulnerable to security threats. Traditional security approaches that implement encryption methods are usually not suitable for all source types from which big data collection takes place because of data diversity. Spoofing is a common practice while acquired data is disguised from an unknown source as being from a known and trusted source. Cybercriminals intentionally put the fabricated data into the actual data that compromises the efficiency of the big data research [16]. The high speed of data acquisition causes difficulty in monitoring traffic in real-time as it is streamed through the storage [17]. The heterogeneous data has discrepancies in data formats, speed, and forms contributing to security risks. In addition, such issues cause persistent threats to be carried in with big data. Since, these threat codes are implicitly present in the acquired data, it is difficult to detect them. Thus, hackers easily attack the data. Therefore, advanced security, authentication, and privacy must be enforced during data acquisition.

Data storage manages and preserves data acquired from distinctive sources. This enables the stakeholders of the organization to have quick access to the data whenever needed. Since, traditional warehouses cannot sufficiently store huge amounts of data,

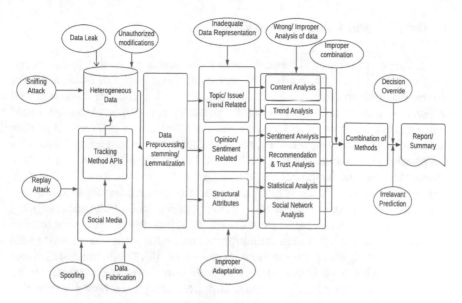

Fig. 2 Security vulnerabilities in social media big data analytics framework

cloud and big data servers are required to cope with the accommodation. Thus, data integrity is put at stake when multiple operations are performed on same data storage in huge quantity and high speed. Conventional encryption measures may not help in such a situation, and sniffers gain entry into the servers exploiting its vulnerabilities. Any data abuse may contribute to privacy breach. Unauthorized metadata modifications lead to inaccurate data sets, which will make it harder to locate the much-needed details. Therefore, it is important to develop new trustworthy data access controls that conform to acceptable security and privacy protection systems [18]. Following the legacy patterns data must be archived at every point of the big data life cycle. Also, good backup and recovery measures must be adopted.

Hackers obfuscate malicious code to prevent detection, and evasion attacks harm the confidentiality of data and result in indiscriminate infringement of consumer policy. Recent studies have shown that during data preprocessing, attackers inject poison into the training system of feature-based machine learning algorithms to influence the collection of features. The injection of classification error deviates user's topic towards the attacker's preference [19]. The interfaces of various stages of analytics framework are targeted to modify the intermediate code and intercept the data approaching the next stage. For example, malicious code like horses or logic bombs can intercept the data generated after preprocessing [20].

Inadequate data representation would lead to its improper adaptation for further analytics steps. The relevance of big data analytics performance is de- pendent on how accurate the data is. If the data arrives from untrustworthy sources or has been tampered in the previous stages, the data analytics would lead to erroneous judgments.

4 Defense and Countermeasures

The evaluation of security vulnerabilities in social media big data analytics framework provides an insight into how to protect different stages of SMA and their intermediate channels from threats and attacks. A variety of countermeasures should be taken as measures for security defense. For example, encryption techniques need to be employed with analytics tool sets and their output data [8]. As well as with traditional large data storage formats, such as relational and non-relational databases and advanced file systems, such as the Hadoop Distributed File System, in order to prevent unauthorized modifications and any possibility of data leak [21]. Centralized key management is the very effective security practice for big data environments [22]. For example, on demand key delivery, policy driven automation, logging, and abstracting key management from key usage. Policy-driven automation handles dynamic user control layers such as multiple administrator configurations that shield the social media big data platforms from insider attacks [8]. The distributed architecture of big data imparts intrusion attempts to itself. Intrusion prevention system helps security admins to defend the big data network from attacks, and intrusion detection system quarantines the intrusion until it does serious harm.

The key concern with phishing attacks is that users might not be able to check the identity of the sender of email messages quickly and accurately. Another issue is that users cannot always correctly distinguish between legal and illegal content. Usually, a phishing attack is the outcome of the user's dependence on a specific web domain, brand, and other trust indicators [23]. One strategy to avoid phishing attacks is to use signature-based anti-spam filters that enable detection and blocking of phishing messages before users view them [24]. In order to alert users of phishing pages, anti-phishing toolbar and browser plug-ins, such as Netcraft or SpoofStick, are used [7]. For example, personalized visual information is an approach used to eliminate the risk of phishing attacks. Using customized pictures to pass online messages or selecting a hidden image to log into a website. By applying this strategy, attackers are unable to send misleading emails because they are unaware of the personalized information selected by the intended user. Message authentication is another approach to phishing attacks that gives an affirmation that messages sent to them come from trustworthy parties [10].

Sybil attacks are based on producing multiple identities through the use of social networks open membership feature [7]. Leveraging one of the main features of social media platforms, which is the trust level established among existing users is one of the defensive strategies for Sybil attacks. While searching for suspicious nodes, network nodes with fewer connections must be considered since a Sybil node cannot have a large number of connections with other network members [25]. Statistical and keyword filtering of messages is one of the most effective methods to detect spam [26]. Statistical filtering like Bayesian filters, computes statistical likelihood to assess whether or not an email is spam, depending on the number of tokens in spam or non-spam messages. Keyword spam filtering uses list of parameters to find suspicious words in the messages for determining if the message is a spam. To detect spam in online social networks, certain algorithms based on machine learning have been designed. Benevenuto has proposed an algorithm to identify video spammers by assessing the users' profiles, social activity, and uploaded videos [27]. In order to make sure that the registered user is an authentic person, there are certain authentication mechanisms. For example, captcha [28], multi-factor identification, and often even requiring the user to submit a copy of the government ID proof [29]. Facebook has recently introduced the feature that lets one know who can view one's post and profile information. It has strengthened our account security by turning on login alerts [30].

Many software vendors provide Internet security solutions, i.e., Kaspersky [31], Avira [32], Symantec [32], Panda [33], and McAfee [34] for social media users. Usually, these security suites provide anti-virus, firewall, and other levels of Internet defense that help social media users defend their computers from threats such as ransomware, clickjacking, and phishing attacks [10]. McAfee Internet security software offers protection for its users against numerous risks, such as botnets, viruses, and unsafe sites [34].

5 Conclusion

Social media platforms have enhanced the disclosure of valuable assets, including individuals' personal information, financial assets, corporate secrets, intellectual property, and digital identity. Irrespective of various protective measures adopted for securing social media big data, it might still be the victim of different kinds of security threats, such as cross-site scripting, spamming, phishing, and clickjacking. We have identified the security vulnerabilities of different stages of social media analytics framework. At all the stages, i.e., data acquisition, preprocessing, data representation, analysis, and presentation, the security risks are inevitable. Hence, an insight on the defense and countermeasures to combat these vulnerabilities in analytics process has also been outlined.

References

1. The impact of big data on innovation management By Jovana, https://innovationcloud.com/blog/the-impact-of-big-data-on-innovation-management.html/. Accessed 16 Nov 2020
2. Social media-Statistics & Facts, https://www.statista.com/topics/1164/social-networks/. accessed 20 Nov 2020
3. Srivastava S, Singh YN (2020) Big social media analytics: applications and Challenges. In: 3rd International conference on computer networks, big data and IoT to be held on 15–16 Dec, 2020, India. To appear in lecture notes on DECT. Springer, pp TBA
4. Number of social network users worldwide from 2017 to 2025, https://www.statista.com/statistics/278414/number-of-worldwide-social-network-users/. Accessed 18 Nov 2020
5. Stiglitz S, Mirbabaie M, Ross B, Neubeger C (2018) Social media analytics–challenges in topic discovery, data collection, and data preparation. Int J Inf Manage 39:156–168

6. Srivastava S, Singh MK, Singh YN (2020) Social media analytics: current trends and future prospects. In: 2nd international conference on communication and intelligent systems to be held on 26–27 Dec, 2020, India. To appear in lecture notes on networks and systems. Springer, pp TBA
7. Deliri S, Albanese M (2015) Security and privacy issues in social networks. In: Colace F, De Santo M, Moscato V, Picariello A, Schreiber F, Tanca L (eds) Data management in pervasive systems. data-centric systems and applications. Springer, Cham, pp 195–209
8. Big Data Security-Issues, Challenges, Tech & Concerns, https://www.rd-alliance.org/group/big-data-ig-data-security-and-trust-wg/wiki/big-data-security-issues-challenges-tech-concerns/. Accessed 23 Nov 2020
9. Venkatraman S, Venkatraman R (2019) Big data security challenges and strategies. AIMS Math 4(3):860–879
10. Fire M, Goldschmidt R, Elovici Y (2014) Online social networks: threats and solutions. IEEE Commun Surv Tutor 16(4):2019–2036
11. Hajli N, Lin X (2016) Exploring the security of information sharing on social networking sites: the role of perceived control of information. J Bus Ethics 133:111–123
12. Das R, Patel M (2017) Cyber security for social networking sites: Issues, challenges and solutions. Int J Res Appl Sci Eng Technol 5(4):833–838
13. Rathore S, Sharma PK, Loia V, Jeong YS, Park JH (2017) Social network security: issues, challenges, threats, and solutions. Inf Sci 421:43–69
14. Singh YN, Singh SK (2013) A taxonomy of biometric system vulnerabilities and defences. Int J Biom 5(2):137–159
15. Damiani E (2015) Toward big data risk analysis. In: IEEE international conference on big data, pp 1905–1909
16. Buried under big data: security issues, challenges, concerns, https://www.scnsoft.com/blog/big-data-security-challenges/. Accessed 24 Nov 2020
17. Kumar BA, Maninder S (2015) Data mining-based integrated network traffic visualization framework for threat detection. Neural Comput Appl 26:117–130
18. Yan Z, Ding W, Niemi V, Vasilakos AV (2016) Two schemes of privacy-preserving trust evaluation. Futur Gener Comput Syst 62:175–189
19. Xiao H, Biggio B, Brown G, Fumera G, Eckert C, Roli F (2015) Is feature selection secure against training data poisoning? In: 32nd international conference on machine learning, vol 37, pp 1689–1698
20. What is a cyber attack?, https://www.ibm.com/services/business-continuity/cyber-attack/. Accessed 28 Nov 2020
21. Bhathal GS, Singh A (2019) Big data: Hadoop framework vulnerabilities, security issues and attacks. Array 1(2):1–8
22. 8 best practices for encryption key management and data security, https://esj.com/articles/2008/07/01/8-best-practices-for-encryption-key-management-and-data-security.aspx/. Accessed 24 Nov 2020
23. Dhamija R, Tygar JD (2005) The battle against phishing: dynamic security skins. In: Proceedings of the symposium on usable privacy and security, Pittsburgh, pp 77–88
24. How to stop phishing attacks, https://www.expertinsights.com/insights/how-to-stop-phishing-attacks/
25. Viswanath B, Post A, Gummadi KP, Mislove A (2011) An analysis of social network-based sybil defenses. ACM SIGCOMM Comput Commun Rev 41(4):363–374
26. Zhang L, Zhu J (2004) An evaluation of statistical spam filtering techniques. ACM Trans Asian Lang Inf Process 3(4):243–269
27. Benevenuto F, Rodrigues T, Almeida V, Almeida J, Zhang C, Ross K (2008) Identifying video spammers in online social networks. In: Proceedings of the 4th international workshop on adversarial information retrieval on the web, pp 45–52
28. Boshmaf Y, Muslukhov I, Beznosov K, Ripeanu M (2011) The socialbot network: when bots socialize for fame and money. In: Proceedings of the 27th annual computer security applications conference, pp 93–102

29. Facebook launches verified accounts and pseudonyms, http://techcrunch.com/2012/02/15/facebook-verified-accounts-alternate-names/. Accessed 25 Nov 2020
30. Starting the decade by giving you more control over your privacy, https://about.fb.com/news/2020/01/data-privacy-day-2020/. Accessed 25 Nov 2020
31. The role of endpoint security in long-term planning, https://media.kaspersky.com/en/business-security/enterprise/kaspersky-security-for-enterprise-catalogue.pdf/. Accessed 27 Nov 2020
32. Compare Avira vs Panda Security, https://crozdesk.com/compare/avira-vs-panda-security/. Accessed 27 Nov 2020
33. WOT partners with Panda Security, https://www.mywot.com/blog/163-wot-partners-with-panda-security/. Accessed 28 Nov 2020
34. Macfee, Macfee Internet Security, http://home.mcafee.com/store/internet-security/. Accessed 26 Nov 2020

Deep Convolutional Neural Network Based Hard Exudates Detection

R. Deepa and N. K. Narayanan

1 Introduction

Sugar patients mainly suffer from a retinal disease called diabetic retinopathy. In this disease when disease starts symptoms may not exist but when disease intensity increases symptoms occurs [1]. There are mainly two stages: Non-Proliferative Diabetic Retinopathy (NPDR), the initial occurrence of Diabetic Retinopathy (DR). The unnatural growth of blood vessels called neovascularization cause Proliferative Diabetic Retinopathy (PDR) is considered as a severe condition [2]. The symptoms of the disease are Microaneurysms, Hard Exudates, Dot and Blot Hemorrhages, Cotton Wool Spots, Neovascularization, etc. In moderate case of the disease, Hard Exudates detection is needed. Hard Exudates appear as yellowish deposits with clear borders. Image without exudates and image with exudates are shown in Fig. 1a and b.

2 Review of Literature

Exudate detection is complicated due to its different types of shapes.

Choudhury et al. [2] suggested an exudate recognition method where feature extraction done by Fuzzy C Means and classification using Support Vector Machine (SVM). Efficacy obtained by the method is 97.6%

R. Deepa (✉)
Department of Information Technology, Kannur University, Kannur, Kerala, India

Department of Computer Applications, College of Engineering, Vadakara, Kozhikode, Kerala 673104, India

N. K. Narayanan
Indian Institute of Information Technology, Kottayam, Valavoor (P.O), Kerala 686635, India
e-mail: nknarayanan@iiitkottayam.ac.in

© The Author(s), under exclusive license to Springer Nature Singapore Pte Ltd. 2021
M. K. Bajpai et al. (eds.), *Machine Vision and Augmented Intelligence—Theory and Applications*, Lecture Notes in Electrical Engineering 796,
https://doi.org/10.1007/978-981-16-5078-9_22

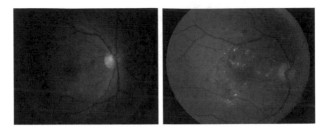

Fig. 1 **a** Image without exudates. **b** Image with exudates

Harangi et al. [3] found out an exudate detection method in which candidate extraction using grayscale morphology. Markovian segmentation is done and classification is done using SVM.

Doaa et al. [4] proposed a feature-oriented technique for exudate detection. All regions similar to exudates are segmented. Then other similar elements are removed. Morphological method for blood vessel extraction. Optic disks are removed by Hough Transform. The last step of exudates estimation is done using morphological reconstruction.

Walter et al. [5] developed exudate detection method in which optic disk was removed by morphological filtering methods and by watershed transformation methods. Sensitivity obtained by this approach is 92.8%. For the experiments, a small database was selected by authors.

Doaa et al. [6] suggested an exudate detection technique in which Hough Transform is used for optic disk removal. The blood vessels that are extracted and the optic disk is eliminated from the total image are segmented to obtain an estimation of exudates. The last step of exudates detection is morphological reconstruction. Sensitivity and specificity obtained are 80 and 100%.

Welfer et al. [7] used a mathematical morphological approach for exudate detection. The dataset used to conduct experiment is DIARET DB1. The sensitivity obtained is 70.48% and specificity is 98.84%.

Zhou et al. [8] suggested an exudate detection approach in which the images are segmented as candidate superpixels. Based on features, the classification performed is supervised multivariable classification. An optic disk detection method is also used. Experiments were done on DIARET DB1 and e-Ophtha EX datasets.

Singh, Anushikha, et al. [9] suggested an exudates detection method that combines thresholding based on intensity and morphology approach for detecting smaller exudates present and removes all false positives. The method has good accuracy.

Syed et al. [10] developed a way for detecting exudates where different combinations of features were used. SVM is used for the segmentation of exudates near the macular region. Databases used are DIARETDB1, MESSIDOR, DRIVE and a local hospital dataset. The average accuracy of all datasets obtained is 95.48%

Huan et al. [11] showed a method for detecting exudates where a combination of median filtering and dynamic clustering analysis was used. The experiments conducted show the algorithm as faster easier and effective.

Bharkad et al. [12] put forward an exudate detection technique where for optic disk (OD) extraction morphological operators are used. OD was masked in the green channel of the image to distinguish OD and exudates. Features from the green plane were taken and using machine learning technique hard exudates are identified.

Dutta et al. [13] showed a technique of exudate detection where a combination of threshold and edge detection will eliminate all noises which lead to false exudates. This method gave accurate results.

Aftab et al. [14] proposed a macular edema detection method where candidate detection is done by a filter bank. A basic exudate property was used for feature extraction and Gaussian mixture model for classification.

Ruba et al. [15] have explained an exudate detection technique where initially image resizing is done and filtered by the median filter. SVM is the classifier that performs exudate, non-exudate classification. Exudate segmentation is done by thresholding and morphological operations.

Sánchez et al. [16] proposed an exudate detection algorithm in which mixture models are used to differentiate exudates and background. Method of edge detection separates hard exudates and cotton wool spots and other artefacts. Sensitivity of 100% and specificity of 90% were obtained.

Eadgahi et al. [17] explained an exudates detection method in which initially retina image preprocessing is done. Blood vessel and optic disk are removed. Segmentation of Hard Exudates was done by a mixture of morphological and reconstruction operations. The experiment was conducted on the DIARETDB1 dataset and 78.28% sensitivity was obtained.

Carrera et al. [18] developed an exudate detection approach, where an image processing method separates blood vessels, hard exudates, and microaneurysms for extracting features which can be used by support vector machine to find out retinopathy grade. The sensitivity obtained is 95%

The already existing exudate detection techniques have performances at the same time they all have drawbacks too. There are many factors like the properties of the device used for taking the image, image modality, contrast difference, illumination, the noises and artefacts also affect accurate detection. In the case of exudates which are in different shapes and scattered everywhere adversely affects the difficulty of detection.

The method proposed in this paper is based on Deep Convolutional Neural Network. In this case, after reading the image it is initially resized. As higher capacity machine needed for processing, original image of size 1500×1152 is resized to 224×224. The preprocessed image is put to a Deep CNN network which is having several hidden layers for training and classification which automatically uses the relevant features for classifying images with exudates and images without exudates.

3 Methodology

The Hard Exudates detection steps used in the proposed method are shown in Fig. 2. To detect Hard Exudates original image is resized as in the case of bigger sized images at the time of processing much computational time and training time are required. The images in the dataset are of size 1500 X 1152 are resized into 224 X 224. The next step is training performed by using Deep CNN on 60% of images from the DIARETDB1 dataset [19]. Classification of images with exudates and without exudates is done using Deep CNN.

Fig. 2 Exudates detection

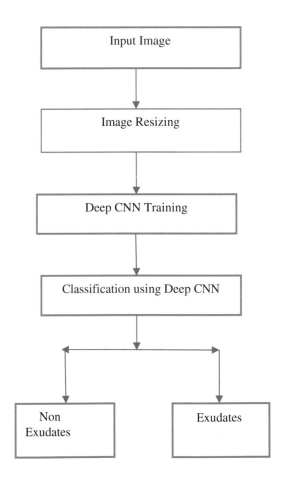

Fig. 3 a Image from
database. **b** Resized Image

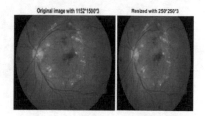

3.1 Image Resizing

The image used for processing and classification is taken from the standard DIARET
DB1 dataset in which the size of the image is 1500 × 1152 and to process it high
capacity machines are needed. So the original image is resized to 224 × 224 for
processing. Figure 3a shows an image from the database and Fig. 3b shows resized
image.

3.2 Deep CNN Training

Convolutional neural networks use convolution in place of multiplication of matrix.
The operation convolution has a linear form. The number of fully connected layers
or hidden layers is more in number in Deep CNN and this helps for feature extraction
on its own. For image classification, Deep CNN is used. The network is trained using
images with exudates and not with exudates. The Deep CNN architecture used in
the proposed method is given in Fig. 4 and the Deep CNN training model is shown
in Fig. 5.

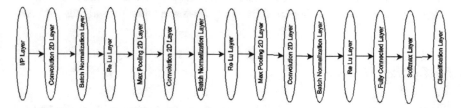

Fig. 4 Deep CNN architecture used in the proposed method

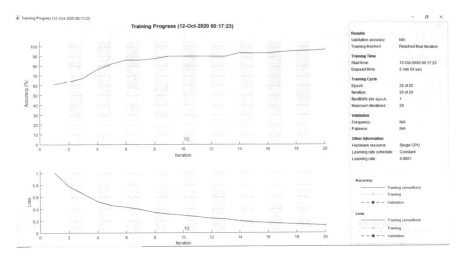

Fig. 5 Deep CNN training model

3.3 *Classification Using Deep CNN*

Deep CNN uses the deep learning method where the relevant features are identified
by the network itself at the time of training and based on the obtained relevant features
classification is performed.

4 Details of Experiments

For conducting experiments, the standard DIARETDB1 dataset which contains 89
images is taken. From the dataset, 60% of images were taken for training purposes.

5 Results Obtained

The accuracy obtained for the exudate detection system is measured by finding out
sensitivity, specificity, etc. The performances of the developed method are given in
Table 1.

The obtained sensitivity is 100%, specificity obtained is 97.87% and accuracy is
98.88%.

Figures 6 and 7 give evaluation measure as graph and bar chart. Figure 8 shows
the CNN Confusion matrix.

Table 1 Performance of the Proposed System

Sensitivity	100%
Specificity	97.87%
Accuracy	98.88%
Error rate	1.1%
Precision	97.67
False positive rate	2.1%

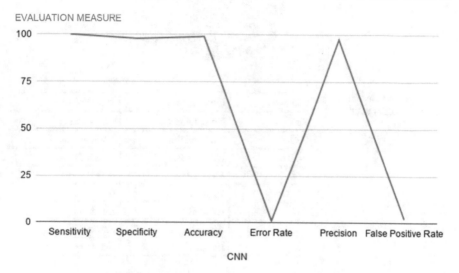

Fig. 6 Deep CNN Based Evaluation

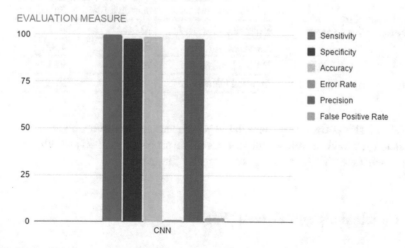

Fig. 7 Evaluation chart

Fig. 8 CNN Confusion
matrix

CNN Confusion Matrix

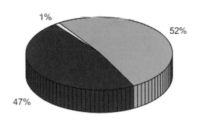

Table 2 Comparison table
showing result obtained and
result predicted

Images	Obtained class	Predicted class
32	No exudates	No exudates
39	No exudates	No exudates
41	No exudates	No exudates
68	Exudates	No exudates
1	Exudates	Exudates
15	Exudates	Exudates
19	Exudates	Exudates
27	Exudates	Exudates

Table 3 Performance
comparisons of the proposed
system and other systems

Different algorithms	Sensitivity%	Specificity%
Walter et al. [5]	92.8%	–
Doaa et al. [6]	80%	100%
Welfer et al. [7]	70.48%	98.84
Proposed method	100	97.87%

Table 2 shows the comparison table which shows the result obtained and result predicted and Table 3 shows comparisons of the proposed method and other methods by exudate detection for classifying diabetic retinopathy.

6 Conclusions and Future Work

The paper presented an automatic Hard Exudate detection technique. In this work as an initial step image resizing is done as a preprocessing step. The proposed paper gives Hard Exudate detection approach which is developed by using the Deep Convolutional Neural Network classifier. For performing experiments publicly available

DIARETDB1 dataset was used. The system gives accurate results compared to the available methods. As a future work, an ensemble method is suggested.

Acknowledgements We are thankful to Dr. Sheeja, Dr. Chandrakanth Eye Hospital, Kozhikode, who helped us for conducting a subjective study

References

1. Deepa R, Narayanan NK (2020, February) Detection of microaneurysm in retina image using machine learning approach. In: 2020 international conference on innovative trends in information technology (ICITIIT). IEEE, pp 1–5
2. Roy A, Dutta D, Bhattacharya P, Choudhury S (2017, April) Filter and fuzzy c means based feature extraction and classification of diabetic retinopathy using support vector machines. In: 2017 international conference on communication and signal processing (ICCSP). IEEE, pp 1844–1848
3. Harangi B, Hajdu A (2014) Detection of exudates in fundus images using a Markovian segmentation model. In: 2014 36th annual international conference of the IEEE engineering in medicine and biology society. IEEE
4. Youssef D et al (2010) New feature-based detection of blood vessels and exudates in color fundus images. In: 2010 2nd international conference on image processing theory, tools and applications. IEEE.
5. Walter T et al (2002) A contribution of image processing to the diagnosis of diabetic retinopathy-detection of exudates in color fundus images of the human retina. IEEE Trans Med Imaging 21(10):1236–1243
6. Youssef D, Solouma NH (2012) Accurate detection of blood vessels improves the detection of exudates in color fundus images. Comput Methods Programs Biomed 108(3):1052–1061
7. Welfer D, Scharcanski J, Marinho DR (2010) A coarse-to-fine strategy for automatically detecting exudates in color eye fundus images. Comput Med Imaging Graph 34(3):228–235
8. Zhou W et al (2017) Automatic detection of exudates in digital color fundus images using superpixel multi-feature classification. IEEE Access 5:17077–17088
9. Singh A et al (2015) Automatic exudates detection in fundus image using intensity thresholding and morphology. In: 2015 7th international congress on ultra modern telecommunications and control systems and workshops (ICUMT). IEEE
10. Syed AM et al (2018) Robust detection of exudates using fundus images. In: 2018 IEEE 21st international multi-topic conference (INMIC). IEEE
11. Wang H, Hsu W, Lee ML (2009) Effective detection of retinal exudates in fundus images. In: 2009 2nd international conference on biomedical engineering and informatics. IEEE
12. Bharkad S (2018) Morphological and neural network based approach for detection of exudates in fundus images. In: 2018 second international conference on computing methodologies and communication (ICCMC). IEEE
13. Dutta MK et al (2015) Exudates detection in digital fundus image using edge based method & strategic thresholding. In: 2015 38th international conference on telecommunications and signal processing (TSP). IEEE
14. Aftab U, Akram MU (2012) Automated identification of exudates for detection of macular edema. In: 2012 cairo international biomedical engineering conference (CIBEC). IEEE
15. Ruba T, Ramalakshmi K (2015) Identification and segmentation of exudates using SVM classifier. In: 2015 international conference on innovations in information, embedded and communication systems (ICIIECS). IEEE
16. Sánchez CI et al (2009) Retinal image analysis based on mixture models to detect hard exudates. Med Image Anal 13(4):650–658

17. Eadgahi MGF, Pourreza H (2012, October) Localization of hard exudates in retinal fundus image by mathematical morphology operations. In: 2012 2nd international econference on computer and knowledge engineering (ICCKE). IEEE, pp 185–189
18. Carrera EV, González A, Carrera R (2017, August). Automated detection of diabetic retinopathy using SVM. In 2017 IEEE XXIV international conference on electronics, electrical engineering and computing (INTERCON). IEEE, pp 1–4
19. Kauppi T, Kalesnykiene V, Kamarainen J, Lensu L, Sorri I, Raninen A, Voutilainen R, Uusitalo H, Kalviainen H, Pietila J (2007) DIARETDB1 diabetic retinopathy database and evaluation protocol. In: 11th conference on medical image understanding and analysis

Transparent Decision Support System for Breast Cancer (TDSSBC) to Determine the Risk Factor

Akhil Kumar Das, Saroj Kr. Biswas, and Ardhendu Mandal

1 Introduction

Breast cancer is a casual malignant growth for ladies; however, seldom in man. BC happens because some breast cells begin to develop strangely. These unusual cells spread through our breast or other organs of the body that are uncontrolled. Every year countless Breast Cancer (BC) patients have passed away across the entire world. After skin malignant growth, breast cancer might be a very normal disease in ladies. Breast cancer has expanded step by step across the entire world since 2000 [1]. As indicated by the World Health Organization (WHO), it 'is seen that 2.1 million ladies are affected every year and 627,000 ladies passed away since 2018. It is around 15% of the deaths among the ladies related to the disease [2]. As per the Centers for Disease Control and Prevention's (CDC's) board, roughly 2,50,000 people have been determined to have breast malignancy disease inside the U.S. Roughly 2300 men and 42,000 ladies have passed away from breast cancer disease every year in the U.S. [3]. As indicated by the Indian Council for Medical Research, 1,50,000 are influenced in breast malignant growth consistently in India, of which 70,000 have passed away. Therefore, breast malignancy is the more dangerous disease in the world. Neural networks can be a computational method in different fields of science, medical and engineering applications. The neural network is used to determine a

A. K. Das (✉)
Department of Computer Science, Gour Mahavidyalaya, Mangalbari, Malda, West Bengal 732142, India

S. Kr. Biswas
Department of Computer Science and Engineering, NIT Silchar, Silchar, Assam 788010, India

A. Mandal
Department of Computer Science and Application, University of North Bengal, Darjeeling, West Bengal 734013, India

© The Author(s), under exclusive license to Springer Nature Singapore Pte Ltd. 2021
M. K. Bajpai et al. (eds.), *Machine Vision and Augmented Intelligence—Theory and Applications*, Lecture Notes in Electrical Engineering 796,
https://doi.org/10.1007/978-981-16-5078-9_23

variety of difficulties, including pattern categorization, clinical diagnosis, and more [4].

This paper has discussed a clinical expert system named Transparent Decision Support System for Breast Cancer (TDSSBC), which created rules that can be utilized in Neural Network. The TDSSBC tunes and prunes the principles to help with settling on a decision support system. The proposed model is an expansion of the Transparent Neural Expert System for Breast Cancer (TNESBC) [5]. The proposed TDSSBC embraces the white-box NN method which is named as "Rule Extraction from Neural Network (NN) applying Classified and Misclassified data" (RxNCM) [6] for rule extraction from the breast cancer dataset. During this framework, the created rules are reasonable from neural networks (NN) for the risk factor of the decision of breast cancer. The dataset has been utilized to check the exhibition of the framework. Tenfold Cross-Validation is utilized to contrast the performance of the framework and the contrary two leaving frameworks (RxNCM and RxREN [7]). The examination has shaped utilizing tenfold Cross-Validation (CV) accuracy, average (Avg) recall rate, average number (AvgNo) of antecedents(Ancent) for each standard rule, and average(Avg) false-positive rate.

2   Background Technology and Basics

2.1   Breast Cancer

Cancer refers to a minimum one lethal disorder that is characterized through the enlargement of unusual cells in the organs. Cancer cells are unsuppressed and destroy the conventional body tissue. breast cancer might be a typical malignancy among ladies, however infrequently in men. Breast cancer is one of the deadly diseases on which cells in the breast are abnormally developed inside the breast. BC have diverse sort that relies upon which cells inside the breast end up having malignant growth. BC have distinct kind that relies upon on which cells in the breast develop to be most cancers. BC begins at any portion of the breast. Normally, breast cancer has 3 primary parts. These are lobules, channels, and connective tissues.

A breast lobule can be a gland. It produces milk. The duct can be a skinny tube that consists of milk from the breast lobules to the nipple. The connective tissue is fabricated from fibrous and fatty tissue that surrounds the lobules and ducts. Normally, BC begins in the ducts channel or lobules. From that point, it 'is spread externally to the breast inside the body [8]. If breast disease is distinguished quickly, it 'is restored before malignant growth starts spreading to different pieces of the body. In any case, regularly, as a rule, breast malignant growth is found at higher stages. Subsequently, it 'is difficult to fix breast disease.

2.2 Causes of Breast Cancer

Breast cancer occurs while breast cells start to develop strangely. These cells are spreading through the breast or different sections of the body that are uncontrolled cells. Typically, breast cancer begins with cells that are delivering milk, i.e. ducts. BC likewise begins inside the glandular tissue, for example, lobules. There is a lot of justification reason for breast cancer. There are two kinds of dangerous risk factors for breast cancer such as changeable risk factors and unchangeable risk factors [2].

Hazard factors like getting more seasoned, hereditary transformation, reproductive history, thick breasts, personal history, family history, and so forth cannot be changed. Some dangerous factors like weight, actual work, liquor utilization, smoking cigarettes, and so forth [2] may be controlled. Hence, the dangerous risk of breast cancer explodes with age. Be that as it may, the danger of bosom disease goes up with age. In this way, breast cancer may be controlled somewhat on the off chance that we have controlled the opportunity of breast malignancy in regular daily existence that is expanded the opportunity of breast cancer disease.

2.3 Neural Network in Breast Cancer

Currently, Neural Networks are often treated collectively of the simplest Machine Learning (ML) method. Neural Network is one of the procedure techniques that rely on the structure and biological NN [9].

NN is a serious application as a decision-support method to look out for disease in our life. Within the NN, information is moving through the network that 'is suffering from the architecture of the NN. NN is that the potential to change the input. Hence, the network generates produces the simplest result while not output condition. It is treated collectively as the simplest machine learning approach because of its universal property. However, the most drawback of NN for taking decisions is their lack of rules and rationalization capability as a result of ANN could be a piece of recording equipment in nature. This recording equipment nature of NN hinders them in several processing tasks.

The proposed system may be a clinical expert system named Transparent Decision Support System for Breast Cancer (TDSSBC). This method has been extracted the rules utilizing the neural network for breast cancer as a result of neural networks has more powerful classifiers. The TDSSBC takes in the white-box NN method which is named "Rule Extraction from Neural Network (NN) applying Classified and Misclassified data" (RxNCM) for rule extraction from the BC dataset. These evaluated rules have been modified and pruned to help in making a decision support system.

3   Literature Survey

Nowadays, a large number of research works have been finished for the identity of the fundamental risk factor of BC along with the prevention of BC applying artificial neural networks (ANN). Jaikrishnan et al. [2] have discussed a method for the prevention of BC utilizing AI. During this characterization method, the accuracy of BC is expanded. In this method, 6 machine learning techniques are explained like Decision Tree (DT), K-Nearest Neighbors (KNN), Gaussian Naïve Bayes (GNB), Support Vector Machine (SVM), Random Forest, and Multilayered Perceptron. Here, they have explained their accuracy. This method is employed the k-fold Cross-Validation (CV) technique for disposing of the bias. Singha et al. [9] have been explained a method for the earliest prediction of BC. They have utilized the data from the UCI machine learning repository for examined and evaluate the accuracy is ninety eight percent with an occasional error rate. It is completed utilized machine learning technique with facilitate of a synthetic Neural Network (NN). Azmi et al. [10] have proposed a new method that classifies the Disease of BC by applying the Neural Network (NN). This approach is economical and easy to address the system. They have been utilized the breast cancer datasets, which have been occupied from UCI machine learning Repository. They have been applied the 70:30 segment for training and evaluating the method. It consists of 2 stages. The input dataset has trained utilized the feed-forward rules in the first stage. The second stage is Neural Network (NN). This method has been applied to categories BC data. Polat et al. [11] have been started a hybrid technique for the recognition of BC dependent on routine blood examination. It is seen that this method is a standardization method. The category accuracy of this approach is 91.37%. Addeh et al. [12] have proposed a shrewd strategy for the location of BC utilizing a Neural Network (NN). The started model comprises 2 sub-modules such as the clustering module and the classifier module. In the clustering module, the input dataset that has been clustered is utilized in the new approach. It 'is anything but an adjusted colonialist serious calculation (MICA) and also K-means method. In this classifier, designs are resolved to utilize a neural network (NN). Sharma et al. [13] analyzed the distinct machine learning (ML) technique for BC prediction like Random Forest, k-Nearest Neighbor and Naïve Bayes. They have observed that every calculation has acquired over ninety-four percent accuracy yet k-NN is the highest accuracy 95.90%. This work has addressed the major risk factors of the BC system through a pedagogical approach.

4   The Proposed Transparent Decision Support System for Breast Cancer

The proposed model is an expansion of the Transparent Neural Expert System for Breast Cancer (TNESBC) [5]. The TDSSBC brings up the white Box Neural Network system which is named "Rule Extraction from Neural Network applying Classified

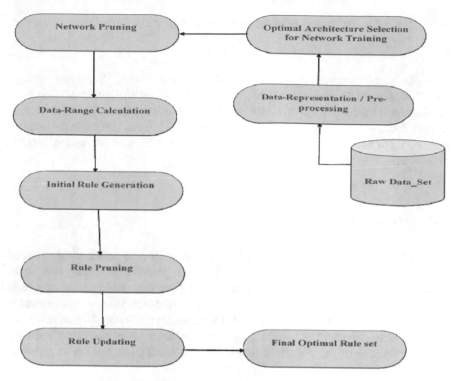

Fig. 1 Layout diagram of TDSSBC system

and Misclassified data" (RxNCM) [6] for rule extraction from the breast cancer dataset. The proposed expert system, TDSSBC, creates IF-THEN-based rules by applying ANN. These rules have been utilized to determine the major feature risk factors of breast cancer. The proposed expert system obeys a pedagogical rule extraction technique. The TDSSBC were utilized each well classified and misclassified style to evaluate the data ranges [6]. The format diagram of TDSSBC is proven in Fig. 1. TDSSBC has seven phases. These are Data-representation/Preprocessing, Optimal Architecture Selection for Network Training (NT), Data-Range Calculation, Rule Pruning, Initial Rule Generation, Rule Updating and Network pruning. A short discussion of all of the segments is given below.

4.1 Data Representation/Pre-processing

Raw data comprise various text and images. It further includes missing values and symbolics as components. Before the training, all missing values are removed and mixed data are converted to numeric values [4]. This altered data set aptly fits as input for Neural Network (NN).

4.2   Data Optimal Architecture Selection for Network Training

Here, the neural network is trained using a Back Propagation (BP) learning strategy with h numbers of hidden neurons and a single hidden layer. The hidden neurons have been selected based on the mean square error of the neural system. This architecture ranges from $l + 1 - 2*l$ neurons, which are hidden [14]. Here, l specifies the number of these input neurons. The least mean square error has been considered for similar processing.

4.3   Network Pruning

A neural network having impertinent information may lead to the diminution of system accuracy. The Neural Network (NN) has been pruned by searching significant input neurons. With every iteration of the Neural Network system, error generated by the input is noted. Subsequently, the input is removed and the mean square error is calculated to achieve the desired outcome. The input having the least calculated error is judged as significant input and the insignificant inputs are eventually removed after each iteration. Here, the sequential floating search mechanism has been applied to the pruned neural network.

4.4   Data-Range Calculation

For each significant input neuron, the data ranges have been evaluated by taking relevant input attributes. The functionality of the significant input neurons is computed using misclassified and correctly classified patterns. Here, the misclassified rate of a particular neuron is evaluated by clearing this neuron and also searching the misclassified styles. Determine correctly classified percentage by searching correctly classified styles utilizing only that neuron. The data range matrix also computes using a combination of the above patterns. The range of data is established utilizing the upper as well as lower limits of the patterns. Here, AT_J is an attribute in class C_M, $MINIMUM_{JM}$ is the lower range, represented by X_{JM} and $MAXIMUM_{JM}$ is the upper range represented by Y_{JM}. Therefore, data range of the attribute AT_J is $[X_{JM}-Y_{JM}]$. In the data matrix, rows indicate the attributes. Here the columns indicate the targets as shown in Fig. 2.

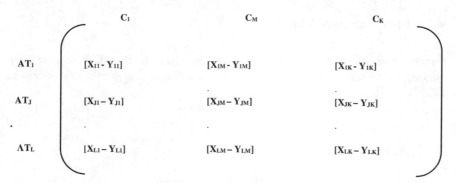

Fig. 2 Data range matrix

4.5 Initial Rule Generation

Here, classification rules have been generated for each class using the above matrix. The classification rules are constructed with help of lower and upper limits as given below.

if (attribute $AT_J >= X_{JM}$ and attribute $AT_J <= Y_{JM}$) then
  class = 'C_M';
else
  class = 'C_F'(say);

4.6 Rule Pruning

These rules may contain certain insignificant attributes. All rules have been pruned to eliminate insignificant attributes in this section. After removing the insignificant attributes from the rules, the rule sets are updated. Then the classification accuracy of the set is measured.

4.7 Rule Updating

After pruning the modified rule-set is examined. The newly updated rules are used to overcome inherent overlapping problems existing in the rule-set. The coinciding values in the lower and upper range of the attribute set are identified for each class and subsequently, the rule-set is updated. Based on the result, the class is modified accordingly. This process is repeated for each attribute.

4.8 Final Optimal Rule Set

Finally, these rule-sets are generated inside the shape of IF-THEN propositional clauses. These rule-sets are utilized the identitication of major risks that prevail in BC.

5 Results and Discussion

Here, the dataset of the BC has been taken from the UCI repository that has been utilized in the test. Six hundred eighty three records have been utilized on this dataset. The dataset comprises 9 attributes and 2 classes.

The outcomes are decided by the usage of tenfold Cross-Validation (CV) to decrease the unfairness associated with random sampling. The overall performance is determined towards the subsequent condition: ten-fold CV accuracy, average (Avg) true positive (TP) rate, average number (AgvNo) of antecedents (Ancet) in keeping for each rule, the average (Avg) false positive (FP) rate.

Two existing rule extraction models based on pedagogical technique, i.e. RxNCM [6] and RxREN [7] are utilized to examine the overall performance of the suggested TDSSBC model which is also an example of a pedagogical technique based rule extraction algorithm.

Table 1 shows the generated rules using the pedagogical technique based rule extraction models, i.e. RxREN, RxNCM and TDSSBC respectively. It represents IF-THEN propositional clauses. It is used only onefold for the superior understanding.

Here, the average no (AvgNo) of the rule antecedents (Avg Antec) is two antecedents for each rule in TDSSBC, 2 for RxNCM. The average no (AvgNo) of these rule antecedents (Avg Antec) is three antecedents in step with a rule for the RxREN. TDSSBC and RxNCM are the equal end result, i.e., two. Therefore, it has concluded that TDSSBC is a higher neighborhood apprehensibility than RxREN due to the fact much less range of rule antecedents (Ancet) on common. The regulations (rules) are proven in Table 1 similar to the fold that generates the best accuracy for the related model. In this fold, the TDSSBC indicates that the Major Factors for breast cancer are Bare_Nuclei > 4.0 and Cell_Size_Uniformity > 5.0.

Table 1 Rules produced for Breast Cancer (BC) from dataset

RxREN	RxNCM	TDSSBC
if (Cell_Size_Uniformity < = 4.0 and Bare_Nuclei < = 5.0 and Normal_Nucleoli < = 6.0) then class = "benign" else: class = "malignant"	if (Bare_Nuclei < = 4.0 and Cell_Size_Uniformity < = 5.0) then class = "benign" else: class = "malignant"	if (Bare_Nuclei < = 4.0 and Cell_Size_Uniformity < = 5.0) then class = "benign" else: class = "malignant"

Table 2 Comparison of results for BC Dataset

Criteria	RxREN	RxNCM	TDSSBC
Accuracy	91.730%	93.160%	93.160%
Avg Antec	3	2	2
Recall	0.90670	0.91830	0.91830
FP rate	0.02540	0.02670	0.02670

Table 2 indicates the overall performance assessment of TDSSBC with two exiting models RxREN and RxNCM. In Table 2, it 'is determined that the TDSSBC plays higher than RxREN; however, tit is identical to RxNCM in all mechanisms for the dataset of BC. The TDSSBC has 93.160% accuracy while RxREN receives 91.730% accuracy and RxNCM has 93.160%. The recall, as well as True Positive (FP) rates of TDSSBC, is higher than RxREN however identical to RxNCM. TDSSBC has a recall value of 0.9183 while the recall of RxNCM and RxREN are 0.9183 and 0.9067 accordingly. TDSSBC is an FT rate value of 0.0267 while the recall of RxNCM and RxREN are 0.0267 and 0.0254 accordingly.

Therefore, it has been found that TDSSBC plays a touch bit higher than the RxREN model for breast cancer dataset however it is identical to RxNCM. The experimental outcomes have a look at that the TDSSBC set of rules is extra essential than RxREN. So, the TDSSBC method is an extra suitable preference for this machine if thinking about all measures. The system has a very slight computational overhead but it produces more accuracy and without difficulty understandable rules.

6 Conclusion

Currently, neural networks systems have achieved a tremendous result because of their widespread estimation property. The main focus is to improve the forecast accuracy of the method. This paper has discussed an expert system named Transparent Decision Support System for Breast Cancer (TDSSBC) to publish the major Risk Factors of breast cancer. The TDSSBC system used the pedagogical rule extraction process that are generated transparent rules. The performance comparison is observed between TDSSBC and two exiting models RxREN and RxNCM. It has been shown that TDSSBC plays barely higher than RxREN; however, it is equal to RxNCM. Hence, the TDSSBC choice gadget is in shape for most breast cancer management. The comparison is utilizes the tenfold CV. The comparison utilized tenfold CV exactness, average number (AvgNo) of antecedents (Antec) for each rule, average (Avg) recall rate, and average false positive (Age) rate. The propositional rules generated by the TDSSBC are tightly packed and comprehensible. Therefore, the IF-THEN propositional policies generated via TDSSBC are clean to give an explanation for and recognize the breast cancer. So, TDSSBC medical expert system will be suitable for most breast cancers management. Therefore, it could be utilized as a decision system for breast cancer in the medical sector.

References

1. Chen W, Zheng R, Baade PD, Zhang S, Zeng H, Bray F, Jemal A, Yu XQ, He J (2016) Cancer statistics in China, 2015, CA. Cancer J Clin 66:115–132. https://doi.org/10.3322/caac.21338.
2. Jaikrishnan SVJ, Chantarakasemchit O, Meesad P (2019) A breakup machine learning approach for breast cancer prediction. In: 2019 11th international conference on information technology and electrical engineering (ICITEE). IEEE, Pattaya, Thailand, pp 1–6. https://doi.org/10.1109/ICITEED.2019.8929977
3. Centers for Disease Control and Prevention's (CDC's), Basic Information About Breast Cancer. https://www.cdc.gov/cancer/breast/basic_info/index.htm. Accessed 14 Nov 2020
4. Bewal R, Ghosh A, Chaudhary A (2015) Detection of breast cancer using neural networks–a review, 6
5. Das AK, Biswas SK, Mandal A, Chakraborty M (2020) A neural expert system to identify major risk factors of breast cancer, 4
6. Biswas SK, Chakraborty M, Purkayastha B, Roy P, Thounaojam DM (2017) Rule extraction from training data using neural network. Int J Artif Intell Tools 26:1750006. https://doi.org/10.1142/S0218213017500063
7. Augasta MG, Kathirvalavakumar T (2012) Reverse engineering the neural networks for rule extraction in classification problems. Neural Proc Lett 35.
8. Centers for Disease Control and Prevention's (CDC's), What is Breast Cancer ? https://www.cdc.gov/cancer/breast/basic_info/what-is-breast-cancer.htm. Accessed 14 Nov 2020
9. Singhal P, Pareek S (2018) Artificial neural network for prediction of breast cancer. In: 2018 2nd international conference on I-SMAC (IoT in Social, Mobile, Analytics and Cloud). IEEE, Palladam, India, pp 464–468. https://doi.org/10.1109/I-SMAC.2018.8653700.
10. Azmi MSBM, Cob ZC (2010) Breast cancer prediction based on backpropagation algorithm. In: 2010 IEEE student conference on research and development (SCOReD). IEEE, Kuala Lumpur, Malaysia, pp 164–168. https://doi.org/10.1109/SCORED.2010.5703994
11. Polat K, Senturk U (2018) A novel ML approach to prediction of breast cancer: combining of mad normalization, KMC based feature weighting and AdaBoostM1 classifier. In: 2018 2nd international symposium on multidisciplinary studies and innovative technologies (ISMSIT). IEEE, Ankara, pp 1–4. https://doi.org/10.1109/ISMSIT.2018.8567245
12. Addeh J, Kalteh A, Zarbakhsh P, Jirabadi M (2013) A research about breast cancer detection using different neural networks and K-MICA algorithm. J Can Res Ther 9:456. https://doi.org/10.4103/0973-1482.119350
13. Sharma S, Aggarwal A, Choudhury T (2018) Breast cancer detection using machine learning algorithms. In: 2018 international conference on computational techniques, electronics and mechanical systems (CTEMS). IEEE, Belgaum, India, pp 114–118. https://doi.org/10.1109/CTEMS.2018.8769187
14. Dattachaudhuri A, Biswas S, Sarkar S, Boruah AN (2020) Transparent decision support system for credit risk evaluation: an automated credit approval system. IEEEHYDCON

Deep-Learning-based Malicious Android Application Detection

Vikas K. Malviya and Atul Gupta

1 Introduction

Android is an operating system developed by Google. It is designed mainly for touchscreen devices such as smartphones and tablets. It is based on the Linux kernel. Java language is primarily used to write Android applications even though the use of other languages is also possible. These applications run on Dalvik virtual machine or Android Run Time (ART). Applications are installed from a single file with the.apk (Android Application Package) file extension. It is the file format used to distribute and install Android applications on the Android operating system.

Android is a privilege-separated operating system. Each app has a unique Linux user ID. It is based on Linux, which helps in isolating applications from each other. An additional permission mechanism is used to enforce restrictions on operations. In this way, Android security architecture ensures that no application has permission to impact other applications, operating system, or user (which includes users' private data such as contacts and e-mails).

The Android security system has two main components. These are the Application Sandbox and Permission models. Android sets up a kernel-level application sandbox that enforces security between applications and the system. Due to this, Android applications cannot interact with each other and have limited access to the operating system. This kernel-level sandbox extends to native code and operating system applications. Application sandbox enforces restrictions on applications to interact with each other and access a limited range of system resources. These restrictions

V. K. Malviya (✉)
NIIT University, Neemrana, Rajasthan, India

A. Gupta
Design and Manufacturing, Indian Institute of Information Technology, Jabalpur, India
e-mail: atul@iiitdmj.ac.in

© The Author(s), under exclusive license to Springer Nature Singapore Pte Ltd. 2021
M. K. Bajpai et al. (eds.), *Machine Vision and Augmented Intelligence—Theory and Applications*, Lecture Notes in Electrical Engineering 796,
https://doi.org/10.1007/978-981-16-5078-9_24

are imposed through a security mechanism known as permissions. In this model, an application has to define permissions which it needs in its manifest file.

We reviewed various approaches proposed by researchers and found that permissions alone are not sufficient to detect malicious intentions of Android applications. We also found that opcodes can be a good candidate for this cause. In this work, analysis of maliciousness detection capability of opcodes is performed with different exercises, and then we performed classification of Android apps using opcode sequences. We used LSTM (Long Short-Term Memory) Networks to detect maliciousness of Android apps.

The rest of the paper is organized as follows. A Review of previous approaches is given in Sect. 2. Section 3 provides details of different exercises and their results. Finally, conclusions from the various exercises are summarized in Sect. 4.

2 Literature Review

Talha et al. [1], Sun et al. [2], and Mahindru and Singh [3] used permissions requested by the application as a feature in their work. Talha et al. [1] and Sun et al. [2] developed an Android malware detection system using machine learning classification named APK Auditor and SIGPID. Bezobrazov et al. [4] also used permissions required by the application in their proposed artificial immune system for Android. Sokolova et al. [5] analyzed co-required permissions by modeling them with graphs and category patterns. Xiong et al. [6] identified contrasting permission patterns that can differentiate between malware and clean applications and used them to develop a framework to detect malware. Wang et al. [7] explored risks associated with the permissions required by the Android apps.

Yerima et al. [8], McWilliams et al. [9], and Yerima et al. [10] combined API calls, system commands, and permissions requested by the app as features in their work. Peiravian and Zhu [11] also combined permissions and API calls to develop a framework for detecting malicious Android apps. Zeng et al. [12] identified the relationship between permissions and API calls and used it to detect malware. Chan and Song [13] compared the classification performance of permissions with the combination of permissions and API calls. Cen et al. [14] combined Android API calls and permissions to develop a probabilistic discriminative model. Qiao et al. [15] detected malware with the combination of patterns of Permissions and API Function calls. Tao et al. [16] used a combination of permission and APIs calls to develop a malware detection system, namely MalPat. Onwuzurike et al. [17] used a call graph created with API calls to detect malware.

Sahs and Khan [18] combined standard Android permissions, user-defined permissions, and a control flow graph generated by raw bytecodes of the methods to detect malware. Canfora et al. [19] proposed a classifier for malicious app detection using occurrences of a specific subset of system calls, a weighted sum of a subset of permissions that the application required, and a set of combinations of permissions.

Aung and Zaw [20] developed a framework for classifying Android applications using features from permissions requested by applications and events obtained from the applications. Yuan et al. [21] proposed a deep-learning-based method combining static and dynamic analysis of Android app for malware detection. Permissions required by the app and sensitive APIs are the features in the static analysis, and the dynamic behavior of the application was considered as features in dynamic analysis. Idrees and Rajarajan [22] combined permissions with intents in the detection of malicious Android apps. Feldman et al. [23] developed a system named analyzer to detect malicious apps using permission requests, high priority receivers, low version number and abuse services. Su and Fung [24] used permissions, sensitive functions applied by the app, native permissions, and intent priority for static analysis to detect malicious apps. Kang et al. [25] proposed an n-opcode-based Android malware classification approach. Their approach provides automated feature discovery, which makes it different from other works. Wang et al. [26] proposed an approach that uses an ensemble of multiple classifiers to detect Android malware. The feature set for this work consists of requested permissions, filtered intents, restricted API calls, code-related information, used permissions, hardware features, and suspicious API calls. Milosevic et al. [27] used permissions and source code-based features separately for the detection of Android Malware. Yang et al. [28] developed a dynamic behavior analysis framework that inspects and records API calls, permission framework, and runtime features of Android applications. Narayanan et al. [29] developed a framework named MKLDroid, which uses a graph kernel to extract information from applications dependency graphs and detect malicious code in different feature sets. Li et al. [30] implemented a clustering system for Android malware. The authors removed third-party libraries from applications and then created fingerprints of the application by feature hashing. Shen et al. [31] used N-gram analysis of information flow for the detection of malicious Android applications. Martinelli et al. [32] developed a framework that combines static and dynamic analysis of Android applications. Static analysis is performed with N-gram analysis. Dynamic analysis is done with the combination of device, user, and application behaviour monitoring. Zhu et al. [33] proposed a deep learning-based malware detection approach. It detects maliciousness by abnormal use of sensitive data by applications. Varsha et al. [34] combined features from hardware, permission, application components, filtered intents, opcodes and strings to detect malicious Android applications.

From this review, we found that permissions alone are not sufficient for understanding application behaviour. The authors combined permissions with other attributes. We found that API calls and intents are major features combined with permissions to detect malicious Android apps. We also found that standard built-in permissions are used by authors as features in their work. The use of developer-defined (nonstandard) permissions is minimal. Opcodes and Java codes are not used much. Opcodes are one such candidate that can be used to identify maliciousness as they show a sequence of operations. Opcode-based techniques have the advantage of learning features from raw data rather than identifying features manually. In other approaches, feature identification and feature selection are needed to find the most effective features. As a result of this scope of machine learning algorithms is limited as some useful features get excluded. It is not the case with opcodes as a sequence of opcodes can indicate the maliciousness of Android applications.

3 Overview of Exercises

We tried to identify the role of opcodes in detecting malicious Android apps. First, we tried to find the role of specific opcode frequency in detecting malicious and benign Android apps. Next, we analyzed opcode sequences frequency to find their role in detecting malicious and benign Android applications. Then we tried to detect maliciousness using opcode sequences using LSTM (Long Short-Term Memory) Networks. We found malicious opcode sequences by comparing opcode sequences from malicious and benign applications. Opcodes appearing in malicious applications but not in benign applications are considered as malicious opcodes.

We used Apktool [35] for reverse engineering apk files of Android apps. Apktool not only unzips files but also converts dex files to smali. These smali files are classes in Android source codes. Each smali file belongs to a class, and it contains opcode sequences of all the methods in that class. We extracted opcodes from these smali files for our analysis. The procedure used for extraction is shown in Fig. 1. Since we have many apps, it was not possible to process each apk file manually. So we wrote a utility in Java for processing bulk apk files. Using this utility, we first extracted all small files. Then we extracted opcode sequences from all the classes of apk files and stored them for further analysis. We performed these exercises with 14,856 malicious apps from virusshare (https://virusshare.com) and 5856 benign apps from playdrone crawler (https://github.com/nviennot/playdrone).

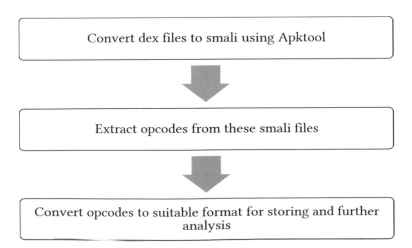

Fig. 1 Extraction procedure of opcodes from smali files

3.1 Analysis of Opcode Occurring Frequency

This exercise is intended to find opcodes that are frequently occurring in malicious apps. We were also interested in comparing the opcodes and their frequency of appearing in both types of apps, so we calculated the number of times a particular opcode is occurring in both types of apps. We obtained a list of opcodes from Reference [36] and Android project website [37] and calculated the count of occurring from smali files. The results are shown in Table 1.

The number of malicious and benign Android applications used in this exercise is not the same, so we calculated the average count of occurrences for comparing them with each other. As shown in Table 1, the frequency of opcodes in malicious and benign apps is almost the same. So, differentiating based only on opcodes frequency is not the right solution. Another important observation we made from this study is that the number of occurrences of a particular opcode in malicious apps is less than its occurrence in benign apps. In our exercise, malicious apps are 14,856, while benign apps are 5856, but still, counts are almost identical in both cases.

Table 1 A comparison of opcodes count in malicious and benign apps

Malicious			Benign		
Opcode	Count	Average	Opcode	Count	Average
Invoke-virtual	160,950,812	10,834.79	Iget-object	137,636,662	23,515.58
Move-result-Object	110,177,887	7416.89	Invoke-virtual	123,900,423	21,168.7
iget-Object	93,639,040	6303.54	Move-result-Object	85,090,145	14,537.87
Const-string	61,925,438	4168.66	iget	64,342,899	10,993.15
Const/4	54,364,700	3659.69	Const/4	46,391,294	7926.07
Invoke-direct	53,619,129	3609.5	Const-string	42,738,305	7301.95
Invoke-static	52,589,324	3540.18	Invoke-direct	42,460,397	7254.47
Move-result	44,199,858	2975.42	Invoke-static	42,405,269	7245.05
New-instance	35,916,622	2417.81	Move-result	37,337,001	6379.12
Return-void	35,262,624	2373.79	Iput	33,102,885	5655.71
Goto	33,520,298	2256.50	return-Void	31,037,379	5302.82
If-eqz	31,423,962	2115.38	Goto	28,727,225	4908.12
const/16	29,304,931	1972.73	New-instance	27,222,577	4651.05
Iput-object	25,934,784	1745.86	If-eqz	25,856,637	4417.67
Iget	24,991,838	1682.39	Invoke-interface	21,314,868	3641.70

3.2 Analysis of Opcode Sequences

This exercise is intended to find opcode sequences that are frequently occurring in malicious apps. We were also interested in comparing opcode sequences and their frequency of appearing in both types of apps. So, we calculated the number of times a particular opcode sequence occurs in both types of apps. We calculated the count of opcode sequences occurring from smali files. The results are shown in Tables 2 and 3.

We calculated average occurrences for opcodes sequences as the number of malicious and benign Android applications used in these exercises are not the same. We have also shown the top 30 sequences whose frequency of occurrence is very high in Table 2. As shown in the table, opcodes' frequency in malicious and benign apps is almost the same. So, differentiating based only on opcodes sequences frequency is not the right solution.

3.3 Classification of Android Applications Using LSTM

Classification of Android applications into malicious and benign is performed in this work. We used LSTM networks for the classification of opcode sequences. The next subsections describe details of the experiment.

Finding Malicious Opcode Sequences. We did this exercise to find malicious opcode sequences from malicious apps. We carried out this study, as shown in Fig. 2. First, we used Apktool [35] to reverse engineer apk files. Each opcode sequence represents a method in smali file. We performed this operation for both the malicious and benign files and then compared these opcode sequences. We listed out those opcodes sequences present in the malicious files but not in benign apk files. These opcode sequences are considered as malicious opcode sequences in this work.

LSTM (Long Short-Term Memory) networks. LSTMs are a special kind of RNN (Recurrent Neural Network). They are capable of learning long-term dependencies. They were introduced by Hochreiter & Schmidhuber [38]. They are now used on a large variety of problems. LSTMs are designed to overcome the long-term dependency problem, which was the shortcoming of RNN. The recurrent neural network is consisting of a chain of repeating neural network units. This repeating unit in simple RNNs is a very simple function. LSTMs also consist of this structure, but the repeating module has a different structure. Instead of having a single neural network layer, there are four, interacting differently.

Experiment Execution. We conducted this experiment to detect malicious Android applications using opcode sequences. Details of experiments are shown in Fig. 3. It was tough to perform this experiment on a single computer, so we deployed Spark's cluster. We used Deeplearning4j [39] library for classification. It is an open-source, distributed deep learning library written for Java and Scala. It can be integrated with Hadoop and Spark.

Table 2 Top 30 most frequently opcode sequences in benign apps

S.No	Opcode	Count	Average
1	Iget-object,return-object	3,695,453	631.38
2	Invoke-direct,return-void	3,626,452	619.59
3	Invoke-virtual,move-result-object,return-object	1,626,034	277.81
4	Return-void	1,221,389	208.68
5	Iput-object,invoke-direct,return-void	1,147,452	196.05
6	Const/4,return	1,072,951	183.32
7	Iget,return	1,012,486	172.99
8	Iget-object,invoke-virtual,return-void	758,907	129.66
9	Iput-object,return-void	746,969	127.62
10	Check-cast,invoke-virtual,return-void	641,819	109.66
11	Invoke-static,return-void	592,379	101.21
12	Iget-boolean,return	517,029	88.34
13	Invoke-static,move-result,return	491,730	84.01
14	New-instance,invoke-direct,return-object	472,787	80.78
15	Invoke-static,move-result-object,return-object	457,969	78.25
16	Invoke-direct,iput-object,return-void	455,713	77.86
17	New-instance,invoke-direct,sput-object,return-void	411,283	70.27
18	Iget-object,invoke-virtual,move-result,return	376,663	64.35
19	Const/4,return-object	361,374	61.74
20	Iget-object,invoke-virtual,move-result-object,return-object	359,007	61.34
21	Iput-object,iput-object,invoke-direct,return-void	355,468	60.73
22	Sget-object,return-object	343,619	58.71
23	New-array,return-object	327,065	55.88
24	Iput-object,return-object	309,869	52.94
25	Invoke-virtual,return-void	302,827	51.74
26	Const/4,invoke-direct,return-void	272,434	46.55
27	Return-object	214,021	36.57
28	Iput,return-void	212,626	36.33
29	Check-cast,invoke-virtual,move-result,return	205,347	35.08
30	Iget-object,invoke-interface,return-void	205,142	35.05

The results of the classification experiment and their comparison with other approaches are shown in Table 4. It is clear from the table that our approach is also achieving the same F1-score as the other approach. Our approach has the benefit of automated feature identification as it is based on deep learning.

Table 3 Top 30 most frequently opcode sequences in malicious apps

S.No	Opcode	Count	Average
1	Invoke-direct,return-void	2,135,251	266.91
2	Iget-object,return-object	2,059,940	257.49
3	Iput-object,invoke-direct,return-void	1,086,247	135.78
4	Iput-object,return-void	798,956	99.87
5	Return-void	770,502	96.31
6	Iget,return	495,805	61.98
7	Const/4,return	412,605	51.58
8	Invoke-virtual,move-result-object,return-object	341,386	42.67
9	Iget-object,invoke-virtual,return-void	323,198	40.40
10	Iget-boolean,return	285,005	35.63
11	Invoke-static,return-void	267,853	33.48
12	Sget-object,return-object	247,029	30.88
13	Check-cast,invoke-virtual,return-void	245,484	30.69
14	Invoke-static,move-result-object,return-object	228,242	28.53
15	Invoke-static,move-result,return	218,860	27.36
16	Iput,return-void	215,076	26.88
17	Iput-object,iput-object,invoke-direct,return-void	199,966	25.00
18	Const/4,return-object	199,614	24.95
19	Invoke-direct,iput-object,return-void	166,019	20.75
20	New-instance,invoke-direct,return-object	165,179	20.65
21	Invoke-virtual,return-void	160,013	20.00
22	Iget-object,invoke-virtual,move-result,return	147,488	18.44
23	Const/4,invoke-direct,return-void	138,106	17.26
24	Check-cast,invoke-virtual,move-result,return	126,543	15.82
25	Iget-object,invoke-virtual,move-result-object,return-object	124,229	15.53
26	Sget-object,iget-object,invoke-interface,return-void	122,453	15.31
27	Iput-object,return-object	120,819	15.10
28	Iput-boolean,return-void	120,257	15.03
29	Invoke-super,return-void	110,195	13.77
30	New-instance,invoke-direct,sput-object,return-void	102,617	12.83

4   Conclusion

In this work, we tried to find possibilities for detection of malicious Android apps using opcodes of applications. We collected malicious and benign applications from different sources and reverse engineered them using apktool for obtaining opcodes of applications. Since our database was huge, so we developed a software utility to automate this process. We conducted three exercises for assessing possibilities. The

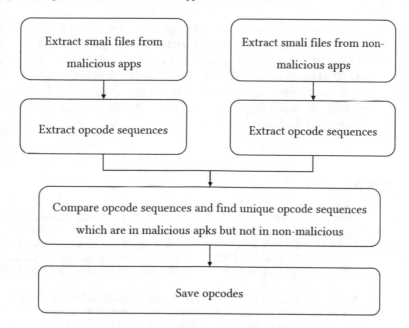

Fig. 2 Steps for obtaining malicious opcodes

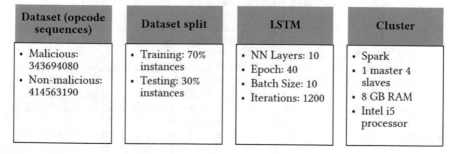

Fig. 3 Details of classification experiment

Table 4 Result of comparison with other approaches with opcode sequence

Approach	Classifier	F1-score	Accuracy
Varsha et al. [34]	SVM	0.72	–
Our approach	LSTM	0.72	0.99

first exercise is done to determine whether opcodes' count is different in malicious and benign apps.

We found that the number of occurrences of a particular opcode is less in malicious apps than in benign apps, and it's not effective in identifying maliciousness alone. The second exercise is done to find whether opcode sequences' frequency can be a candidate for detecting malignancy. We found that this is also not effective in doing this. Then we identified malicious opcode sequences by finding opcodes present only in malicious apps. With these malicious and benign opcode sequences, we performed a classification experiment with LSTM. We found that these opcode sequences are very much effective in differentiating malicious apps from benign apps. The results of exercises done in this work will help researchers focus intensely on opcode sequences for detecting malicious Android applications.

References

1. Talha KA, Alper DI, Aydin C (2015) APK auditor: Permission-based Android malware detection system. Digit Investig 13:1–14. https://doi.org/10.1016/j.diin.2015.01.001
2. Sun L, Li Z, Yan Q, Srisa-an W, Pan Y (2016) SigPID: significant permission identification for Android malware detection. In: 2016 11th International Conference on Malicious and Unwanted Software (MALWARE). IEEE, pp 1–8. https://doi.org/10.1109/MALWARE.2016.7888730
3. Mahindru A, Singh P (2017) Dynamic permissions based Android malware detection using machine learning techniques. In: Proceedings of the 10th innovations in software engineering conference, pp 202–210. https://doi.org/10.1145/3021460.3021485
4. Bezobrazov S, Sachenko A, Komar M, Rubanau V (2015) Artificial immune system for Android OS. In: Proceedings of the 2015 IEEE 8th international conference on intelligent data acquisition and advanced computing systems: technology and applications. IDAACS 2015, vol 1, pp 403–407. https://doi.org/10.1109/IDAACS.2015.7340767
5. Sokolova K, Perez C, Lemercier M (2017) Android application classification and anomaly detection with graph-based permission patterns. Decis Support Syst 93:62–76. https://doi.org/10.1016/j.dss.2016.09.006
6. Xiong P, Wang X, Niu W, Zhu T, Li G (2014) Android malware detection with contrasting permission patterns. China Commun 11:1–14. https://doi.org/10.1109/CC.2014.6911083
7. Wang W, Wang X, Feng D, Liu J, Han Z, Zhang X (2014) Exploring permission-induced risk in Android applications for malicious application detection. IEEE Trans Inf Forensics Secur 9:1869–1882. https://doi.org/10.1109/TIFS.2014.2353996
8. Yerima SY, Sezer S, McWilliams G, Muttik I (2013) A new Android malware detection approach using Bayesian classification. In: 2013 IEEE 27th international conference on advanced information networking and applications, pp 121–128. https://doi.org/10.1109/AINA.2013.88
9. McWilliams G, Sezer S, Yerima SY (2014) Analysis of Bayesian classification-based approaches for Android malware detection. IET Inf Secur 8:25–36. https://doi.org/10.1049/iet-ifs.2013.0095
10. Yerima SY, Sezer S, Muttik I (2014) Android malware detection using parallel machine learning classifiers. In: 2014 8th international conference on next generation mobile apps, services and technologies, pp 37–42. https://doi.org/10.1109/NGMAST.2014.23
11. Peiravian N, Zhu X (2013) Machine learning for Android malware detection using permission and API calls. In: Proceedings-International conference on tools with artificial intelligence. ICTAI, pp 300–305. https://doi.org/10.1109/ICTAI.2013.53
12. Zeng H, Ren Y, Wang QX, He NQ, Ding XY (2014) Detecting malware and evaluating risk of app using Android permission-API system. In: 2014 11th international computer conference on wavelet active media technology information process. ICCWAMTIP 2014, pp 440–443. https://doi.org/10.1109/ICCWAMTIP.2014.7073445

13. Chan PPK, Song WK (2014) Static detection of Android malware by using permissions and API calls. In: Proceedings-International conference on machine learning and cybernetics, vol 1, pp 82–87. https://doi.org/10.1109/ICMLC.2014.7009096
14. Cen L, Gates CS, Si L, Li N (2015) A probabilistic discriminative model for Android malware detection with decompiled source code. IEEE Trans Dependable Secur Comput 12:400–412. https://doi.org/10.1109/TDSC.2014.2355839
15. Qiao M, Sung AH, Liu Q (2016) Merging permission and api features for Android malware detection. In: Proceedings-2016 5th IIAI international congress on advanced applied informatics, IIAI-AAI 2016, pp 566–571. https://doi.org/10.1109/IIAI-AAI.2016.237
16. Tao G, Zheng Z, Guo Z, Lyu MR (2017) MalPat: mining patterns of malicious and benign Android apps via permission-related APIs. IEEE Trans Reliab 1–15. https://doi.org/10.1109/TR.2017.2778147
17. Onwuzurike L, Mariconti E, Andriotis P, De Cristofaro E, Ross G, Stringhini G (2017) MaMaDroid: detecting Android malware by building markov chains of behavioral models (extended version). https://doi.org/10.14722/ndss.2017.23353
18. Sahs J, Khan L (2012) A machine learning approach to Android malware detection. In: 2012 European intelligence and security informatics conference, pp 141–147. https://doi.org/10.1109/EISIC.2012.34
19. Canfora G, Mercaldo F, Visaggio CA (2013) A classifier of malicious Android applications. In: Proceedings-2013 2013 International conference on availability, reliability and security ARES 2013, pp 607–614. https://doi.org/10.1109/ARES.2013.80
20. Aung Z, Zaw W (2013) Permission-based Android malware detection. Int J Sci Technol Res 2
21. Yuan Z, Lu Y, Wang Z, Xue Y (2015) Droid-Sec: deep learning in Android malware detection. Comput Commun Rev 44:371–372. https://doi.org/10.1145/2619239.2631434
22. Idrees F, Rajarajan M (2014) Investigating the Android intents and permissions for malware detection. In: International conference on wireless and mobile computing, networking and communications, pp 354–358. https://doi.org/10.1109/WiMOB.2014.6962194
23. Feldman S, Stadther D, Wang B (2015) Manilyzer: automated Android malware detection through manifest analysis. In: Proceedings-11th IEEE international conference on mobile ad hoc and sensor systems MASS 2014, pp 767–772. https://doi.org/10.1109/MASS.2014.65
24. Su MY, Fung KT (2016) Detection of Android malware by static analysis on permissions and sensitive functions. In: International conference on ubiquitous and future networks, ICUFN, 2016-August, pp 873–875. https://doi.org/10.1109/ICUFN.2016.7537161
25. Kang BJ, Yerima SY, McLaughlin K, Sezer S (2016) N-opcode analysis for Android malware classification and categorization. In: 2016 international conference on cyber security and protection of digital services, cyber security 2016, pp 13–14. https://doi.org/10.1109/CyberSecPODS.2016.7502343
26. Wang W, Li Y, Wang X, Liu J, Zhang X (2018) Detecting Android malicious apps and categorizing benign apps with ensemble of classifiers. Futur Gener Comput Syst 78:987–994. https://doi.org/10.1016/J.FUTURE.2017.01.019
27. Milosevic N, Dehghantanha A, Choo KKR (2017) Machine learning aided Android malware classification. Comput Electr Eng 61:266–274. https://doi.org/10.1016/j.compeleceng.2017.02.013
28. Yang M, Wang S, Ling Z, Liu Y, Ni Z (2017) Detection of malicious behavior in Android apps through API calls and permission uses analysis. Concurr Comput Pract Exp 29:e4172. https://doi.org/10.1002/cpe.4172
29. Narayanan A, Chandramohan M, Chen L, Liu Y (2017) A multi-view context-aware approach to Android malware detection and malicious code localization. Empir Softw Eng 1–53. https://doi.org/10.1007/s10664-017-9539-8
30. Li Y, Jang J, Hu X, Ou X (2017) Android malware clustering through malicious payload mining. Lecture notes in computer science (including Subser. Lect. Notes Artif. Intell. Lect. Notes Bioinformatics). 10453 LNCS, pp 192–214. https://doi.org/10.1007/978-3-319-66332-6_9
31. Shen F, Del Vecchio J, Mohaisen A, Ko SY, Ziarek L (2017) Android malware detection using complex-flows. In: 2017 IEEE 37th international conference on distributed computing systems, pp 2430–2437. https://doi.org/10.1109/ICDCS.2017.190

32. Martinelli F, Mercaldo F, Saracino A (2017) BRIDEMAID: an hybrid tool for accurate detection of Android malware. In: Proc. 2017 ACM Asia conference on computer and communications security-ASIA CCS'17, pp 899–901. https://doi.org/10.1145/3052973.3055156

33. Zhu D, Jin H, Yang Y, Wu D, Chen W (2017) DeepFlow: deep learning-based malware detection by mining Android application for abnormal usage of sensitive data. In: Proceedings-IEEE symposium on computers and communications, pp 438–443. https://doi.org/10.1109/ISCC.2017.8024568

34. Varsha MV, Vinod P, Dhanya KA (2017) Identification of malicious Android app using manifest and opcode features. J Comput Virol Hacking Tech 13:125–138. https://doi.org/10.1007/s11416-016-0277-z

35. Apktool-A tool for reverse engineering 3rd party, closed, binary Android apps. https://ibotpeaches.github.io/Apktool/. Accessed 29 Nov 2020

36. Dalvik opcodes. http://pallergabor.uw.hu/androidblog/dalvik_opcodes.html. Accessed 29 Nov 2020

37. Dalvik bytecode|Android Open Source Project. https://source.android.com/devices/tech/dalvik/dalvik-bytecode. Accessed 29 Nov 2020

38. Hochreiter S, Urgen Schmidhuber J (1997) Long short-term memory. Neural Comput 9:1735–1780

39. Deeplearning4j: Open-source, Distributed Deep Learning for the JVM. https://deeplearning4j.org/. Accessed 29 Nov 2020

A New Adaptive Inertia Weight Based Multi-objective Discrete Particle Swarm Optimization Algorithm for Community Detection

Ashutosh Tripathi, Mohona Ghosh, and Kusum Kumari Bharti

1 Introduction

Complex systems are present all around us. They can be seen in the social groups of people, power distribution, neurons in the brain, bonds in chemicals and many more fields. Researchers have shown keen interest in the study of complex networks and their characteristics in recent years since many complex systems such as Online Social Media, World Wide Web, etc. can be modeled as complex networks. There are many characteristics of complex networks which can be studied to gain a better understanding of these networks. Some of these characteristics are centrality measures [1] (between-ness, closeness, degree centralities), characteristic motifs [2], clusters and communities, modularity, etc. A network can be modeled as a graph which is a set of nodes and the corresponding edges which connect nodes with each other. The graphs which consist of all the unique edges possible between the available set of nodes are called complete graphs. However, in the real world, most of the networks are not complete graphs. Moreover, the distribution of edges in the network is also non-uniform. This uneven distribution gives rise to interesting modules in the networks which are known as communities. Communities in a network are such partitions of the network, where the number of connections (edges) between different partitions is sparse as compared to the connections within the nodes of a single partition.

A. Tripathi · K. K. Bharti
PDPM Indian Institute of Information Technology Design and Manufacturing, Jabalpur, India
e-mail: ashutosht@iiitdmj.ac.in

K. K. Bharti
e-mail: kusum@iiitdmj.ac.in

M. Ghosh (✉)
Indira Gandhi Delhi Technical University for Women, Delhi, India
e-mail: mohonaghosh@igdtuw.ac.in

© The Author(s), under exclusive license to Springer Nature Singapore Pte Ltd. 2021
M. K. Bajpai et al. (eds.), *Machine Vision and Augmented Intelligence—Theory and Applications*, Lecture Notes in Electrical Engineering 796,
https://doi.org/10.1007/978-981-16-5078-9_25

A complex optimization problem may require optimization of more than one objective function to reach near optimum solutions. Such problems are known as multi-objective optimization problems as opposed to single-objective optimization problems which require optimization of a single objective. In multi-objective optimization problems, improving solutions based on one objective function may result in the deterioration of other objective functions. In such cases, the concept of Pareto dominant [3] sets is considered to find the best possible optimal solutions. A Pareto-optimal set is a set of solutions in which no single solution is better or dominant than any other solution in the set with respect to all the objective functions. Community detection in complex networks can be formulated as a multi-objective discrete optimization problem. Many network clustering and community detection techniques have been developed in recent years to solve this problem. Nature-inspired optimization algorithms are a class of optimization algorithms that take inspiration from nature. Iteratively find better solutions to an optimization problem based on some techniques which take inspiration from nature. Some examples of nature-inspired optimization algorithms are Particle Swarm Optimization [4], Artificial Bee Colony [5], Genetic Algorithm [6], etc.

Particle Swarm Optimization [4] (PSO) algorithm is a metaheuristic optimization algorithm that works on the natural phenomenon of bird flocking. Each bird in a flock takes the decision to move in a direction based on its own experience and the experience of its neighbor while searching for a food source. The information passing by birds is done by the loudness of their shrieking sound while they all fly together forming beautiful patterns without colliding with each other. In PSO, different particles are randomly generated in the search space of our problem at hand. The particles update their position based on three factors, current position, the best-known direction of a particle, and the best-known direction of a group These different factors are given different weightages according to the problem. The particles update their position based on three factors, current position, the best-known direction of a particle, and the best-known direction of a group.

A complex optimization problem may require optimization of more than one objective function to reach near-global optimum solutions. Such problems are known as multi-objective optimization problems as opposed to single-objective optimization problems which require optimization of a single objective function. Community detection in complex networks can be formulated as a multi-objective discrete optimization problem. With the use of intelligent inertia weight strategies, these algorithms can be improvised to perform better by adjusting the step size of the flight of the particle to a new position.

In this work, we present a new Adaptive Inertia Weight based MODPSO for Community Detection. In [7], two objective functions have been taken for optimization which are kernel k-means (KKM) and ratio cut (RC) which we consider for our work as well. We evaluate different inertia weights techniques with MODPSO [7] algorithm for community detection in complex networks. We show that while adaptive inertia weight based MODPSO gives consistently the best results for all benchmark datasets by maximizing the modularity of the real-world networks taken in our analysis, the same uniformity in delivering the best results was not observed in others. The rest of the paper is presented as follows. In Sect. 2, we present some of the earlier works mainly in the field of Discrete PSO and various inertia weight techniques. In Sect. 3, we discuss our contribution to this work. In Sect. 4, an adaptive inertia weight based Multi-Objective Discrete Particle Swarm Optimization for community detection in complex networks is presented. This section also mentions other inertia weight techniques which are known to perform well with PSO. These strategies have been compared with adaptive inertia based MODPSO, which is the main objective of this study. In Sect. 5, we discuss the results obtained along with their analysis. Finally, Sect. 6 concludes the paper with a discussion about future work.

2 Related Work

PSO has emerged as one of the most popular nature inspired optimization algorithms for solving continuous search space optimization problems. Researchers have made further efforts to improvise the PSO for solving discrete search space optimization problems too. These improvised algorithms can be termed as Discrete PSOs (DPSOs). Kennedy and Eberhart in [8] presented Binary PSO (BPSO), which made use of binary coding schemes. Sha and Hsu in [9] solved the job shop scheduling problem using DPSO. In their work, they used space transformations to map continuous search space to discrete search space. Newman [10] proposed a matrix eigenvector-based solution for community detection. A Genetic Algorithm based solution known as GA-Net was proposed by Pizzuti et al. [11] for social networks. Bandyopadhyay et al. [12] proposed a multi-objective community detection algorithm (AMOSA) for complex network using the simulated annealing method. Gupta and Kumar [13] proposed a rough set-based community detection algorithm known as LUAMCOM in which they used link upper approximation method along with mutual link reciprocity threshold criteria to identify communities in complex networks.

Most of the algorithms in community detection work on the optimization of network modularity. However, modularity-based approaches suffer from a drawback of resolution limit as pointed out by Fortunato and Barthlemy [14]. In a network, community structures smaller than a certain scale are not detected, depending upon the network size and the interconnectedness of the network. Gong et al. [7] proposed a decomposition-based multi-objective DPSO known as MODPSO for community detection in complex networks. They worked on optimization of two different mutually competing objectives which are kernel k-means (KKM) and ratio cut (RC). Thus, the problem of resolution limit can be overcome by using KKM and RC as objectives for optimization instead of modularity. In MODPSO, the particles are represented as a vector of node labels. Initialization of particles in the population is done using the Label Propagation Algorithm. Population diversity is promoted by choosing a random neighbor as the leader for the particle in place of *gbest* as used in the conventional PSO algorithm. To further promote population diversity, a turbulence operator is used. This turbulence operator mutates the particle positions by a small amount based on a small probability value which is simply a random number. Any PSO algorithm updates the particle velocities based on current velocity and best-known positions of the particle as well as the group. The current velocity factor in the PSO velocity update helps in further exploration of the search space. Factors of the best-known position of a particle and the best-known position of the population as a whole help in the exploitation of the information known beforehand. To balance exploration and exploitation, the different factors are multiplied by some weights. This weight is called as inertia weight in a PSO.

In MODPSO, random inertia weights are used. However, some previous works have illustrated that random inertia weight strategy may not always be the best strategy to be used in a PSO algorithm. Researchers have explored a number of inertia weight techniques in PSO which can very well be applied to Discrete PSO problems with slight improvisations. Bansal et al. [15] in their work explored 15 different inertia weight techniques in their work. They tested their approach by applying different inertia weight techniques in complex optimization objective functions. In their results summary, they present 4 such inertia weight techniques which perform best in their results. These inertia weight techniques are chaotic inertia weight, random inertia weight, constant inertia weight and linearly decreasing inertia weight. Li et al. [16] applied adaptive inertia weight technique in discrete PSO in which they regulated particle velocity according to the difference between the particle's current position and the global best position. They used various techniques to promote particle diversity so that the objective function search space is thoroughly explored. Their results clearly show that the DPSO-PDM algorithm presented by them performs better than other discrete PSO algorithms like MOGA-Net, LPA, GA-Net, and CNM.

3 Our Contribution

A multi-objective community detection overcomes the resolution limit problem of a modularity optimized community detection. In the velocity update equation of any PSO-derived algorithm, it is important to choose inertia weight carefully as it guides the particles while balancing the exploration and exploitation capability of the algorithm. Thus, an inertia weight strategy that intelligently chooses the inertia weight according to the position of the particle in the search space can help the particle to reach the optimum position. Our contributions in this paper are as follows:

1. We present a new Adaptive Inertia Weight based Multi-Objective Discrete Particle Swarm Optimization algorithm for community detection in complex networks. We utilize the global best solutions to calculate particle diversity. This particle diversity is utilized to calculate the inertia weight for the velocity update rule. A low particle diversity indicates that the particle is close to the global optimum solution. In such a case, the adaptive inertia weight reduces, hence the particle's inertial velocity component is reduced. Similarly, a high particle diversity indicates that the particle is far away from the global optimum.

In such a case, the particle's inertial velocity is increased and the particle flies with greater inertial velocity to explore the search space. Thus, adaptive inertia weight strategy intelligently calculates the inertia weight balancing the exploration of the search space and the exploitation of the information available about it.

2. We study various inertia weight techniques such as chaotic, random, constant and linearly decreasing inertia weights, which are known to perform better with PSO [16], and apply them in the MODPSO algorithm.

3. We present a comparative analysis of these inertia weight strategies with our new Adaptive Inertia Weight based MODPSO. Our analysis shows that an Adaptive Inertia Weight based MODPSO algorithm delivers consistently best results on all the benchmark real-world datasets with maximum Q values of 0.457, 0.527728 and 0.60457 for Zachary's Karate Club, Bottlenose Dolphins and American College Football datasets, respectively. On the other hand, the same uniformity in delivering the best modularity score values for all datasets is not observed with the other inertia weight strategies evaluated in this work.

4. To the best of our knowledge, this work is the first attempt towards analyzing the effect of adaptive inertia weight strategy in a multi-objective community detection optimization problem.

4 An Adaptive Inertia Weight Based Multi-objective Discrete Particle Swarm Optimization for Community Detection in Complex Networks

In this section, we discuss MODPSO along with the concepts of modularity optimization and multi-objective optimization techniques. Five different inertia weight techniques are also explored which are as follows: chaotic inertia weight, random inertia weight, constant inertia weight, linearly decreasing inertia weight.

4.1 Modularity

Modularity is an important network characteristic that helps in gaining information regarding the network structure. It is defined as the difference between the fraction of edges that fall within network clusters and the fraction of edges that could be expected in a random network with the same number of nodes and edges as the network under consideration. The former statement simply means that a network with some clustered structures will have higher modularity than a random network with the same number of nodes and edges.

A measure of modularity known as modularity function or Q value is mentioned in above cited works. The networks with better partitioning structures will have greater modularity. Assume a network $G(V,E)$ where $V = \{v_i \mid i = 1,2,3,...,n\}$ with n nodes is the vertex set of G and $E = \{e_i \mid i = 1,2,3,...,m\}$ with m edges is the edge set of the network. The adjacency matrix Adj of the network G is a $n \times n$ matrix which can be defined as

$$Adj_{ij} = \begin{cases} 1, & where\ node\ i\ connects\ with\ j \\ 0, & otherwise \end{cases} \tag{1}$$

For the network G the modularity Q if G is defined as

$$Q = \frac{1}{2m} \sum_{ij} Adj_{ij} - \frac{k_i k_j}{2m} \times \delta(C_i, C_j) \tag{2}$$

Here, k_i and k_j are the degrees of node i and node j, respectively. $\delta(C_i, C_j)$ represents whether or not i and j are in the same community with a value 1 for the same community and 0 for different communities.

In community detection problems, the modularity function is a very popular choice for the objective function, since networks with higher modularity have more distinct communities. However, modularity measure suffers from a problem of resolution limit. According to the resolution limit, depending upon the network size and the interconnectivity among the nodes, communities below a certain size are not detected. Due to this, a PSO algorithm may get stuck in a local optima and may not reach the global optimum solution. The direct use of modularity measure as an objective function in a PSO algorithm should be avoided in favor of any better objective function. A community detection can be framed as a multi-objective optimization using two such optimization objectives other than modularity using which the community structure of a network can be explained. These measures are kernel k-means and ratio cut.

4.2 Kernel K-Means (KKM) and Ratio Cut (RC)

In MODPSO algorithm, the objective of the algorithm is the minimization of KKM and RC functions. For the graph $G(V,E)$, with $|V| = n$ nodes and $|E| = m$ edges and the adjacency matrix given as A_{ij}, assume a partition of G into k clusters given as $\Omega \neg = \{c_1, c_2,...,c_k\}$. For $V_1, V_2 \in \Omega \neg$, $L(V_1, V_2) = \sum_{i \in V_1, j \in V_2} A_{ij}$ and $L(V_1, \bar{V}_2) = \sum_{i \in V_1, j \in \bar{V}_2} A_{ij}$ where $\bar{V}_2 = \Omega \neg V_2$. The kernel k-means (KKM) for a network is given as

$$KKM = 2(n - k) - \sum_{i=1}^{k} \frac{L(V_i, V_i)}{|V_i|} \tag{3}$$

The ratio cut for a network is defined as

$$RC = \sum_{i=1}^{k} \frac{L(V_i, \overline{V_i})}{|V_i|} \qquad (4)$$

These two functions follow opposite trends with respect to the number of communities. The KKM is a decreasing function of the number of network communities whereas the opposite is true for RC. Thus, both these objectives conflict with each other. We can consider the right operand of KKM as the sum of intracommunity link densities. On the other hand, RC can be considered as the sum of inter-community link densities. Minimization of KKM and RC ensures dense intracommunity link densities and sparse intercommunity link densities. Due to this, the minimization of these objectives can result in better community partitions.

4.3 Adaptive Inertia Weight Strategy Based Multi-objective Discrete Particle Swarm Optimization Algorithm

The Particle Swarm Optimization algorithm is used for finding the optimal solution of an objective function by defining multiple particles which move around the search space of the objective function while sharing function information among themselves. A particle is an object which has a position in search space and respective objective function evaluation at that position. The set of particles is termed as the population. Particles are initialized with some velocity, which results in the change of particle position iteration after iteration. The velocity of the particles can be modified according to the velocity update equation, which consists of a summation of three factors in traditional PSO. The velocity update equation for a particle is given as

$$V_i = \omega V_i + rc_1(pbest_i - x_i) + rc_2(gbest - x_i) \qquad (5)$$

Here V_i denotes the current particle velocity, $pbest_i$ denotes the best-known position encountered by the particle i, and $gbest$ denotes the best-known position encountered by the whole particle swarm till update. ω denotes the inertia weight of the particle which is very important in deciding how much weightage to the current velocity must be given in determining the updated velocity. The second term in the update equation guides the particle towards the best-known particle position till the time of update. Similarly, the third factor is used to guide the particle towards the best-known position encountered by the swarm. Here, r is a random number between 0 and 1. Whereas c_1 and c_2 are two constant values known as cognitive and social components respectively, which help in the exploitation of the best-known particle position and the best-known position of the particle swarm in guiding the particle. The velocity guides the particle in its flight to reach the optimal solution. Eventually, the particles should converge towards a single position which is called the optimal solution. The discrete particle swarm optimization works on a similar concept, although it requires some adaptation in the definition of particle position and particle velocity.

In a discrete PSO-based complex network community detection problem, a particle is coded as a vector of nodes with the community label of the node as the value at the position in the array corresponding to that node. A particle represents a potential solution for the optimization problem. A change in particle position simply means the change of community label for one or more nodes. It is represented as $X_i = \{x_i | i \in [1, n]\}$. Here, n is the total number of nodes in the network. If $x_i = x_j$, i and j belong to the same community. The discrete velocity of a particle i is given as $V_i = \{v_i | i \in [1, n]\}$. It is binary-coded such that the value 0 shows that the community label of the node in the particle should remain unchanged, and the value 1 shows that the community label of the node may be changed. The update equation for the discrete particle velocity is given as:

$$V_i = sig(\omega V_i + rc_1(pbest_i \oplus x_i) + rc_2(gbest \oplus x_i)) \tag{6}$$

Here ω, r, c_1, c_2, $pbest_i$ and $gbest$ have their usual meanings as in the case of conventional PSO. The $\oplus$ is defined as an XOR operator. Also, $sig()$ is the sigmoid function given by

$$sig(x) = \frac{1}{1 + e^x} \tag{7}$$

The sigmoid function is defined for the vectors in discrete PSO as

$$Y_i = sig(X_i) = \begin{cases} y_i = 1 \ if \ rand(0, 1) < sigmoid(x_i) \\ y_i = 0 \ if \ rand(0, 1) \geq sigmoid(x_i) \end{cases} \tag{8}$$

Here, $Y_i = (y_1, y_2,...,y_n)$ and $X_i = (x_1, x_2,..., x_n)$.

We use the updated velocity after each iteration to update the particle position. We define the discrete position update rule as

$$x_i^t = x_i^t \otimes v_i^t \tag{9}$$

For $X_2 = X_1 \otimes V_i$, the updated position obtained by moving from X_1 with velocity V_i using operation $\otimes$ is given as

$$\begin{cases} x_{2i} = x_{1i} if \ v_i = 0 \\ x_{2i} = Nbest_i if \ v_i = 1 \end{cases} \tag{10}$$

Here, $Nbest_i$ is the label identifier that is possessed by most of the neighbors of node i in the network. $Nbest_i$ is calculated as

$$Nbest_i = arg \max_r \sum_{j \in N} \varphi(x_{ij}, r) \tag{11}$$

where $\varphi(i,j) = 1$ if $i = j$ and 0 otherwise.

To promote population diversity, the MODPSO algorithm uses a random approach to select *Nbest,* and particle mutation strategy with a small probability. Thus, *Gbest* is replaced by *Nbest.* The personal best of a particle is stored using the concept of Pareto dominance in which a random solution out of a number of mutually non-dominating multi-objective solutions is chosen.

In the next section, we have discussed different inertia weight strategies. One of these strategies is adaptive inertia weight. Using this strategy, we propose a new Adaptive Inertia Weight based MODPSO algorithm. In adaptive inertia weight strategy, we first calculate the particle diversity, which is defined as

$$Div(X_i) = \frac{Count(P_i, P_g)}{n} \qquad (12)$$

The particle diversity is the ratio of the number of community labels of the nodes which are different between the current particle and the global best-positioned particle. The inertia weight for a particle is given as

$$w_i = w_{min} + (w_{max} - w_{min}).Div(X_i) \qquad (13)$$

In our algorithm, we make one more change, i.e., including the global best particle position in the calculation of particle velocity. The particle velocity update equation used in our algorithm is given by

$$V_i = sig(\omega V_i + rc_1(pbest_i \oplus x_i) + rc_2(Nbest \oplus x_i) + rc_3(Gbest \oplus x_i)) \qquad (14)$$

Usually, the values of c_1 and c_2 are taken as 1.494. In our algorithm, since we need to accommodate for c_3 too, we take c_1, c_2, c_3 as 1.367, 1.367, and 0.31 to keep the sum of constants with and without c_3 almost equal.

4.4 Inertia Weight Strategies

Inertia weight is very important in guiding a particle with weightage to its current velocity. Thus, it helps in more and more exploration of the particle in the search space. In this work, we have applied different inertia weight strategies in MODPSO to examine how a change in inertia weight strategy results in a change in the performance of the algorithm.

Chaotic inertia weight strategy involves a chaotic random number in generating the inertia weight for the current iteration. A random inertia weight strategy is a very simple strategy involving a random number. A constant inertia weight technique takes a constant value of inertia weight for all the iterations. The linearly decreasing inertia weight technique takes larger inertia weights in the starting iterations. This is done to ensure that enough search space is explored before convergence so that the possibility of local optima convergence is decreased. Gradually, the inertia weights for further iterations are reduced following a linear function. Toward the end of the algorithm, small inertia weights are taken to avoid major flights of the particles and let them converge to an optimal position.

Adaptive inertia weight strategy, using which we have proposed our algorithm in this work uses a diversity function in determining the inertia weight for a particle. Unlike other inertia weight strategies discussed in this section before, the inertia weight is different for each particle in each iteration. The inertia weight strategies used and their equations are given below.

5 Experiments and Results

We used these inertia weight strategies as given in Table 1 with MODPSO. Three popular undirected real-world labeled datasets were taken for the analysis. These datasets are Zachary's Karate Club dataset, Bottlenose dolphin dataset, and American college football dataset. The network diagrams of the datasets [16] are shown in Figs. 1, 2, and 3. Table 2 mentions the structure of these datasets. Normalized Mutual Information (NMI) metric is used to calculate how well the network labels are assigned by the algorithm as compared to the true labels of the nodes. For a network with two partitions A and B, let an element C_{ij} of the confusion matrix C

Table 1 Different inertia weight strategies used in this paper

Name of inertia weight	Formula
Chaotic	$z = 4 \times z \times (1 - z)$
	$w = (w_1 - w_2) \times \frac{MAXiter - iter}{MAXiter} + w_2 \times z$
Random	$w = 0.5 + \frac{Rand()}{2}$
Constant	$w = c$
	$c = 0.7$ (considered for experiments)
Linearly decreasing	$w_k = w_{max} - \frac{w_{max} - w_{min}}{iter_{max}} \times k$
Adaptive	$Div(X_i) = \frac{Count(P_i, P_g)}{n}$
	$w_i = w_{min} + (w_{max} - w_{min}).Div(X_i)$

Fig. 1 Zachary's Karate Club dataset showing two different communities in the network as per the true labels. Different colors signify members of different communities

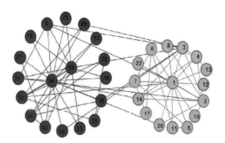

Fig. 2 Bottlenose Dolphin dataset showing two different communities in the network as per the true labels. Different colors signify different communities

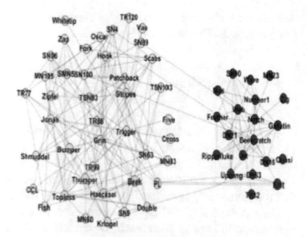

Fig. 3 American College Football dataset showing 12 different communities in the network as per the true labels. Different colors signify different communities

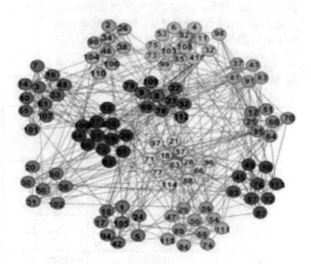

Table 2 Three popular undirected real-world labeled datasets

Network	Nodes	Edges	Number of communities
Zachary's Karate club	34	78	2
Bottlenose Dolphins	62	159	2
American College Football	115	613	12

denotes the number of common nodes of community i in partition A and community j in partition B. The $NMI(A,B)$ is given as

$$NMI = \frac{-2\sum_{i=1}^{C_A}\sum_{j=1}^{C_B} C_{ij}\log\left(C_{ij}N/C_iC_j\right)}{\sum_{i=1}^{C_A} C_i\log\left(C_i/N\right) + \sum_{j=1}^{C_B} C_j\log\left(C_j/N\right)} \tag{15}$$

Here, C_A and C_B are the number of communities in partitions A and B, respectively. C_i is the sum of elements in row i of C and C_j is the sum of elements in column j of C. N is the total number of nodes present in the network. An $NMI(A,B)$ value of 1 shows that the partitions in A, and B are identical. A value 0 of $NMI(A,B)$ shows that the community partitions in A and B *are* completely different.

We ran the MODPSO algorithm on these real-world unlabeled datasets for 30 iterations with 75 generations each. We calculated the maximum Q value and average Q value for all the inertia weight strategies. Similarly, maximum and average NMI is also recorded for each dataset and inertia weight strategy. The results obtained are shown in Table 3.

Table 3 Experimental results of the application of various inertia weight techniques in MODPSO

Name of inertia weight		Karate Club	Dolphin	Football
Chaotic	Max Q	**0.41979**	0.525315	**0.60457**
	Avg Q	0.417735	0.521334	0.604196
	Max NMI	1	1	0.928143
	Avg NMI	0.985394	1	0.927638
Random	Max Q	**0.41979**	0.522428	0.601009
	Avg Q	0.418754	0.516093	0.593385
	Max NMI	1	1	**0.936064**
	Avg NMI	1	0.988338	0.926687
Constant	Max Q	**0.41979**	0.524643	**0.60457**
	Avg Q	0.419477	0.524596	0.603237
	Max NMI	1	1	0.926879
	Avg NMI	1	0.981624	0.923778
Linearly decreasing	Max Q	**0.41979**	0.525315	0.603204
	Avg Q	0.419592	0.525083	0.602455
	Max NMI	1	1	0.928943
	Avg NMI	0.989102	1	**0.927612**
Adaptive	Max Q	**0.41979**	**0.527728**	**0.60457**
	Avg Q	**0.419633**	**0.526166**	**0.604287**
	Max NMI	1	1	0.926879
	Avg NMI	0.989142	1	0.926879

The results of the experiments as given in Table 3 clearly show that adaptive inertia weight performs better than other inertia weight techniques almost every time. This is evident from both the maximum and average Q values. The main reason behind the consistent results of the adaptive inertia weight strategy can be attributed to its adaptability to the particle drifts from the global best solutions. When a particle is farther from the global best solution, it increases the inertia weight of the velocity update equation, thereby increasing the step length. On the other hand, when the particle is closer to the global best solution, it decreases the step length. Thus, it strikes a balance between the local and global search by adapting to the distance of the particle from the currently known optimal solution.

For Zachary's Karate Club dataset, our algorithm finds the max and average Q values as 0.41979 and 0.419633. All the other algorithms also find the same value of max Q but the average Q value is greatest in the case of adaptive inertia weight strategy. For the Bottlenose Dolphin dataset, the max and average Q values found by adaptive inertia weight based MODPSO are 0.527728 and 0.526166, respectively. It is greatest among the max and average Q values found by other strategies. In the American College Football dataset, chaotic, random, and adaptive inertia weight strategies with MODPSO find the max Q value of 0.60457, which is greatest among all the inertia weight strategies used in this paper. However, the average Q value found by our approach is 0.604297 which is close to the maximum Q score and greatest among all the other average Q values for the American College Football dataset. Thus, it is clear that our algorithm performs consistently better than other inertia weight approaches in maximizing the Q value of the real-world networks. In NMI calculations, we see that other algorithms also perform equally good, still max and average NMI scores calculated by our algorithms are also very close to the best results. Max NMI scores of 1 are found for Zachary's Karate Club dataset and Bottlenose Dolphin dataset by our algorithm as well as other inertia weight strategies. The convergence plots for the three datasets Karate Club, Bottlenose Dolphin, and American College Football are shown in Figs. 4, 5 and 6 respectively.

6 Conclusion and Future Work

From the experiments done on three real-world labeled datasets, it can be concluded that adaptive inertia weight strategy works better than other inertia weight strategies given in this paper in maximizing the modularity scores of the real-world networks in community detection problems. It strikes a balance between global and local search by adapting to the distance of the particle from the optimal solution. Although other inertia weight strategies which are known to perform well with PSO have also been tested, our algorithm is the most consistent one, giving the best results for maximum and average Q values for all the datasets considered in this paper. In the future, we will try to explore the best exploration–exploitation balance strategies from other nature-inspired algorithms which could help us to quickly escape locally optimum solutions and help in converging to globally optimal solutions efficiently.

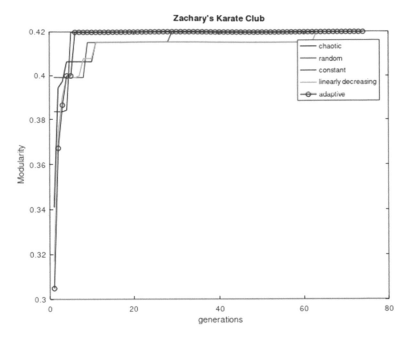

Fig. 4 Zachary's Karate Club convergence plot using different inertia weight strategies with MODPSO

Fig. 5 Bottlenose Dolphin convergence plot using different inertia weight strategies with MODPSO

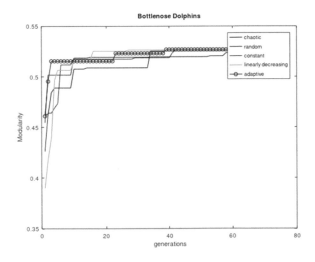

Fig. 6 American College Football convergence plot using different inertia weight strategies with MODPSO

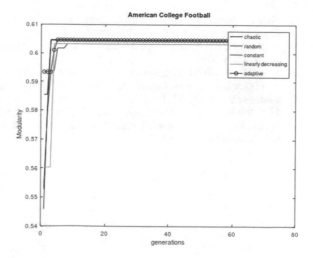

References

1. Hansen DL, Schneiderman B, Smith MA, Himelboim I (2011) Social network analysis: measuring, mapping, and modeling collections of connections. In: Analyzing social media networks with NodeXL: insights from a connected world. Elsevier Inc., Burlington, pp 31–52
2. O'Callaghan D, Harrigan M, Carthy J, Cunningham P (2012) Network analysis of recurring youtube spam campaigns. In: Sixth international AAAI conference on weblogs and social media
3. Brisset S, Gillon F (2015) Approaches for multi-objective optimization in the ecodesign of electric systems. In: Eco-friendly innovation in electricity transmission and distribution networks, Elsevier, pp 83–97
4. Kennedy J, Eberhart R (1995) Particle swarm optimization. In: Proceedings of ICNN'95-international conference on neural networks, vol 4. IEEE
5. Dervis K, Basturk B (2007) Artificial bee colony (ABC) optimization algorithm for solving constrained optimization problems. In: International fuzzy systems association world congress. Springer, Berlin, Heidelberg
6. Horn J, Nafpliotis N, Goldberg DE (1994) A niched Pareto genetic algorithm for multiobjective optimization. In: Proceedings of the first IEEE conference on evolutionary computation. IEEE world congress on computational intelligence. IEEE
7. Gong M, Cai Q, Chen X, Ma L (2014) Complex network clustering by multiobjective discrete particle swarm optimization based on decomposition. IEEE Trans Evol Comput 18(1)
8. Kennedy J, Eberhart R (1997) A discrete binary version of the particle swarm algorithm. In: Proceedings of IEEE international conference on systems, man and cybernetics, vol 5. Oct 1997, pp 4104–4108
9. Sha DY, Hsu CY (2006) A hybrid particle swarm optimization for job shop scheduling problem. Comput Ind Eng 51(4):791–808
10. Newman MEJ (2006) Finding community structure in networks using the eigenvectors of matrices. Phys Rev E 74(3):036104. (Sept 2006)
11. Pizzuti C (2008) GA-Net: a genetic algorithm for community detection in social networks. In: Proceedings of parallel problem solving nature, vol 5199, pp 1081–1090
12. Bandyopadhyay S, Saha S, Maulik U, Deb K (2008) A simulated annealing-based multi-objective optimization algorithm: AMOSA. IEEE Trans Evol Comput 12(3):269–283. (Jun 2008)

13. Gupta S, Kumar P (2020) An overlapping community detection algorithm based on rough clustering of links. Data Knowl Eng 125:101777
14. Fortunato S, Barthelemy M (2007) Resolution limit in community detection. Proc Natl Acad Sci 104(1):36–41
15. Bansal JC, Singh PK, Saraswat M, Verma A, Jadon SS, Abraham A (2011) Inertia weight strategies in particle swarm optimization. In 2011 Third world congress on nature and biologically inspired computing. IEEE
16. Li X, Wu X, Xu S, Qing S, Chang PC (2019) A novel complex network community detection approach using discrete particle swarm optimization with particle diversity and mutation. Appl Soft Comput 81:105476

Automatic Diagnosis of Covid-19 Using Chest X-ray Images Through Deep Learning Models

Siddharth Gupta, Palak Aggarwal, Sumeshwar Singh,
Shiv Ashish Dhondiyal, Manisha Aeri, and Avnish Panwar

1 Introduction

As stated by the World Health Organization (WHO), disease generated by the virus continues to develop and produce a severe concern for mankind. In the past 20 years, various viruses such as Severer Acute Respiratory Syndrome (SARS) in 2002–2003, HINI influenza in 2009, Middle East Respiratory Syndrome (MERS) in 2012 have been identified [1]. In December 2019, a new type of human virus called Coronavirus or Covid-19 that belongs to a family of RNA viruses in the Nidovirales order was originated from Wuhan, Hubei, China [2]. The Basic Respiratory Number (BRN) for coronavirus (SARS-COV2 virus) is 2 to 3, that is, every one individual is responsible for spreading this virus to two other individuals [3]. The symptoms observed in the infected patient are cold, cough, fever, and deficiency in breathing (dyspnea). However, if the infection becomes too severe it may result in multiple organ failures. After observing the high number of active cases and deaths due to this virus, the WHO declared it as "WORLDWIDE PANDEMIC" [4].

The drastic rise in the number of patients infected by Covid-19 has brought down the best medical facilities to the point of failure all over the world. Table 1 shows the total number of positive cases, active cases, and total deaths for the top 15 countries across the world [5]. The rise in the number of cases for Covid-19 has increased the cost of diagnosis in private sectors and still, it is a very big issue especially for under developing countries where the medical facilities are very poor [6]. The research carried out shows radiological image based detection of Covid-19 is relatively faster than PCR testing [7]. In March 2020, when a pandemic spread in the entire world,

S. Gupta (✉) · P. Aggarwal · S. A. Dhondiyal
Graphic Era Deemed to be University, Dehradun, India

S. Singh · M. Aeri · A. Panwar
Graphic Era Hill University, Dehradun, India

© The Author(s), under exclusive license to Springer Nature Singapore Pte Ltd. 2021
M. K. Bajpai et al. (eds.), *Machine Vision and Augmented Intelligence—Theory and Applications*, Lecture Notes in Electrical Engineering 796,
https://doi.org/10.1007/978-981-16-5078-9_26

Table 1 Top 15 Countries covid-19 positive cases as of 1 August 2020 [5]

S.No	Country names	Total cases	Active cases	Death cases
1	USA	4,706,180	2,220,971	156,764
2	Brazil	2,666,298	689,679	92,568
3	India	1,701,532	568,047	36,587
4	Russia	845,443	184,861	14,058
5	South Africa	493,183	159,007	8,005
6	Mexico	424,735	99,331	46,688
7	Peru	414,735	108,391	19,217
8	Chile	355,667	17,883	9,457
9	Spain	335,602	NA	28,445
10	Iran	306,752	23,940	16,982
11	UK	303,181	NA	46,119
12	Colombia	295,508	131,016	10,105
13	Pakistan	278,305	25,177	5,951
14	Saudi Arabia	275,905	37,381	2,866
15	Italy	247,537	12,422	35,141

there is a rapid increase in the chest X-ray images for Covid-19, therefore, a motivation for finding a pattern for automatic detection and diagnosis of Covid-19 is carried out this research. The total number of positive Covid-19 cases of several countries that exist all across the world can be extracted from [8].

The advancement of Deep Learning (DL) [9] based applications for medical image classification make it possible to classify Covid-19, normal, and pneumonia images into the right category. In this work, several CNN models are fed with CT scan images of a chest X-ray. The features are extracted from images and finally with the help of various Machine Learning (ML) classifiers several input images are classified as Covid-19 positive, pneumonia images, or normal images with no infection. The obtained results are inspiring and represent the advantage of using DL techniques.

The next section in the paper represents the various research works carried out by several researchers for the detection and classification of Covid-19 images. Section 3 includes the description of the dataset, preprocessing of the dataset, the architecture used, and several parameters that measure the performance of several DL models and ML classifiers. Section 4 includes the result which determines the performance measurement of several classifiers and finally, the paper is concluded by relating all the observations.

2 Related Work

Apostolopoulos et al. [10] used 1427 X-ray images from patients suffering from common bacterial pneumonia, positive Covid-19, and normal images. Several deep learning architectures are used to train dataset images. The obtained results show accuracy, sensitivity, and specificity of 96.78%, 98.66%, and 96.46%. Farooq and Hafeez [11] have built the open-source dataset and applied various CNN frameworks to diagnose Covid-19 and pneumonia images. The input images are preprocessed and fed to pretrained Res-Net 50 architecture. The accuracies obtained by applying Res-Net50 architecture is 96.23% and with this model the Covid-19 images can be easily and early detected. Feng et al. [12] used 1658 patients' X-ray images of Covid-19, and 1027 patients of CAP images were captured. An infection size aware random forest (iSARF) method was proposed where infected lesions are categorized based on the size where the random forest is used for classification. The result shows that the accuracy of 87.9% is obtained, specificity is 83.3% and sensitivity of 90.7% is obtained. Wang et al. [13] have used 453 CT images of Covid-19 positive cases were collected. Out of these 217 images were used as training sets. The algorithm used for classification is the inception migration learning model. The results obtained show internal validation achieve an accuracy of 82.9%, with a specificity of 80.5% and a sensitivity of 84% and the external validation dataset shows a total accuracy of 73.1% with a specificity of 67% and sensitivity of 74%. The results indicate a high value of deep learning methods to extract radiographical features for Covid-19 diagnosis. Shan et al. [14] used the dataset used that comprised 300 CT images used for validation. 249 Covid-19 positive images were used as training images. Several image acquisition parameters are used for image preprocessing. Obtained images are fed to the VB-Net model for the classification of Covid-19 images from the dataset. The system obtained dice coefficients of 91.6%.

3 Methodology

3.1 Dataset Description

The dataset is publically available and comprises 400 images [15]. These images are divided into training and testing datasets. The images used are from the training set. There are totals of three classes of images, first-class consists of positive Covid-19 chest X-ray images, the second class comprises normal chest X-ray images without any infection and the third class of images are the patients suffering from pneumonia. A detailed description of the dataset can be extracted from Table 2.

Table 2 Dataset description for COVID-19, pneumonia, and normal images

Dataset/classes	Covid19	Normal	Pneumonia	Total
# of images in training set	61	69	70	200
# of images in testing set	61	69	70	200
Total	122	138	140	400

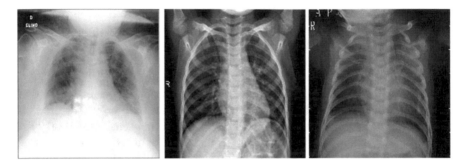

Fig. 1 Dataset Images for **A** Covid-19 positive case. **B** Normal chest X-ray image. **C** Pneumonia infected image

3.2 Dataset Pre-processing

A lot of images are collected for creating a dataset. The size of every image has a variable length and height. Also, the images are captured from different devices; therefore, the resolution of every image is also different. To classify the images the size of every image should be equal. To provide an efficient dataset all the images are pre-processed. For preprocessing the images, several preprocessing techniques such as image cropping and resizing are performed. By applying these techniques all the images in the dataset are set to the same standard size. Figure 1 shows the dataset images of Covid-19 positive patient chest X-ray, normal chest X-ray images of the patient, and pneumonia chest X-ray image.

3.3 Architecture Used

The recommended framework for accurate detection of Covid-19 chest X-ray images using deep learning model and machine learning classifiers consists of VGG16 [16], VGG19 [16], and Inception v3 [17] architecture for training the images and then using several ML classifiers such as KNN [18], Tree [19], RF [20], NN [21], LR [22], and AdaBoost [23] for classification chest X-ray images. Figure 2 describes the overall architecture.

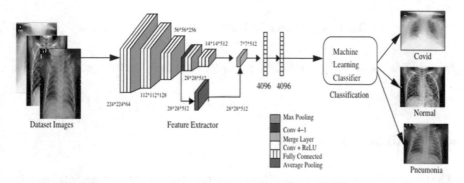

Fig. 2 Overall architecture for detection of Covid-19 positive cases images from chest X-ray images

- Different dataset images including positive Covid-19, pneumonia, and normal chest X-ray are taken. Every image is pre-processed and converted to the standard size.
- The dataset images are fed to various powerful DL models for extracting the features. VGG16, VGG19, and Inception v3 models are used. Out of these VGG16 and Inception v3 performed well. Inception v3 has simple architecture and has the ability for tackling the problem of overfitting. Finally, this model is capable to train many features which enhances its power for classification purposes. Another model that performs fine for feature training is VGG16. This model comprises 13 convolutional filter layers along with 3 fully connected layers and 5 max-pool layers. The filter size used is 3 × 3 with stride one and padding of one pixel is done, respectively.
- Once the processing is finished the extracted images are used for classification of Covid-19 positive cases images, pneumonia images, and normal images without any infection with the help of several Machine Learning classifiers such as KNN, Tree, RF, NN, LR, and AdaBoost.

Once the training part is finished, several machine learning classifiers such as KNN, Tree, RF, NN, AdaBoost is used to classify the images as positive Covid-19, pneumonia, and normal images without any infection. Once the classification has been performed the results obtained are evaluated based on several parameters such as AUC [24], Accuracy [25], F1 score, Precision, and Recall [26]. The obtained parameters can be calculated using Eqs. (1), (2), (3), and (4).

$$\text{Accuracy} = (\text{TN} + \text{TP}) / (\text{TN} + \text{TP} + \text{FN} + \text{FP}) \tag{1}$$

$$\text{Recall} = \text{TP} / (\text{TP} + \text{FN}) \tag{2}$$

$$\text{Precision} = \text{TP} / (\text{TP} + \text{FP}) \tag{3}$$

$$F1 \text{ Score } = 2 * (\text{Recall} * \text{Precision}) / \text{Recall} + \text{Precision} \qquad (4)$$

where TP is True Positive, TN is True Negative, FP is False Positive, and FN is False Negative.

4 Result and Discussions

The proposed architecture is fed with 400 images. These images comprise Covid-19 positive chest X-ray images infected pneumonia images and normal images without any infection. To classify these images, several deep learning models such as VGG16, VGG19, and Inception v3 are used. According to the results obtained in Tables 3, 4 and 5, VGG16 and Inception v3 are selected as benchmark models for the feature extraction and Random Forest ML classifier outperformed the rest of the classifiers. The result in Table 3 shows the performance of the VGG16 model along with KNN, Tree, RF, NN, LR, and AdaBoost classifiers. Out of all the classifiers, Logistic Regression gives the best result of 97%.

The results in Table 4 show the performance of the VGG19 model along with respective classifiers such as KNN, Tree, RF, NN, LR, and AdaBoost. The results show that logistic regression gives the best result with an accuracy of 96%.

Table 3 Performance metrics for VGG16 model and respective classifiers

Method	AUC	Accuracy	F1 score	Precision	Recall
KNN	0.987	0.940	0.940	0.945	0.940
Tree	0.876	0.870	0.870	0.871	0.870
RF	0.980	0.905	0.906	0.908	0.905
NN	0.967	0.935	0.935	0.935	0.935
LR	0.991	**0.970**	0.970	0.970	0.970
AdaBoost	0.887	0.850	0.850	0.851	0.850

Table 4 Performance metrics for VGG19 model and respective classifiers

Method	AUC	Accuracy	F1 score	Precision	Recall
KNN	0.987	0.930	0.930	0.936	0.930
Tree	0.813	0.770	0.771	0.772	0.770
RF	0.982	0.915	0.915	0.916	0.915
NN	0.957	0.925	0.925	0.926	0.925
LR	0.997	**0.960**	0.960	0.960	0.960
AdaBoost	0.869	0.825	0.825	0.826	0.820

Table 5 Performance metrics for Inception V3 model and respective classifiers

Method	AUC	Accuracy	F1 score	Precision	Recall
KNN	0.985	0.920	0.921	0.927	0.920
Tree	0.775	0.705	0.706	0.710	0.705
RF	0.973	0.890	0.890	0.891	0.890
NN	0.995	**0.970**	0.970	0.970	0.970
LR	0.992	0.940	0.940	0.941	0.940
AdaBoost	0.796	0.730	0.729	0.730	0.730

Table 6 Confusion matrix for logistic regression classifier and VGG16 model

		Predicted			
Actual		Covid19	Normal	Pneumonia	Σ
	Covid-19	58	0	3	61
	Normal	1	67	1	69
	Pneumonia	1	3	66	70
	Σ	60	70	70	200

The result shows that the Inception V3 model and VGG16 model outperformed several other models. The highest scores obtained are using Inception V3 and VGG16 model along with logistic regression classifier. The accuracies obtained are 97% for both the models. The results show that whenever a new chest X-ray image is fed into the proposed model based on the ability to extract the features, it will easily classify the input image into Covid-19 positive category or pneumonia-infected category or no infection category.

Another parameter used to depict the performance of various DL models and several ML classifiers is the ROC curve. The ROC curve is a graph plotted between the true positive rate and the false positive rate at several threshold values. The biggest advantage of using the ROC curve is that it has the ability to determine the performance of several binary classifiers. Figure 3 shows the ROC curve for comparing the performance of several ML classifiers. It can be easily observed that Logistic Regression outperforms the rest of the classifiers to classify the Covid-19, normal, and pneumonia images [27, 28].

Figure 4 shows the performance of the VGG19 model and several ML classifiers. The obtained observations verify that Logistic Regression classifiers outperform the other classifiers for classifying the Covid-19, normal, and pneumonia images.

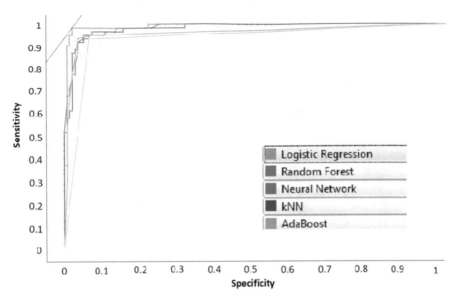

Fig. 3 ROC curve for VGG16 model along with several ML classifiers with respect to Covid-19, pneumonia, and normal chest X-ray images

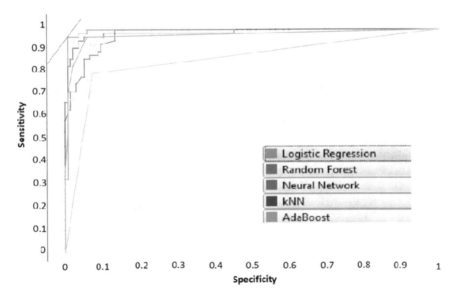

Fig. 4 ROC curve for VGG19 model along with several classifiers with respect to Covid-19, pneumonia, and normal chest X-ray images

5 Conclusion

The current pandemic situation of Covid-19 has been termed as a worldwide health emergency due to the immense contagiousness of the infection. At the time of writing this paper, no clinically approved vaccine is out to control the pandemic situation therefore early detection of Covid-19 is a must. The only approach to protect the non-infected person from the infected patient is to quarantine or isolate the infected patient. Therefore, the detection and diagnosis of Covid-19 infected patients bear foremost importance. Modern techniques such as chest X-ray and CT are playing a major role in the early diagnosis of the Covid-19 infection. In this work, we have taken the dataset that comprises Covid-19 positive, normal, and pneumonia chest X-ray images, and after preprocessing the images are passed to several feature extraction deep learning models and finally to the several machine learning-based classifiers for the classification of the chest X-ray images into Covid-19 positive or not positive classes, respectively. The experimental results obtained by VGG16 and Inception V3 model and Logistic Regression and Neural Network classifier obtained an accuracy of 97% to correctly identify the Covid-19 patient.

References

1. Cascella M, Rajnik M, Cuomo A, Dulebohn SC, Di Napoli R (2020) Features, evaluation and treatment coronavirus (COVID-19). In Statpearls [internet]. StatPearls Publishing.
2. Dhama K, Sharun K, Tiwari R et al (2020) Coronavirus disease 2019–COVID-19 preprints, April 2020
3. Zhao S, Lin Q, Ran J et al (2020) Preliminary estimation of the basic reproduction number of novel coronavirus (2019-nCoV) in China, from 2019 to 2020: A data-driven analysis in the early phase of the outbreak. Int J Infect Dis 92:214–217
4. Al-Shamsi HO, Alhazzani W, Alhuraiji A et al (2019) A practical approach to the management of cancer patients during the novel coronavirus disease 2019 (COVID-19) pandemic: an international collaborative group. Oncologist 25(6):e936
5. Worldometers: COVID-19 Coronavirus Pandemic. https://www.worldometers.info/coronavirus/. Accessed 1 Aug 2020
6. Choo EK, Rajkumar SV (2020) Medication shortages during the COVID-19 crisis: what we must do. Mayo Clinic Proc 95(6):1112–1115. (June 2020)
7. Ucar F, Korkmaz D (2020) COVIDiagnosis-Net: deep Bayes-SqueezeNet based diagnostic of the coronavirus disease 2019 (COVID-19) from X-ray images. Med Hypotheses 109761
8. World Health Organization; Coronavirus disease 2019 (COVID-19) situation report–83. https://www.who.int/docs/default-source/coronaviruse/situationreports/20200412-sitrep-83-covid-19.pdf?sfvrsn=697ce98d_4. Accessed 1 Aug 2020.
9. LeCun Y, Bengio Y, Hinton G (2015) Deep learning. Nature 521(7553):436–444
10. Apostolopoulos ID, Mpesiana TA (2020) Covid-19: automatic detection from X-ray images utilizing transfer learning with convolutional neural networks. Phys Eng Sci Med
11. Farooq M, Hafeez A (2020) Covid-resnet: A deep learning framework for screening of covid19 from radiographs. arXiv:2003.14395. (March 2020)
12. Shi F, Xia L, Shan F et al (2020) Large-scale screening of covid-19 from community acquired pneumonia using infection size-aware classification. arXiv:2003.09860. (March 2020).
13. Wang S, Kang B, Ma J et al (2020) A deep learning algorithm using CT images to screen for Corona Virus Disease (COVID-19). MedRxiv. (January 2020)

14. Shan F, Gao Y, Wang J et al (2020) Lung infection quantification of covid-19 in CT images with deep learning. arXiv:2003.04655. (March 2020)
15. Publically available dataset on github. https://github.com/vj2050/Transfer-LearningCOVID19/tree/master/dataset_3_classes/train
16. Simonyan K, Zisserman A (2014) Very deep convolutional networks for large-scale image recognition, pp 1409–1556. (Sept 2014)
17. Szegedy C, Vanhoucke V, Ioffe S, Shlens J, Wojna Z (2016) Rethinking the inception architecture for computer vision. In: Proceedings of the IEEE conference on computer vision and pattern recognition, pp 2818–2826
18. Altman NS (1992) An introduction to kernel and nearest-neighbor nonparametric regression. Am Stat 46(3):175–185
19. Tsipouras MG, Tsouros DC, Smyrlis PN, Giannakeas N, Tzallas AT (2018) Random forests with stochastic induction of decision trees. In: 2018 IEEE 30th international conference on tools with artificial intelligence (ICTAI), pp 527–531. (Nov 2018)
20. Denisko D, Hoffman MM (2018) Classification and interaction in random forests. Proc Natl Acad Sci 115(8):1690–1692
21. Schmidhuber J (2015) Deep learning in neural networks: an overview. Neural Netw 61:85–117
22. Gasso G (2019) Logistic regression.
23. Zhou S, Yin K, Liu Z, Fei F, Guo J (2017) sEMG-based hand motion recognition by means of multi-class adaboost algorithm. In 2017 IEEE international conference on robotics and biomimetics (ROBIO), pp 1056–1061. (Dec 2017)
24. Zweig MH, Campbell G (1993) Receiver-operating characteristic ROC) plots: a fundamental evaluation tool in clinical medicine. Clin Chem 39(4):561–577
25. Panwar A, Semwal G, Goel S, Gupta S (2020) Stratification of the lesions in color fundus images of diabetic retinopathy patients using deep learning models and machine learning classifiers. In: 26th annual international conference on advanced computing and communications (ADCOM 2020), Silchar, Assam, India. (in press).
26. Gupta S, Panwar A, Goel S, Mittal A, Nijhawan R, Singh AK (2019) Classification of lesions in retinal fundus images for diabetic retinopathy using transfer learning. In: 2019 international conference on information technology (ICIT), Bhubaneswar, India, 2019, pp 342–347. https://doi.org/10.1109/ICIT48102.2019.00067
27. Gupta S, Panwar A, Aggarwal P, Chaubey N (2020) Accurate prognosis of covid19 using CT scan images with deep learning model and machine learning classifiers. In: 2nd national conference on communication systems (NCOCS), NIT, Punducherry, Karaikal. (in press).
28. Gupta S, Panwar A, Chauhan A (2020) Automatic detection and classification of pneumonia chest x-ray images using transfer learning methods. In: 9th world conference on applied sciences, engineering and management (WCSEM 2020) at Paris. (Dec 2020, in press).

Density-Assessment for Breast Cancer Diagnosis Using Deep Learning on Mammographic Image: A Brief Study

Shaila Chugh, Sachin Goyal, Anjana Pandey, Sunil Joshi, and Mukesh Azad

1 Introduction

Collectively, India, China, and the United States have approximately one-third of the global breast cancer burden. The signs of breast cancer are anomalies such as the presence of breast mass, changes in the form and dimension of the breast, variations in breast skin color, breast ache, etc. Diagnosis of cancer is carried out on the basis of non-molecular parameters, such as the form of tissue, pathological properties, and clinical location. The unregulated division of one cell starts with cancer and occurs in the form of a tumor. There are many imaging methods, such as magnetic resonance imaging, ultrasound imaging, X-ray imaging, for breast examination. Mammography is the most powerful early breast cancer diagnosis technique that uses a low-dose X-ray radiation method for routine screening for breast cancer.

Deep Learning based Computer Aided Diagnosis (CAD) systems allow anomalies in mammography images to be examined (e.g., micro-calcification, masses, and distortions). Mammogram preprocessing, enhancement, region of interest (mass) assessment, two-stage mass classification (normal /abnormal then abnormal is labeled as benign/malignant) are usually the complete mammogram-based CAD system.

The most prevalent mammography findings like abnormal mass fields, micro-calcifications (MCs), architectural areas distortion, and asymmetry are associated with breast density [1]. It has proven to be one of the most accurate screening tools and a primary approach for screening and detection of breast cancer at an early stage. The breast density BI-RADS (Breast Imaging Reporting and Data System) are considered as the primary factor for breast cancer diagnosis.

The constraints of the current CAD suggest that machine learning and image processing advances techniques and mammographic image prevalence have opened

S. Chugh (✉) · S. Goyal · A. Pandey · S. Joshi · M. Azad
Samrat Ashok Technological Institute, Vidisha, India

© The Author(s), under exclusive license to Springer Nature Singapore Pte Ltd. 2021 313
M. K. Bajpai et al. (eds.), *Machine Vision and Augmented Intelligence—Theory and Applications*, Lecture Notes in Electrical Engineering 796,
https://doi.org/10.1007/978-981-16-5078-9_27

up a chance to fix the difficult problem using deep learning methods for early detection of breast cancer [2, 3].

The aim of the survey was to highlight the challenges of applying deep learning to early breast cancer detection using digital multi-view mammographic data on the basis of breast density. In the multi-view digital mammographic results, the current deep learning literature can be defined for discrimination against breast density, identification, and classification of lesions in breast cancer. The remainder of this analysis is structured as follows. A general breast density assessment/estimation for CAD system of breast cancer using deep learning consists of three basic stages:

(I)   Selection of a breast mammogram image dataset.
(II)   Enhancement, Segmentation, Feature calculation.
(III) Classification.

2 Deep Neural Network for Breast Density Assessment Literature Survey

Using a Deep CNN, the author in [6] suggests extraction of features to classify breast density in to BIRADS Classes of breast density. They used 307 Mammographic Images. To train a CNN and feature extraction from a deep layer, they normalized images to 260 × 200 pixels. CNN is used for feature extraction and multilayer perceptron neural networks are used to classify the density category-wise. This work suggests that the actual entities that assess the breast density classes are global features and the image normalization by reducing the size has no great impact on the classification results. To assess mammographic density, the author in [7] introduced ResNet18 and implemented the deep mammographic density classification for the first time on clinical application and the validated learning-based model by radiologists for acceptance of its evaluation. A deep CNN was trained to estimate the breast density of based on an experienced radiologist's initial understanding of 414,799. Digital screening mammograms were collected from January 2009 to May 2011 for 27,684 patients checking the resulting algorithm on a sample of 8677 mammograms in 5741 women on a held-out test set. In addition, a reader analysis of 500 mammograms randomly selected from the test collection was conducted by five radiologists. Finally, in routine clinical practice, the algorithm was applied, where eight radiologists examined 10,763 consecutive mammograms using this model.

Deep neural network was explored to (i) separating fatty breasts (A and B) from dense ones (C and D), (ii) assessing the low-dense group into (A and B) (iii) classifying the high-dense group into C and D. To achieve this, nearly four thousands images acquired were used to train Inception-V3 network architecture from nine mammography units and three manufacturers. On the ImageNet data collection, the network was pre-trained and the author trained it on a private dataset using transfer learning. Evaluated network output on a blinded test range of one hundred fifty mammograms acquired from fourteen mammography units installed. Based on the consensus of three radiologists, a reference density value was obtained for these images. In the high versus low-risk classification, the network achieved an accuracy of 92.0%. The overall accuracy was 85.9 and 86.1% for the second and third classification tasks [5].

Discrimination against breast densities serves as a predictor for breast cancer, and the findings can be visually accessed by radiologists. The research focuses on the distinction of 2 challenging categories: BIRADS II(or B) and BIRADS III (or C) of breast tissues density, not all four categories. Their methodology shows promising outcomes with a huge dataset of size 200,00 images with AlexNet [8].

Li et al. [9] presents a strategy for the mammographic density classification task focused on dilated and attention-guided residual learning. With two datasets, one private dataset and one public dataset, the proposed approach was instantiated and assessment accuracies of 88.7% and 70% were achieved, respectively. Though the accuracy of the public dataset classification was lower than that of the private dataset, which was most likely due to the scale of the dataset. An efficient result than the simple residual networks and many other deep learning-based approaches are obtained by the proposed model. In addition, a multi-stream network architecture was developed primarily aimed at analyzing multi-view mammograms. Li et al. [9] presented ResNet50 with dilated convolutions (DC) and attention modules (CA) achieved the best assessment results in comparison to other presented works [5, 6, 8].

Ahn et al. [10] proposed a CNN with transfer learning to assess breast density. CNN has been qualified to extract visual features from the ROI of the image derived from all the mammograms and describe them as density A, B, C, or D (BIRADS) classification. This approach achieves a 96% coefficient of correlation on 397 mammographic images belongs to a private dataset.

The application was submitted by [11] for the classification of breast densities, using deep neural network (DNN), in Mammographic Images. The report consisted of 20,000 diagnostic mammograms, Labeled as breast densities of four classes (i.e., A: fatty, B: fibro-glandular Dense, C: heterogeneously dense, D: exceedingly dense). A dense convolutional layer of scratch-based CNN was used in the multi-view Mammographic Image, to classify breast densities.

In a related analysis, the breast density was classified by [12] the method of estimation using Residual CNN. Their research was aimed at the use of the residual CNN to assess the density of BI-RADS into four groups. There were seventy layers of residual CNN with seven residual learning blocks with two additional thirty six and forty eight weighted networks. The cross-entropy loss could be reduced by the ResNets in order to increase the precision of classification. Their findings revealed with an increased residual layer, the precision of the classification increased. The cost of computation however has been raised.

An unsupervised deep learning technique was suggested by [13]. Breast density and risk score assessment in the ROI using the technique conventional sparse autoencoder (CSAE) in order to learn the features. For density assessment throughout mammography, score was used for categories labels: pectoral muscle, density-A tissues, and the density-D tissues of breast. Score of mammographic image texture is calculated to mark two labels regarded as cancerous and normal patches. The score was used as a threshold for the segmentation of the tissue from the Mammographic Image. The Dice score measure the segmentation quality. The CSAE (conventional sparse auto encoder) has been modeled for three private separate datasets, and the findings derive good result's relationship with the results collected by experts manually.

A CNN-based assessment of density was proposed by [14]. Method is used for assisting the radiologist in scoring risk. CNN is the one that is Learn from unseen images to determine the visual analogue score. A good correlation and match concordance was shown by the process in a comparison with 2 independent readers in a clinical setting.

Author in [15] used deep convolutional neural neurons in their research. Network is model for multi view data prediction of breast densities. Breast density was predicted by the method and categorized into three types: BI-RADS-0, BI-RADS-1, and BI-RADS-2, respectively. Furthermore, the anomalies from the ROIs derived from these categories, have been classified as Benign and Malignant images. The research discussed the effect on the assessment of density class of the dataset size and Mammographic Image resolution for training–testing. In addition, the rescaling of the image size did not have any effect on the method's assessment accuracy. Findings prove to be good agreement with specialist radiologists' manual ratings.

3   Dataset for Mammogram Images

In training and testing, mammographic databases play a significant role to assessment of methods of DL. There is a massive data required to train a deep learning network. The availability of detailed databases with annotations is Important to the advancement of deep learning growth in medical imaging. Bilateral craniocaudal (CC) and mediolateral oblique (MLO) are standard views which are key part of routine screening mammography [4].

There are popular publicly accessible Mammographic Image databases in Table 1:

4   Summary of Brief Study Shown in Table 2

See (Table 2).

The density of the breast is a proven a risk marker for developing cancer of the breast. It essentially tests in the breast, the volume of dense/fibro glandular tissue. Breast density clinical assessment is visually conducted by the four qualitative BI-RADS definitions are used by radiologists of Breast density range from A to D. In some paper it refers as BIRADS I to BIRADS IV. Breast density four categories described as First - Almost entirely fatty, Second - Scattered areas of fibro glandular density, Third - Heterogeneously dense, which may obscure small masses, Fourth - Extremely dense, which lowers the sensitivity of mammography. The assessment of

Table 1 Public datasets for mammographic images

DM dataset	Number of patient	Number of images	Available classes	Image format	Image view
DDSM	2620	10,480	Normal, Benign & Malignant	JPEG	CC,MLO
CBIS-DDSM	6775	10,239	Normal, Benign & Malignant	DICOM	CC,MLO
MIAS	161	322	Normal, Benign & Malignant	PGM	MLO
Inbreast	115	410	Normal, Benign & Malignant	DICOM	CC,MLO
BCDR	1734	3703 FM -3612 DM	Normal, Benign & Malignant	TIFF	CC,MLO
mini-MIAS	161	322	Normal, Benign & Malignant	PGM	CC,MLO

first and forth is highly consistent and relatively easy, there is greater variability in distinguishing second from third. Since the guidelines for additional screening and risk management can differ by breast density, it is particularly effective to have a consistent breast density assessment, reducing the risk of mislabels when assigning classes of BIRADS density (i.e., I, II, III, IV) [5].

5 Performance of Breast Density Assessment

Figure 1 shows two dimensional representation of two class assessment experiments. The (i,j)th cell of the confusion table give value, the number of times that the ith density class is classified as the j th density class [1].

Among the different performance measures of Breast Density Class Assessment, this table used to calculate various performance measures like:

(i)   Recall value is formulated as Recall = TruePositive/(TruePositive + FalseNegative).

(ii)   Precision value is formulated as Precision = TruePositive /(TruePositive + FalsePositive).

(iii)   Specificity value is formulated as Specificity = TrueNegative/(TrueNegative + FalsePositive).

(iv)   Accuracy value is formulated as ACC = (TruePositive + TrueNegative)/(TruePositive + TrueNegative + FalsePositive + FalseNegative).

(v)   F1 score value is formulated as F1 = (2 × Recall)/(2 × Recall + FalsePositive + FalseNegative).

Table 2 Brief study

References	Year	Method	Dataset numbers/type	Conclusion
[6]	2017	CNN + (MLP-NN)	307/Public INbreast/ Mammographic images multiview	Global Acc = 98.4%
[9]	2020	Deep Residual CNNs (ResNet50 + DC + CA)	1985/Private &410/Public-INbreast-Mammographic images multiview	Acc = 88.7% /70.0%
[7]	2018	Deep CNN + ResNet18	1985/Private &410/Public INbreast-Mammographic images multiview	Acc = 87.1/63.8
[5]	2019	CCN + Inception-V3 + transfer Learning	1985 multiview/Private &410/Public INbreast-multiview	Acc = 86.2/63.9
[8]	2018	CNN (AlexNet; transfer learning)	200,00/Private Mammographic images (multiview)	AUC = (0.98)Acc = 82
[11]	2018	CNN (transfer learning)	201,179/Private Mammographic images (multiview)	Mean AUC (0.934)
[12]	2018	CNN (scratch based)	410/Public Mammographic Image(multiview)/INbreast	Acc = (92.63%)
[13]	2016	CNN + stacked autoencoder	493 + 668/Private Mammographic images (multiview)	AUC (0.61)
[14]	2019	CNN	67,520/Private Mammographic Image(multiview)	Average match concordance index of 0.6
[15]	2017	Multi view deep neural network	886,000/Private Mammographic image(multiview)	Mean AUC (0.735)

	Estimated Density Class	
Actual Density Class	TruePositive	FalseNegative
	FalsePositive	TrueNegative

Fig. 1 Confusion table

6 Conclusion

The contribution of deep learning models to the assessment of breast density helped doctors greatly by offering a second opinion to establish the final report, which increased patients' satisfaction and trust. However, our research indicated that the mammographic image is the most efficient and accurate instrument used for breast cancer CAD system. As a result of an understanding survey from the existing literature the number of image dataset and the size or dimension of mammographic image play important role to achieve higher density assessment accuracy. By measuring the categories of breast density, it gained more prominent attention in providing significant details for early diagnosis of breast irregular tissues. Due to Global Feature extraction capabilities, the state-of-the art Deep Neural Networks, particularly CNN, have recently advanced breast density classification. The kernel, as the centre of the CNN model, provides actual entities that assess the breast density classes are global features, it also allows the CNN model to extract more hidden structures from the images. This gives some excellent results for a breast density assessment or classification.

References

1. Dhungel N, Carneiro G, Bradley A (2017) A deep learning approach for the analysis of masses in mammograms with minimal user intervention. Med Image Anal 37:114–128. https://doi.org/10.1016/j.media.2017.01.009
2. LeCun Y, Bengio Y, Hinton G (2015) Deep learning. Nature 521:436–444. https://doi.org/10.1038/nature14539
3. Lee J, Jun S, Cho Y, Lee H, Kim G, Seo J, Kim N (2017) Deep learning in medical imaging: general overview. Korean J Radiol 18:570. https://doi.org/10.3348/kjr.2017.18.4.570
4. Hamed G, Marey M, Amin S, Tolba M (2020) Deep learning in breast cancer detection and classification. Adv Intell Syst Comput 322–333. https://doi.org/10.1007/978-3-030-44289-7_30
5. Gandomkar Z, Suleiman M, Demchig D, Brennan P, McEntee M (2019) BI-RADS density categorization using deep neural networks. In: Medical imaging, 2019 image perception, observer performance, and technology assessment. https://doi.org/10.1117/12.2513185
6. Thomaz R, Carneiro P, Patrocinio A (2017) Feature extraction using convolutional neural network for classifying breast density in mammographic images. In: Medical Imaging 2017: Computer-Aided Diagnosis. https://doi.org/10.1117/12.2254633
7. Lehman C, Yala A, Schuster T, Dontchos B, Bahl M, Swanson K, Barzilay R (2019) Mammographic breast density assessment using deep learning: clinical implementation. Radiology 290:52–58. https://doi.org/10.1148/radiol.2018180694
8. Mohamed A, Berg W, Peng H, Luo Y, Jankowitz R, Wu S (2017) A deep learning method for classifying mammographic breast density categories. Med Phys 45:314–321. https://doi.org/10.1002/mp.12683
9. Li C, Xu J, Liu Q, Zhou Y, Mou L, Pu Z, Xia Y, Zheng H, Wang S (2020) Multi-view mammographic density classification by dilated and attention-guided residual learning. IEEE/ACM Trans Comput Biol Bioinf 1–1. https://doi.org/10.1109/tcbb.2020.2970713
10. Ahn C, Heo C, Jin H, Kim J (2017) A novel deep learning-based approach to high accuracy breast density estimation in digital mammography. In: Medical Imaging 2017: Computer-Aided Diagnosis. https://doi.org/10.1117/12.2254264
11. Wu N, Geras K, Shen Y, Su J, Kim S, Kim E, Wolfson S, Moy L, Cho K (2018) Breast density classification with deep convolutional neural networks. In: 2018 IEEE international conference on acoustics, speech and signal processing (ICASSP). https://doi.org/10.1109/icassp.2018.8462671
12. Xu J, Li C, Zhou Y, Mou L, Zheng H, Wang S (2018) Classifying mammographic breast density by residual learning. Cornell University

13. Kallenberg M, Petersen K, Nielsen M, Ng A, Diao P, Igel C, Vachon C, Holland K, Winkel R, Karssemeijer N, Lillholm M (2016) Unsupervised deep learning applied to breast density segmentation and mammographic risk scoring. IEEE Trans Med Imaging 35:1322–1331. https://doi.org/10.1109/tmi.2016.2532122

14. Ionescu G, Fergie M, Berks M, Harkness E, Hulleman J, Brentnall A, Cuzick J, Evans D, Astley S (2019) Prediction of reader estimates of mammographic density using convolutional neural networks. J Med Imaging 6:1. https://doi.org/10.1117/1.jmi.6.3.031405

15. Geras K, Wolfson S, Shen Y, Kim S, Moy L, Cho K (2017) High-resolution breast cancer screening with multi-view deep convolutional neural networks. Cornell University

Classification of Land Cover and Land Use Using Deep Learning

Suraj Kumar, Suraj Shukla, K. K. Sharma, Koushlendra Kumar Singh, and Akbar Sheikh Akbari

1 Introduction

In the classification of land cover and land use, each image is assigned a class label indicating the physical material of the object surface (e.g. *grass, residential, agricultural, asphalt,* etc.). Land cover refers to the surface cover on the ground, whether vegetation, grass, water bodies, bare land or other. Land use refers to the purpose the land serves, for example, residential, wildlife habitat or agriculture. This task is quite challenging due to the heterogeneous appearance and high intra-class variance of objects. A land cover image can contain many different land cover elements and form complex structures, and a specific land cover type can be a part of a different land use image. The information about land use and land cover is stored in geospatial databases, typically acquired and maintained by national mapping agencies. Such databases consist of class labels indicating the images' land use and land cover.

The classification of land cover and land use has mainly been tackled by supervised methods. A large variety of features and classifiers have been applied for that purpose. We are going to use convolutional neural networks (CNN) for the classification of Land use and Land cover as recent works on the classification of images have focused on CNN.

CNNs have outperformed other classifiers for pixel-based classification by a large margin if a sufficient amount of training data is available. We compare the dependence of land use and land cover classification based on different variants, related works and future scope of our work based on the proposed methodology.

S. Kumar · S. Shukla · K. K. Sharma · K. Kumar Singh (✉)
National Institute of Technology Jamshedpur, Jamshedpur, Jharkhand, India
e-mail: koushlendra.cse@nitjsr.ac.in

A. S. Akbari
Leeds Beckett University, Caedmon, 207, Headingley Campus, Leeds, UK

© The Author(s), under exclusive license to Springer Nature Singapore Pte Ltd. 2021
M. K. Bajpai et al. (eds.), *Machine Vision and Augmented Intelligence—Theory and Applications*, Lecture Notes in Electrical Engineering 796,
https://doi.org/10.1007/978-981-16-5078-9_28

We start this review with a discussion of ResNet architecture which we have used for the classification of land cover and land use. In the second part, we discuss different CNN architectures used for land use and land cover classification from satellite image data, focusing on the overall strategy and the way in which land cover and land use are integrated into the process. Then, we have discussed the effect of changing parameters on our result.

Traditional methods based on CNN that were used for classification have certain shortcomings when the number of layers, i.e., depth of the network is increased. The problems that may have occurred by increasing the number of layers is of vanishing/exploding gradient or the model may be overfitting resulting in high test error. The problem with vanishing/exploding gradient can be solved by batch normalization to some extent. However, the problem of overfitting still persists with the increasing depth of the network. ResNet eliminates the case of overfitting by using identity mapping and residual learning. Hence, we have used ResNet for the classification of land cover and land use classification and the architecture and methodology used by ResNet is reviewed in further discussion.

There have been various algorithms proposed and developed for the classification of land cover and land use. EuroSAT is a novel dataset and deep learning benchmark for land use and land cover classification [1], which consists of 27,000 labeled images with 10 different land use and land cover classes. There have been comparisons made between different Convolution Neural Networks that were used for the classification of land use and land cover. The method of bypassing and deep residual learning for image classification [2] led to the development of architectures that provided a means to effectively train end-to-end networks with more than 50–100 layers without the case of overfitting and vanishing or exploding gradient. ResNet is a CNN that has an architecture based on highway networks [3] and works on identity mapping and deep residual learning approach [2].

Kaiming et al. have used Deep residual learning for image recognition [2]. C. yang et al. proposed a convolution neural network based classification of land cover as well as land use [4]. The simultaneous classification of land cover use based on higher-order conditional random field model has been proposed by Lena Albert et. al. [5]. The land cover and land use classification with the help of remote sensor data has been given by James et al. [3]. The case study of land use of Burdhman town is given by Gupta et al. [6]. P. K. Malupatta proposed a system for the analysis of land use using remote sensing and GIS data. Y. Lu uses multi-resolution remote sensing data for purpose of Land use classification [7, 8].

The present approach is to determine land cover and to classify land use objects based on convolution neural networks (CNN) and to study the effects of changing a parameter on the results. The input data for the proposed approach are aerial images from Sentinel-2 satellite images. Land cover and land use for each image have been determined with the use of CNN. The present work also describes the effect of changing parameters on our results and output generated in each case. Comparisons of our results with different existing algorithms have also been analysed.

2 Proposed Methodology

2.1 Environmental Setup

The operating system to be used as the environment for the project is Ubuntu. Next, we need a browser; in this case, we have used Google Chrome. We have used Google Colab, which is a cloud platform provided by Google for free and it comes with 12.72 gigabytes of GPU and 358.27 GB of storage for free. It has various inbuilt libraries and provides integration with various other libraries. It provides iPython notebook for writing codes. The only other requirement apart from having a browser and internet connection is to have a Google account. The rest of the requirements are fulfilled by Google Colab over the cloud.

2.2 Dataset

The dataset used for classification of land cover and land use is of Sentinel 2 satellite that is freely available and can be used for different purposes. The data consists of 27,000 labeled images in 10 classes. The dataset is separated into training data, validation data and test data.

2.3 Data Preprocessing

The dataset consists of large number of images and supplying all those images as one set without any preprocessing will increase the time taken to train the model and may result in overfitting, vanishing gradient or exploding gradient. Thus, we need to preprocess the data in order to normalize it and divide it into different batches so as to input the data in batches and not as set of whole. The batch size can be of anything between 1 to 2000. We are taking a batch size of 224. Then we apply batch normalization over the set of data.

Input: Values of x over a mini-batch: $\beta = \{x_{1...m}\}$;
Parameters to be learned: γ, β
Output: $\{y_i = BN_{\gamma,\beta}(x_i)\}$
$\mu_\beta \leftarrow 1/m\sum_{i=1}^{m} x_i$// mini-batch mean
$\sigma^2_\beta \leftarrow 1/m\sum_{i=1}^{m} (x_i - \mu_\beta)^2$ //mini-batch variance
$\hat{X}_i \leftarrow (x_i - \mu_\beta)/\sqrt{(\sigma^2_\beta + \varepsilon)}$ //normalize
$y_i \leftarrow \gamma \hat{X} + \beta \equiv BN\gamma,\beta(x_i)$ //scale and shift

Once the data is normalized, it will become easy to train the model. The other significances of batch normalization are it reduces the size of data and bring the variants or parameters of images in a range.

2.4   Model Training and Implementation

We have used fastai library for the classification of land cover and land use and trained our model using the same. Once the preprocessing is done and we have normalized data (it is represented by a variable named data). We provide this data along with other parameters such as CNN we are going to use and what will be metrics to display the result to a function provided by fastai library named cnn_learner. Cnn_learner takes these data and matrices pass them to the layers of ResNet. We can vary the number of layers by passing different parameters such as ResNet18, ResNet 34 or ResNet50. Using the training data, the weights of different layers of ResNet are adjusted. Once the weights are updated using training data, validation data is used to validate the network and adjust the weights further. By implementing the above steps, we have prepared the model for our dataset. Now, this model can be used for different purposes and we are using this for the classification of land cover and land use. The weights are updated using backpropagation and each weight is updated by derivation of total error with weights [9]. The equation of weight updating is represented in the figure (Fig. 1).

3   Testing and Results

Using the ResNet model with 18 layers, we get an accuracy of 93–95% and an error of 5–7% for our test dataset for classification of land use and land cover (Table 1).

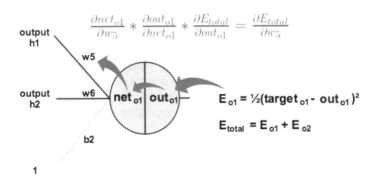

Fig. 1   Updating weight in backpropagation

Table 1   Error rate of ResNet18 for land cover and land use classification

Epoch	Train_loss	Valid_loss	Error_rate	Time
0	0.335153	0.189856	0.062730	52:57
1	0.246830	0.155434	0.049008	02:53

This accuracy is much more than that can be obtained using a traditional dataset that doesn't implement the concept of highway networks. Even, this result can be further improved by increasing the number of layers, changing learning rates and increasing the number of epochs.

In analysis of our model, we are going to check the result of changing variants on our model and how the accuracy can be further improved. The result of our model is displayed in the form of a confusion matrix that shows the number of images in class predicted truly and falsely among all the classes. The confusion matrix has been shown in Fig. 2.

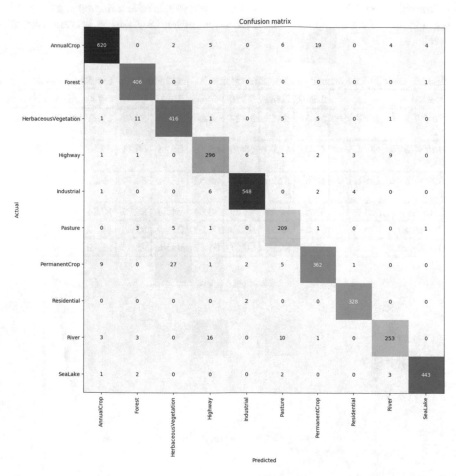

Fig. 2 Confusion matrix

3.1   Analysis and Comparison

The comparison of ResNest with traditional CNNs shows that it has higher accuracy from all of them for the same set of data [1]. The comparison statistics show at training and test split of 80/20 the ResNet gives the best result. However, we have further improved this accuracy by 1–2% and tested our results to show that it doesn't result in overfitting.

Table 2 shows the classification accuracy, in percentage for different training sets on the EuroSAT data set. Learning rate plays a vital role in determining the accuracy of classification. We analysed the loss at different values of learning rate and plotted a graph for the same. Figure 3 shows the effect of learning rate on loss at different levels.

Table 2 Classification accuracy (%) of different training-test splits on the EuroSAT dataset

Method	10/90	20/80	30/70	40/60	50/50	60/40	70/30	80/20	90/10
BoVW(SVM, SIFT, k = 10)	54.54	56.13	56.77	57.06	57.22	57.47	57.71	58.55	58.44
BoVW(SVM, SIFT, k = 100)	63.07	64.80	65.50	66.16	66.25	66.34	66.50	67.22	66.18
BoVW(SVM, SIFT, k = 500)	65.62	67.26	68.01	68.52	68.61	68.74	69.07	70.05	69.54
CNN (two layers)	75.88	79.84	81.29	83.04	84.48	85.77	87.24	87.96	88.66
ResNet 50	75.06	88.53	93.75	94.01	94.45	95.26	95.32	96.43	96.37
GoogleNet	77.37	90.97	90.57	91.62	94.96	95.54	95.70	96.02	96.17

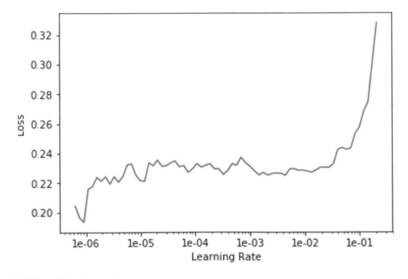

Fig. 3 Effect of learning rate

Increasing the number of layers further increases our accuracy and we can achieve an accuracy of 97–99% in the classification of land use and land cover using ResNet 34 and limiting the range of learning rate to lower values.

4 Conclusions

The proposed approach to determine land cover and to classify land use objects based on Convolution Neural Networks (CNN) and to study the effects of changing a parameter on the results. The proposed approach has been validated with the input aerial images from Sentinel-2 satellite images. We have used ResNnet18 model for the classification of land cover based on aerial images and derived data. Land cover and land use for each image have been determined with the use of CNN. The present work also successfully describes the effect of changing parameters on our results and output generated in each case. Comparisons of our results with different existing algorithms have also been analysed. Experiments show that the overall accuracy of the proposed approach is 93–95% for land cover and land use. The classification of land cover and land use has a positive contribution towards the utilization of land by humans.

References

1. Helber P, Bischke B, Dengel A, Borth D (2017) EuroSAT: a novel dataset and deep learning benchmark for land use and land cover classification. IEEE J Sel Top Appl Earth Obs Remote Sens
2. He K, Zhang X, Ren S, Sun J (2016) Deep residual learning for image recognition. In: IEEE conference on computer vision and pattern recognition CVPR. IEEE, pp 770–777
3. Anderson JR, Hardy EE, Roach JT, Richard E (1976) Witmer. A land use and land cover classification system for use with remote sensor data. Prof Pap
4. Yang C, Rottensteiner F, Heipke C (2018) Classification of land cover and land use based on convolutional neural networks, ISPRS annals of the photogrammetry. Remote Sens Spat Inf Sci
5. Albert L, Rottensteiner F, Heipke C (2015) A higher order conditional random field model for simultaneous classification of land cover and land use. ISPRS
6. Srimanta G, Moupriya R (2012) Land use /land cover classification of an urban area-a case study of Burdwan municipality, India. ISSN-2012
7. Mallupattu PK, Sreenivasula Reddy JR (2013) Analysis of land use/land cover changes using remote sensing data and GIS at an urban area. Sci World J
8. Liu Y, Pei Z, Wu Q, Guo L, Zhao H, Chen X (2011) Land use/land cover classification based on multi-resolution remote sensing data. In: Li D, Chen Y (eds) Computer and computing technologies in agriculture V. CCTA. IFIP Advances in Information and Communication Technology, p 369
9. Badrinarayanan V, Kendall A, Cipolla R (2017) SegNet: a deep convolutional encoder-decoder architecture for image. IEEE Trans Pattern Anal Mach Intell 39(12):2481–2495

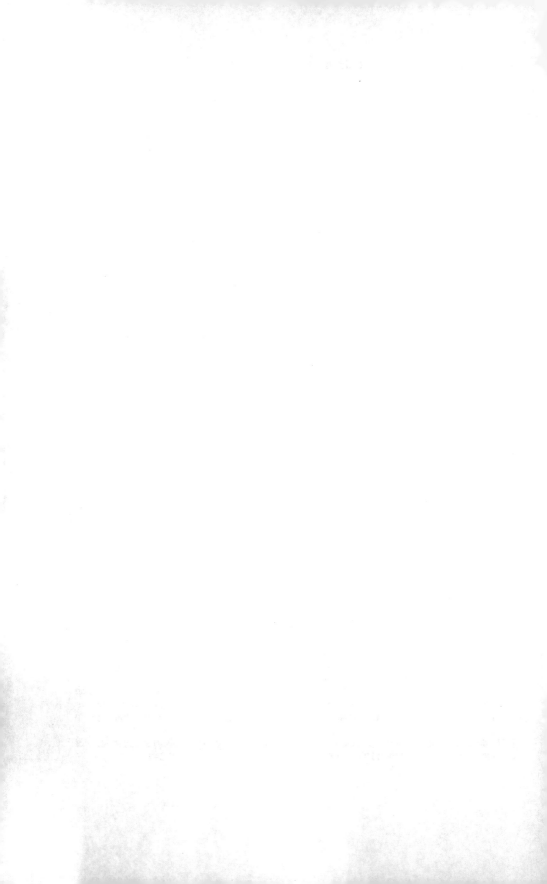

Three-Dimensional Fractional Operator for Benign Tumor Region Detection

Saroj Kumar Chandra, Abhishesk Shrivastava, and Manish Kumar Bajpai

1 Introduction

Computer-aided diagnostic (CAD) models have shown outstanding performance in the diagnosis of critical diseases such as cancer. It helps clinical professionals to identify suspicious regions in the images obtained using imaging techniques. These imaging techniques are popular in visualizing the internal structure of the human body. It has several members such as X-ray imaging, computed tomography (CT), magnetic resonance imaging (MRI), and positron emission tomography (PET) [1]. These techniques can produce the internal structure of the human body. The images obtained by these techniques are used to inspect suspected regions for the presence or absence of cancerous cells. Image processing techniques are useful in detecting and segmenting suspicious regions. Boundary detection and segmentation are the most useful techniques in this category. The segmentation technique separates the image into different regions by using color, texture, contrast, brightness, and gray level [2]. It is used in cancer detection to separate the cancerous region from non-cancerous regions [3]. The brain tumor is one kind of cancer in which cancerous or tumor cells are automatically generated inside the human brain and disrupt the functioning of the human brain [4]. It has been further classified into benign (grade I and II) and malignant (grade III and IV). The benign brain tumor is the initial stage of a brain tumor and it can be diagnosed without internal surgery. It is very difficult to locate benign brain tumors due to low-intensity variation to their surrounding non-tumorous

S. K. Chandra (✉)
Computer Science and Engineering, OP Jindal University, Raigarh, India

A. Shrivastava
Computer Science and Engineering, National Institute of Technology, Raipur, Raipur, India

M. K. Bajpai
Computing Science and Engineering, Indian Institute of Information Technology Design and Manufacturing Jabalpur, Jabalpur, India

© The Author(s), under exclusive license to Springer Nature Singapore Pte Ltd. 2021
M. K. Bajpai et al. (eds.), *Machine Vision and Augmented Intelligence—Theory and Applications*, Lecture Notes in Electrical Engineering 796,
https://doi.org/10.1007/978-981-16-5078-9_29

healthy cells. It has been investigated that benign brain tumor leads to malignant brain tumor if not detected. Hence, a suitable approach is required to detect these benign brain tumor cells accurately. Segmentation is used as the primary tool for detecting and segmenting brain tumors. It includes contour and shape-based methods [5–7], multi-resolution analysis based [8], machine learning-based [9], statistical-based methods [10], and boundary and region-based methods [11].

Boundary-based detection methods use either the first or second gradient to detect cancer boundary [2, 12]. It has been found that these methods are highly responsive in the cases where intensity variation is high enough to be detected. hence, these methods fail to detect low variational regions such as being region. The cancer data are obtained by imaging techniques and hence undesired noises come along with data. It has been found that the second-order gradient methods are highly sensitive to noise. Hence, these are not suitable for detecting benign regions. The response of region growing methods is highly dependent on seed selection which delimits its performance. Watershed-based methods suffer pixel overlapping at boundaries of two regions [13, 14]. Level-set methods are highly dependent on curve initialization [15, 16]. The fuzzy-c-means method is computationally inefficient [17, 18]. However, it has been observed the existing techniques are unable to detect benign region boundaries due to similarity with the surrounding noncancerous cells. Hence, the present work targets the development of a novel method for detecting and segmenting the benign region. Fractional-calculus-based methods are more immune to noise and preserve texture details in smooth areas. The fractional-calculus-based method can detect small intensity variation, which is a desired property for tumor detection in the early stage. A comparative study has also been performed with the proposed methods available in the literature.

The organization of the manuscript is articulated as follows. The proposed methodology has been presented in Sect. 2 along with the algorithm. This section also presents the proposed numerical head phantom that has been used for validation of the proposed work has been presented. The result and discussion are presented in Sect. 3.

2 Proposed Methodology

Because the left and the right Riemann–Liouville Fractional Derivative (RLFD) of a constant is nonzero, they are widely used in image processing. A digital image is defined as a two-dimensional function $\mathbf{u}(\mathbf{x}, \mathbf{y}, \mathbf{z})$, where $\mathbf{x}$, $\mathbf{y}$, and $\mathbf{z}$ are spatial coordinates and represent grid point. The image is defined with a grid size equal to **1**. The value of $\mathbf{u}(\mathbf{x}, \mathbf{y}, \mathbf{z})$ is called the color intensity of the image at point $(\mathbf{x}, \mathbf{y})$. The derivative of an image is used to get the boundary of the object present in the image. In the present work, both left and right RLFD have been used to design fractional operators for benign brain tumor detection in the proposed work. However, the left RLFD of a constant at the left boundary is not defined but it does not affect the performance since the derivative is defined inside the pixel only.

Fractional derivative of an image function $\mathbf{u}\ (\mathbf{x},\ \mathbf{y},\ \mathbf{z})$, can be calculated using Grunwald–Letnikov fractional derivative definition for $\mathbf{X}, \mathbf{Y}$, and $\mathbf{Z}$ directions [19]. $\mathbf{X}$-directional forward and backward derivatives can be obtained as

$$D_{GL+x}^{\alpha}u(x, y, z) = u(x, y, z) + (-\alpha)u(x - 1, y, z) +$$
$$\frac{(-\alpha)(-\alpha + 1)}{2!}u(x - 2, y, z) + \dots + \frac{\Gamma(k - \alpha - 1)}{((k - 1)!(\Gamma - \alpha))}u(x - (k - 1), y, z) \tag{1}$$

$$D_{GL-x}^{\alpha}u(x, y, z) = u(x, y, z) + (-\alpha)u(x + 1, y, z) +$$
$$\frac{(-\alpha)(-\alpha + 1)}{2!}u(x + 2, y, z) + \dots + \frac{\Gamma(k - \alpha - 1)}{((k - 1)!(\Gamma - \alpha))}u(x + k - 1), y, z) \tag{2}$$

Similarly, $\mathbf{Y}-$ and $\mathbf{Z}$-directional gradients can be obtained as

$$D_{GL+y}^{\alpha}u(x, y, z) = u(x, y, z) + (-\alpha)u(x, y - 1, z) +$$
$$\frac{(-\alpha)(-\alpha + 1)}{2!}u(x, y - 2, z) + \dots + \frac{\Gamma(k - \alpha - 1)}{((k - 1)!(\Gamma - \alpha))}u(x, y - (k - 1), z) \tag{3}$$

$$D_{GL-y}^{\alpha}u(x, y, z) = u(x, y, z) + (-\alpha)u(x, y + 1, z) +$$
$$\frac{(-\alpha)(-\alpha + 1)}{2!}u(x, y + 2, z) + \dots + \frac{\Gamma(k - \alpha - 1)}{((k - 1)!(\Gamma - \alpha))}u(x, y + k - 1, z) \tag{4}$$

$$D_{GL+z}^{\alpha}(x, y, z) = u(x, y, z) + (-\alpha)u(x, y, z - 1) +$$
$$\frac{(-\alpha)(-\alpha + 1)}{2!}u(x, y, z - 2) + \dots + \frac{\Gamma(k - \alpha - 1)}{((k - 1)!(\Gamma - \alpha))}u(x, y, z - (k - 1)) \tag{5}$$

$$D_{GL-z}^{\alpha}u(x, y, z) = u(x, y, z) + (-\alpha)u(x, y, z + 1) +$$
$$\frac{(-\alpha)(-\alpha + 1)}{2!}u(x, y, z + 2) + \dots + \frac{\Gamma(k - \alpha - 1)}{((k - 1)!(\Gamma - \alpha))}u(x, y, z + k - 1) \tag{6}$$

Central difference can be calculated as:

$$D_{GLx}^{\alpha}u(x, y, z) = D_{GL+x}^{\alpha}u(x, y, z) - D_{GL-x}^{\alpha}u(x, y, z) \tag{7}$$

$$D_{GLy}^{\alpha}u(x, y, z) = D_{GL+y}^{\alpha}u(x, y, z) - D_{GL-y}^{\alpha}u(x, y, z) \tag{8}$$

$$D_{GLz}^{\alpha}u(x, y, z) = D_{GL+z}^{\alpha}u(x, y, z) - D_{GL-z}^{\alpha}u(x, y, z) \tag{9}$$

Here, $\mathbf{0 < k < n, 0 < \alpha < 1}$. Mask of any order, i.e., $\mathbf{3 \times 3 \times 3, 5 \times 5 \times 5} \dots$ can be calculated by Eqs. (7), (8), and (9).

2.1   Algorithm Design for the Proposed Fractional Operator

The algorithm for designing of fractional order mask and benign brain tumor detection is shown in Algorithms **1**.

Algorithm **1** has been designed to detect the boundary of the tumor region. In algorithm **1**, $\mathbf{Mask_X}^\alpha$, $\mathbf{Mask_Y}^\alpha$, and $\mathbf{Mask_Z}^\alpha$ are directional fractional derivative masks or operators. They are used to obtain the boundary of the benign region by using Eqs. (7), (8), and (9). Both masks stores fractional coefficients for calculating the directional derivative of the image. In algorithm **1**, $\mathbf{k}$ is used to store fractional coefficient values at a particular position in the marks. Suppose, $k = \left(floor\left(\frac{Size}{2}\right)\right) - (j-1)$ is used to get fractional coefficient at the center of the mask, $\mathbf{k > 0}$ and $\mathbf{k < 0}$ are used to obtain left and right side of fractional coefficients from the center position of the mark. The designed directional masks are convolved in the image get boundary. In algorithm **1**, Thresh is the optimal threshold, it is being used for the categorization of image pixels. It has been calculated using Otsu's method [2]. $\mathbf{I}$ is the input image. **GradX** stores **X**-directional boundary information by convolving image $\mathbf{I}$ with $\mathbf{X}$ directional fractional mask $\mathbf{Mask_X}^\alpha$, here, * is convolution operator. Similarly, **GradY** and **GradZ** store **Y**- and **Z**-directional boundary information by convolving image $\mathbf{I}$ with $\mathbf{Y}-$ and **Z**-directional fractional masks $\mathbf{Mask_Y}^\alpha$ and $\mathbf{Mask_Z}^\alpha$, respectively. Gradmag stores combined boundary information by calculating $\sqrt{GradX^2 + GradY^2 + GradZ^2}$. Finally, image edge information $\mathbf{I_{edge}}$ has been obtained by thresholding. The thresholding with condition **Gradmag (i, j, k) < = Thresh** has been used to store only non-spurious edges.

Algorithm 1 $(Size, \alpha, Mask_X^\alpha, Mask_Y^\alpha)$

Input: U, α
Output: I_{edge}
　　I_{edge}: Calculated edge pixel
　　begin
　　$Thresh \leftarrow OTSU$
　　$GradX \leftarrow U * Mask_X^\alpha$
　　$GradY \leftarrow U * Mask_Y^\alpha$
　　$GradZ \leftarrow U * Mask_Z^\alpha$
　　$Gradmag \leftarrow \sqrt{GradX^2 + GradY^2 + GradZ^2}$
　　$i \leftarrow 1; j \leftarrow 1$
　　while $i \leq Size$ **do**
　　　　while $j \leq Size$ **do**
　　　　　　while $k \leq Size$ **do**
　　　　　　　　if $Gradmag(i, j) \geq Thresh$ **then**
　　　　　　　　　　$I_{edge}(i, j, k) = Gradmag$
　　　　　　　　else
　　　　　　　　　　$I_{edge}(i, j, k) = 0$
　　　　　　　　end if
　　　　　　　　$j = (k + 1)$
　　　　　　end while
　　　　　　$j = (j + 1)$
　　　　end while
　　　　$i = (i + 1)$
　　end while
　　end

Table 1 Hardware configuration used

Hardware	Capacity
CPU clock speed	2.27 Ghz
RAM	32 GB
LI cache memory	256 KB
L2 cache memory	1 MB
L3 cache memory	4 MB

2.2 Experimental Work

All experimental works have been performed in MATLAB. The hardware configuration used for implementing algorithms is shown in Table 1.

Boundary-based segmentation methods, i.e. Sobel, Prewitt, Canny, and Laplacian of Gaussian (LoG) [20–23] have been evaluated by the proposed numerical head phantom of size **1024 × 1024 x 1024** based on the specification proposed by Shepp-Logan [24]. The original numerical head phantom has ten ellipsoids. The proposed head phantom has introduced a new ellipsoid, which acts as a benign region. The new ellipsoid has very low intensity with its surrounding ellipsoid. The proposed numerical head phantom is shown in Fig. 1 The tumorous region has been marked by a red circle for visual understanding only. The parameters used for numerical phantom design are shown in Table 2. Here, **A** represents the intensity of ellipsoid, *a, b,* and *c* represents axes along X and Y and Z directions, respectively. The values of x_0, y_0, and z_0 are the centers of the ellipsoid. The values of ϕ, θ, and ψ in Table 2 represent the rotation angle of the ellipsoid along **X** and **Y** and **Z** directions, respectively.

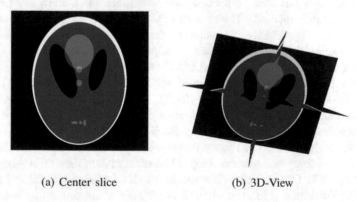

(a) Center slice   (b) 3D-View

Fig. 1 Numerical head phantom

Table 2 3D Numerical head phantom parameters

"A"	"a"	"b"	"c"	"x0"	"j/0"	"z0"	"ϕ"	"θ"	"ψ"
255	353	471	414	512	512	512	0	0	0
−200	339	447	399	512	528	512	0	0	0
−50	56	158	112	740	250	512	5	0	10
−50	81	209	153	220	550	512	−10	0	−10
50	107	128	209	512	300	512	0	0	0
50	23	23	23	512	430	512	0	0	0
50	23	23	23	512	530	512	0	0	0
50	23	11	23	480	820	512	0	0	0
50	12	12	11	525	820	512	0	0	0
50	11	23	11	555	820	512	0	0	0
03	23	11	23	655	655	512	0	0	0

3 Results and Discussion

The validation of the proposed method has been done on the numerical head phantom designed in Fig. 1. The benign region has been marked with a red circle in the center slice of the numerical head phantom. As it can be observed from Fig. 1, there is a very small intensity variation with its neighboring regions. The marked region acts as a benign region in the current work. A fractional-order mask of size **3 × 3 × 3** and of order **0.5** has been designed. OTSU optimal threshold has been used for experimental purposes. Results are shown in Fig. 2. It can be easily observed that the proposed fractional method gives a more accurate boundary of the benign region. A visual comparative study has been performed with Sobel, Prewitt, Canny, and Laplacian of Gaussian (LoG) methods. It has been observed that the Canny and Laplacian of Gaussian (LoG) methods are unable to detect benign regions. Connectionless boundary pixels are obtained using these methods. Although some benign boundary pixels have been detected by the Sobel and Prewitt methods, they are not connected.

Quantitative evaluation of the proposed work with other state-of-the-art methods has been done by Detect Error Ratio (DER), Detect Common Ratio (DCR), and Detect Common Similarity (DCS) techniques [25]. It can be observed from Table 3 that the proposed method is able to detect **100%** benign region pixels as represented by DCR value. It has also been found that if we implement the Canny method with modification of fractional operator in gradient computation then noise suppression can be avoided in Canny. This will result in a reduction in computational requirements. The DER value represents boundary pixels that are present in one method and absent in another one. Its value is high in all cases because other methods are unable to detect benign region boundary pixels. The validation of the proposed work has been also done performed on the brain tumor dataset [26]. This dataset has 3064 T1-weighted contrast-enhanced images of 233 patients with 3 kinds of brain tumor: meningioma (708 slices), glioma (1426 slices), and pituitary tumor (930 slices). Four

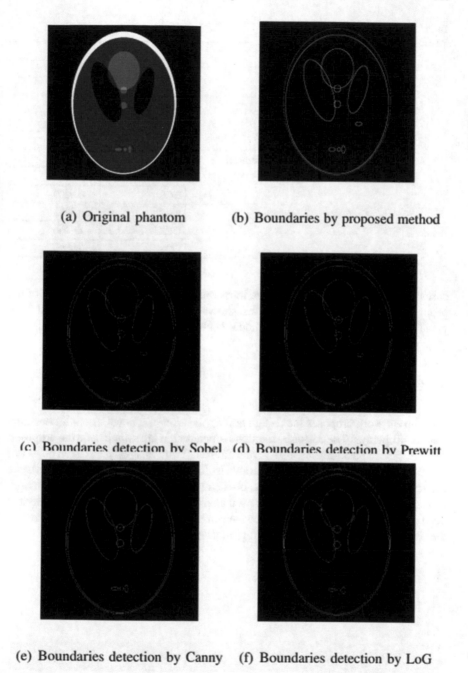

(a) Original phantom   (b) Boundaries by proposed method

(c) Boundaries detection by Sobel   (d) Boundaries detection by Prewitt

(e) Boundaries detection by Canny   (f) Boundaries detection by LoG

Fig. 2 Detection of tumorous region by various methods

Table 3 Comparative study
with existing methods

	Measures	a = 1.5
Sobel	DER	47.7957
	DCR	1.00000
	DCS	0.0209
Prewitt	DER	47.7957
	DCR	1.00000
	DCS	0.0209
Zucker Hummel	DER	47.7957
	DCR	1.00000
	DCS	0.0209
Laplacian	DER	100.8233
	DCR	1.00000
	DCS	0.0099

cases of meningioma have been taken into consideration for visual validation of the proposed work. the results obtained are shown in Fig. 3. It has been observed from visual inspection that the proposed model is able to detect the cancer region.

4 Conclusion

The current work proposes the design and application of a novel three-dimensional fractional operator. The designed fractional operator has been applied on the proposed numerical head phantom and also on real database brain images. It has been observed that the proposed fractional operator is able to detect boundary or benign regions more accurately as compared to other state-of-the-art methods considered for evaluation. A quantitative comparative study has been also performed on the proposed numerical head phantom and higher performance measurement has been obtained. In the future, the work can be extended to benign region detection in mammograms.

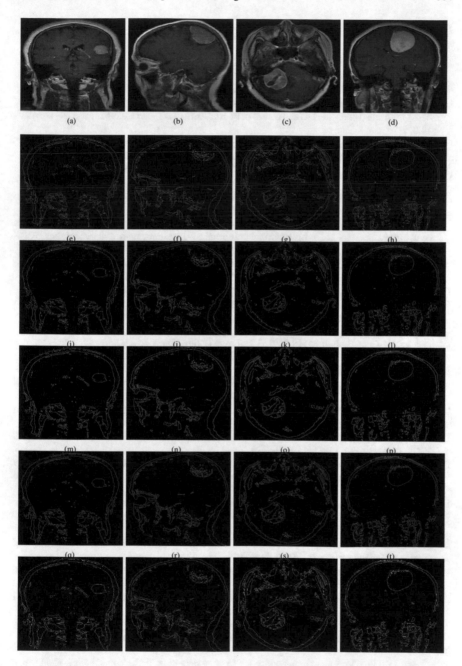

Fig. 3 In first row, original imagex have been shown. Second, third, fourth, fifth and sixth rows show results obtained by Sobel, Prewitt, Canyy, Laplacian and proposed method, respectively

References

1. Andersen AH (1989) Algebraic reconstruction in ct from limited views. IEEE Trans Med Imaging 8(1):50–55
2. Gonzalez RC, Woods RE (2014) Digital image processing, 3rd edn. Pearson
3. Demirhan A, Toru M, Guler I (2015) Segmentation of tumor and edema along with healthy tissues of brain using wavelets and neural networks. IEEE J Biomed Health Inform 19(4):1451–1458
4. American brain tumor association. http://www.abta.org
5. Terzopoulos D, Fleischer K (1988) Deformable models. Vis Comput 4:306–331
6. Kassa M, Witkin A, Terzopoulos D (1987) Snakes: active contour models. Int J Comput Vis 4:321–331
7. Osher S, Sethian JA (1988) Propagating with curvature dependent speed: algorithms based on Hamilton–Jacobi formulations. J Comput Phys 19:12–49
8. Shi Z, Shibasaki R (1999) An approach to image segmentation using multiresolution analysis of wavelets. In: 1999 IEEE international conference on systems, man, and cybernetics, IEEE SMC '99 Conference Proceedings, vol 6. IEEE, pp 810–815
9. Ren X, Malik J (2003) Learning a classification model for segmentation. In: Proceedings ninth IEEE international conference on computer vision, vol 1. IEEE, pp 10–17
10. Pieczynski W (1992) Statistical image segmentation. Mach Graph Vis 1:261–268
11. Kaganami HG, Beiji Z (2009) Region-based segmentation versus edge detection. In: 2009 Fifth international conference on intelligent information hiding and multimedia signal processing. IEEE, pp 1217–1221
12. Aslam A, Khan E, Beg MMS (2015) Improved edge detection algorithm for brain tumor segmentation. Second Int Symp Comput Vis Internet 58:430–437
13. Tian X, Yu W (2016) Color image segmentation based on watershed transform and feature clustering. In: 2016 IEEE advanced information management, communicates, electronic and automation control conference (IMCEC). IEEE, pp 1830–1833
14. Kumar PS, Kumar PG (2015) Computer aided brain tumor detection system using watershed segmentation techniques. Int J Imaging Syst Technolgy 25(4):297–301
15. Wang T, Cheng I, Basu A (2009) Fluid vector flow and applications in brain tumor segmentation. IEEE Trans Biomed Eng 56(3):781–789
16. Marsousi M, Plataniotis KN, Stergiopoulos S (2017) An automated approach for kidney segmentation in three-dimensional ultrasound images. IEEE J Biomed Health Inform 21(4):1079–1094
17. Dash AK, Majhi B (2015) Image segmentation using fuzzy based histogram thresholding. In: 2015 IEEE international conference on signal processing, informatics, communication and energy systems (SPICES). IEEE, pp 1–5
18. Abdel-Maksoud E, Elmogy M, Al-Awadi R (2015) Brain tumor segmentation based on a hybrid clustering technique. Egypt Inform J 16(1):71–81
19. Oldham KB, Spanier J (2006) The fractional calulus theory and applications of differentiation and integration of arbitrary order. Academic Press, New York, first edition
20. Duda RO, Hart PE (1971) Pattern classification and scene analysis. Wiley, New York, first edition
21. Prewitt JMS (1970) Object enhancement and extraction. In: Lipkin BS, Rosenfeld A (eds) Picture processing and psychopictorics, 1st edn. Academic Press, New York
22. Marr D, Hildreth E (1980) Theory of edge detection. Proc R Soc Lond 207:187–217
23. Canny J (1986) A computational approach to edge detection. IEEE Trans Pattern Anal Mach Intell 8:679–714
24. Shepp LA, Logan BF (1974) The fourier reconstruction of head section. IEEE Trans Nucl Sci 21:21 43

25. Chandra SK, Bajpai MK (2019) Mesh free alternate directional implicit method based three-dimensional super-diffusive model for benign brain tumor segmentation. Comput Math Appl
26. Cheng J (2017) Brain tumor dataset. https://figshare.com/articles/dataset/brain_tumor_dataset/1512427

Hybrid Features Enabled Adaptive Butterfly Based Deep Learning Approach for Human Activity Recognition

Anagha Deshpande◉ and Krishna K. Warhade

1 Introduction

In recent years, human activity recognition has pulled in an expanding measure of consideration from exploration and industry networks [1]. It takes up a significant part in video surveillance, frameworks that track anomalous occasions, and human-machine collaboration [2]. Human function authentication has been used in a variety of areas, e.g., human–PC collaboration, game control, and intelligence monitoring [3]. The increase in cases of burglary and defacing has expanded the requirement for 24×7 visual surveillance in the living premises, business regions, and thick traffic zones [4]. Current surveillance frameworks contain surveillance cameras and it requires enormous labor to deal with the camera yield [5]. HAR is the ever-sprouting investigation territory as it discovers magnificent applications in surrounding helped living frameworks, medical precaution, observation frameworks for inside and outside exercises, video order, computer-generated reality innovation, and so on [6].

For effectual human activity recognition, researchers worked on the human motions captured by a single camera or multiple camera environment [7]. In particular, there is a huge literature on human activity but still a challenging issue because of the enormous variety of in-person appearance, occlusion, variation in scale and different variables, camera motion. Thermal infrared (IR) cameras are not affected by external illumination since they generate images based on the heat radiated by the body. IR cameras are used for human action recognition in the context of elderly care and supervision [8]. Feature extraction is the principal vision task in real-life recognition and comprises of separating stance and movement signals from the video that are

A. Deshpande (✉) · K. K. Warhade
School of Electronics & Communication Engineering, Dr. Vishwanath Karad MIT World Peace University, Pune, Maharashtra, India
e-mail: anagha.deshpande@mitwpu.edu.in

© The Author(s), under exclusive license to Springer Nature Singapore Pte Ltd. 2021
M. K. Bajpai et al. (eds.), *Machine Vision and Augmented Intelligence—Theory and Applications*, Lecture Notes in Electrical Engineering 796,
https://doi.org/10.1007/978-981-16-5078-9_30

discriminative concerning human activities. Low dimension images are represented using skeleton poses and their motions [9].

Skeletal features are fragmented into various body parts based on the similarity measure between neighbor pixels in the diffusion tensor field [10]. View angle change, shadow challenges in the HAR is addressed by considering the complement of human silhouette [11]. In feature extraction, multiple features fusion techniques perform superior based on have superior performance to techniques of individual features. Thus, the descriptor formed by the amalgamation of the motion and appearance characteristics makes human activity recognition more efficient and robust [12].

In recent years, the Deep neural network (DNN) technique is largely used for video classification tasks [12–14]. There are a few lacunae of DNN that it still faces issues like structural complexity, gradient-based backpropagation suffers local minima, computational cost, training time, and amount of data required to avoid overfitting. Genetic algorithms to some extent can address a few DNN issues by optimum weight initialization and selection of correct hyperparameters [15].

Monarch butterfly optimization (MBO) is the nature-inspired genetic algorithm proposed by Wang [16] based on the study of the monarch butterflies' migration behavior. Researchers have shown a comparative study of the performance of MBO with other metaheuristic algorithms, which has shown promising results [17]. MBO algorithm needs a simple calculation process, requires fewer computational parameters. It is with great ability to deal with the issue of exploration and exploitation. has given strength to the choice. This has motivated and strengthened the choice of MBO, to optimize the DNN to improve the performance of Human Activity Recognition. This study also emphasizes on Adaptive Monarch Butterfly Algorithm (AMBO) to overcome the problems like search strategy, premature convergence, and poor performance on complex optimization problems in MBO.

The paper is organized as follows: Sect. 2 presents the review of related work, Sect. 3 contains the problem definition of human activity recognition and Sect. 4 contains the proposed method. Section 5 provides the experimental result and the discussion of the technique. Here the data set parameters are analyzed and the experimental results are noted. Finally, the conclusion of the proposed method is given in Sect. 6.

2 Literature Review

Several methodologies have been suggested for the detection of human activity in the literature survey. Recently published works are those existing as follows among the most.

In 2019 Wang and Chen [18] have developed a multi-label zero-shot human action via joint ranking embedding. Their system comprehensively handles the problems of obscure fleeting limits between various factions inside a video clip for multi-label learning and adventures the side data with respect to the semantic connection between various human actions for zero-shot learning. In particular, the structure comprises two-segment neural networks for visual and semantic embedding separately. The exploratory outcomes on two feebly commented on multi-label human activity datasets exhibit the viability of their system. Human action recognition using two-stream attentions based LSTM was evaluated by Dai et al. [19] in 2019. This paper uses the visual attention mechanism and a two-stream consideration-based LSTM network. This work specifically considered the connection between two profound feature transfers, and modify the profound learning network boundary dependent on the connection judgment. The test result shows that it can accomplish the best in class execution in normal situations. In 2019, Chaudhary and Murala [20] have analyzed a deep network for human action recognition using weber motion. In this paper, an incredibly quick algorithm was created for HAR utilizing WMHI, present data, and convolutional neural networks. For continuous implementation, the two essential rules on which an algorithm can be dissected were reality and intricacy. The recognition results beat the current outcome by a critical edge. Multiple streams deep learning models for HAR were analyzed by Gu et al. [21] in 2019. This paper describes the features of the global and local motion. 3-channel-based designs run deep global operating effectively and the local spatial and fleeting examples were extricated from the skeleton diagram. The structure was assessed on two RGB-D datasets. The exploratory outcomes show the viability of their strategy. In 2019 Arivazhagan et al. [22] have analyzed HAR since RGB-D data. A multiclass SVM classifier was utilized for grouping the features into different activity classifications. Algorithm trial reported with MSR Daily Activity 3D dataset and UDT-MHAD action database and got authentication speed of 98.75 and 84.12%. Learning multi-learning features for sensor-based human action recognition using a single body-worn inertial sensor was analyzed by Xu et al. [23] in 2017. The structure comprises three stages, low-level features catch the time and frequency area property while midlevel portrayals gain proficiency with the arrangement of the activity. The technique accomplishes cutting edge exhibitions, 88.7, 98.8, and 72.6% (weighted F1 score) individually, on Skoda, WISDM, and OPP datasets. In 2017 Liu et al. [24] have developed a skeleton visualization for view-invariant HAR. Initially, a grouping depends view-invariant change was created to dispense with the impact of view minor departure from spatiotemporal distributions of skeleton joints. Second, shadow images of skeletal progression were altered, as skeletal joints, spatial–temporal data illustrate. Besides, visual and motion enhancement techniques were used for shadow images to enhance their local patterns. The experimental result shows that the consistency of the dataset demonstrates the superiority of their method.

Additionally, Human action recognition in video scenes from multiple camera viewpoints was analyzed by Itano et al. [25] in 2019. This exploration advances by decreasing the input dimensionality to the recognition framework, and by utilizing a Multilayer Perceptron Artificial Neural Network whose hyper boundaries were streamlined by a Genetic Algorithm. Critical enhancements in the recognition rate have been acquired.

3 Problem Definition

Human Activity Recognition (HAR) is identifying and classifying different human activities from a video sequence based on actions and environmental conditions. In HAR abnormal activity recognition aims to ensure immediate intervention, by humans or machines, in case of danger or necessity. The development of an intelligent surveillance system that automatically detects human motion or actions from video and categorizes it as normal or abnormal is a need for both the commercial and public sector surveillance industry. Several strategies have been implemented by the researchers, still, a few issues need to be addressed. These are recorded underneath:

- The existing techniques are inadequate in identifying imperfectly performed activities due to appearance, occlusion, camera motion, light effects.
- Recognition of human activity is a highly challenging problem due to the large variations in in-person appearance, backgrounds, challenges in scale, and other factors.
- In the existing method [22], the human action recognition is not efficient because of inter and intra-class variation in RGB local binary pattern.
- An area of research in detecting the event or activity by single or multiple humans as the normal or abnormal activity is still untouched by researchers.

The objective of this work is to develop an effective algorithm for human activity recognition to automatically identify an event or activity as a normal or an abnormal human activity from the video sequences.

4 Proposed Human Activity Reorganization

The main objective of the proposed method is to identify the normal or abnormal human activity from video sequences in challenging environmental conditions. First, the input videos are converted into a number of frames. After that, the proposed method selects the keyframe from the number of frames by using a structural similar method (SSIM). Next, the important features are extracted from the input keyframe. Finally, the selected features are fed to the classifier for identifying human activity. Here the suggested method utilizes optimal deep learning techniques for identifying human activity. In the proposed method, the traditional deep learning algorithm is improved utilizing optimization techniques. Here the Adaptive Monarch Butterfly optimization algorithm (AMBO) is used to improve the performance in the traditional deep learning algorithm. The overall diagram of the proposed method is given below.

As shown in Fig. 1, the input video frames are converted into several frames. After converting video sequences into video frames, selects the keyframe from the number of video frames by using Structural Similarly Measure (SSIM). The detailed description of keyframe extraction is given below.

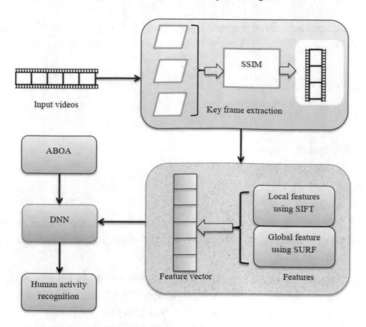

Fig. 1 An overall diagram of the proposed method

4.1 SSIM-Based Key Frame Extraction

The main objective of this section is to separate the keyframe from the video. Consider the video V^i which consists of several frames $V_i^F (i = 1, 2, ..., n)$. So, we have converted the video into several video frames F^i. After converting video footage into video frames, we select the keyframe from the number of video frames using the Structural Similarly Measure (SSIM). It is used to reduce the amount of video information as the location of physical memory. Therefore, it is necessary to extract keyframes from videos to effectively recognize human activities.

Let V_i^F denote the sequence of video frames in a sample video sequence, and is represented in Eq. (1)

$$V_i^F = \{V_1^F, V_2^F, V_j^F, \wedge V_n^F\} \tag{1}$$

where
$n \rightarrow$ Number of frames in the video sequences.
$V_j^F \rightarrow j$th frame of the video.

The SSIM Index is a strategy used to decide the nature of videos and computerized images by estimating the comparability concerning images. It is based on a conceptual model that uses luminosity and contrast information and uses perceived change in structural information. The idea behind the configuration information provides significant information about the spatial structure of an object close-pixels high with cross-function calls. The SSIM between two frames is calculated using Eq. (2).

$$SSIM\left(V_j^F, V_{j+1}^F\right) = \frac{(2\vartheta_j\vartheta_{j+1} + X_1)(2\sigma_{j,j+1} + X_2)}{(\vartheta_j^2 + \vartheta_{j+1}^2 + X_1)(\sigma_j^2 + \sigma_{j11}^2 + X_2)} \tag{2}$$

where,

$\vartheta_j \rightarrow$ Average of frames in V_j^F

$\vartheta_{j+1} \rightarrow$ Average of V_{j+1}^F

$\sigma_j^2 \rightarrow$ Variance of V_j^F

$\sigma_{j+1}^2 \rightarrow$ Variance of V_{j+1}^F

X_1 and X_2 denote the two variables, they are defined as $X_1 = (a_1d)^2$ and $X_2 = (a_2d)^2$, where $a_1 = 0.01$, $a_2 = 0.03$ and d represents the dynamic range. The dynamic range has the value of $2^{bits\ per\ pixel-1}$.

The comparability estimation is accomplished for all the sets of frames. A predefined threshold is set for the determination of keyframes. The frames, for which the SSIM index is not exactly the threshold, are considered as the keyframes. This indicates that the activity in the $(j + 1)$th frame is different from that in the jth frame then the $(j + 1)$th frame is measured as the keyframe.

The similarity measurement is done for all pair frames. The defined threshold is set before the mainframes are selected. Frames, where the SSIM score is less than the threshold, are considered as a keyframe. This indicates that the function of the $(j + 1)$th frame is different from the jth frame, and therefore the $(j + 1)$th frame is considered the mainframe. Thus, the keyframes, denoted as K^F, which are selected based on the SSIM measure from m frames, are represented in Eq. (3)

$$K_i^F = \{K_1^F, K_2^F, K_j^F, \wedge K_n^F\} \tag{3}$$

where K_i^F represents the ith keyframes selected from m frames and n denotes the total number of keyframes selected. SSIM index is a promising technique utilized for comparable estimation by reducing the computational intricacy.

4.2 Feature Extraction

After the keyframe extraction process, important features are extracted from each frame. Feature extraction is one of the important steps in image processing. Feature extraction includes lessening the number of assets expected to describe an enormous video outline. When performing complex frames examination, huge intricacy emerges from the number of factors included. Examination with countless factors ordinarily requires a lot of memory and computational force. Feature extraction is an overall cycle for making calculations of factors to manage these issues while representing the image with adequate accuracy.

4.2.1 Scale-Invariant Feature Transform (SIFT)

This algorithm is used to extract the local feature such as video frame rotation, scaling, viewpoint change, and noise. SIFT algorithm has four steps such as detection of scale space, localization of key points, orientation assignment, and generation of descriptors.

Detection of scale-space extrema: Initial production scale-space model of the building to find interesting points to be considered. To create space in scale, the original video frame is considered and blurred frames are created. In this way, many numbers of the original video frames are achieved. The size of each number is half of the previous video frames. In each octave, the frames are blurred using a Gaussian blur operator. Gaussian ambiguity is applied to every pixel of each octave. The mathematical operation of the scale-space extreme is given in Eq. (4):

$$B(p, q, \vartheta) = B^G(p, q, \vartheta) * V(p, q) \tag{4}$$

Here B is represented as the blurred video frames, B^G denotes the Gaussian blur video frames, V represents the video frames, p and q is the location of the coordination, ϑ represents the scale parameters, and $*$ represents the convolution operation of p and q.

The image is convolved with Gaussian filters at different scales, and then the difference of successive Gaussian-blurred images is taken. Key points are then extracted as local maxima/minima of the Difference of Gaussians (DoG) that occur at multiple scales. This is fast and efficient because the Gaussian difference is a simple subtraction.

Localization of key points: The previous step makes a lot of important points. These key points are on an edge or they are not differentiated enough. In both cases, features are not useful. For less varied features, the intensities are checked. If the intensity level is less than a threshold value, it is discarded. Therefore, the main point candidates are localized and refined by eliminating the key points based on peak and edge thresholding.

Orientation Assessment: The main point orientation is done by providing rotational variation. The gradient size and orientation are grouped in advance using pixel differences. The orientation assessment mathematical expression is given in Eqs. (5) and (6)

$$a(p, q) = \sqrt{(B(p + 1, q) - B(p - 1), q)^2 + (B(p, q + 1) - B(p, q - 1)} \tag{5}$$

The orientation angle δ is given by

$$\delta(p, q) = \tan^{-1} \frac{(B(p, q + 1) - B(p, q - 1)}{(B(p + 1, q) - B(p - 1, q)} \tag{6}$$

After the measurement, a 360-degree view of the break histogram made up of 36 bins, each trough covers 10 degrees. The main point of this type of orientation histogram surrounding pixels is counted. 1.5* Size of the video frames to be blurred and the window size should be equal to $1.5*\vartheta$.

Generation of Descriptors: The gradient magnitude and orientation calculate the local video frame interpretation for each of the key points. To get the local image interpretation, a key point descriptor for each key point is created. A 16×16 neighborhood around the key point is taken which is divided into 16 sub-blocks of 4×4 size. For each sub-block, 8 bin orientation histograms are created. So, a total of 128 bin values are available. These 128 numbers form a vector number. This feature vector is now uniquely used to identify a specific key point.

4.2.2 Speed Up Robust Features (SURF)

The global features are extracted using SURF techniques. SURF algorithm is utilized by its powerful attributes, which are the size of the variation; translation variation, variation in lighting, the rotational variation which can be detected in images taken under. This algorithm consists of four main steps: Integral image generation, Fast-Hessian detector (interest point detection), Descriptor orientation assignment (optional), Descriptor generation.

The Integral Image is used to accelerate speed by reducing the computational complexity considerably, Eq. (7) shows an integral image. In an integral image, each pixel represents the cumulative sum of a corresponding input pixel with all pixels above and to the left of the input pixel.

$$I \sum (y, z) = \sum_{j=0}^{y} \sum_{k=0}^{z} I(j, k) \tag{7}$$

Metrics Hessian finds significant points of the image using the SURF decide. Equation (8) shows a typical two-dimensional function of the original limit. The determinant of the Hessian matrix is calculated by first applying convolution with Gaussian kernel and then second-order derivatives with approximate Gaussian kernels. 9X9 box filters are further used for approximation. Equation (9) is used to compensate for this approximation.

$$H_{(y,z)} = det \begin{pmatrix} \frac{\partial^2 f}{\partial y^2} & \frac{\partial^2 f}{\partial y \partial z} \\ \frac{\partial^2 f}{\partial y \partial z} & \frac{\partial^2 f}{\partial y^2} \end{pmatrix} \tag{8}$$

$$H(\overline{y}) = D_{yy}(\overline{y})D_{zz}(\overline{y}) - (0.9D_{yz}(D_{yy}(\overline{x}))^2 \tag{9}$$

The third parameter is determined by measuring using Eq. (10); this creates a parameter for determining the three-dimensional location of the results, which is commonly referred to as scale-space. Size varies according to octaves and spacing.

$$H(y) = H + \frac{\partial H^T}{\partial y} y + \frac{1}{2} y^T \frac{\partial^2 H}{\partial y^2} y \tag{10}$$

$$\hat{y} = \frac{\partial^2 H^{-1}}{\partial y^2} \frac{\partial H}{\partial y} \tag{11}$$

SURF algorithm is used; all the representative points are considered with the same weight. This can be represented by relegating dynamic loads to the agent focuses. Naturally, genuine agent focuses will show up in pictures in the preparation set and bogus delegate focuses will show up once in a while. Based on this intuition, the weight of each representative point can be defined as in Eq. (12):

$$W_p = \frac{Number\ of\ detected\ images\ with\ respect\ to\ point\ P}{number\ of\ training\ images\ in\ the\ object} \tag{12}$$

4.3 Deep Neural Network Based Recognition

After completing the feature extraction, the local and global features are fed to the classifier. Here, we are utilizing a deep neural network classifier. DNN is an artificial neural network (ANN) between the input and output layers include a number of hidden units. Deep learning techniques are highly effective when the quantity of available samples amid the training stage is vast. During ordinary DNN preparation, loads of the neurons are refreshed at every redundancy until there is a blunder among yield and input is inside resistance. In this work, optimized DNN was used to classify human activity from the input videos. For this identification, the performance parameters such as accuracy, sensitivity, specificity, area under region of conversion are considered. DNN includes two phases: pre-training (utilizing generative deep belief network) and fine-tuning stages.

4.3.1 DNN Pre-training

A DNN is the quintessential deep learning (DL) model. The engineering of the DNN has generally included three sections, in particular, the input layer, shrouded layer, and yield layer, in which each layer has a few interconnected preparing units. In the DNN, each layer uses a nonlinear change on its input and gives a representation in its output. In this work, the DNN is analyzed utilizing different parameters for example accuracy, sensitivity, and specificity of video frames.

Consider $[f_m]$ being the input features where $1 \leq m \leq N$ and O denotes the output data sets. A brief model of the neural network can be given as O the number of times for the yield of the entire network and O_H the time for the yield of the hidden layer. The first hidden element releases the second hidden layer, multiplied by another set of weights.

In the first hidden layer, the weighted values of the information are enhanced with the ability to add to the neuron's gradient as in Eq. (13):

$$O_{H\_1}(x = 1, 2.., K) = \left(\sum_{m=1}^{M} w_{xm} f_m \right) + B_x \tag{13}$$

where B_x represents the constant value is known as bias, w_{xm} is the interconnection weight connecting the first hidden layer and input feature with M and K denote the quantity of hidden and input nodes in the main hidden layer. The activation function of the first hidden layer output is denoted as

$$F\left(O_{H\_1}(x)\right) = \frac{1}{\left(1 + e^{-O_{H\_1}(x)}\right)} \tag{14}$$

The output of nth the hidden layer can be specified as Eq. (15)

$$O_{H\_n}(q) = \left(\sum_{z=1}^{K} w_{qx} F\left(O_{H\_(n-1)}(x)\right) \right) + B_q \tag{15}$$

where B_q specify the bias of qth the hidden node, w_{qx} is the interconnection weight between the (n)th hidden layer and $(n-1)^{th}$ hidden layer with K hidden nodes. The actuation work which is the yield of the nth hidden layer is explained as

$$F\left(O_{H\_y}(q)\right) = \frac{1}{\left(1 + e^{-O_{H\_n}(q)}\right)} \tag{16}$$

At the output layer, the output of nth the hidden layer is again duplicated with the interconnection weights (i.e., weight between the nth output layer and hidden layer) and afterward summarized with the bias B_p as

$$O(p) = F\left(\sum_{p=1}^{K} w_{pq} F\left(O_{H\_n}(q)\right) + B_p \right) \tag{17}$$

where w_{pq} represents the interconnection weight at the nth hidden layer and output layer having pth and qth individually. The initiation work at the yield layer goes about as the yield of the entire model.

Currently, the model differs from the target output and the output of the model is achieved to improve the error. The calculation of the error is defined in Eq. (18)

$$Error = \frac{1}{M} \sum_{m=1}^{M} (Actual(O_m) - T \arg et(O_T))^2 \qquad (18)$$

where $Target(O_T)$ denotes the target output and $Actual(O_m)$ is the real output. The error must be decreased to attain an improved DNN. As a result, the weight values must be balanced until the error in each iteration decreases.

4.3.2 Fine Turning Phase

At this point, the weight parameter of the DNN is adjusted or improved by using AMBO. The optimization algorithm is used to find the optimum weights to provide the best error rate and performance accuracy. The monarch butterfly optimization (MBO) algorithm is the latest metaheuristic algorithm presented by Wang et al. [26]. It simulates the migration behaviors of monarch butterflies in nature. MBO algorithm is tested through thirty-eight benchmark problems and performance is compared with the other five metaheuristic algorithms [27].

MBO algorithm is mainly determined by the migration operator and butterfly adjusting operator. The migration operator and Butterfly adjusting operator can be implemented simultaneously. Therefore, the MBO method is ideally suited for parallel processing. MBO algorithm has a simple calculation process, requires less computational parameters. The mathematical equations and formulas proposed for this algorithm are given as follows:

Step 1: Initialization.

The initialization is an important process for all the optimization algorithms. Here, the different positions of weights are considered as the initial solution. The initial solution is randomly generated. The weight parameters are initialized as follows:

$$S = (S_1, S_2, K, S_i) \qquad (19)$$

where S_i represents the ith solution and it can be defined as follows:

$$S_i = \{w_{xm}, w_{qx}, w_{pq}\}_i \qquad (20)$$

where w_{xm} represents the interconnection of weight between the input feature and hidden layer, w_{qx} represents the interconnection weight between the nth hidden layer $n - 1$th hidden layer, and w_{pq} denotes the interconnection weight at the nth output layer and the hidden layer having qth and pth nodes separately (Fig. 2).

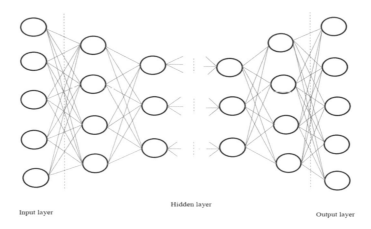

Fig. 2 Structure of deep neural network

Step 2: Fitness calculation.

After initialization, the fitness of each value is calculated. The determination of fitness is a vital part of the BOA algorithm. It is utilized to assess the inclination (integrity) of arrangements. Here, classification accuracy is the principal rule used to plan fitness work. Every time the fitness of each solution is calculated. The mathematic expression of fitness calculation is given by

$$fitness = max(Accuracy) \tag{21}$$

$$Accuracy = \frac{TN + TP}{(TN + TP + FN + FP)} \tag{22}$$

where TP represents the true positive, TN denotes the true negative, FP represents the false positive, and FN denotes the false negative.

Step 3: Updation.

After completing the fitness calculation, we update the solution based on the BOM algorithm. Here, two operators are repeated until the termination process. The detailed description of the two operators is given below.

Migration process:

In BOA, the number of butterflies in subpopulation 1 and subpopulation 2 is ceil $(P * NP)(NP_1)$ and $(NP - NP_1)(NP_2)$, respectively. Here, ceil (y) rounds y to the nearest integer or greater than or equal to y: NP represents the number of population; P represents the ratio of butterflies in the subpopulation. The mathematical expression of the migration process is given below.

$$y_{i,k}^{t+1} = y_{n1,k}^{t} \tag{23}$$

where $y_{i,k}^{t+1}$ represents the kth element of yi at generation $t+1$ that presents the position of the butterflies i. Similarly, $y_{n1,k}^{t}$ denotes the kth element of $yn1$, which is the newly generated position of butterfly $n1$, t represents the current generation number. The butterfly $n1$ is randomly selected from subpopulation 1. When $n \leq P$ the element k in the newly generated butterfly and it can be calculated by

$$n = rand * period \tag{24}$$

where rand is a random number obtained from a uniform distribution. In the contrast, if $n > P$, the element k is newly generated is given by

$$y_{i,k}^{t+1} = y_{n2,k}^{t} \tag{25}$$

where $y_{i,k}^{t+1}$ represents the kth element of $yn2$, which is the newly generated position of the butterfly $n2$. The butterfly $n2$ is randomly selected from subpopulation 2.

Butterfly Adjusting Operator:

For all the elements in butterfly j, if a randomly generated number $rand$ is smaller than or equal to P, it can be updated as,

$$y_{j,k}^{t+1} = y_{best,k}^{t} \tag{26}$$

where $y_{j,k}^{t+1}$ represents kth element of yj at the generation of $t+1$ that presents the of the butterfly j. Similarly, $y_{best,k}^{t}$ represents the kth element of y_{best} which is the best butterfly in subpopulation 1 and subpopulation 2. t represents the current generation number. In the contrast, if $rand$ is bigger than the p, it can be updated by

$$y_{j,k}^{t+1} = y_{n3,k}^{t} \tag{27}$$

$y_{n3,k}^{t}$ represents the kth element of y_{n3} that is randomly selected in subpopulation 2. Here $n_3 \in \{1, 2, 3, .., NP_2\}$. Under this condition, if $rand > BAR$, it can be further updated as follows:

$$y_{j,k}^{t+1} = y_{j,k}^{t+1} + \alpha(dy_k - 0.5) \tag{28}$$

$$\beta = \frac{s_{max}}{t^2} \tag{29}$$

A. Deshpande and K. K. Warhade

where *BAR* represents the butterfly adjusting rate, β represents the weighting factor and s_{max} maximum walk step that the butterfly can move in one step and t represents the current generation. dy represents the walk step of butterfly j that can be calculated by performing the levy flight.

$$dy = Levy(y_j^t)$$ (30)

Step 5: Termination.

The algorithm stops its implementation just if a maximum number of emphases are accomplished and the arrangement which contains the best weight esteem is picked.

The problems in MBO algorithms are fixed population size during the entire optimization process, population degradation, and slow convergence speed of algorithms. These are addressed using Adaptive Monarch Butterfly Algorithm(AMBO) by adaptively adjusting the value of P and by applying a greedy strategy to find the fitness of the newly generated butterfly.

5 Results and Discussion

In this paper, human activity recognition is implemented using three classifiers DNN, DNN optimization using the MBO algorithm, and DNN optimization using the AMBO algorithm. The experimentation is done using the MATLAB platform and conducted on an Intel i5 machine with 12 GB of RAM. The performance of the proposed method is evaluated by accuracy, sensitivity, specificity, FRR, FNR, FDR, PPV, NPV, and region of curve (ROC). A comparison between the three approaches is carried out. The evaluation matrices of the proposed method are described as follows,

5.1 Evaluation Matrices

The evaluation matrices accuracy, sensitivity, specificity, FRR, FNR, FDR, PPV, NPV, and region of curve (ROC) are used for the evolution of the comparative methods. The performance evaluation matrices are defined as follows:

Sensitivity: Some real positives to the sum of true positive and false negative rate sensitivity are called sensitivity. The mathematical expression of sensitivity is given as

$$Sensitivity = \frac{T^P}{T^P + F^N} \times 100$$ (31)

Specificity: Specificity is the ratio of several true negative to the sum of a true negative and false positive.

$$Specificity = \frac{T^P}{T^P + F^P} \times 100 \tag{32}$$

Accuracy: Accuracy is calculated by the measures of sensitivity and specificity. It is denoted as follows:

$$Accuracy = \frac{T^P + T^N}{T^P + F^P + T^N + F^N} \times 100 \tag{33}$$

Positive Predictive Value (PPV): The fraction of positive experiment consequences which are considered as the Positive Predictive Value.

$$PPV = \frac{T^P}{T^P + F^P} \times 100 \tag{34}$$

Negative Predictive Value (NPV): The fraction of negative experiment consequences which are considered as the Negative Predictive Value.

$$NPV = \frac{T^N}{T^N + F^N} \times 100 \tag{35}$$

False Positive Rate (FPR): FPR is calculated as the number of incorrect positive predictions divided by the total number of negatives. It can also be calculated as 1 − specificity.

$$FPR = \frac{T^P}{T^N + F^P} \times 100 \tag{36}$$

False Negative Rate (FNR): FNR is calculated as the number of incorrect negative predictions divided by the total number of negatives.

$$PPV = \frac{F^N}{T^P + F^N} \times 100 \tag{37}$$

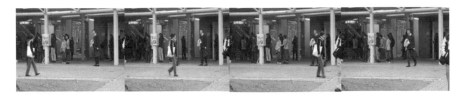

Fig. 3. Sample data set for Video 1

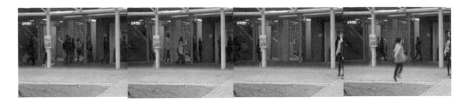

Fig. 4 Sample data set for Video 2

5.2 Data Description

To testify the effectiveness of the proposed method, the video sequence contains the avenue data set. Avenue Dataset contains 16 training and 21 testing video clips. The total numbers of training frames are 15,328 with a resolution of each frame of 640 × 360 pixels. There are 14 unusual events including strange actions like running, throwing objects and loitering, unusual objects, wrong direction, etc. Challenges in the Avenue dataset are camera shake, few outliers, some normal patterns rarely appear in training data [28]. The sample video sequence are given below (Figs. 3 and 4).

5.3 Experimental Result

In this section, the experimental results of the proposed method are discussed. The testing of the proposed method is done on 12 testing videos. This proposed method is used to predict normal or abnormal human activity. Human activity recognition is used in video surveillance systems that track abnormal events, and human–machine interaction. Table 1 demonstrates the results of the proposed method for the classification of activity.

Table 1 Experimental results of video 1 and video 2 frames

Predicted image for Input video 1	Normal/Abnormal activity	Predicted image for input video 2	Normal/Abnormal activity
	Normal		Normal
	Abnormal		Abnormal
	Abnormal		Normal
	Abnormal		Abnormal

Table 2 Comparative analysis video 1

	Sensitivity	Specificity	Accuracy	PPV	NPV	FPR	FNR	FDR
ABO-DNN	0.9214	0.9158	0.9190	0.9347	0.8990	0.8411	0.0785	0.0652
BO-DNN	0.9	0.9065	0.9025	0.9264	0.8738	0.0934	0.1	0.0735
DNN	0.8857	0.8971	0.8906	0.9185	0.8571	0.1028	0.1142	0.0814

Table 3 Comparative analysis video 2

	Sensitivity	Specificity	Accuracy	PPV	NPV	FPR	FNR	FDR
ABO-DNN	1	0.9584	0.9666	0.8601	1	0.0415	0	0.1398
BO-DNN	0.9918	0.9189	0.9337	0.7577	0.9977	0.0810	0.0081	0.2422
DNN	0.9268	0.8939	0.9006	0.6909	0.9794	0.1060	0.0731	0.3090

5.4 Comparative Analysis

This section shows, comparative analysis of the proposed and the existing methods. To prove the effectiveness of the proposed method, we have compared the proposed method with the existing methods such as Monarch Butterfly Optimization with Deep Neural Network (MBO-DNN) and DNN. Here, the performance parameters analyzed are accuracy, sensitivity, specificity, FRR, FNR, FDR, PPV, NPV, and region of curve (ROC). The comparative analysis of the proposed method is given in Tables 2 and 3.

Figure 5 represents the comparative analysis of the proposed method against the existing method for video file 1. In video file 1, the accuracy of the proposed method is 91%; the existing methods are 90% and 89% respectively. The comparison shows that the Accuracy, Sensitivity, Specificity results of the proposed method are better than the existing method.

Figure 6 demonstrates the comparative analysis of the proposed method against the existing method in video 2. Comparing the proposed and existing method as shown in Table 4, the proposed method is much better than the existing methods.

Figure 7 shows the recognition accuracy chart for the 12 different testing videos for three classifiers DNN, MBO, AMBO. The recognition accuracy plot shows that AMBO algorithms performance is better compared to MBO and DNN. Feature Extraction time recorded is four frames per second. Prediction time recorded is 0.22 frames per second.

5.5 Comparative Analysis of the Published Paper

In this section, the comparative analysis of the proposed method and the currently published paper is carried out. To prove the effectiveness of the proposed method, we compare the three published papers. In this published paper [28], the abnormal

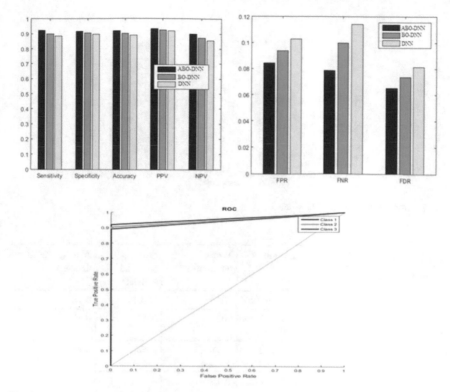

Fig. 5 Comparative analysis of video 1

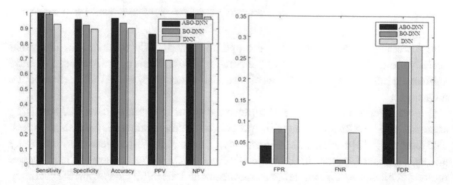

Fig. 6 Comparative analysis of video 1

event detection was implemented using sparse combination learning. In the existing method [29], implementation is done using discriminative frameworks for large video detection using spatiotemporal descriptors with SVM as a classifier. The abnormal video detection form videos using two-stream recurrent variational autoencoder [30].

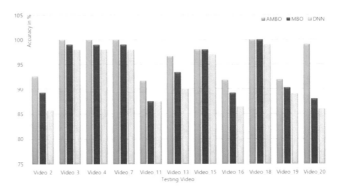

Fig. 7 Comparative analysis of video 1

Table 4 Comparative analysis of the proposed and the published papers

Method	Year of publication	Accuracy (Avenue dataset)	AUC (Avenue dataset)
Lu et al. [28]	2013	92.9%	0.78
Giorno et al. [29]	2016	91%	0.80
Yan et al. [30]	2018	93%	0.80
Trong et al. [31]	2019	–	0.87
Proposed method		**96%**	**0.95**

The methodology used by [31] is the optical flow and CNN Model for abnormal activity recognition. Table 4 shows the comparative analysis of the proposed method against the published paper in terms of recognition accuracy and AUC for the Avenue dataset.

Figure 8 represents a graphical representation of the comparative analysis using accuracy and AUC parameters of the proposed method against the published papers. The reference [28] contains 92.9% accuracy, Giorno et al. [29] achieves 91% accuracy and the published paper [30] contains 93% accuracy. The accuracy of the proposed method achieves 96%. Comparing the proposed and the published paper, the accuracy and AUC of the proposed method are very much better than the published paper.

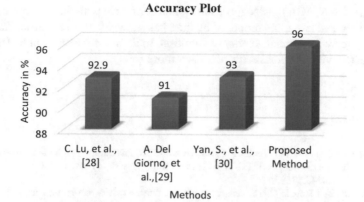

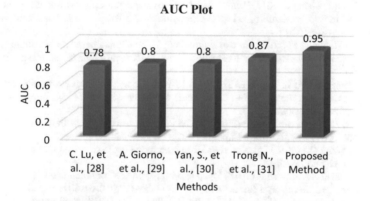

Fig. 8 Comparative analysis of the proposed method against the published papers

6 Conclusion

This paper presented a framework for human activity recognition using an adaptive deep neural network. The key aim was to detect anomalous activity in the video sequences. In this method, the input videos are converted into a number of frames. After that, the keyframes are extracted by using SSIM measures. The features from keyframes are extracted using the local and global feature methods. Here, the local features are extracted using the SIFT method, and the global features are extracted using the SURF method. After completing the feature extraction, the selected features are fed to the classifier for identifying human activity. This work proposed a novel method of optimizing DNN using the Monarch Butterfly algorithm and Adaptive Monarch Butterfly algorithm for human activity classification. The performance evaluation was conducted on the Avenue datasets to obtain the FRR, FNR, FDR, PPV, NPV, Accuracy, and AUC results. The adaptive butterfly monarch optimization algorithm (AMBO) shows improvement in the recognition accuracy compared to the traditional DNN, MBO-DNN approach. When compared with the existing methods for the Avenue dataset, the proposed method has shown better recognition accuracy and AUC score for human activity recognition. In the future model can be tested on real-time test videos to make this approach more robust.

References

1. Ramanathan M, Yau WY, Teoh EK (2014) Human action recognition with video data: research and evaluation challenges. IEEE Trans Human-Mach Syst 44(5):650–663. https://doi.org/10. 1109/thms.2014.2325871
2. Li K, Liu Z, Liang L (2016) Ampyanan song: human action recognition using associated depth and skeleton information. In: 2nd IEEE international conference on computer and communications (ICCC)
3. Wei S, Song Y, Zhang Y (2017) Human skeleton tree recurrent neural network with joint relative motion feature for skeleton-based action recognition. In: IEEE international conference on image processing (ICIP)
4. Su B, Wu H, Sheng M (2017) Human action recognition method based on hierarchical framework via Kinect skeleton data. In: International conference on machine learning and cybernetics (ICMLC)
5. Cai X, Zhou W, Wu L, Luo J, Li H (2016) Effective active skeleton representation for low latency human action recognition. IEEE Trans Multimed 18(2):141–154. https://doi.org/10. 1109/tmm.2015.2505089
6. Diraco G, Leone A, Siciliano P (2013) Human posture recognition with a time of flight 3D sensor for in-home applications. Expert Syst Appl 40(2):744–751
7. Lin Y-L, Wang MJ (2012) Constructing 3D human model from front and side images. Expert Syst Appl 39(5):5012–5018
8. Akula A, Shah AK, Ghosh R (2018) Deep learning approach for human action recognition in infrared images. Cognit Syst Res 50:146–154. https://doi.org/10.1016/j.cogsys.2018.04.002
9. Pham HH, Khoudour L, Crouzil A, Zegers P, Velastin SA (2018) Exploiting deep residual networks for human action recognition from skeletal data. Comput Vision Image Underst 170:51–66. https://doi.org/10.1016/j.cviu.2018.03.003
10. Yoon SM, Kuijper A (2013) Human action recognition based on skeleton splitting. Expert Syst Appl 40(17):6848–6855. https://doi.org/10.1016/j.eswa.2013.06.024
11. Rahman SA, Leung MKH, Cho SY (2013) Human action recognition employing negative space features. J Vis Commun Image Represent 24(3):217–231
12. Zhao D, Shao L, Zhen X, Liu Y (2013) Combining appearance and structural features for human action recognition. Neurocomputing 113:88–96
13. Ijjina EP, Mohan CK (2016) Hybrid deep neural network model for human action recognition. Appl Soft Comput 46:936–952. https://doi.org/10.1016/j.asoc.2015.08.025
14. Ahad MAR (2013) Smart approaches for human action recognition. Pattern Recogn Lett 34(15):1769–1770
15. Sheeba PT, Murugan S (2018) Hybrid features-enabled dragon deep belief neural network for activity recognition. Imag Sci J 66:6:355–371. https://doi.org/10.1080/13682199.2018.148348
16. Wang GG, Deb S, Cui Z (2015) Monarch butterfly optimization. Neural Comput Appl 1–20
17. Sankalap Arora, Satvir Singh.: Butterfly optimization algorithm: a novel approach for global optimization, Springer-Verlag GmbH Germany, part of Springer Nature, (2018) https://doi.org/ 10.1007/s00500-018-3102-4
18. Wang Q, Chen K (2020) Multi-label zero-shot human action recognition via joint latent ranking embedding. Neural Netw 122:1–23
19. Dai C, Liu X, Lai J (2020) Human action recognition using two-stream attention-based LSTM networks. Appl Soft Comput 86:105820–105820. https://doi.org/10.1016/j.asoc.2019.105820

20. Chaudhary S, Murala S (2019) Deep network for human action recognition using Weber motion. Neurocomputing 367:207–216. https://doi.org/10.1016/j.neucom.2019.08.031
21. Gu Y, Ye X, Sheng W, Ou Y, Li Y (2019) Multiple stream deep learning model for human action recognition. Image Vision Comput
22. Arivazhagan S, NewlinShebiah R, Harini R, Swetha S (2019) Human action recognition from rgb-d data using the complete local binary pattern. Cognitive Syst Res
23. Xu Y, Shen Z, Zhang X, Gao Y, Deng S, Wang Y, Chang C, E I (2017) Learning multi-level features for sensor-based human action recognition. Pervasive Mobile Comput 40:324–338
24. Liu M, Liu H, Chen C (2017) Enhanced skeleton visualization for view-invariant human action recognition. Pattern Recogn 68:346–362
25. Itano F, Pires R, de Abreu de Sousa MA, Del-Moral-Hernandez E (2019) Human action recognition in video scenes from multiple camera viewpoints. Cognitive Syst Res 56:223–232. https://doi.org/10.1016/j.cogsys.2019.03.010
26. Wang G, Deb S, Cui Z (2015) Monarch butterfly optimization. Neural Comput Appl
27. Hu H, Cai Z, Hu S, Cai Y, Chen J, Huang S (2018) improving monarch butterfly optimization algorithm with self-adaptive population, algorithms
28. Lu C, Shi J, Jia J (2013) Abnormal event detection at 150 fps in MatLab. In: Proceedings of the IEEE international conference on computer vision, pp 2720–2727
29. Giorno A, Bagnell JA, Hebert M (2016) A discriminative framework for anomaly detection in large videos. In: European conference on computer vision, pp 334–349
30. Yan S, Smith JS, Lu W, Zhang B (2018) Abnormal event detection from videos using a two-stream recurrent variational autoencoder. IEEE Trans Cognitive Dev Syst
31. Nguyen T, Meunier J (2019) Anomaly detection in video sequence with appearance-motion correspondence. IEEE/CVF International Conference on Computer Vision (ICCV)

A Secure Color Image Encryption Scheme Based on Chaos

Rajiv Ranjan Suman, Bhaskar Mondal, Sunil Kumar Singh, and Tarni Mandal

1 Introduction

The Internet is spreading overwhelmingly every day. Due to its easy connectivity through smartphones, people of all professions, age groups, geographical locations are becoming connected. A huge population performs countless kinds of activities including entertainment, social media, business, banking, academics, etc. [11]. In all these activities, sensitive personal information is transmitted and shared over the Internet which is an insecure channel. Most often, such information includes color images of persons, groups, medical data, business data, government, or enterprise documents, etc. Disclosure of such data may lead to significant loss of property, reputation, credential, or even claim life. Hence, assurance of privacy and integrity of such data over the Internet is a tough challenge for the researchers [2, 8].

Data encryption is widely used to protect confidentiality as well as the integrity of data. An image encryption technique transforms the plain text image to some unrecognizable and noise-like format with the help of an encryption algorithm and

R. R. Suman (✉) · T. Mandal
Department of Mathematics, National Institute of Technology Jamshedpur, 831014 Jamshedpur, India
e-mail: rrsuman.cse@nitjsr.ac.in

T. Mandal
e-mail: tmandal.ath@nitjsr.ac.in

B. Mondal
Department of Computer Science and Engineering, National Institute of Technology Patna, Patna, India
e-mail: bhaskar.cs@nitp.ac.in

S. K. Singh
School of Computer Science and Engineering, VIT-AP University, Near Vijayawada, Amaravati, Andhra Pradesh, India

© The Author(s), under exclusive license to Springer Nature Singapore Pte Ltd. 2021
M. K. Bajpai et al. (eds.), *Machine Vision and Augmented Intelligence—Theory and Applications*, Lecture Notes in Electrical Engineering 796,
https://doi.org/10.1007/978-981-16-5078-9_31

a secret key [10]. During the past two decades, many algorithms were reported to encrypt images efficiently [5]. Slow speed of encryption and scalability are the major limitations of most of the reported algorithms when used to encrypt many color images of large size and high resolution.

Color image encryption proposed by Broumandnia [3] is a five-step procedure in 3-D space. It implements diffusion and confusion of pixels using substitution and permutation operations, respectively. They used a function based on modular arithmetic along with operations reversible for multiplication to implement 3D modular confusion. Speed of key generation, period of keys, and size of keyspace of the encryption scheme were increased due to the use of 3D modular chaotic arithmetic. However, its computations are not free from high overhead.

Valandar et al. [13] presented an encryption technique that uses a 3-D chaotic map containing six keys. Interval of control parameters is shown with the help of bifurcation diagrams and Lyapunov exponent to realize the chaotic nature of their proposed map. The randomness of the generated numbers was verified by the cobweb plot, cross coloration, and statistical tests (ENT, NIST, and DIEHARD). Hence, the implemented map could be used as a pseudonumber generator. An image encryption presented by Mondal et al. [7] used a new sin-cos cross chaotic map. In [9], they presented one more scheme in which genetic operations were used for encrypting images.

Chai et al. [4] proposed a cryptosystem for color images. It uses a dynamic DNA sequence and four-wing hyper-chaotic system for encryption. Encoding as well as decoding rules were chosen based on input unencrypted images. It uses a novel diffusion procedure to diffuse the DNA sequence of the input image. The method provides good security performance.

Kovalchuk et al. [6] used the RSA algorithm to develop a new encryption-decryption algorithm for grayscale as well as color images. Encryption or decryption was applied on each row of the input image matrix with and without use of additional noise-mixing. The effectiveness of this scheme was tested and verified by conducting several experiments with grayscale as well as color images. Bit-wise binary operations gave low computational overhead and faster speed to this technique.

A DNA-based multi-channel chaotic encryption scheme was reported by Wang et al. [14] for colored images. It generates six sets of chaotic key sequences. Then RGB components of the input image are extracted and DNA matrix are generated from DNA coding. Three equal size sub-matrices are obtained after scrambling the DNA matrix using XOR with chaotic key matrices. Finally, multiple diffusion operations are performed to encrypt the colored image.

1.1 Objective and Contribution

This paper proposes a color image encryption scheme based on a chaotic Duffin map. The scheme works in two steps (i) first it permutes pixel positions and then (ii) performs diffusion of pixel values. The scheme permutes the pixels of all three components red, green, and blue based on the random number obtained from the chaotic Duffin map. Then it changes the pixel values using the same series of pseudorandom number. The initial state along with parameters of the Duffin map becomes the key for the encryption scheme.

The scheme was tested with security parameters like histogram analysis, correlation coefficient, PSNR, entropy, UACI, and NPCR. The experimental results demonstrate that the scheme is secure and robust against different security attacks.

The next section discusses the chaotic Duffin map followed by the proposed method in Sect. 3. Experimental results are given in Sect. 4. Finally, in Sect. 5, the conclusion is given.

2 Chaotic Duffing Map

The Duffing map or Holmes map is a discrete chaotic dynamical system. In chaotic map, point (x_k, y_k) on the Cartesian plane is mapped to a new location using Eqs. 1 and 2. The generated (x_i, y_i) are plotted for the map in Fig. 1a and the bifurcation diagram is shown in Fig. 1b, which shows the chaotic nature of the map. The series of (x_i, y_i) are the pseudorandom number sequence (PRNS) that is used for the encryption.

$$x_{k+1} = y_k \tag{1}$$

$$y_{k+1} = \beta x_k + \alpha y_k - y_k^3 \tag{2}$$

The behavior of the map is determined by two parameters α and β, which are set near to $\alpha = 2.75$ and $\beta = 0.2$ to get a good chaotic nature.

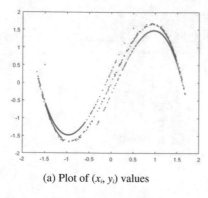
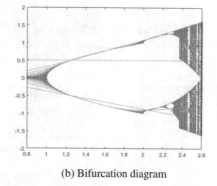

(a) Plot of (x_i, y_i) values   (b) Bifurcation diagram

Fig. 1 Chaotic nature of Duffin map

3 The Proposed Scheme

The proposed scheme takes a color image I of size $r \% c$ as input and encrypts the
image based on pseudorandom number sequence (PRNS) generated by the chaotic
Duffin map. This map generates two PRNS represented as R_r and R_y. The initial
conditions x_k and y_k and the chaotic parameters α and β of the Duffin map are the
secret key $K = (x_k, y_k, \alpha, \beta)$ for the proposed cryptosystem. The overall representation of the scheme is presented in Fig. 2. The algorithm has two main steps (i)
permutation and (ii) diffusion. The algorithm is given below.

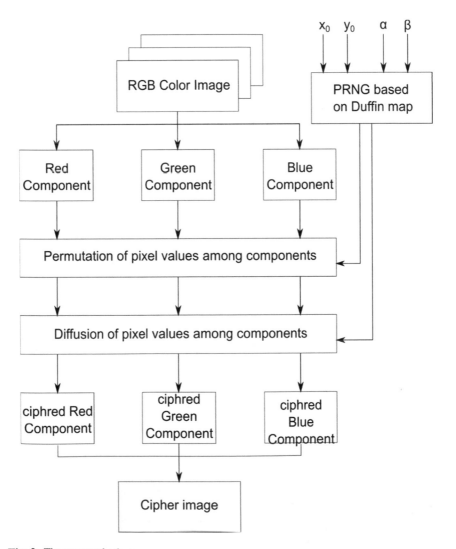

Fig. 2 The proposed scheme

1. Read a color plain image I of size $r \% c$.
2. Generate two PRNS R_x and R_y using the Duffin map each of size $r \% c$.
3. Permute the position of the pixel of Red (R), Green (G), and Blue (B) components of the RGB image using Eq. 3.

$$I_p\big(R_x(m,n), R_y(m,n), 1\big) = I(m,n,1)$$
$$I_p\big(R_x(m,n), R_y(m,n), 2\big) = I(m,n,2)$$
$$I_p\big(R_x(m,n), R_y(m,n), 3\big) - I(m,n,3) \qquad (3)$$

4. The pixel values of the permuted image I' are modified using Eq. 4.

$$I_c(m,n,1) = I_p(m,n,1) \oplus \big((R_x(m,n) + R_y(m,n))\bmod 256\big)$$
$$I_c(m,n,2) = I_p(m,n,2) \oplus \big((R_x(m,n) + R_y(m,n))\bmod 256\big)$$
$$I_c(m,n,3) = I_p(m,n,3) \oplus \big((R_x(m,n) + R_y(m,n))\bmod 256\big) \qquad (4)$$

5. The I_c is produced as the encrypted image.

4 Security Test Results

The proposed scheme was evaluated with different images for many security metrics. Experimental results are presented in this section. Four color images of different sizes and types were chosen namely (i) Lena (512 × 512), (ii) Airplane (256 × 256), (i) Fruits (350 × 350), and (iv) Peppers (400 × 400) for evaluating the algorithm. The results depict that the proposed algorithm is promising and secure against attacks.

4.1 Analysis of Histogram

The histogram analysis visualizes the pixel frequencies in an image. The uniformity in the histogram of the cipher image shows the good quality of the cryptosystem. The plain color image and its histogram are presented in Fig. 3a, b whereas the cipher image and its histogram are shown in Fig. 3c, d. From Fig. 3, it can be well noticed that the histogram of the cipher image is changed drastically from the plain image, which depicts the good quality of the proposed system. Further, the component-wise histogram of the plain image and the cipher image are presented in Fig. 4.

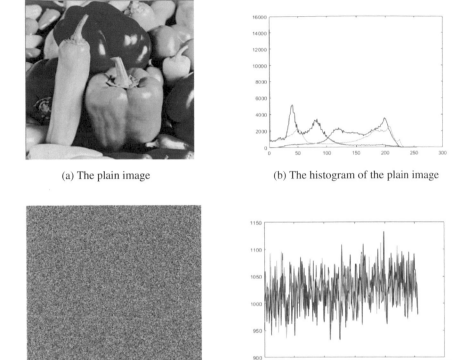

(a) The plain image

(b) The histogram of the plain image

(c) Encrypted image

(d) The histogram of the encrypted image

Fig. 3 Experimental results on the Pepper image

4.2 Correlation Coefficient

The correlation among the adjacent pixels in the plain image is remarkably high due to the redundancy of information in the images. The high correlation needs to be broken and should be near to zero in the cipher image to resist any statistical attacks. The calculated values of each component of the plain images and the cipher images are placed in Table 1. It can be noticed that correlation among pixels in the cipher images is drastically reduced as compared with that in the plain images. Comparison of correlation values Lena image is shown in Table 2. The correlation coefficient CC is given by Eq. 5.

$$CC = \frac{E[(A_1 - \mu A_1)(A_2 - \mu A_2)]}{\sigma A_1 \sigma A_2} \qquad (5)$$

where A_1 and A_2 are sets of selected adjacent pixels and σA_1 and σA_2 are respective standard deviations.

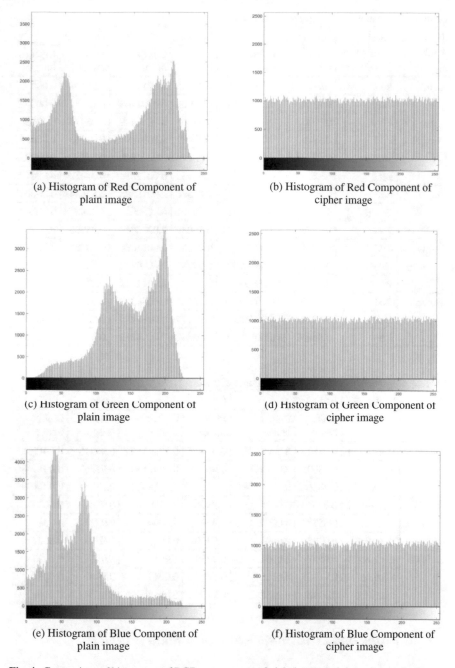

(a) Histogram of Red Component of
plain image

(b) Histogram of Red Component of
cipher image

(c) Histogram of Green Component of
plain image

(d) Histogram of Green Component of
cipher image

(e) Histogram of Blue Component of
plain image

(f) Histogram of Blue Component of
cipher image

Fig. 4 Comparison of histograms of RGB components of plain image and cipher image for Pepper image

Table 1 Correlation test results and comparison

Image name	Image compo-nent	Horizontal		Vertical		Diagonal	
		Plain image	Cipher image	Plain image	Cipher image	Plain image	Cipher image
Lena	Red	0.9754	0.00030215	0.98695	0.0013188	0.96368	0.000130
	Green	0.97445	0.00084163	0.98685	0.00014687	0.96251	0.002563
	Blue	0.95315	0.0019335	0.97367	0.0016489	0.93374	0.001889
Air-plane	Red	0.97264	0.0016611	0.95681	0.00078998	0.93433	0.000005
	Green	0.95778	0.00074349	0.96775	0.0024013	0.93259	0.002038
	Blue	0.96398	0.00082967	0.93532	0.001291	0.91458	0.000426
Baboon	Red	0.92307	0.0011754	0.86596	0.0018598	0.85434	0.000062
	Green	0.86548	0.0010952	0.76501	0.002992	0.7348	0.002674
	Blue	0.90734	0.00020721	0.88089	0.0028424	0.83986	0.002927
Fruits	Red	0.9726	0.0025169	0.97282	0.0031644	0.95226	0.001203
	Green	0.97738	0.0014982	0.9778	0.00067421	0.962	0.003654
	Blue	0.98025	0.00099807	0.9807	0.0047153	0.96572	0.003574
Peppers	Red	0.96352	0.00077369	0.96634	0.0034343	0.95638	0.001613
	Green	0.98112	0.00080362	0.98177	0.0039453	0.96866	0.001750
	Blue	0.96652	0.0010569	0.96642	0.0036216	0.94779	0.001057

Table 2 Comparison of Correlation test results with Refs. [1, 12]

Scheme	Direction	Red		Green		Diagonal	
		Plain image	Cipher image	Plain image	Cipher image	Plain image	Cipher image
Our's	Horizontal	0.9754	0.00030215	0.97445	0.00084163	0.95315	0.0019335
	Vertical	0.98695	0.0013188	0.98685	0.00014687	0.97367	0.0016489
	Diagonal	0.96368	0.00013044	0.96251	0.0025632	0.93374	0.0018893
Ref. [1]	Horizontal	0.9794	0.0024	0.9806	0.0009	0.9604	0.0032
	Vertical	0.9574	0.0052	0.9593	0.0004	0.9237	0.0017
	Diagonal	0.9363	0.0003	0.9400	0.0012	0.8898	0.0027
Ref.[12]	Horizontal	0.9647	0.0091	0.9730	0.0012	0.9484	0.0223
	Vertical	0.9639	0.0123	0.9407	0.0047	0.8907	0.0057
	Diagonal	0.9143	0.0258	0.9186	0.0188	0.8434	0.0142

4.3 Entropy and Peak Signal-To-Noise Ratio (PSNR)

The entropy of an image represents the randomness of pixel values. One of the cryptographic objectives is to increase the randomness in pixels of the produced cipher image. The results in Table 3 show that the entropy values of cipher images are increased (near to 8) as compared to entropy values of corresponding plain images. The entropy is given by Eq. 6.

$$H(m) = \sum_{k=0}^{2^N-1} p(m_k) \times \log_2 \left[\frac{1}{p(m_k)} \right] \tag{6}$$

where p is the probability of each gray-scale value. If a cipher image becomes completely random then the entropy becomes very near to 8.

The PSNR is the ratio between the power of the plain image and the cipher image. A higher value of PSNR depicts the potential of the cryptosystem. The calculated values of PSNR are shown in Table 3.

4.4 UACI and NPCR

The unified average changed intensity (UACI) and number of changing pixel rates (NPCR) are the two important measurements of the quality of a cryptosystem. The calculated values are presented in Table 3 which shows that the proposed scheme is strong enough against attacks. UACI calculates the average difference of intensities between two cipher images C and C' given by Eq. 7. A value of UACI around 30 is

Table 3 Test values of Entropy, PSNR, UACI, and NPCR

Image name	Image Compo-nent	Entropy		PSNR	MSE	UACI	NPCR
		Plain image	Cipher image				
Lena	Red	7.2625	7.9994	46.294	106.51	33.034	99.927
	Green	7.5902	7.9993	45.585	90.464	30.584	99.904
	Blue	6.9843	7.9992	44.553	71.326	27.669	99.917
Air-plane	Red	6.7178	7.9993	45.985	99.192	31.908	99.911
	Green	6.799	7.9993	46.304	106.74	33.057	99.902
	Blue	6.2138	7.9994	46.204	104.32	32.703	99.887
Baboon	Red	7.7067	7.9992	45.381	86.301	29.96	99.926
	Green	7.4744	7.9993	44.919	77.597	28.615	99.911
	Blue	7.7522	7.9993	45.81	95.271	31.353	99.906
Fruits	Red	7.0556	7.9993	46.485	111.28	33.757	99.904
	Green	7.3527	7.9993	45.986	99.206	31.909	99.905
	Blue	7.7134	7.9992	45.613	91.047	30.686	99.899
Peppers	Red	7.3388	7.9994	45.043	79.845	28.953	99.886
	Green	7.4963	7.9993	46.54	112.71	34.003	99.909
	Blue	7.0583	7.9991	46.533	112.52	34.023	99.934

acceptable in encryption.

$$UACI = \sum_{m,n} \frac{|C(m, n) - C'(m, n)|}{F \times T} \times 100\% \tag{7}$$

where F is the maximum possible pixel value of the image and T is the total number of pixels in the image.

NPCR calculates the percentage of differences among pixels of two cipher images C and C' whose plane images have only one to few bits difference. The NPCR is given by Eq. 8.

$$D(m, n) = \begin{cases} 0, & if \ C(m, \ n) = C'(m, \ n) \\ 1, & if \ C(m, \ n) \neq C'(m, \ n) \end{cases}$$

$$NPCR = \sum_{m,n} \frac{D(m, n)}{T} \times 100\% \tag{8}$$

where T is the total number of pixels in the image.

5 Conclusion

The security of color images is a warranting requirement in current days. This paper proposed a secure encryption algorithm for color images based on the Duffin map. The proposed algorithm is robust and secure, which is easily observable from the results generated and presented in this paper. The algorithm shows good and acceptable results in security metrics like histogram analysis, correlation coefficient, entropy, PSNR, UACI, and NPCR. The algorithm may be used for real communication and storage of color images over the Internet. It can also be implemented on hardware to improve the performance.

References

1. Ali TS, Ali R (2020) A new chaos based color image encryption algorithm using permutation substitution and boolean operation. Multimedia Tools and Applications
2. Arpacı B, Kurt E, C̦ elik K, Ciylan B (2020) Colored image encryption and decryption with a new algorithm and a hyperchaotic electrical circuit. J Electr Eng Technol 1–17
3. Broumandnia A (2019) The 3D modular chaotic map to digital color image encryption. Futur Gener Comput Syst 99:489–499
4. Chai X, Fu X, Gan Z, Lu Y, Chen Y (2019) A color image cryptosystem based on dynamic DNA encryption and chaos. Signal Process 155:44–62

5. Hasanzadeh E, Yaghoobi M (2019) A novel color image encryption algorithm based on substitution box and hyper-chaotic system with fractal keys. Multimed Tools Appl 1–19
6. Kovalchuk A, Lotoshynska N, ml MG, Izonin I, Berezko L (2019) An approach towards an efficient encryption-decryption of grayscale and color images. Procedia Computer Science 155, 630–635 (2019), the 16th International Conference on Mobile Systems and Pervasive Computing (MobiSPC 2019),The 14th International Conference on Future Networks and Communications (FNC-2019),The 9th International Conference on Sustainable Energy Information Technology.
7. Mondal B, Behera PK, Gangopadhyay S (2020) A secure image encryption scheme based on a novel 2d sine-cosine cross-chaotic (sc3) map. J Real-Time Image Process
8. Mondal B, Mandal T (2017) A light weight secure image encryption scheme based on chaos & DNA computing. J King Saud Univ-Comput Inf Sci 29(4):499–504
9. Mondal B, Mandal T (2020) A secure image encryption scheme based on genetic operations and a new hybrid pseudo random number generator. Multimed Tools Appl 79:17497–17520
10. Mondal B, Singh S, Kumar P (2019) A secure image encryption scheme based on cellular automata and chaotic skew tent map. J Inf Secur Appl 45:117–130
11. Mondal B, Sinha D, Gupta NK, Kumar N, Goyal P (2012) An optimal (n, n) secret image sharing scheme. UACEE Int J Comput Sci Appl 2(3):61–66
12. Sun Yj, Zhang H, Wang Xy, Wang Mx (2020) Bit-level color image encryption algorithm based on coarse-grained logistic map and fractional chaos. Multimed Tools Appl 1–19
13. Valandar MY, Barani MJ, Ayubi P (2019) A fast color image encryption technique based on three dimensional chaotic map. Optik 193, 162921
14. Wang Y, Wu C, Kang S, Wang Q, Mikulovich VI (2020) Multi channel chaotic encryption algorithm for color image based on DNA coding. Multimed Tools Appl 18317–18342

Simulation of Groundwater level by Artificial Neural Networks of Parts of Yamuna River Basin

Saad Asghar Moeeni, Mohammad Sharif, Naved Ahsan, and Asif Iqbal

1 Introduction

Groundwater is the most important source of natural resources. It is a vital source of industries, agriculture, and domestic requirements which want to be carefully managed for hard rock and drought-prone areas [1]. It has become a reliable source of water in all climatic regions of the world [2]. Groundwater is the largest available freshwater resource in the whole world. Aquifer wells provide potable water to 50% of the world's population and record 43% of overall irrigation water consumption. In addition, worldwide 2.5 billion citizens depend entirely on groundwater supplies in order to meet their everyday needs [3]. In arid and semi-arid climates, with frequent dry spells and sometimes erratic surface waters (Liamasand Martínez-Santos, 2005), groundwater is significant. Groundwater is an important medium of water supply in different regions of the world, as a result, several studies highlighted different features of groundwater such as storage potential, hydrogeology, water quality , exposure, and so on [4–7]. Furthermore, groundwater simulation has become an essential tool among scientists and engineers working on water management for optimizing and protecting the development of groundwater. Physically, during the past few years, simulations have been implemented to simulate and analyze the groundwater environment and then take remedial steps in order to allow effective use of the control of water supplies. These models act as a hydrological variableness framework and

S. Asghar Moeeni (✉) · M. Sharif · N. Ahsan
Department of Civil Engineering, Jamia Millia Islamia, New Delhi, India
e-mail: smoeeni@gmail.com

A. Iqbal
Piro Tech, New Delhi, India

© The Author(s), under exclusive license to Springer Nature Singapore Pte Ltd. 2021   377
M. K. Bajpai et al. (eds.), *Machine Vision and Augmented Intelligence—Theory
and Applications*, Lecture Notes in Electrical Engineering 796,
https://doi.org/10.1007/978-981-16-5078-9_32

understand the physical processes within the aquifer. Hydrologists, mechanics, and environmental engineers use this frequently in computer applications but challenges range from aquifer protection yield to soil quality and clean-up. Although such models use data in highly intense, laborious, and expensive ways. As a consequence, physical models in developed countries are significantly limited because of the lack of appropriate and high-quality data.

In this paper, we have used ANN for groundwater prediction of four Blocks of the BANDA District of UP. Prediction of groundwater is very important for planning groundwater administration and water resources in any river basin. Physical-based models are widely used in groundwater simulation. Wide numbers of numerical models have already been developed for different areas with different objectives such as to express provincial groundwater behavior and to understand local hydrological processes [8–10]. The relevance of the ANN technique in water management ranges from event-based simulation to real-time simulation. It has been used for rainfall-runoff simulation, precipitation simulation as well as for stream flows simulation, evapotranspiration, water quality as well as groundwater [11–13]. In the literature, comparatively less research on the ANN-based approach in groundwater hydrology has been used in comparison to surface water hydrology. Neural networking practises are used in groundwater hydrology for the evaluation of the aquifer parameters [14–20], groundwater quality predictions [17, 21, 22].

2 Study Area

Banda district lies between latitude 25°00′00″ and 25°59′00″ north and longitude 80°06′00″ and 81°00′00″. The district's total area is 4460 km². Baberu is one block of the Banda district. It consists of 570.41 km². The area geologically comprises Precambrian Bundelkhand granites overlain by Vindhyan and quaternary alluvium. The area is roughly plain apart from some isolated granitic hillocks and the division of point bars natural levees, and flood plain. It is made up of unconsolidated deposits of Indo-Gangetic alluvium of recent age comprising silt clay, silt, Kankar, sand and their admixtures of various grades.

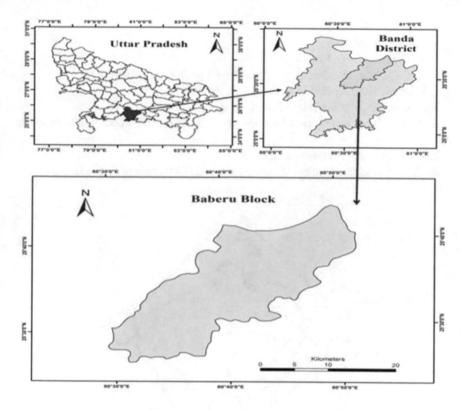

3 Study Period

The periods for study depend from the time of minimum to the time of maximum water table elevation as the non-monsoon period and from the time of minimum to the time of maximum water table elevation as monsoon period. For this purpose, data have been taken from 1995 to 2016 in northern India and the water year is considered from November 1 to October 31 next year. The study periods are taken as non-monsoon periods for the duration of November to May.

4 Materials and Methods

4.1 Ground Water Balance Equation

$$R_c + R_i + R_r + R_t + S_i + I_g = E_t + T_p + S_e + O_g + \Delta S \qquad (1)$$

where

R = Rainfall Recharge;

R_c = Canal seepage Recharge;

Rr = Field irrigation Recharge; Rt = Recharge from pond storage

I_g = inflow from blocks; Et = Evapo-transpiration;

T_p = Groundwater discharge from tube well;

S_i, S_e = influent and effluent seepage from rivers; Og = outflow to other blocks;

and

ΔS = change in groundwater storage.

All these parameters are calculated by Central Groundwater norms [Ref].

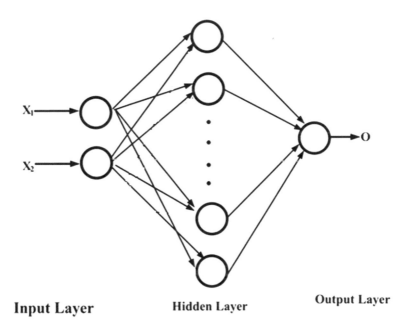

Input Layer   **Hidden Layer**   **Output Layer**

ANN Architecture

For the prediction of groundwater resources, ANN model is proposed the proposed models have been built using MATLAB The proposed ANN model consists of only a hidden layer in between input and output layers. Transfer function used on behalf of the hidden layer is sigmoid whereas used for output layer it is linear. Four different algorithms Levenberg Marquardt, Gradient Descent, Scaled Conjugate Gradient, and Bayesian Regularization backpropagation algorithm are used for training. The proposed model has been trained, tested, and validated with recharge and discharge and groundwater level data. The block diagram of the proposed two inputs and one output ANN model is shown in Fig. 1. The structure of an ANN is usually prejudiced by the nervous structure of humans.

Fig. 1 Actual and predicted groundwater level through Levenberg–Marquardt for Non-Monsoon season

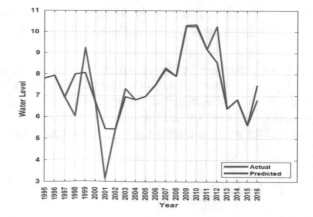

4.2 Levenberg–Marquardt (LM)

The Levenberg–Marquardt technique is a modification of the typical Newton algorithm for ruling an optimum answer to minimize complexity. It employs approximation to the Hessian matrix in the subsequent Newton-like weight update

$$x_{k+1} = x_k - \left[J^T J + \mu I \right]^{-1} J^T e \qquad (2)$$

when neural network x is the weights, J of Jacobian matrix minimizes the presentation criterion, μ of a scalar emphasizes the phase of learning, and e is the vector of the residual error. When μ is bigger, Eq. 1 is decent in the gradient for a limited stage scale. The Newton method is faster and more reliable, near to minimum error, because the objective is to change size. The scalar μ is zeros equation 1 automatically is the Newton method. Newton's method is quick and more accurate because of the shifting toward the Newton method quickly. Levenberg–Marquardt has computational requirements so it can be used for small networks [23].

4.3 Bayesian Regularization (BR)

The Bayesian regularization is an algorithm that mechanically sets optimum standards in support of the parameter of the point function. The weight and bias of the network be understood to be a random variable with specified circulation. The benefit of Bayesian control is that the feature should not surpass the scale of the network. The effective usage of Bayesian regularization in literature [24].

4.4 Gradient Descent by Means of Momentum and Adaptive Learning Rate Back Propagation (GDX)

In order to measure the derivative of the output cost function according to the arbitrary weights and bias of the network, this technique utilizes a standard back propagation algorithm. This strategy utilizes gradient descent with momentum to control each variable. With each level of shift, the learning rate is increased if efficiency declines, one of the simplest and most popular ways to train a network [25].

4.5 Scaled Conjugate Gradient (SCG)

The scaled conjugate gradient (SCG) algorithm [26] determines the quadratic error calculation in the neighborhood. Moller [26] proved this hypothetical base work to be the primary order approach for the primary derivative, such as regular back propagation, and found an important way to obtain a local minimum of second-order technique in the second derivatives. SCG is a second-order combination of gradient algorithms that has helped to reduce a multidimensional target function. SCG is a simple algorithm and employs a scaling method that holds the search through information iteration away from the time-consuming line [26, 27] has shown that the SCG approach presents super linear convergence for major problems.

4.6 Criteria for Evaluation

The following statistical indices such as R^2 efficiency criteria, root mean square error (RMSE), Mean Absolute Error (MAE), Mean Square Error (MSE), and coefficient of correlation (r) were used to evaluate the performance.

5 Results and Discussion

In Babeu Block of BANDA, part of the Yamuna river basin, the purpose of ANN is to measure the capacity to predict a fluctuation of the groundwater level. The network has the following input parameters, Recharge and Discharge. In recharge all the parameters are included like recharge from rainfall, recharge from canal seepage, recharge from field irrigation, recharge from pond storage and in discharge all the parameters are included like groundwater discharge from tube well, influent and effluent seepage from rivers, and for the output parameters, groundwater levels were taken. The four wells' groundwater levels were estimated by using the feed-forward network with a back propagation algorithm. Minimum errors were saved in the trained networks. The neural networks of each wells producing maximum value for R^2. was selected as the best network.

For ALIHA well LAT = 25.495 LONG = 80.525

Year	Recharge in Ham	Discharge in Ham	Groundwater level in MBGL
1995	2776.139	74.557	6.53
1996	2594.47	74.63	5.09
1997	2488.79	71.615	5.1
1998	2903.234	71.610	5.28
1999	2352.035	80.709	5.33
2000	3168.478	80.704	7.43
2001	3436.0.904	80.700	4.08
2002	3435.626	80.695	5.73
2003	3137.422	80.535	1.83
2004	4802.41	81.270	5.23
2005	1735.716	81.717	5.3
2006	3301.524	82.368	5.91
2007	2686.633	82.156	5.5
2008	3983.97	82.704	6.09
2009	3155.92	83.233	8.03
2010	3077.607	83.802	7.02
2011	3556.657	109.231	6.05
2012	3294.387	109.784	8.02
2013	3152.837	111.968	6.11
2014	2603.938	113.001	6.5
2015	3019.837	114.034	6.8
2016	3593.046	114.146	8.3

HAM = Hectare Metre, MBGL = Metre Below Groundlevel
For Mural well LAT = 25.51, LONG = 80.562

Year	Recharge in HAM	Discharge in HAM	Groundwater level in MBGL
1995	7082.457428	190.2115222	4.3
1996	6618.994941	190.410659	3.9
1997	6349.392655	182.7041859	2.1
1998	7406.700558	182.6928576	4.7
1999	6000.488148	205.9046163	3.1
2000	8083.388163	205.8932881	2.42
2001	8768.194147	205.8819598	2.6
2002	8764.93384	205.8706316	9.65

(continued)

(continued)

Year	Recharge in HAM	Discharge in HAM	Groundwater level in MBGL
2003	8004.157891	205.4621211	0
2004	12,251.87134	207.3352643	1.33
2005	4428.140221	208.4777991	2.87
2006	8422.813025	210.1386775	8.52
2007	6854.111735	209.5955874	5.97
2008	10,163.88281	210.9957958	5.95
2009	8051.360821	212.3960043	5.36
2010	7851.559325	213.7962128	6.3
2011	9073.706649	278.6707427	6.13
2012	8404.605956	280.0800508	3.6
2013	8043.484473	285.6519149	2.34
2014	6643.138717	288.287559	3.31
2015	7704.17571	290.923203	5.33
2016	9166.541755	291.2091086	2.26

For Patwan well LAT = 25.59 LONG = 80.56

Year	Recharge in HAM	Discharge in HAM	Groundwater level in MBGL
1995	13,691.21989	367.7011551	4.3
1996	12,795.29261	368.0861097	7.2
1997	12,274.11981	353.1885944	6.5
1998	14,318.01985	353.1666955	7.9
1999	11,599.64652	398.0377444	6.3
2000	15,626.13626	398.0158455	6.52
2001	16,949.94645	397.9939467	7.87
2002	16,943.64389	397.9720479	8.74
2003	15,472.97486	397.1823492	0
2004	23,684.30256	400.8033545	7.93
2005	8560.113787	403.012008	11.66
2006	16,282.28428	406.2226805	11.05
2007	13,249.80092	405.1728238	16.6
2008	19,647.97613	407.8795908	17.35
2009	15,564.22365	410.5863577	17.52
2010	15,177.98396	413.2931247	17.5
2011	17,540.5379	538.7031909	14.8
2012	16,247.08788	541.4275485	11.3
2013	15,548.99775	552.1986145	5.67

(continued)

(continued)

Year	Recharge in HAM	Discharge in HAM	Groundwater level in MBGL
2014	12,841.96536	557.2936233	10.25
2015	14,893.07416	562.3886321	15.55
2016	17,719.99904	562.9413209	13.65

For Baberu well LAT $= 25.54$ LONG $= 80.71$

Year	Recharge in HAM	Discharge in HAM	Groundwater level in MBGL
1995	4581.922195	123.0553666	3.15
1996	4282.089958	123.1841961	1.95
1997	4107.673562	118.1985734	2.5
1998	4791.687917	118.1912447	2.05
1999	3881.953419	133.2078507	2.15
2000	5229.463927	133.200522	2.89
2001	5672.492038	133.1931933	2.65
2002	5670.382817	133.1858646	1.85
2003	5178.206727	132.921583	1.45
2004	7926.220778	134.1333936	1.95
2005	2864.739275	134.8725445	3.46
2006	5449.051313	135.9470325	5.62
2007	4434.196323	135.595686	5.2
2008	6575.418306	136.5015363	6.37
2009	5208.744171	137.4073867	5.5
2010	5079.484671	138.313237	5.25
2011	5870.140175	180.2831396	2.75
2012	5437.272439	181.1948768	3.65
2013	5203.64865	184.7995363	2.84
2014	4297.709523	186.5046389	3.93
2015	4984.136373	188.2097414	4.45
2016	5930.198882	188.394705	4.32

For ALIHA Well, all recharge and discharge data were calculated according to the groundwater estimation committee norms. In the year 2002, recharges were the most, i.e., 3435.626 and the discharges were the most in the year 114.146. For Murwal well, maximum recharge was found in the year 2008, that is, 10,163.88281 HAM and maximum discharge was found in the year 2016 that is 291.2091086 HAM. For Patwan well, maximum recharge was found in the year 2004, that is, 23,684.30256 HAM and maximum discharge was found in the year 2016, that is, 562.9413209 HAM. For Baberu well, maximum discharge was found in the year 2016, that is,

188.394705. HAM and maximum recharge were found in the year 2004 that is 7926.220778 HAM.

For ALIHA Well

See Figs. 1, 2, 3 and 4.

Fig. 2 Scatter diagram for actual and predicted groundwater level for $R^2 =$ 0.88 for testing

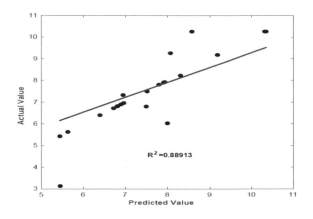

Fig. 3 Actual and predicted groundwater level through Bayesian Regularization for Non-Monsoon season

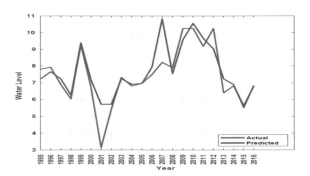

Fig. 4 Scatter diagram for actual and predicted groundwater level for $R^2 =$ 0.85 for testing

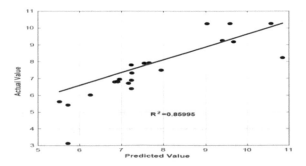

For Baberu well

See Figs. 5 and 6.

For Murwal Well

See Figs. 7 and 8.

For Patwan Well

See Figs. 9 and 10.

Fig. 5 Actual and Predicted groundwater level through Bayesian Regularization for Non-Monsoon season

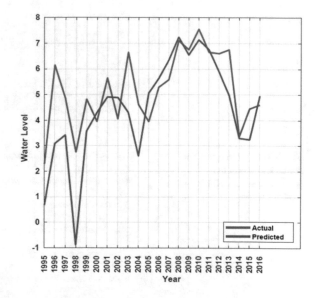

Fig. 6 Scatter diagram for actual and predicted groundwater level for $R^2 = 0.77$ for testing

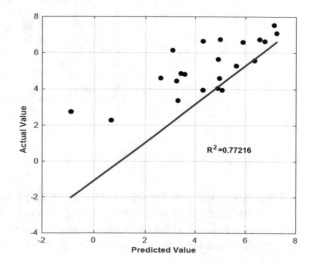

Fig. 7 Actual and predicted
groundwater level through
Levenberg- Marquardt for
Non-Monsoon season

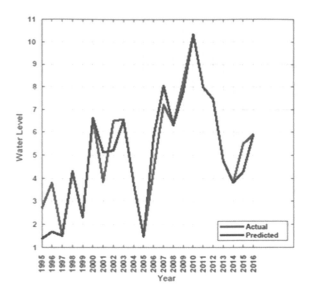

Fig. 8 Scatter diagram for
actual and predicted
groundwater level for $R^2 =$
0.94 for testing

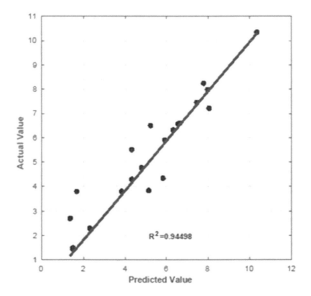

6   Conclusion

The function of the artificial neural network of feed-forward back propagation into
groundwater prediction has been investigated in this research paper. Input and output
data are grouped into hydro-geological well classes and the LM, SCG, BR and GD
have been trained for each well sheet. The findings demonstrate explicitly that the

Fig. 9 Actual and predicted groundwater level through Levenberg--Marquardt for Non-Monsoon season

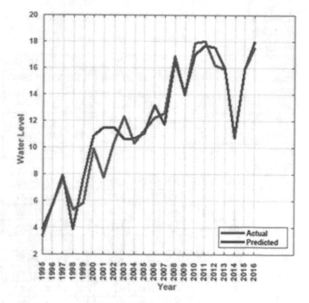

Fig. 10 Scatter diagram for actual and predicted groundwater level for $R^2 = 0.96$ for testing

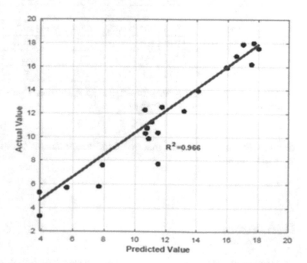

LM algorithm works well for all four wells. Results demonstrate that the ANN model is capable of predicting the virtual physical structure's complex response. A major advantage of this ANN technique is that it can provide good predictions by means of limitations of groundwater data (Table 1).

Table 1 Comparison of performance of models developed for all wells, training, testing and validation

For Aliha well

Evaluation criteria	Epoch	LM			BR			GDX			SCG		
		TRNG	TST	VALI	TRNG	TST	VALI	TRNG	TST	VALI	TRNG	TST	VALI
R^2	2000	0.88	0.85	0.85	0.85	0.83	0.54	0.34	0.22	0.16	0.86	0.83	0.72
MAE	2000	0.38	0.40	0.41	0.55	0.67	1.0	5.18	7.37	13.2	0.66	0.74	0.79
MSE	2000	0.64	0.79	0.77	0.80	0.90	4.29	39.31	81.27	205.9	1.24	1.18	1.73
RMSE	2000	0.80	0.89	0.81	0.89	0.95	2.07	6.27	9.01	14.3	1.17	1.08	1.31
For Murawal well													
R^2	2000	0.94	0.74	0.73	0.88	0.71	0.7	0.88	0.87	0.8	0.77	0.7	0.69
MAE	2000	0.45	0.14	0.14	0.85	1.17	1.32	0.89	0.78	1.71	2.56	1.17	1.4
MSE	2000	0.64	8.6	8.6	1.16	4.02	2.6	1.26	1.16	4.32	10.5	2.8	8.6
RMSE	2000	0.8	2.9	2.9	1.08	2.0	1.6	1.12	1.07	2.09	3.17	1.69	2.9
For Baberu well													
R^2	2000	0.82	0.78	0.73	0.77	0.78	0.70	0.57	0.51	0.34	0.72	0.67	0.63
MAE	2000	0.59	0.51	0.71	1.11	1.15	0.52	1.77	1.17	9.9	0.67	0.83	0.84
MSE	2000	0.85	0.87	0.97	2.1	2.5	1.38	6.81	2.13	14.0	0.97	1.31	1.47
RMSE	2000	0.92	0.93	0.98	1.4	1.6	1.17	2.6	1.46	11.9	0.98	1.14	1.21
For Patwan Well													
R^2	2000	0.98	0.96	0.75	0.722	0.721	0.51	0.67	0.455	0.44	0.88	0.86	0.84
MAE	2000	0.41	0.80	1.55	2.40	0.51	5.18	24.39	4.47	5.5	1.57	1.9	1.71
MSE	2000	0.89	1.36	15.9	9.39	0.87	50.3	8.8	105.7	66.3	4.2	6.62	6.1
RMSE	2000	0.94	1.16	3.9	3.06	0.93	7.09	29.78	1.46	8.14	2.0	2.57	2.4

LM = Levenberg Marquardt Algorithm, BR = Bayesian Regularization Algorithm, GDX = Gradient Discent Algorithm, SCG = Scaled Conjugate Gradient Algorithm

Acknowledgements The authors would like to specially thank to the Banda irrigation department to provide all necessary data.

References

1. Selvam S (2012a) use of remote sensing and GIS techniques for land use and land cover mapping of tuticorin coast, Tamil Nadu. Univ J Environ Res Tech V.2(4):233–241
2. Todd DK, Mays LW (2005) Groundwater hydrology, 3rd edn. Wiley, Hoboken
3. UNESCO (2015) Water for a sustainable world. Facts and figures. The United Nations World Water Development Report 2015. United Nations World Water Assessment Programme Programme Office for Global Water Assessment, Division of Water Sciences, Perugia, Italy, p 12
4. Pandey VP, Kazama F (2011) Hydrogeologic chararacteristics of groundwater aquifers in Kathmandu Valley, Nepal. Environ Earth Sci 62(8):1723–1732
5. Pandey VP, Kazama F (2012) Groundwater storage potential in the Kathmandu Valley's shallow and deep aquifers. In: Shrestha S, Pradhananga D, Pandey VP (eds) Kathmandu valley groundwater outlook, AIT/SEN/CREEW/ICRE-UY, pp 31–38

6. Pandey VP, Shrestha S, Kazama F (2012) Groundwater in the Kathmandu Valley : development dynamics, consequences and prospects for sustainable management. European Water 37:3–14

7. Pandey VP, Shrestha S, Kazama F (2012) A framework for measuring groundwater sustainability. Environ Sci Policy 14(4):396–407

8. Matej G, Isabelle W, Jan M (2007) Regional groundwater model of north-east Belgium. J Hydrol 335:133–139

9. Pool DR, Blasch KW, Callegary JB, Leake SA, Graser LF (2011) Regional groundwater-flow model of the redwall-muav, coconino, and alluvial basin aquifer systems of Northern and Central Arizona: USGS Scientific Investigation Report 2010–5180, v. 1.1, 101

10. Yao Y, Zheng C, Liu J, Cao G, Xiao H, Li II, Li W (2015) Conceptual and numerical models for groundwater flow in an arid inland river basin. Hydrol Proc 29:1480–1492

11. ASCE Task Committee (2000) Artificial neural networks in hydrology—I: preliminary concepts. J Hydrol Eng ASCE 5(2):115–123

12. ASCE Task Committee (2000) Artificial neural networks in hydrology—II: hydrologic applications. J Hydrol Eng ASCE 5(2):124–137

13. Gobindraju RS, Ramachandra Rao A (2000) Artificial neural network in hydrology. Kluwer, Dordrecht

14. Aziz ARA, Wong KFV (1992) Neural network approach to the determination of aquifer parameters. Ground Water 30(2):164–166

15. Balkhair KS (2002) Aquifer parameters determination for large diameter wells using neural network approach. J Hydrol 265(1):118–128

16. Garcia LA, Shigdi A (2006) Using neural networks for parameter estimation in ground water. J Hydrol 318(1–4):215–231

17. Hong YS, Rosen MR (2001) Intelligent characterization and diagnosis of the groundwater quality in an urban fractured-rock aquifer using an artificial neural network, Urban Water 3(3):193–204

18. Karahan H, Ayvaz MT (2008) Simultaneous parameter identification of a heterogeneous aquifer system using artificial neural networks. Hydrogeol J 16:817–827

19. Samani M, Gohari-Moghadam M, Safavi AA (2007) A simple neural network model for the determination of aquifer parameters. J Hydrol 340:1–11

20. Shigdi A, Garcia LA (2003) Parameter estimation in groundwater hydrology using artificial neural networks. J Comput Civ Eng ASCE 17(4):281–289

21. Kuo V, Liu C, Lin K (2004) Evaluation of the ability of an artificial neural network model to assess the variation of groundwater quality in an area of blackfoot disease in Taiwan. Water Res 38(1):148–158

22. Milot J, Rodriguez MJ, Serodes JB (2002) Contribution of neural networks for modeling trihalomethanes occurrence in drinking water. J Water Resour Plan Manage ASCE 128(5):370–376

23. Maier HR, Dandy GC (1998) Understanding the behavior and optimizing the performance of back- propagation neural networks: an empirical study .Environ Modell Softw 13:179–191

24. Anctil F, Perrin C, Andressian V (2004) Impact of the length of observed records on the performance of ANN and of conceptual parsimonious rainfall- runoff forecasting models. Environ Model Softw 19(4):357–368

25. Haykin S (1999) Neural networks :a comprehensive foundation. 2nd ed. Prentice Hall, New Jersey, p 823

26. Moller MF (1993) A scaled conjugate gradient algorithm for fast supervised learning. Neural Netw 6(4):525–533

27. Karmokar BC, Mahmud MP, Siddique MK, Nafi KW, Kar TS (2012) Touchless written english characters recognition using neural network. Int J Comput Org Trends 2(3):80–84

Diabetes Prediction Using Deep Learning Model

Nishq Poorav Desai, Utkarsha, Avanish Sandilya, Krishna Kalpesh Patel, and Kanchan Lata Kashyap

1 Introduction

Diabetes disease occurs due to the inability of enough insulin production by pancreas or inability to consume the produced insulin properly by the human body. Blood sugar is controlled by the insulin which is a type of hormone. The result of uncontrolled diabetes is hyperglycaemia which damages the human nerves system. The World Health Organization (WHO) evaluated the worldwide regularity of diabetes among matured people as 8.5% in 2014. A total of 72.96 million diabetes instances are observed in the grown-up population of India [1]. The commonness in urban regions ranges approximately between 10.9 and 14.2%. Diabetes can be vanquished by following healthy diet and improving lifestyle.

The clinical expenses of diabetic individuals are also high [2]. In the on-going diabetes review in America led by Health Union, 74 and 32% of overview respondents have a yearly family unit income below $75 K, and $30 K, respectively. A segment of the expenses of clinical supplies and specialist visits is secured by protection. Medicare covers 35% of the respondents. Present work provides the automatic diabetes prediction which depends on the different features of a person. This diabetes prediction system determines whether the person is suffering from diabetic or not. The deep learning-based model is trained in the present work for diabetic prediction.

This work is structured in the following sections. The literature review is discussed in Sect. 2. The proposed model is described in Sect. 3. Experimental results are discussed in Sect. 4. Conclusions are discussed in Sect. 5.

N. P. Desai · Utkarsha · A. Sandilya · K. L. Kashyap (✉)
VIT University, Bhopal, Madhya Pradesh, India
e-mail: kanchan.k@vitbhopal.ac.in

K. K. Patel
Pioneer Pharmacy Degree College, Vadodara, Gujarat, India

M. K. Bajpai et al. (eds.), *Machine Vision and Augmented Intelligence—Theory and Applications*, Lecture Notes in Electrical Engineering 796,
https://doi.org/10.1007/978-981-16-5078-9_33

393

2 Related Work

Various algorithms of diabetes prediction are already implemented by different authors. Calisir et al. automate the diagnosis system of diabetes by applying Linear Discriminant Analysis (LDA) technique [3]. The highest 89.74% of accuracy is achieved by using the Support Vector Machine (SVM) classifier with Morlet wavelet. Zou et al. have applied various machine learning techniques which are decision tree, random forest, and neural network to predict diabetes mellitus. Dimensionality reduction is done by feature selection techniques which are principal component analysis and minimum redundancy maximum relevance and achieved 80.84% accuracy [4]. Tigga et al. used logistic regression, K-nearest neighbor, SVM, naïve Bayes, decision tree, and random forest for the classification of diabetic and non-diabetic [5]. The highest 90% accuracy is achieved by the random forest classifier. Sisodia et al. applied decision tree, naïve Bayes, and SVM for prediction of diabetes. The highest 76.30% accuracy is achieved by the naïve Bayes classifier [6]. Wu et al. obtained 95.42% accuracy by utilizing improved k-NN and logistic regression techniques to predict diabetes mellitus of Type 2 [7]. Meng et al. achieved 73.23 and 77.87% classification accuracies by implementing neural network and decision tree (C.5) model, respectively [8]. Choubey et al. used genetic algorithm- and radial basis function-based neural network techniques for feature selection and diabetes classification. The highest 76.087% classification accuracy is achieved on PIMA dataset [9]. Haung et al. obtained the highest 95% accuracy on Ulster Community and Hospitals Trust (UCHT) dataset by applying naïve Bayes, IB1, and decision tree classifier for diabetes prediction [10]. Perveen et al. applied naïve Bayes and decision tree techniques for diabetes prediction and achieved 81 and 80% true positive rates, respectively [11]. The various supervised and unsupervised machine learning models are implemented by various authors in existing work. Deep learning-based algorithm is implemented in the proposed work to improve the diabetes detection accuracy.

3 Methodology

The graphical representation of the proposed work is depicted in Fig. 1. This work consists of normalization of the raw input data followed by training as well as testing of the deep learning model. Each step is briefly outlined in subsequent sections.

3.1 Raw Data Input

The validation of the proposed model is done by using PIMA diabetes dataset [12]. This dataset is taken from the National Institute of Diabetes, Digestive, and Kidney

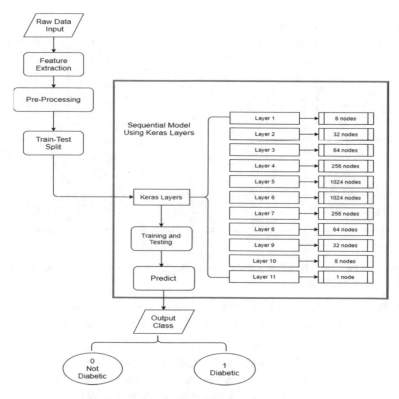

Fig. 1 Block diagram of automatic diabetic prediction model

Diseases which consists of various attributes collected from 768 people. The dataset includes eight independent variables which are pregnancies, plasma glucose concentration in 2 h in an oral glucose tolerance test, diastolic blood pressure (mm Hg), triceps skinfold thickness (mm), 2 h serum insulin (mu U/ml), body mass index (weight in kg/(height in m)^2), and diabetes pedigree function. Sample records of the PIMA dataset are listed in Table 1. A brief description of each feature of the dataset is presented as follows:

Pregnancies: During pregnancy, blood glucose level increases due to the hormones created by the placenta. Although, the pancreas consumes enough insulin but sometimes human body unable to prepare enough insulin which increases the glucose levels and results in gestational diabetes.

Glucose: Diabetes increases the glucose levels which is higher than ordinary also known as hyper-glycemia. Sudden change in the glucose level can be subjected to diabetes. **Blood Pressure (BP)**: Type 2 diabetes attributable due to impedance from insulin that is kind of a hormone in the human body that utilizes glucose for energy. Over the long run, diabetes harms the little veins in the human body and makes the

Table 1 Samples of PIMA dataset

S no.	Pregnancies	Glucose	BP	ST	Insulin level	BMI	DPF	Age	Outcome
1	6	148	72	35	0	33.6	0.627	50	1
2	1	85	66	29	0	26.6	0.351	31	0
3	8	183	64	0	0	23.3	0.672	32	1
4	1	89	66	23	94	28.1	0.167	21	0
5	0	137	40	35	168	43.1	2.288	33	1
6	5	116	74	0	0	25.6	0.201	30	0
7	3	78	50	32	88	31	0.248	26	1
8	10	115	0	0	0	35.3	0.134	29	0
9	2	197	70	45	543	30.5	0.158	53	1
10	8	125	96	0	0	0	0.232	54	1

walls of veins which builds pressure and prompts hypertension. So, blood pressure is associated with diabetes.

Skin Thickness (ST): It is dictated by collagen content and expanded in insulin-subordinate diabetes mellitus (IDDM). Skin thickness of triceps skinfold is connected with diabetes.

Insulin Level: Wrecked insulin-delivering cells also create insulin. Insulin should be incumbent to transfer glucose into cells all through the body. The subsequent insulin lack leaves an excessive amount of glucose in the blood and insufficient in the cells for energy and thus causes diabetes.

Body Mass Index (BMI): Overweight (BMI > 25) burdens the internal parts of individual cells. Insulin obstruction and high centralizations of the sugar glucose in the blood are definite indications of diabetes.

Diabetes Pedigree Function (DPF): It is a function that scores the expectation of having diabetes depending on family ancestry and genetics.

Age: It is an important factor for the development of type 2 diabetes due to the joined impacts of expanding insulin opposition and debilitated pancreatic islet work with aging.

3.2 Pre-processing

Data standardization is a process of tuning and rescaling features in such a manner that the resulting attribute has 0 mean and the standard deviation of 1. The dataset is normalized by implementing the Z-score method to ensure its uniform-ness. Mathematically this method is defined as follows:

$$z = \frac{(x - u)}{S^1} \tag{1}$$

Here, u and s denote the average and standard deviation of each feature, respectively.

3.3 Deep Learning Model

The basic sequential model is given as an interconnection of dense layers which can be trained for deep learning system. Keras is one of the examples of deep learning framework implemented in the proposed work for diabetes prediction.

Keras Layers (for Neural Network)

Keras is minimal structure and open-source deep learning framework implemented in Python. It provides a simple way to construct deep learning models depending on TensorFlow [13]. Keras layers are the fundamental units of neural networks. A layer comprises a tensor-input, tensor-output computation function, and a state, which is saved in TensorFlow variables. Tensors are multidimensional arrays with a same data type and also immutable. Tensors contain basic data types such as floats, integers, complex numbers, and strings along with special tensors with different shapes known as (i) ragged tensors and (ii) sparse tensors. The input parameters set for the Keras model are given as [14] follows:

- The first parameter denotes the number of neurons.
- *input_shape* denotes the input data shape.
- *kernel_initializer* is resolute as a uniform function.
- *kernel_regularizer* denotes the regularizer to be applied.
- *kernel_constraint* is initialized as a *MaxNorm* function.
- *activation function* is initialized as Relu function.

This model contains total of 11 layers which include 9 hidden layers. Out of 9 hidden layers, the first 10 layers include Rectified Linear Activation (Relu) with 8, 32, 64, 256, 1024, 1024, 256, 64, 32, and 8 nodes, respectively. The last layer has a single node with Sigmoid Activation function which classifies output as diabetes and non-diabetes. Keras have two types of models, namely, (i) Keras sequential model and (ii) Keras functional model.

Keras Sequential Model

It is the basic sequential model with many layers and sustaining the balance of all the layers [14]. This model is proper with plain set of layers and each layer is having only single input and output tensor.

Keras Functional Model

The Keras functional API is more flexible than the Keras sequential API [14]. It can deal with the models having non-linear topology, shared layers, and even multiple inputs or outputs.

4 Experimental Results

Keras deep learning model is trained by applying the train-test split and tenfold cross-validation method. The dataset has been divided as 25 and 75% testing and training set, respectively. Training of the model is performed with binary cross-entropy loss function with Stochastic Gradient Descent (SGD) optimizer. SGD updates the parameter value for every training data sample (x^i), and output label (y^i) which are defined as follows:

$$\theta = \theta - \eta \nabla_\theta J(\theta; x^i; y^i) \tag{2}$$

The classification is done by binary cross-entropy loss function which is mathematically represented as follows:

$$H_p(q) = -1/N \left(\sum_{i=1}^{N} (y_i \cdot \log(p(y_i)) + (1 - y_i) \cdot \log(1 - p(y_i))) \right) \tag{3}$$

Here, y_i represents the predicted output. The training and testing set is compiled with 220 epochs with batch size and verbose assigned as 1. The performance results of the proposed model are computed in terms of sensitivity, specificity, accuracy, precision, and F1-score [15]. All the performance matrices are computed using a confusion matrix which is depicted in Table 2. For two output class, the predicted outcome can be categorized as false negative when the person is diabetic and model prediction is non-diabetic, false positive when the person is non-diabetic and model prediction is diabetic, true negative when the person is non-diabetic and model prediction is non-diabetic, and true positive when the person is diabetic and model prediction is also diabetic. The model predicts as non-diabetic or outcome is predicted as 0 and model predicts as diabetic or outcome is predicted as 1.

The sensitivity, specificity, accuracy, precision, recall, and F1-score are defined as follows:

Table 2 Confusion matrix

	Predicted output	
Actual output	True	False
True	True Positive (TP)	False Positive (FP)
False	False Negative (FN)	True Negative (TN)

$$\text{Sensitivity:} \quad \frac{TP}{TP + FN} \tag{4}$$

$$\text{Specificity:} \quad \frac{TN}{TN + FP} \tag{5}$$

$$\text{Precision:} \quad \frac{TP}{TP + FP} \tag{6}$$

$$\text{Accuracy:} \quad \frac{TP + TN}{TP + TN + FP + FN} \tag{7}$$

$$\text{F1 - score:} \quad \frac{2 * TP}{2 * TP + FP + FN} \tag{8}$$

The experiment has been done with various numbers of dense layers. Total of six deep learning models are structured with different dense layers as given in Table 3. The performance results obtained with each model by train-test split method are analyzed in Table 4. The highest value of 96.108, 96.06, 93, 98, 95, and 94% training accuracy, testing, sensitivity, specificity, precision, and F1-score is obtained, respectively, by the proposed model. Training model accuracy and loss of each model are depicted in Fig. 2.

Table 3 Input parameters of the proposed deep learning model (number of input nodes = 8 and number of output node = 1)

Model number	Type	Number of dense layers	Epochs	Batch size
1	Functional	8/32/64/128/512/1024/1024/512/128/64/32/8	140	27
2	Functional	8/32/64/256/1024/1024/256/64/32/8	45	5
3	Functional	8/32/64/128/512/1024/512/128/64/32/8	15	10
4	Sequential	-8/32/64/256/256 /1024/1024/256/256/32/8	232	18
5	Sequential	8/32/64/256/1024 /256/64/32/8-	1670	227
6	Sequential	8/32/64/256/1024 /1024/256/64/32/8-	1670	215

Table 4 Validation results (by train-test split method) obtained from the proposed model

Model number	Training accuracy (%)	Testing accuracy (%)	Sensitivity (%)	Specificity (%)	Precision (%)	F1-score (%)
1	88.91	71.65	50	85	68	58
2	91.25	72.83	56	83	65	60
3	93.39	66.14	52	75	55	53
4	83.07	72.05	41	88	64	50
5	92.80	73.23	72	74	58	65
6	**96.11**	**96.06**	**93**	**98**	**95**	**94**

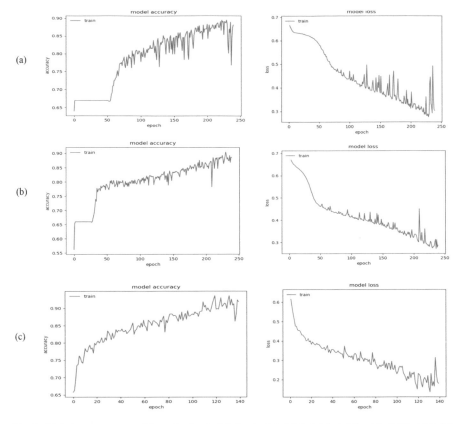

Fig. 2 Training accuracy and loss obtained of defined **a** Model 1, **b** Model 2, **c** Model 3, **d** Model 4, **e** Model 5, **f** Model 6

Performance of the proposed model is also compared with the various machine learning techniques, namely, logistic regression, random forest, SVM, and k-NN (with $k = 3, 4, 5$, and 6) [15] which is depicted in Table 5. Results of the proposed model along with traditional machine learning are also measured by applying 10-fold cross-validation techniques which are listed in Table 6. It can be observed that the testing results of the proposed deep learning model is better than the traditional machine learning techniques.

5 Conclusions

This endeavor presents an automatic diabetes prediction system by implementing a deep learning model. The experiment is performed on the publicly available PIMA

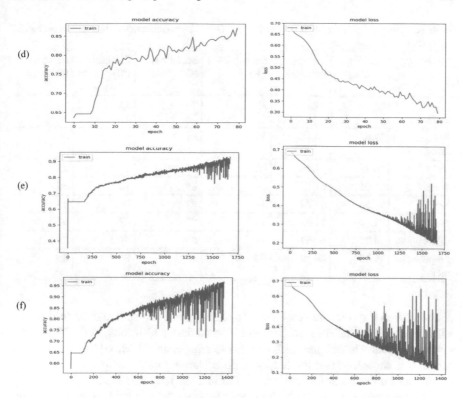

Fig. 2 (continued)

Table 5. Comparison of the obtained results (by train-test split method) of proposed model with traditional machine learning models

Model type	Training accuracy (%)	Testing accuracy (%)	Sensitivity (%)	Specificity (%)	Precision (%)	F1-score (%)
Logistic regression	79.38	72.44	65	75	65	57
Random forest	100	79.53	63	89	76	69
SVM	78.82	72.40	49	86	67	57
KNN-3	85.02	70.47	50	81	57	53
KNN-4	81.52	70.47	37	88	60	46
KNN-5	82.10	69.69	50	80	56	53
KNN-6	75.68	75.59	44	92	73	55
Proposed model	**96.108**	**96.06**	**93**	**98**	**95**	**94**

Table 6. Comparison of the obtained results (by 10-fold cross-validation) of the proposed model with machine learning models

Model type	Training accuracy (%)	Testing accuracy (%)	Sensitivity (%)	Specificity (%)	Precision (%)	F1-score (%)
Logistic regression	78.79	74.41	75	74	75	60
Random forest	77.63	74.41	52	86	67	59
SVM	76.37	77.78	80	76	71	75
3-NN	73.93	69.69	44	83	58	50
4-NN	73.54	69.29	33	89	60	43
5-NN	71.79	74.02	50	87	67	57
6-NN	74.32	69.69	44	83	58	53
Proposed model	**79.05**	**89.29**	**92**	**87**	**86**	**89**

dataset. Testing results are obtained by applying train-test split and 10-fold cross-validation techniques. The results of proposed model are also compared with various machine learning techniques such as logistic regression, SVM, k-NN, and random forest. It is concluded that the proposed deep learning model outperforms than the traditional machine learning methods. In future, the proposed model will be tested on a new diabetes dataset and deployment of this model will be done in the website for the diabetes prediction.

References

1. Julio V, Santiago JE, Davis F, Hemoglobin F (1978) A1c levels in a diabetes detection program. J Clin Endocrinol Metabol 47(3):578–580
2. Carr DB, Steven G (1998) Gestational diabetes: detection, management, and implications. Clin Diab 16(1):4–6
3. Çalişir D, Doğantekin E (2011) An automatic diabetes diagnosis system based on LDA-Wavelet Support Vector Machine classifier. Expert Syst Appl 38(7):8311–8315
4. Zou Q, Qu K, Luo Y, Yin D, Ju Y, Tang H (2018) Predicting diabetes mellitus with machine learning techniques. Front Genet 9:515
5. Tigga NP, Garg S (2021) Predicting type 2 diabetes using logistic regression. In: Nath V, Mandal JK (eds) Proceedings of the fourth international conference on microelectronics, computing and communication systems. Lecture notes in electrical engineering, vol 673
6. Sisodia D, Sisodia DS (2018) Prediction of diabetes using classification algorithms. Procedia Comput Sci 132:1578–1585
7. Wu H, Yang S, Huang Z, He J, Wang X (2018) Type 2 diabetes mellitus prediction model based on data mining. Inform Med Unlocked 10:100–107
8. Meng X, Huang Y, Rao D, Zhang Q, Liu Q (2013) Comparison of three data mining models for predicting diabetes or prediabetes by risk factors. Kaohsiung J Med Sci 29(2):93–99

9. Choubey DK, Paul S (2017) GA_RBF NN: a classification system for diabetes. Int J Biomed Eng Technol 23(1):71–93
10. Huang Y, McCullagh P, Black N, Harper R (2007) Feature selection and classification model construction on type 2 diabetic patients' data. Artif Intell Med 41(3):251–262
11. Perveen S, Shahbaz M, Keshavjee K, Guergachi A (2019) Metabolic syndrome and development of diabetes mellitus: predictive modeling based on machine learning techniques. IEEE Access 7:1365–1375
12. http://networkrepository.com/pima-indians-diabetes.php
13. https://www.tensorflow.org/guide/intro_to_modules
14. https://keras.io/guides/sequential_model/
15. Duda RO, Hart PE, Stork DG (2001) Pattern classification. Wiley, New York. ISBN: 978-0-471-05669-0

Object Detection Using YOLO Framework for Intelligent Traffic Monitoring

I. C. Amitha⬤ and N. K. Narayanan

1 Introduction

Traffic management is the arrangement and control of both static and dynamic traffic components, including pedestrians, bicyclists, and vehicles. The main goal of this study is to provide a better and safe movement of pedestrians and vehicles. The usual action of traffic lights needs additional Machine Intelligence than meager control and coordination to guarantee that traffic and pedestrians move as smoothly, and safely as possible. Traffic management systems in cities facing some sort of challenges due to the rapid advancement of urbanization, traffic blockage, and various circumstances. Intelligent Transportation Systems (ITS) combine various latest technologies to provide intelligence for the system to monitor and coordinate transportation activities smoothly. Video-based surveillance arrangements became an essential part of ITS. This arrangement acquires the vehicle's presence and excerpts additional details regarding their detection, tracking, recognition, and behavior analysis of vehicle movement. A present surveillance arrangement is a static approach that accumulates traffic flow details that generally includes traffic constraints and traffic occurrence detection. The static time setting on each lane will lead to unnecessary waiting thereby losing one's precious minutes. We propose a system that could get the count of vehicles present in each lane thereby we could get a clear picture of the traffic flow on each lane thus developing a dynamic system that can control the traffic based on the count obtained from each lane. The common approach to get the number of vehicles and their categorization can be approximately partitioned into

I. C. Amitha (✉)
Department of Information Technology, Kannur University, Kannur, Kerala, India
e-mail: amithaic@gmail.com

N. K. Narayanan
Indian Institute of Information Technology, Kottayam, Kerala, India
e-mail: nknarayanan@iiitkottayam.ac.in

hardware and software resolutions. Even though the hardware solution is fast and has better accuracy than the software methods. But the maintenance cost of hardware solutions is more expensive than the software resolutions [1–3].

The advancements in computing techniques and the rapid improvement in the recognition of objects from image and video lead to a hassle-free recognition of vehicles passing over a surveillance screen. Once the vehicles are recognized by a model, the method needs to determine the pertinence of the vehicle that is identified from distinct frames to accomplish the vehicle counting task. Once the vehicle count is obtained, it will be used for controlling the traffic signals, thereby avoiding unwanted delays in the lane [2].

2 Related Work

Object detection and retrieval in images or video plays an important role in our daily life. Various vehicle detection, counting, and tracking techniques have been reported in the literature. Asha and Narasimhadhan [4] have proposed a system that can detect and count vehicles in diverse circumstances. They have used the YOLO structure to identify the vehicles and the exact tracking is done by correlation filters. Their method precisely counts the number of vehicles in the preferred videos. In Zaatouri and Ezzedine [5] recommend a system to get better performance in an intelligent transport system by establishing an algorithm to control road traffic based on deep learning. To get real-time traffic conditions, they have used a YOLO network and it is passed to an embedded controller. Huang et al. [6] have reported a feature-oriented technique that analyses and counts the vehicles on a two-way road. They have categorized the vehicles from the input video according to their extracted features.

In Liu et al. [7] described a procedure to discover and track moving objects through background deduction accompanying a fixed camera. Their method shows strength against noise, luminance variation, shadows, and obstructions. Lai et al. [8] efficiently extract the vehicle areas through a combined methodology. They also contributed to the reduction of computational time through the introduction of overlapping ratio. They efficiently classified the vehicles into three classes, viz.: truck, car, and bus according to compactness and aspect ratio. Song et al. [9] have used an efficient object detection method YOLOv3 for their end-to-end vehicle detection from an annotated vehicle dataset. Their empirical outcome shows that the prospective vehicle detection and tracking technique is best suited for intelligent traffic management. In Gao and Li [10] have proposed vehicle detection through a convolutional neural network based on SSD. The excision analysis determines the efficiency of those arrangements. Dai et al. [11] have described a system for counting vehicles for video input and it is validated through different traffic scenes. They can achieve great accuracy using YOLOv3 with their dataset even though in complex traffic situations.

Fang et al. [12] have presented a novel vehicle tracking scheme and its performance is reported to be equivalent to state-of-the-art techniques. Their proposed algorithm is capable to track even if there is some obstruction or aspect ratio change. In Scheel and

Dietmayer [13] suggested a method to track multiple vehicles by utilizing an alternative radar model. Empirical results show that their approach can beat the manually designed model. Zhang et al. [14] have proposed one fusion-based method for the discovery and acceleration estimation of vehicles. A color faster R-CNN was used to detect the vehicles and the acceleration estimations are done by Kalman filter. Amitha and Narayanan [15, 16] proposed an efficient object detection method using SIFT and R-CNN. Farhodov et al. [17] have explained the use of Discriminative Correlation Filter (with Channel and Spatial Reliability) (CSRT) tracker for drone data. Emami et al. [18] uses Continuously Adaptive Mean-Shift (CAMSHIFT) tracker for object detection and tracking in a fault-free manner. Henriques et al. [19] explained a Kernel Correlation Filter (KCF) which is useful for visual object tracking. The usefulness of these three trackers for road vehicle tracking is studied in this paper and it is found that KCF provides the best results for our experiment.

3 Methodology

The present system of traffic monitoring is a static time-based system, in which the traffic signal changes according to the time assigned. The present hardware solution involves the use of inductive loop detectors, piezoelectric sensors, microwave radar detectors, infrared detectors, but the implementation and maintenance of all these detectors is hard and expensive. We aim to develop a software solution that is a dynamic adaptive system that could work in real time by considering the count of vehicles. The system works using the YOLO tool, a deep learning approach that would take in the video streams as the input to the system. The system then takes the count of vehicles in each frame, thereby determining the number of vehicles in each lane. Thus, an adaptive decision regarding the present situation could be made. The proposed solution would be much cheaper and easier to implement just with the help of monitoring cameras. Since we already have monitoring cameras in most of the cities, just an up-gradation would be enough for the implementation. Thus, the system could save the precious time of each one's life wasted in traffic jams. The proposed technique is capable of achieving greater accuracy and fast results.

Object detection using the YOLO framework for intelligent traffic monitoring is a dynamic real-time system for controlling road traffic. The whole system can be divided into two phases; in the first phase, it is to obtain the count of vehicle present in each lane. The architecture of object detection using the YOLO framework for intelligent traffic monitoring is illustrated in Fig. 1. The vehicle counting arrangement is made up of three elements such as detector, tracker, and counter. The detector recognizes vehicles from a given video frame and it produces a set of bounding boxes all over the vehicles and it is fed to the tracker. The tracker makes use of the bounding boxes to track the vehicles in consecutive frames. On the other hand, the detector is again utilized to amend trackers regularly to guarantee that they are still tracking the vehicles properly. The counter maintains a counting line over the road. When a vehicle passes the line, the vehicle count is updated.

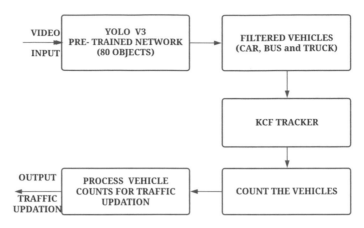

Fig. 1 Proposed system architecture

During the second phase, the system involves the count processing algorithm to which the count obtained from similar lanes in a junction is processed. In the second phase system, we have the input as the number of vehicles on each lane in the corresponding junction. These counts depict the current real-time traffic condition of the lane. Thus, as we get the traffic condition on each lane, we get a clear picture of the traffic in real time; thus, the algorithm in the second phase could make a dynamic decision to control the traffic by giving maximum priority to the lane having maximum traffic. Thus, the dynamic system could act adaptively very well with satisfying results and accuracy. The overall architecture comprises a detector that produces a vehicle's bounding box area, a tracker to track the vehicles entering the region specified by open CV, the counter responsible for vehicle counting, and the count processing algorithm whose results would give the output of the traffic signals in the junction.

Initially, video input is fed to the YOLO framework for intelligent traffic monitoring. The vehicle detector framework carries out the initial eradication and processing of the video for consecutive applications. The prospective method employs the prepared YOLO setup as the fundamental structure of the vehicle detector. Apart from the moving vehicles, some other classes of objects too in the traffic specifically pedestrians, bicycles, and animals, so for counting purpose vehicles should be extracted [2]. The trained YOLO framework can recognize 80 various objects. Object detection using the YOLO framework for intelligent traffic monitoring systems detects three classes of vehicles such as trucks, cars, and buses. To process only the three classes, we modify the actual YOLO code [2]. For this, a region is specified to the input video frame with the help of an open CV. This is done so that only those vehicles entering this region would be detected by the detector so that we could restrict and be confident only relevant vehicles are detected so that we get the optimized results.

The tracker is used to track the vehicles upon detection by the detector. For that, a region will be specified in the video frame with the help of OpenCV. The vehicles would get starting detected once it starts entering the region thereafter the vehicles will be tracked by a tracker with the help of the coordinates of the bounding boxes. This will be done to those vehicles that correspond to the determined region only. To perform this tracking operation, we have used the KCF tracker. From the outset, we select a reference point. After the reference point is chosen, the counter will check each frame one by one if there is a vehicle passing the checkpoint. For every vehicle co-ordinate in the current frame, we have to discover the pair which has the shortest separation between this co-ordinate and all vehicle co-ordinates in the past frame. At that point, we utilize a threshold to eliminate the accompanying scenarios.

4 Experimental Results

Our proposed method is implemented and tested with three different publicly available standard video inputs of vehicle lanes in various conditions. In our proposed system, we have experimented with three different object detection and tracking mechanism. Firstly, with SIFT and RCNN [15] combined with KCF tracker. Secondly, with MSER and faster RCNN, our newly implemented object retrieval framework combined with the KCF tracker. Finally, with our proposed system, YOLO with KCF tracker. The resultant accuracy and performance comparisons with other methods are shown in Tables 1, 2, and 3, and their graphical representations are shown in Fig. 2. Three different sized video sequences are used in our experiment.

Table 1 Detection accuracy of SIFT and RCNN with KCF tracker

Video sequence	Number of frames	Total no. of vehicles in the ground-truth	Total no. of vehicles detected using SIFT and RCNN with KCF	Detection accuracy (%)
1	400	8	6	75
2	780	14	10	71.42
3	2100	19	15	73.68

Table 2 Detection accuracy of MSER and faster RCNN with KCF tracker

Video sequence	Number of frames	Total no. of vehicles in the ground-truth	Total no. of vehicles detected using MSER and faster RCNN with KCF	Detection accuracy (%)
1	400	8	6	75
2	780	14	11	78.57
3	2100	19	16	84.21

Table 3 Detection accuracy of the proposed method (YOLO and KCF tracker)

Video sequence	Number of frames	Total no. of vehicles in the ground-truth	Total no. of vehicles detected using the proposed method (YOLO and KCF)	Detection accuracy (%)
1	400	8	8	100
2	780	14	13	92.85
3	2100	19	17	89.47

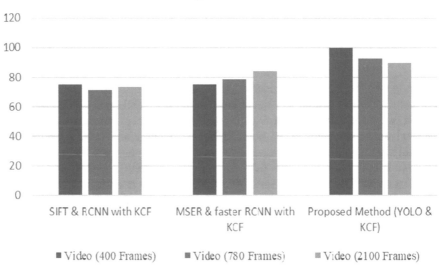

Fig. 2 Performance comparison of various vehicle detection mechanisms (using a clustered column chart)

For video the sequence with 400 frames has achieved a detection accuracy of 75% in the first two methods and 100% in our proposed method. For video sequence with 780 frames have achieved a detection accuracy of 71.42% in the first method, 78.57% in the second method, and 92.85% in our proposed method. For video sequence with 2100 frames has achieved a detection accuracy of 73.68% in the first method, 84.21% in the second method, and 89.47% in our proposed method.

Our experimental results show that the proposed method gives us the most accurate result comparing to other methods. Our system, thus developed gives us the most accurate and it gives the best results. The correctly detected vehicles are properly classified and the count is generated by the tracker in the most accurate form. This count is then processed by the thus called count by processing algorithm which compares the count obtained from the different lanes of the junction and analyses which lane is having the most traffic and the traffic signals updated in real-time accordingly. Traffic signals are changed according to the number of vehicles in each lane from a red signal to a green signal.

Prospective method is compared with state-of-the-art methods and the experimental results have shown our system performs well with the combination of tasks such as vehicle detection, counting, tracking, and generate signals for intelligent traffic monitoring system. Unlike proposed method, Lin and Sun [2] presented a YOLO-based system which is mainly applied for vehicle counting in road traffic, they have tested their system with their own traffic dataset. Asha and Narasimhadhan [4] proposed a method which is suitable for traffic management, they have achieved the vehicle counting task by the help of YOLO framework and correlation filter. Their experimental results compared with the manual vehicle count. Compared with the similar framework, our method outperforms in the overall traffic monitoring and management.

5 Conclusion

An intelligent transportation framework guarantees a protected transportation condition. Profiting by the fast improvement of object detection, it can accomplish a thorough assignment like traffic stream counting without any problem. Our studies show that the proposed software solution is more flexible, easy to maintain and implement, and much cheaper than the aforementioned hardware solutions. Thus, a dynamic system is being developed that could control the traffic signals based on the present traffic conditions by obtaining the count of the traffic present in each lane associated with a traffic junction and then after processing these counts by the so developed traffic processing algorithms. By trying with different trackers, the accuracy and general efficacy of the framework are illustrated. The currently developed system is very easy for its implementation of the present system. An up-gradation to present monitoring cameras is to be done and a central server at the nearest traffic station would facilitate the control and processing of the system. Thus, the proposed system ensures saving precious minutes in each person's life. In the future, the system can be further developed into a fully dynamic system that could enable a dynamic traffic lane for ambulances or other emergencies. This would enable the control of any rapid traffic situations even in case of any emergencies within the control room itself.

References

1. Olariu S, Weigle MC (eds) (2009) Vehicular networks: from theory to practice. CRC Press
2. Lin JP, Sun MT (2018, November) A YOLO-based traffic counting system. In: 2018 conference on technologies and applications of artificial intelligence (TAAI). IEEE, pp 82–85
3. Redmon J, Farhadi A (2018) Yolov3: an incremental improvement. arXiv preprint arXiv:1804.02767

4. Asha CS, Narasimhadhan AV (2018, March) Vehicle counting for traffic management system using YOLO and correlation filter. In: 2018 IEEE international conference on electronics, computing and communication technologies (CONECCT). IEEE, pp 1–6
5. Zaatouri K, Ezzedine T (2018, December) A self-adaptive traffic light control system based on YOLO. In: 2018 international conference on internet of things, embedded systems and communications (IINTEC). IEEE, pp 16–19
6. Huang DY, Chen CH, Hu WC, Yi SC, Lin YF (2012) Feature-based vehicle flow analysis and measurement for a real-time traffic surveillance system. J Inform Hiding Multimedia Signal Process 3(3):279–294
7. Liu Y, Ai H, Xu GY (2001, September) Moving object detection and tracking based on background subtraction. In: Object detection, classification, and tracking technologies, vol 4554. International Society for Optics and Photonics, pp 62–66
8. Lai JC, Huang SS, Tseng CC (2010, June) Image-based vehicle tracking and classification on the highway. In: The 2010 international conference on green circuits and systems. IEEE, pp 666–670
9. Song H, Liang H, Li H, Dai Z, Yun X (2019) Vision-based vehicle detection and counting system using deep learning in highway scenes. Eur Transp Res Rev 11(1):51
10. Gao H, Li X (2020) Vehicle detection in high resolution image based on deep learning. Int Arch Photogrammetry Remote Sens Spat Inform Sci 43:49–54
11. Dai Z, Song H, Wang X, Fang Y, Yun X, Zhang Z, Li H (2019) Video-based vehicle counting framework. IEEE Access 7:64460–64470
12. Fang Y, Wang C, Yao W, Zhao X, Zhao H, Zha H (2019) On-road vehicle tracking using part-based particle filter. IEEE Trans Intell Transp Syst 20(12):4538–4552
13. Scheel A, Dietmayer K (2018) Tracking multiple vehicles using a variational radar model. IEEE Trans Intell Transp Syst 20(10):3721 3736
14. Zhang Y, Song B, Du X, Guizani M (2018) Vehicle tracking using surveillance with multimodal data fusion. IEEE Trans Intell Transp Syst 19(7):2353–2361
15. Amitha IC, Narayanan NK (2020, February) Object retrieval in images using SIFT and R-CNN. In: 2020 international conference on innovative trends in information technology (ICITIIT). IEEE, pp 1–5
16. Amitha IC, Narayanan NK (2018) Image object retrieval using conventional approaches: a survey. Int J Eng Technol Sci—IJETS V(IX), September 2018. ISSN(P) 2349-3968, ISSN(O) 2349-3976
17. Farhodov X, Kwon OH, Kang KW, Lee SH, Kwon KR (2019, November). Faster RCNN detection based OpenCV CSRT tracker using drone data. In: 2019 international conference on information science and communications technologies (ICISCT). IEEE, pp 1–3
18. Emami E, Fathy M, Kozegar E (2013, September) Online failure detection and correction for CAMShift tracking algorithm. In: 2013 8th Iranian conference on machine vision and image processing (MVIP). IEEE, pp 180–183
19. Henriques JF, Caseiro R, Martins P, Batista J (2014) High-speed tracking with kernelized correlation filters. IEEE Trans Pattern Anal Mach Intell 37(3):583–596

A Convolutional Neural Network Model to Predict Air and Water Hazards

A. Akshayarathna, K. Divya Darshini, and J. Dhalia Sweetlin

1 Introduction

Water and air Pollution are considered to be amongst the main dangers to the health of living beings and the planet. It can potentially affect all the organ systems of a living being, can cause degradation of the ecosystem and food resources. It also affects crop quality and agriculture. Hence, it trickles down to all aspects of life on Earth. It is a major problem in "developing" countries/third-world countries such as India [1], mainly due to the dumping of waste onto their shores and lands by "developed", industrialized countries [2], by products of resource extraction or through the exporting of trash to be recycled [3].

Large industries owned by investors in developed nations face environmental restrictions in these developed nations due to rising concerns, but flourish with profitable gains in Third World nations [4] due to planned negligence in implementing environmental policies in these countries [5]. As a result of market expansion techniques and the constant search for cheap labor in Third World countries, these countries face grave environmental dangers.

"Now, in addition to worrying about the environmental implications of *deforestation*, *desertification*, and *soil erosion*, developing countries are facing threats of pollution that come from development, industrialization, poverty, and war" [6]. As the World Health Organization (WHO) points out, outdoor air pollution contributes as much as 0.6–1.4 percent of the burden of disease in developing regions, and other pollution, such as lead in water, air, and soil, may contribute 0.9 percent. Estimates indicate that the proportion of the global burden of disease associated with environmental pollution hazards ranges from 23% as in [7] to 30% as in [8]. These estimates include infectious diseases related to drinking water, sanitation, and food hygiene;

A. Akshayarathna · K. Divya Darshini · J. Dhalia Sweetlin (✉)
Anna University, MIT Campus, Chennai, India
e-mail: jdsweetlin@mitindia.edu

© The Author(s), under exclusive license to Springer Nature Singapore Pte Ltd. 2021 413
M. K. Bajpai et al. (eds.), *Machine Vision and Augmented Intelligence—Theory and Applications*, Lecture Notes in Electrical Engineering 796,
https://doi.org/10.1007/978-981-16-5078-9_35

respiratory diseases related to severe indoor air pollution from biomass burning; and vector-borne diseases with a major environmental component, such as malaria. These three types of diseases each contribute approximately 6 percent to the updated estimate of the global burden of disease as mentioned in [9].

Air pollution is caused by a whole host of factors, a major contributor being emissions. Unrefined emission of gases and pollutant particles without following environmental regulations, or perhaps even due to the lack of appropriate norms is a major factor. The amounts and types of emissions change every year. These changes are caused by changes in the nation's economy, industrial activity, technology improvements, traffic, and by many other factors. Water pollution is also caused by various issues, unrestrained flow of untreated water from production plants is cited to be a significant factor in increasing pollution, especially with regard to public water bodies that are accessed by all. The problems regarding environmental norms or the lack of them apply here as well. Therefore, in the face of such grave effects, while the policies and the actions to be taken in order to repair the situation and ensure environmental safety are the way to go in the long-run, preventive measures for the short-term are also required, as there is no guarantee of safety for the water or air we consume.

Many studies have been conducted on accurate prediction of air pollution and water pollution levels, as well as prediction of breathability of air and drinkability of water. These studies have been conducted in various fields using a whole variety of techniques. In the purview of this project, many of the models proposed in these studies have been implemented using Machine Learning or Deep Learning, involving image processing. Numerous comparative studies have been performed to find a low-cost, high-efficiency technique for pollution prediction as opposed to traditional meteorological methods that are expensive as well as inefficient in view of public's current needs. This project's aim is to create a small simulation of what could be a large-scale and more complex image processing model to detect basic drinkability/breathability of water/air on the basis of images sent in by the end user.

2 Literature Review

Various studies on different already existing models have been made to get a better understanding. One such study [10] has provided an alternative/addition to traditional methods of Air Quality Estimation. Qiang Zhang et al. explained the various shortcomings in these methods and have conducted a comprehensive study of the history of this field. They have used a Convolutional Neural Network-based ResNet model for this purpose and have created AQC-Net from it. A self-supervision module designed by the authors called Spatial and Contextual Attention block (SCA) module was employed to the third block of Residual Neural Network structure (ResNet18) to create CNN-residual network-based AQC-Net to make the image-detection more sensitive and the coverage of sample area wider. Their dataset size is 1241 images and was built from scratch: "a multi-scenario air-quality image database" NWNUAQI.

They compared their model against other deep learning models on the same dataset: traditional SVM which had an accuracy of 60%, the parent model ResNet had an accuracy of 70.1%, and the VGG16 model which had an accuracy of 68.3%. However, the authors' VGG16 AQC-Net model outperformed all of the above with 74% accuracy for data with wide coverage. The study had a few drawbacks mainly owing to its small scale: dataset size, inclination toward daylight images, and regional data as opposed to a more generalized data collection.

Liu et al. [11] proposed an image processing technique that exclusively focuses on detecting air-quality levels, based on the fact that changes or fluctuations in certain parameters: contrast, blur, and noise across time series of images (in different atmospheric conditions) indicate a change in the air-quality levels indirectly. They isolate these images on the basis of these parameters and Detrended Fluctuation Analysis technique is performed on them through detecting trends in the image series. They have used the fluctuation mode of detecting trends, as they profess it to be the best among the three (mixed, fluctuation and draw-up modes) for short as well as long-range time series. They have tested this method against the rescale-range method (R/S). Gaussian white noise is created and added into the original sequence, which is then analyzed by DFA and R/S and scaling exponent α is plotted. From the plots, the authors have deduced that R/S is better for short series but inclines toward the peaks, however, DFA works for both long- and short-range series and that the latter's scaling exponent is more stable when the noise is increased in the samples. The model is not devoid of shortcomings, owing to its extensive computation, however the authors have presented a low-cost alternative to expensive but inefficient traditional meteorological detection.

Ameer et al. [12] have performed a comparative analysis of four different machine learning advanced regression techniques—Decision Tree regression, Random Forest regression, Multi-Layer Perceptron regression, and Gradient Boosting regression—to determine the best model for predicting air-quality levels (Air Quality Index). The basis on which they have determined it is the size of the dataset and processing speed. Mean Absolute Error (MAE) and Root Mean Square Error (RMSE) have been used for this comparative evaluation and the models have been employed on ApacheSpark. Their dataset was generated through sensors placed in 5 different cities in China, to obtain real-time information. In order to judge the prediction performance of the four models, models were evaluated on datasets of different sizes and that of different regions. They have created correlation matrices of PM2.5 levels (on which AQI is calculated) with other meteorological parameters, for each of the five cities. Across different dataset sizes and regional variations, Random Forest regression was found by the authors to be the best among the four, in terms of speed, accuracy, and identification of peak values, whereas Gradient Boosting regression was found to be the worst among the four in terms of the same factors.

Rahman et al. [13] have analyzed the possibility of usage of the neural networks in prediction of the air pollution on example of the industrial city of Sterlitamak (Russian Federation). At the first stage of scientific research, the authors developed a neural network model for short-term prediction of air pollutants, specific for the city with developed chemical and petrochemical industry, such as dust, ammonia, hydrogen sulfide, phenol, vinyl chloride, nitrogen dioxide. The offered model provides forecasts with an advance up to several days depending on the meteorological characteristics of the following days. For ammonia the best adequacy of the short-term prediction model is the one achieved in the feedforward neural network with the learning algorithm based on Conjugate Gradient Backpropagation with Powell-Beale restarts. The second stage of scientific research of the authors was the development of a neural network model describing the air pollution index in any given point of the city, taking into account its local orographic characteristics. The different kinds of the neural networks were probed by the authors. As a result the Elman neural network showed the best adequacy of air pollution index prediction. However, variation of the number of the neurons in the hidden layer did not lead to a significant change in the quality of the neural network model. Using the developed software in the Sterlitamak city shows that it is quite an effective prediction tool. The accuracy of the forecasts is more than 83%.

Toivanen et al. [14] identify clean water by measuring water transparency (Secchi depth) and turbidity by monitoring using mobile phones and a small device designed for water quality measurements. The main algorithm behind the process is concerned with working of mobile phones and Secchi3000 and the water quality analysis. The mobile phone application that the users can use to gather observations is called EnviObserver. It is a tool for participatory sensing which utilizes people as sensors by enabling them to report environmental observations with a mobile phone. The user sends the data collected to a central server for automatic water quality analysis. The water quality analysis deals with automatic detection of the locations of the tags in the picture and extracts pixel RGB values for the black, gray, and white areas of the two tags and then carries out the actual water quality analysis based on the RGB values extracted by the tag recognition algorithm. The detection process was first to locate the surrounding areas of the lower and upper tags by the template matching method. The second step is to use a contour-based approach to look into the surroundings found by the template matching method. Overall, the variation of the measurements at each site was <10% of the reference value.

Jonna et al. [15] used digital image processing methods supplemented by visual interpretation which will be useful for effective utilization of Remote Sensing data to determine quality of water. The primary indicative signal that is useful for water quality studies is the volume reflectance and backscattered energy caused by the impurities in water. However, in addition to this signal, radiation reflected by the water surface and bottom (depending upon the depth of water) would reach the sensor. For digital image processing various image enhancement techniques such as contrast stretch, band rationing, principal component analysis are used. The FCC of principal component bands does not show any betterment in land cover depiction. Though the individual bands showed good variation in gray levels, the density sliced images of band 5 and band 6 showed better variation within the reservoir.

Chakma et al. [16] go for image-based air-quality analysis particularly to predict the concentration estimation of particulate matter with diameters <2.5 μm (PM2.5) which are very hazardous to humans to inhale. A deep Convolutional Neural Network (CNN) is used to classify natural images into different categories based on their

PM2.5 concentration using a dataset which contains sample images to find the pollution. They only need cameras, without the need of an expensive setup. The image-based haze level analysis methods are mainly inspired by the dehazing algorithms. The adopted model is CNN imagenet-matconvnet-very deep model. This model achieved very high performance on ImageNet dataset, which has over 15 million high resolution images from 1000 categories. This CNN model has 8 convolutional layers with max pooling and Relu and the last three are full connection layers (FC6, FC7, and FC8). The output of the last FC layer is input to the softmax to produce the classification results. The input to the CNN is the RGB three color channels of an image with size 24 × 224. CNN is used for PM2.5 concentration estimation and two transfer learning methods, CNN fine-tuning and random forest classification using image features extracted by CNN are used. The final algorithm used is transfer learning.

Shafi et al. [17] propose Internet of Things (IoT) which is used to measure the quality of water. A real-time embedded prototype has been built to record the water quality parameters from the water samples collected from various sources across the study area. Data is sent to the cloud for real-time storage and processing. The processed data can be remotely monitored and water flow can be controlled using developed software solution comprising of mobile app and a dashboard. In addition to the water quality monitoring and control system, the predictive analysis of the collected data has been performed. Machine learning algorithms have been applied for the classification of water quality and the experimental results indicate that deep neural networks outperform all other algorithms with an accuracy of 93%. The sensing module consists of three most influencing water quality measuring sensors, i.e., pH sensor, turbidity sensor, and temperature sensor. These sensors are connected to an Arduino board, for collecting data. The second module is a data analytics module in which predictive analysis is performed on the dataset. The water samples are used for training purposes in machine learning algorithms such as SVM, NN, and kNN. The third module is the actuator module which provides a remote water flow control system along with remote monitoring. A mobile app has been developed so that the end user can remotely monitor the water quality parameters as the updated readings are continuously being transmitted to the cloud after every 30 seconds.

Joans [18] proposed idea of obtaining the images from environment and monitoring the pollutants present in the environment using image processing method as an alternative to camera-based smoke and exhaust detection system. Traditional systems measuring the HSU grade are implemented with mobile units. The major advantage of this paper is detecting the smoke exhaust in any environment. Experimental results show that the proposed algorithm can produce the AQI evaluation with a considerable accuracy 93.78%. The key idea of the study was to investigate a means to detect and identify smoke-exhausting vehicles from the traffic flow. They need to implement smoke detection analysis software (SDAS) that includes an algorithm for image processing. The algorithm is based on image analysis from thermal and visible wavelength cameras. Edges are boundaries between different textures or the change of intensity. Edge also can be defined as discontinuities in image intensity from one pixel to another. Edge detection uses a canny edge detector which is an edge detection operator that uses a multistage algorithm to detect a wide range of edges in images.

Shonono et al. [19] are concerned with image processing to detect water quality. Most wastewater quality indicators are not visible and can only be detected in laboratories using reagents or high definition microscopic devices. The quality of wastewater is assessed by looking at both its chemical and physical compositions, as well as its micro-bacterial constituents. It requires the services of an artisan trained personnel to perform the assessment using the appropriate standardized instruments. There are four phases of image processing techniques, namely the image acquisition, pre-processing (noise removal and image enhancement), image segmentation, and image analysis. Each of the mentioned phases has enhanced techniques to ensure high-quality image. A typical image processing block diagram is outlined in detail. In this system, MATLAB software was used to recognize the protozoa and metazoa and the image analysis program written in MATLAB has proven to be adequate in doing the identification job.

Comparing all the works done previously it could be noted that many authors conducted studies focussing only on a single locality. Few authors chose other more complex methods to determine pollution such as Secchi depth measurements, IoT, remote sensing data, and many other techniques. This project's idea was to minimize the complexity of the method used to detect pollution to a simple CNN model. This project also focusses on creating a model to predict pollution worldwide without restricting the detection to a single locality.

3   Proposed Work

Machine Learning is a study of algorithms which provides systems the capability to automatically learn and improve from experience without being explicitly programmed. In machine learning computers programs are trained to access data and use it to learn for themselves. Supervised Learning has been used in this project because the dataset is confined and non-expandable. Machine learning algorithms and Deep learning algorithms are both widely used in the field today. The shift over from ML to DL that is "The deep learning revolution", as it is called, is taking place because of 2 main differences amongst many others: 1. Learning Classification functions. 2. Model-building process. 1. Machine learning algorithms cannot learn non-linear decision boundaries, unlike Deep learning algorithms. It is also not capable of learning all the kinds of functions used in dividing data into classes. This gives Deep learning algorithms an upper hand. 2. The model-building process is different in deep learning and machine learning and requires an in-depth explanation. However, to be concise, Deep learning can learn complex features in an incremental and automated manner, unlike Machine Learning which requires domain expertise and requires a breakdown of the problem statement data to make it simpler in order to solve it as described in [20].

Neural Networks are of many types, and many new kinds of neural networks are being developed right now. To compare three of the most common kinds which include Artificial Neural Network (ANN), Recurrent Neural network (RNN), and Convolutional Neural Network (CNN) many aspects were studied. To make a brief comparison, ANN reduces a 2-dimensional image to a 1-dimensional vector, compromising on spatial details. It also requires a very high number of trainable parameters even for small images. RNN is a modified ANN. It trains sequential data well, unlike ANN, in that it learns successive data in the training dataset with a dependency on the preceding data. It performs parameter sharing as well, reducing the computational cost RNN is apt for time-series data, therefore it does not apply to the aim of this project. Vanishing and exploding gradients are an issue with both RNN and ANN. CNN uses filters/kernels to perform feature extraction from the dataset, and it learns these filters in an automated manner without having to provide explicit instructions to the model. CNN also recognizes and learns spatial features from an image unlike RNN and ANN, which makes it relevant in image and video processing models. Like RNN, it performs parameter sharing, i.e., it applies the given parameters/filters to different parts of each input data producing feature maps.

Hence in this project Convolutional Neural Networks concepts have been chosen over other Supervised Learning techniques because it has the capability to provide high accuracy with minimal datasets as in [21]. The core concept of CNN is it uses convolution of image and filters to generate invariant features which are passed onto the next layer. These invariant features being passed to the next layer are convoluted with different filters to generate more invariant and abstract features and the process continues till one gets final feature/output which is invariant to occlusions. The proposed work can be well understood from the architecture diagram given in Fig. 1.

3.1 Architecture Diagram

Data Layer

In this layer, the air and water data that have been acquired from various online sources have been stored and classified into the training and validation datasets. For air 200 images were collected from online sources and classified into a 80:20 ratio for training and validation. For water 400 images were collected from online sources and classified them into a 70:30 ratio for training and validation. There are two classes in corresponding to air and water. For water the two classes were clean and polluted. For air the two classes were Breathable and hazardous. Two different models one training on air dataset and another training on water dataset were built. Both the models were build based on CNN concepts and the air model has a prediction accuracy of 82.50% and water model that has an accuracy of 90%.

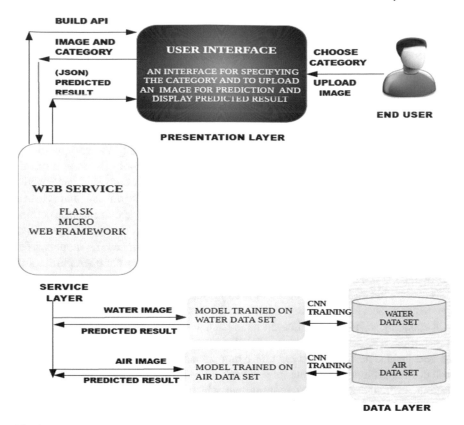

Fig. 1 Architecture diagram

Models

Building of a convolutional model for both the prediction of air pollution and water pollution is based on inference obtained from the literature survey and understanding the basic working of a CNN model.

Convolutional Layer

This layer is a mandatory for all CNN-based models. This project uses 3 layers of Conv2D for both the models. The first Convolutional layer has been implemented with 16 convolutional filters and the no. of filters have been increased in multiples of 2 in successive convolutional layers in both the models, i.e., the 2nd Convolutional Layer has 32 filters and the last Convolutional layer has 64. All of these filters are used to convolve with each of the input channels/batches. Stride has been given as 3×3, which specifies the block/window size by which the convolution is performed by the filter with each input channel matrix. Input shape is chosen as rows $\times$ columns $= 200 \times 200$ in input batches of 3. The padding is given as "same" for all 3 convolutional layers in order to prevent loss of data in the images.

Pooling Layers

It is used to reduce the dimensions while maintaining the input shape ratio given in Convolutional Layers. A 2 × 2 pooling function has been used in order to reduce the dimensions of the Convolved output channels by half to help increase the processing and computational efficiency in the two models.

Dropout

This has been used to reduce overfitting in the models. It has been applied after every ReLU activation layer. This "drops out" a few nodes during every stage in the training process to prevent the air and water models fitting the images provided in the training datasets too closely that would make them incapable of predicting hazards in any new images sent in by the end user.

Flatten Layer

Flatten layer and a type of fully connected layer (here Dense has been used) are basic layers present in all models across the spectrum. Flatten converts the pooled channel to a single column that is to be passed to a fully connected layer, such as a Dense layer. The 2-dimensional channels are converted to single-dimensional nodes, from which the predictions are made for both the air and the water models.

Dense Layer

It has been used as the last layer. This is a type of fully connected layer to which the flattened channels are sent. Activation Layers have been applied to Convolutional Layers and to the last Dense Layer. Before any activation layer this formula is performed for the preceding layer.

$$x = (\text{weight} * \text{input node}) + \text{bias} \tag{1}$$

Bias is not used in this model, as there was no need for it. These values of x found as given in (1) for each node are inputted to Activation Layers. Both the activation layers used are non-linear.

ReLU

Mathematical function of ReLU is shown in (2).

$$f(x) = \max(0, x) \tag{2}$$

All the neurons are not activated at the same time, which contributes to relative computational efficiency as well as reduction of overfitting. It reduces vanishing gradients and expanding gradients. It doesn't saturate for very high or very low inputs of x, if a neuron is activated its value will be close to 1. Working of ReLU could be understood from Fig. 2 referred from [22]. From the graph it is seen that ReLU function returns zero for negative input and returns the input in case of a positive input.

Fig. 2 ReLU activation [22]

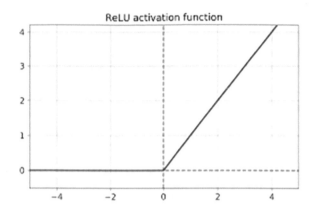

Sigmoid

Mathematical function of sigmoid is given in (3).

$$f(x) = 1/\left(1 + e^{(-x)}\right) \tag{3}$$

It transforms the range of values between 0 and 1 as shown in Fig. 3 referred from [23]. Since the classification required is a binary classification sigmoid is used at the output layer to reduce the range between 0 and 1. This is applied on the last (dense) layer. It is applied for binary classifications. In the MNIST AND CIFAR models that had been referred to as part of the research, a softmax activation layer had been applied on the last dense layer, but as the model performs a binary classification instead of categorical/multiple classes unlike MNIST and CIFAR, softmax was replaced with sigmoid.

Fig. 3 Sigmoid activation [23]

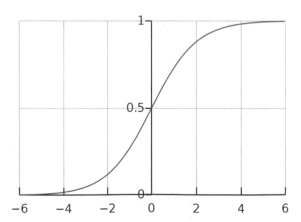

Batch Normalization

Batch normalisation has been used in this project. Oftentimes, either Batch Normalization or Dropout is used in a model, but this project has made use of both these layers in both of its models. This layer is applied to each batch (batch specifies the number of samples that are image processed before the model is updated each time during training). The batch number inputted in this project is 3. Batch normalisation is a layer that is used to prevent overfitting, increase processing efficiency, and the independence of each layer in performing its functions. It does this by subtracting the mean value of all the input nodes in each batch to bring it to zero mean, and by dividing their standard deviation to bring it to one. This is called "transformation" or "normalization" of inputs. This project makes use of this layer to reduce the variance shift in successive layers, standardizing the data to better prediction performance as explained in [24].

Backpropagation

When the neural network is initialized, each element of the layer that is neuron is initialized with a given weight. When input images are loaded, they are passed through the network of neurons and based on the weights the network provides an output for each. Backpropagation helps to adjust the weights of the neurons so that the result comes closer and closer to the known true result. The structure of backpropagation is explained clearly in Fig. 4 referred from [25]. There is a travel back from the output layer to the hidden layer to adjust the weights such that the error is decreased. As inferred from [26] to [27], based on how the alteration of weights takes place there are several optimizers available. It was seen that by using adam optimizer and rmsprop optimizer the highest accuracy is obtained with minimal training. Thus rmsprop optimizer is chosen.

Due to backpropagation, if a network has n hidden layers, n derivatives will be multiplied together. If the derivatives are large then the gradient will increase exponentially leading to a large value gradient and this is what is called the problem of exploding gradient. Alternatively, if the derivatives are small then the gradient will

Fig. 4 Backpropagation [25]

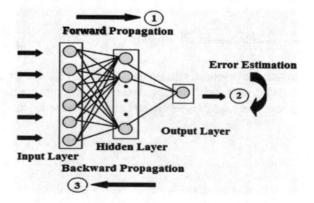

decrease exponentially as there is propagation through the model until it reaches is a very small value and vanishes and this is the vanishing gradient problem. There are various ways to solve this problem as explained in [28, 29]. ReLU activation has a gradient slope of 1. During backpropagation, there are not any gradients passed back that are progressively getting smaller and smaller, but instead the gradients stay the same. ReLU solves the vanishing gradient problem. Hence ReLU activation is found to be the solution of this problem.

Cross-Entropy

Cross-entropy is the default loss function to use for binary classification problems as explained in [30]. It is used where the target values are in the set $\{0, 1\}$. As a model has to be build to predict between 2 classes, namely, polluted/non-polluted binary cross-entropy was chosen.

Service Layer

Flask micro web framework as explained in [31] is launched for building an API built based on HTML. The two models which had undergone CNN training on water dataset and air dataset have already been loaded and is ready for prediction in this layer.

Essentially, this layer serves as an intermediate between Data layer and Presentation layer. It receives the category of pollution user wishes to detect that is air or water and the image provided for prediction from the presentation layer with the help of json request and then sends them to the loaded model for prediction and return the result to the presentation layer.

Presentation Layer

This is the outermost layer of this project through which the end user can communicate with the model. The user has to specify whether they wish to detect hazards in air or water. Then they can upload the image in JPEG format. The image is passed on to the service layer and given to the respective model for prediction. The result of the prediction is shown to the user in the presentation layer.

4 Results and Discussion

In order to practically understand the layers used in a typical Convolutional Neural Network and their working, apart from general research, 2 popular CNN image processing models were studied and applied to the dataset.

4.1 MNIST

MNIST model was created to train the system in image processing to recognize handwritten digits. The accuracy on applying this model to dataset of the project was minimal around 11.67%.

4.2 CIFAR-10

CIFAR-10 model was created to train the system in image processing to classify the image into one of 10 classes of ordinary things. The accuracy on applying this model to the dataset was minimal and around 50%.

4.3 Inference

On application of these models, following were inferred: (1) They do not apply Dense layers in the beginning, nor do they include fully connected layers in the beginning. Instead a Convolutional Layer is usually applied. (2) Classification based on categorical labels can cause errors as machine learning algorithms relatively understand integer values better as they have an ordered relationship. Hence, either of two methods-Integer Encoding and One-Hot Encoding is used to convert categorical labels to numerical labels. In both the models, One-Hot Encoding is used. (3) Padding is used as "same" in CIFAR-10 and "valid" in MNIST, thus in the latter the dimensions are preserved throughout in order to not lose information, however the former doesn't face loss of information problem. (4) MaxPooling Layer is always used in Convolutional Neural Networks to aid better processing. (5) Dense Layer is used as the last layer to act as a fully connected layer. (6) Flatten Layer is usually used before the last Dense Layer.

4.4 Building of the Model

Originally when the model was being built each Convolutional Layer was added one-by-one until the training accuracy improved. 4 Conv2D layers showed the maximum training accuracy, anything less brought the accuracy value down. The parameters were tweaked and adjusted appropriately (as explained in the previous section) as the model was being built. Initially the model built for water pollution prediction could not reach an accuracy more than 78% due to overfitting. The training accuracy reached up to 99.6% but the validation accuracy kept flickering between 73 and 78%. Increasing Dropout values of the layers helped in bridging the gap between validation accuracy and training accuracy. But a higher value of Dropout such as 0.1 resulted in underfitting that is the training accuracy began to fall under 80%. Considering that unnecessarily deeper networks for small datasets could contribute to poor prediction performance and therefore accuracy, upon reducing the Convolutional Layers and their subsequent Pooling, Activation and Dropout layers to 3 sets instead of 4, in both the Air and Water models, the accuracy improved by around 2 or 3 values.

After this, understanding that tackling overfitting would handle the root of this issue, two dropouts 0.05 and 0.02 were fixed, upon numerous trials-and-errors. Then additionally, Batch Normalization was chosen to fix this issue in a more drastic manner. Batch Normalization was applied thrice after the Activation and Dropout layers of each Convolutional layer in the Water model. This aided in boosting the performance accuracy.

Similarly the model built for air hazard prediction could not reach an accuracy more than 72% due to overfitting. The training accuracy reached up to 98% but the validation accuracy kept flickering between 65 and 72%. The Dropout values were changed to 0.1 and 0.02 after which additionally, Batch Normalization was applied 3 times in the model after the Activation and Dropout layers of each Convolutional layer in the Air model to improve accuracy.

This improved accuracy of the Water model to around 83% and the Air model to around 70%. However, upon performing trial-and-error on the position of the Batch Normalization layers in the model, the accuracy value showed changes. Initially, the position was changed from post-Activation and Dropout layers to pre-Activation and Dropout layers at all 3 points, in both the models. This did not show any significant improvements.

Instead, through trial-and-error, when the Batch Normalization was applied only once in the Water model after the 2nd Conv2D Layer and twice in the Air model after the 2nd and 3rd Conv2D Layers, there was a drastic improvement in the prediction performance/accuracy of the Air and Water models.

4.5   Air Model

Accuracy of air model is 82.5% as shown in Fig. 5. The x-axis represents the number of epochs and y-axis represents the accuracy obtained. The loss that occurred during training is shown in Fig. 6. The x-axis represents the number of epochs and the y-axis represents the corresponding loss. The predictions made by the air model are explained in Figs. 7 and 8. Whenever an image is provided the model predicts the pollution level and provides the result.

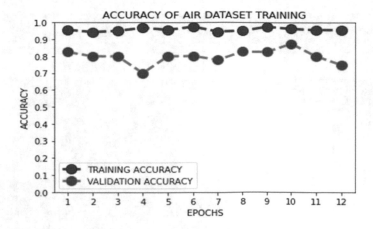

Fig. 5 Accuracy of air model

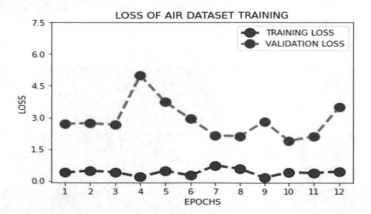

Fig. 6 Loss of air model

4.6 Water Model

Accuracy of water model is 90.00% as shown in Fig. 9. The x-axis represents the number of epochs and y-axis represents the accuracy obtained. The loss occurred during training is shown in Fig. 10. The x-axis represent the number of epochs and y-axis represent the corresponding loss. The predictions made by the air model are explained in Figs. 11 and 12. Whenever an image is provided the model predicts the pollution level and provides the result.

The accuracy of the air model is lesser than the water model due to the comparatively smaller size of the air dataset. Moreover the models have not been trained with datasets pertaining to any specific locality or region. This model is designed to predict hazardous air or water irrespective of the locality, based only on the image

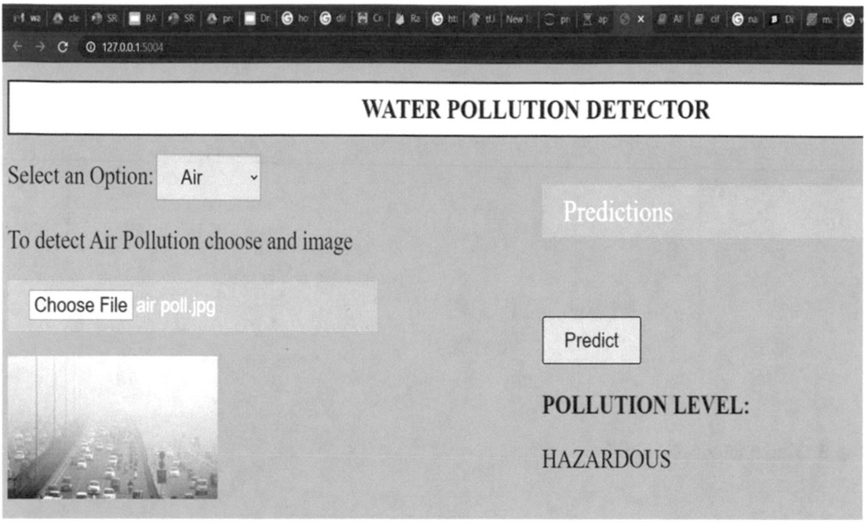

Fig. 7 Air pollution detection (1)

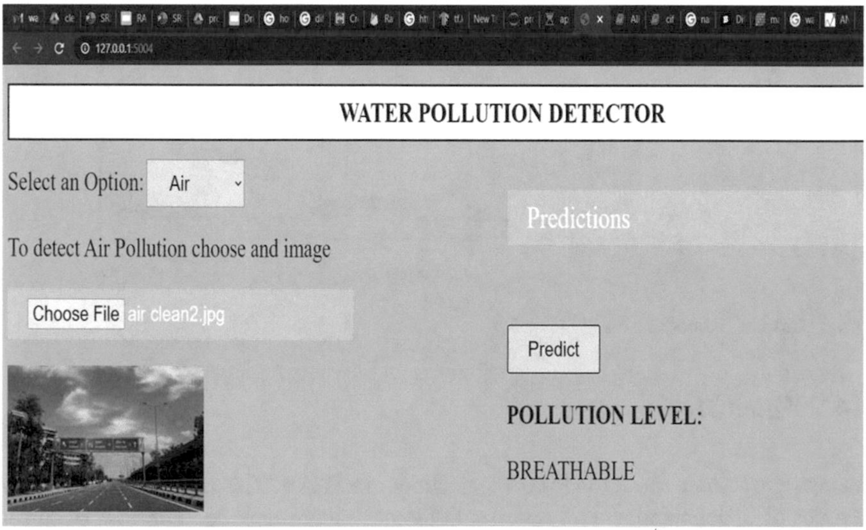

Fig. 8 Air pollution detection (2)

being provided. It can detect hazardous air from any region with an accuracy of 82.5% and polluted water from any region with an accuracy of 90%. Using batch normalization to obtain high accuracy with a relatively small dataset and building a CNN model that is not location-specific are being proposed to be novel about this project.

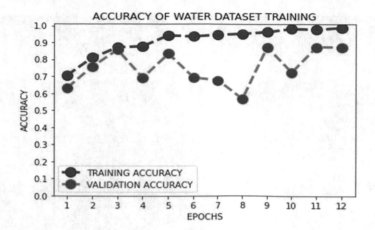

Fig. 9 Accuracy of water model

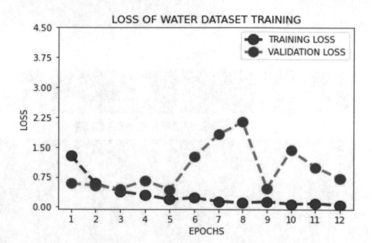

Fig. 10 Loss of water model

5 Hardware and Software Components

The entire project was developed based on Jupyter Notebook available in Anaconda Navigator using modules such as Keras, Tensorflow, and Flask.

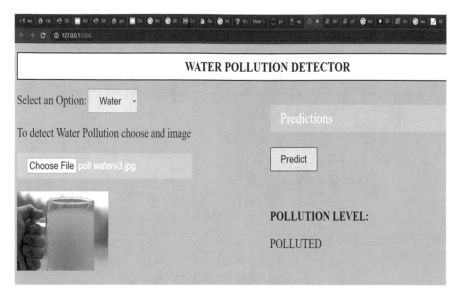

Fig. 11 Water pollution detection (1)

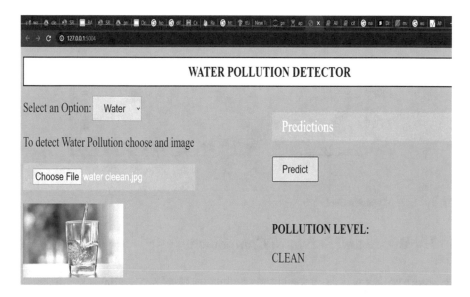

Fig. 12 Water pollution detection (2)

6 Conclusion

Many techniques can be opted for determining the quality of air and water accurately and extensive research material exists for the same. This project makes use of Convolutional Neural Networks to build a model to predict if the water or air/atmosphere was hazardous through images provided by the end user. Flask Framework has been used to deploy these two models into a single user-friendly interface for the end user. The user needs to simply take a photo of the air or water in question to know if it is drinkable/safe for use/breathable or hazardous and send it to the model through the webpage framework. This is an attempt to increase the accessibility to such information, as well as a small-scale project to experiment using image processing and deep learning to make pollution detection efficient and low cost.

References

1. Pollution and the Poor. Economist 322(February 15, 1992):18–19
2. Kumar P (1992) Stop dumping on the South. World Press Review (June 1992):12–13
3. CNN International https://edition.cnn.com/
4. LaDou J (1991) Deadly migration: hazardous industries' flight to the third world. Technol Rev (July 1991):47
5. Collins C, Darch C (1992) Summit sets a rich table, but Africa gets the crumbs. Nat Catholic Reporter 29(July 3, 1992):12
6. Third World Pollution. Environmental encyclopedia. Encyclopedia.com, 16 Oct. 2020. https://www.encyclopedia.com
7. World Health Organization Office of Global and Integrated Environmental Health. https://www.who.int/
8. National Center for Biotechnology Information. https://www.ncbi.nlm.nih.gov/
9. World Health Organisation. https://www.who.int/
10. Zhang Q, Fu F, Tian R (2020) A deep learning and image-based model for air quality estimation. Sci Total Environ 724:138178. ISSN 0048-9697 (Elsevier)
11. Liu H, Li F, Lu H (2010) Imaging air quality evaluation using definition metrics and detrended fluctuation analysis. In: IEEE 10th international conference on signal processing proceedings, Beijing, pp 968–971. https://doi.org/10.1109/ICOSP.2010.5655838
12. Ameer S et al (2019) Comparative analysis of machine learning techniques for predicting air quality in smart cities. IEEE Access 7:128325–128338. https://doi.org/10.1109/ACCESS.2019.2925082
13. Rahman P, Panchenko A, Safarov A (2017) Using neural networks for prediction of air pollution index in industrial city. IOP Conf Ser: Earth Environ Sci 87:042016. https://doi.org/10.1088/1755-1315/87/4/042016
14. Toivanen T, Koponen S, Kotovirta V et al (2013) Water quality analysis using an inexpensive device and a mobile phone. Environ Syst Res 2:9
15. Jonna S, Badarinath KVS, Saibaba J (1989) Digital image processing of Remote Sensing data for water quality studies. J Indian Soc Remote Sens 17:59–64
16. Chakma A, Vizena B, Cao T, Lin J, Zhang J (2017) Image-based air quality analysis using deep convolutional neural network. In: 2017 IEEE international conference on image processing (ICIP), Beijing, 2017, pp 3949–3952. https://doi.org/10.1109/ICIP.2017.8297023
17. Shafi U, Mumtaz R, Anwar H, Qama, A, Khurshid H (2018) Surface water pollution detection using Internet of Things, 92–96. https://doi.org/10.1109/HONET.2018.8551341

18. Joans (2017) Air pollution monitoring through image processing. Int J Res Appl Sci Eng Technol 1377–1382. https://doi.org/10.22214/ijraset.2017.10200
19. Shanono I, Sapiee M, Aziz A, Azha K, Suleiman N, Gomes A, Gomes C (2018) Image processing techniques applicable to wastewater quality detection: towards a hygienic environment. J Mater Environ Sci 9:2288–2303
20. Nielsen MA (2015) Neural networks and deep learning. Determination Press
21. Lai Y (2019) A comparison of traditional machine learning and deep learning in image recognition. 2019/10. IOP Publishing. SP- 012148. VL 1314. SN 1742–6588. SN 1742-6596
22. Activation functions in neural networks. https://debuggercafe.com/activation-functions-in-neural-networks/
23. Sigmoid function. https://en.wikipedia.org/wiki/Sigmoid_function
24. Ioffe S, Szegedy C (2015) Batch normalization: accelerating deep network training by reducing internal covariate shift. In: ICML'15: Proceedings of the 32nd International Conference on Machine Learning, vol 37. pp 448–456
25. Beginner into neural networks. https://medium.com/@purnasaigudikandula/a-beginner-intro-to-neural-networks-543267bda3c8
26. LeCun YA, Bottou L, Orr GB, Müller KR (2012) Efficient BackProp. In: Montavon G, Orr GB, Müller KR (eds) Neural networks: tricks of the trade. Lecture notes in computer science, vol 7700. Springer, Berlin, Heidelberg. https://doi.org/10.1007/978-3-642-35289-8_3
27. Ruder S (2016) An overview of gradient descent optimization algorithms. arXiv PrePrint arXiv:1609.04747
28. Machine Learning Mastery. https://machinelearningmastery.com/
29. Nielsen MA (2015) Why are deep neural networks hard to train? In Nielsen MA (ed) Neural networks and deep learning. Determination Press
30. Zhu H, Kaneko T (2018) Comparison of loss functions for training of deep neural networks in Shogi. In: 2018 conference on technologies and applications of artificial intelligence (TAAI), Taichung, pp 18–23. https://doi.org/10.1109/TAAI.2018.00014
31. Smyth P (2018) Creating web APIs with Python and Flask. Programming Historian 7. https://doi.org/10.46430/phen0072

Deep Learning in Quadratic Frequency Modulated Thermal Wave Imaging for Automatic Defect Detection

G. T. Vesala, V. S. Ghali, R. B. Naik, A. Vijaya Lakshmi, and B. Suresh

1 Introduction

Non-destructive testing (NDT) techniques promise to improve the quality and produce defect-free products in various industries. Over the other conventional NDT techniques, active infrared non-destructive testing (IRNDT) is gaining interest due to its subsurface analysis characteristics with the whole field, non-contact, and remote inspection capabilities [1]. Active thermography (AT) uses the heat map over the test object surface to distinguish the subsurface anomalies under a controlled external stimulus. However, deeper defect detection and depth resolution characteristics promote quadratic frequency modulated optical stimulus as a viable excitation scheme in AT over other conventional stimulation mechanisms [2]. The recent trend in post-processing research introduced fascinating feature extraction methodologies in quadratic frequency modulated thermal wave imaging (QFMTWI) for efficient defect detection [3]. Though these techniques feature an enhanced detection, they require human expertise for qualitative and quantitative assessment which is prone to human errors. Besides, the present trend in the industrialization and NDT techniques are enabling with artificial intelligence and deep learning based techniques to automate the defect detection, without human intervention.

Machine learning has been introduced in conventional thermography in the late 1990s, but extensive research on deep learning was initiated in the recent past with

G. T. Vesala (✉) · V. S. Ghali · A. Vijaya Lakshmi · B. Suresh
Infrared Imaging Center, Department of ECE, Koneru Lakshmaiah Educational Foundation, Vaddeswaram, Guntur, India

R. B. Naik
Naval Materials Research Laboratory, Ambernath (E), Thane, Maharashtra, India

A. Vijaya Lakshmi
Department of ECE, Amrita Sai Institute of Science and Technology, Paritala, Andhra Pradesh, India

© The Author(s), under exclusive license to Springer Nature Singapore Pte Ltd. 2021   433
M. K. Bajpai et al. (eds.), *Machine Vision and Augmented Intelligence—Theory and Applications*, Lecture Notes in Electrical Engineering 796,
https://doi.org/10.1007/978-981-16-5078-9_36

an initiation by Yousefi [4] with transfer learning for automatic defect detection in pulsed thermography. Later, Saeed in [5] used three object localization deep convolution neural network (CNN) models to locate defects in observed thermograms. A similar approach is presented in [6], but the author used principal component analysis as a pre-processing and data augmentation strategy to overcome over-fitting problems. In contrast, the defect detection is treated as schematic segmentation problem in [7] and CNN based U-net and long short term memory (LSTM) based networks are used to achieve it in PT. On the other hand, the scarcity in the thermographic data is addressed and achieved a significant augmentation through deep CNN based generative adversarial networks (GAN). The augmented thermal response is validated using principal component and independent component analysis techniques, respectively [8, 9]. However, the defect depth estimation remains a challenging task and is recently achieved using LSTM based regression models [10, 11] by training on the thermal contrast curves of defects in pulsed thermographic inspection.

In contrast, Cao introduced a 2-stream deep CNN architecture as a similarity prediction network between the thermal profiles in lock-in thermography [12] for defect classification. However, the present article deals with non-stationary stimulus based QFMTWI modality in which artificial neural network and decision trees have been introduced in the recent past as automatic defect detection networks [13, 14]. But, deep learning through CNN or LSTM is still a novel concept in QFMTWI. On the other hand, the introduction of one-dimensional CNN gained interest in the recent past for various signal classification tasks [15] with various architectures. Inception based GoogleNet is imported and modeled with 1D-CNN to classify different signals in structural health monitoring [16, 17] in the recent past.

The present article introduces a 1D-CNN based GoogleNet architecture for automatic defect detection in QFMTWI. Experimentation is carried out over a mild steel sample with flat bottom holes, and few profiles from defective and non-defective regions are extracted as a training set. Cross-validation is employed to monitor the training performance of the proposed network and tested with the entire sample thermal response to automatically visualize the classified defects. Further, the classification performance is validated through machine learning and thermographic metrics by comparing with the conventional and state of the art feature based defect detection techniques.

2 Automatic defect detection in QFMTWI

In QFMTWI, a low power optical stimulus modulated by a band of low frequencies is imposed on the test sample with a set of halogen lamps. The illuminated stimulus heats the sample surface and generates thermal waves that propagate into the subsurface layers through diffusion phenomenon. Any inhomogeneity underneath the surface disturbs the thermal wave propagation, reflects, and further heats up the respective location on sample surface. An infrared camera captures this heat map

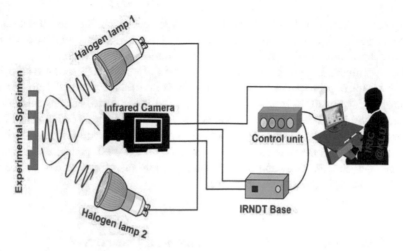

Fig. 1 Schematic of the experimental setup of QFMTWI

over the sample surface, which is further processed with various processing techniques for defect detection. Figure 1 presents the schematic of the experimentation of QFMTWI [2].

2.1 Feature Extraction in QFMTWI

Various processing techniques have been introduced in QFMTWI as feature extraction techniques for efficient defect detection. A polynomial fitting procedure is used to remove the mean raise in each temporal thermal profile as a pre-processing step. Then the resultant dynamic temporal thermal profile is subjected to various feature separation techniques. Fourier transform based phase analysis (FFT phase), principal component analysis (PCA), and random projection transform (RPT) are efficient feature separation techniques in QFMTWI [3]. In FFT phase, Fourier transform is employed over each temporal thermal profile, and respective phase components are derived. Further, the phase contrast is used to distinguish defective and sound regions. This phase contrast and blind frequencies derived from the phase profiles favor the quantitative assessment of defect depths [18].

In contrast, statistical techniques like Principal component analysis (PCA) and random projection transform (RPT) became efficient feature separation techniques in QFMTWI. PCA projects the high dimensional thermal response into a lower-dimensional subspace through orthogonal projection using Eigenvalue or singular value decomposition. On the other hand, RPT performs the orthonormal projection through Gram-Schmidt orthogonalization. In both cases, the initial step is to reshape the three-dimensional thermal response to a 2D vector. Then the covariance vector is computed in PCA, which is further applied to Eigen decomposition to extract Eigenvectors and Eigen Values. The most significant components are sorted by arranging Eigenvectors in descending order to the corresponding Eigenvectors.

Few dominant Eigenvectors are selected and projected back to the data-driven vector to form principal components which are further converted into 3D and visualized for enhanced defect detection. On the other hand, RPT employs QR-decomposition on 2D thermal response vector that is resulting in orthonormal basis vectors with lower dimension. These low dimension features are further visualized, and defect enhancement is analyzed. Compared to the FFT phase, the statistical parameter-dependent PCA and RPT efficiently dilute the effects of non-uniformity and other noises in the thermal response.

2.2 Automatic Defect Detection Through GoogleNet

GoogleNet is a deep convolutional neural network architecture introduced in 2014 to meet image classification and object localization for computer vision applications. It is a 22 layer deep network with intermediate decision layers named as Inception modules. Unlike sequential alignment of hidden layers, inception modules use a parallel arrangement of convolution layers with different kernel sizes to extract distinct features in a single layer. These extracted features are fused at the end and fed to consecutive inception layers for high level feature extraction. This parallel arrangement extensively reduces the number of trainable parameters compared to sequential networks and learns different features of the input simultaneously [19].

Apart from computer vision tasks that operate on image features, recent introduction of compact 1D-CNN model favored the application of this inception module driven deep learning model to various signal classification problems in a straight forward approach [16, 17]. The theoretical generalization of 1D-CNN's is similar to that of the 2D-CNN's except that 1D-CNN's works on signal's temporal variations [15]. In the present case, thermographic signals extracted from the test sample belong to either defective region or non-defective regions. Defect detection through feature extraction methods recommends an experienced observer to investigate on few frames which leads to human errors. To avoid such human errors and provide automatic defect detection, a deep GoogleNet architecture, as shown in Fig. 2, is introduced in this article.

The model consists of different layers like 1D-convolutional layer, max-pooling layer, inception layer, dropout layer, and fully connected network. The input is fed to the first hidden layer having 1D-convolutional filters with large kernel size to significantly reduce the dimensionality of the subsequent layers for faster computations at hidden layers. The inception layer comprises of convolution layers with different kernel sizes (1, 3, 5) as shown in Fig. 2 that simultaneously extract different features from the input features and finally fuses to create a compact feature vector which is fed to the next inception layer. A dropout layer between the final fully connected layer and inception module is used to overcome the over-fitting phenomenon. Finally,

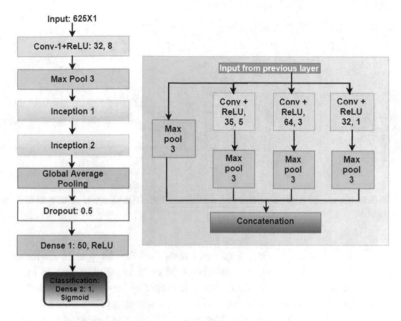

Fig. 2. 1D-CNN based GoogleNet architecture (left) and the inception module (right)

the fully connected network presents the classified result. The hidden layers are activated with Rectified linear unit (ReLU) activation, and the final classification layer in fully connected network is activated with sigmoid activation function. The network is trained on a few selected thermal profiles and in the testing phase, and the entire sample thermal response is fed to classify defective and non-defective thermal profiles using a loss function given by

$$L = \sum_{i=1}^{n} y_i \le \log \hat{y}_i, \tag{1}$$

where L is the loss, n is the number of classes, and y_i is the probability of a given thermal profile to be classified as class i.

3 Experimentation and Data Preparation

Experimentation is carried over a mild steel specimen with flat bottom holes of different sizes with varying depths. The schematic layout of the test sample is shown in Fig. 3a. The front surface of the test sample is excited with a 2 kW quadratic frequency modulated optical heat flux modulated by a band of 0.01–0.1 Hz by a set of halogen lamps for 100 s. The resultant thermal response is recorded in a FLIR

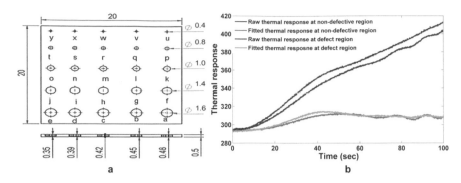

Fig. 3. **a** Schematic layout of mild steel sample (dimensions in cm) and **b** extraction of dynamic thermal profile

A655SC thermal camera having a spectral range of 7.5–14 μm at 25 frames per seconds. A black paint having an emissivity of 0.95 is painted on the inspecting side of the test sample to maintain uniform emissivity [20]. The recorded thermal response covers a thermogram cube of 2500 frames with a resolution of 450×450 after removing the extra background. The mean raise in the temporal thermal profile of each pixel in view is removed through a proper fitting technique to extract the dynamic thermal profiles as shown in Fig. 3b.

Each linear fitted temporal thermal profile is down-sampled at a factor of 4 to get a reduced feature-length of 625 samples to reduce the computation complexity of the network. The down-sampled thermal profiles are associated with respective labels where thermal profiles at defective, and non-defective regions are associated with 1 and 0, respectively, by mapping with the physical locations of the test sample. This results in 22,845 defective and 179,655 non-defective pixel locations, out of which, 8 k defective and 12 k non-defective thermal profiles are extracted to prepare a training dataset. The testing dataset is the available, total thermal response that is reshaped to form a 2D vector with pixels along rows and their respective temporal evolution in columns.

4   Results and Discussion

Initially, the training and testing data (temporal thermal profiles) are normalized with respect to their standard deviation as a pre-processing step used in machine learning. Though CNN architectures require high configuration GPU to train, 1D-CNN's proved to be simple enough to train in CPU based hardware [15]. Hence, the proposing architecture is trained with 20 k thermal profiles on an Intel i3 CPU with 8 GB RAM and 2 TB memory in Python 3.6.10 environment. During the training process, binary cross-entropy is used as a loss function that is given in Eq. (1) and

Adam with default hyper-parameters is used as optimizer. The batch size is set to 64 and the networks trained for 500 back-propagation iterations for 9.025 h.

A 20% of training data is splitted and validated on the model simultaneously during the training, and the loss curves from Fig. 4 suggest that the model is training properly without over-fitting and saturated at 120 epochs with a validation loss of 0.008. Further, the entire sample thermal response is fed to the trained model for defect classification, and the final classification result is compared with the conventional feature extraction techniques and is presented in the left side of Fig. 5. Figure suggests that the deep learning based network offers automatic and efficient defect detection in mild steel sample than the conventional feature extraction techniques. The time elapsed for testing is 19.8 min. In addition, the proposed methodology is compared with the decision tree and ANN based defect classification approaches [13, 14]. The

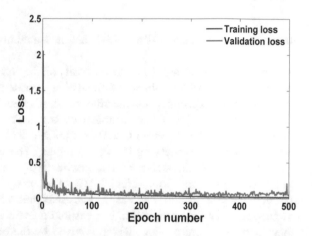

Fig. 4 Training validation of the proposed network

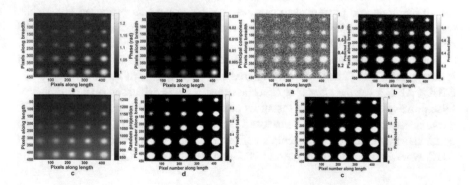

Fig. 5 Comparison of defect detection in mild steel sample using feature extraction methods such as **a** FFT phase at 0.05 Hz, **b** 2nd PCA, **c** 1st RPT, and d. proposed deep learning architecture (in left) and **a** decision tree, **b** ANN, and **c** proposed deep learning architecture (in right)

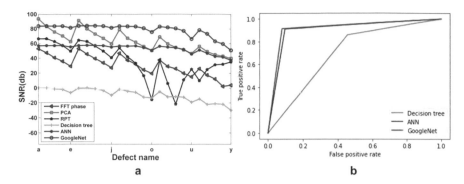

Fig. 6 a Signal to noise ratio comparison of mild steel sample and **b** comparison of defect classification performance using AUC

defect classification performances using DT and ANN are presented in right side of Fig. 5.

One can observe from the results that DT is able to classify all the defects but most of the non-defective region is classified as defective one which is due to the attributes in thermal response of mild steel specimen. On the other hand, ANN and GoogleNet learn the distinct features in each hidden layer and able to classify defects accurately. However, one can observe that the proposed GoogleNet present less false alarms compared to ANN by efficiently classifying the sound region. The classification performance of the machine learning models is compared with the pre-defined ground truth. It is observed that the proposed GoogleNet 94.83% of accuracy in predicting the exact ground truth of the pixel profile, whereas DT and ANN present 56.86% and 90.30% accuracy. However, the defect signature is measured using signal to noise ratio (SNR) in thermographic point of view, which is given by the ratio between the mean difference in the defective region to non-defective region and the standard deviation of the non-defective region [13, 14]. The SNR of each defect is computed for all methods and presented in Fig. 6a. It is observed that proposed GoogleNet presents high SNR compared to other conventional feature extraction methods and defect classification techniques.

Further, the classification performance of proposed 1D-CNN based GoogleNet is compared with DT and ANN using area under the region of interest (ROI) curve (AUC). AUC gives the efficiency of a classification network based on the number of false positive and true positive instances observed in a classification task. The AUC curve between DT, ANN, and proposed GoogleNet is presented in Fig. 6b, which concludes that GoogleNet presents an efficient defect classification with 91.66% of AUC, whereas DT and ANN present 70.1 and 90.65% of AUC.

5   Conclusion

The present article introduces a 1D-CNN based deep GoogleNet architecture for automatic defect detection in QFMTWI. Experimentation is carried out over a mild steel sample and training and testing datasets prepared from the generated thermal response. The proposed architecture trained on the training set and the entire sample response fed to test the network for automatic defect detection in the mild steel sample. The defect classification performance of proposing deep learning architecture is compared with the conventional feature extraction methods. Comparative analysis using classified result and respective SNR's suggests that the proposed deep learning architecture provides automatic defect detection without human intervention. The researches will be extending to study and introduce more deep learning architectures in QFMTWI.

Acknowledgements This work is supported by Naval Research Board, India, under the grant no. NRB-423/MAT/18-19.

References

1. Maldague XPV (2001) Theory and practice of infrared thermography for nondestructive testing. Wiley, New York
2. Ghali VS, Mulaveesala R (2012) Quadratic frequency modulated thermal wave imaging for non-destructive testing. Prog Electromagn Res M 26:11–22
3. Ghali VS, Subhani S, Mulaveesala R (2013) Applications of feature separation based subsurface analysis for frequency modulated thermal wave imaging. Proc APCNDT, CP-65
4. Yousefi, Bardia,: Application of deep learning in infrared non-destructive testing. QIRT 2018 Proc
5. Saeed N, King N, Said Z, Omar MA (2019) Automatic defects detection in CFRP thermograms, using convolutional neural networks and transfer learning. Infrared Phys Technol 102:103048
6. Fang Q, Nguyen BD, Castanedo CI, Duan Y, Maldague II X (2020) Defects detection in infrared thermography by deep learning algorithm. In: Thermosense: thermal infrared applications XLII, vol 11409, p 114090T. International Society for Optics and Photonics
7. Luo Q, Gao B, Woo WL, Yang Y (2019) Temporal and spatial deep learning network for infrared thermal defect detection. NDT & E Int 108:102164
8. Liu K, Li Y, Yang J, Liu Y, Yao Y (2020) Generative principal component thermography for enhanced defect detection and analysis. IEEE Trans Instrument Measur
9. Liu K, Tang Y, Lou W, Liu Y, Yang J, Yao Y (2020) A thermographic data augmentation and signal separation method for defect detection. Measur Sci Technol
10. Fang Q, Maldague X (2020) A method of defect depth estimation for simulated infrared thermography data with deep learning. Appl Sci 10(19), 6819
11. Wang Q, Liu Q, Xia R, Li G, Gao J, Zhou H, Zhao B (2020) Defect depth determination in laser infrared thermography based on LSTM-RNN. IEEE Access 8:153385–153393
12. Cao Y, Dong Y, Cao Y, Yang J, Ying Yang M (2020) Two-stream convolutional neural network for non-destructive subsurface defect detection via similarity comparison of lock-in thermography signals. NDT&E Int 112:102246
13. Vijaya Lakshmi A, Gopi Tilak V, Parvez MM, Subhani SK, Ghali VS (2019) Artificial neural networks based quantitative evaluation of subsurface anomalies in quadratic frequency modulated thermal wave imaging. Infrared Phys Technol 97:108–115

14. Vijaya LA, Ghali VS, Subhani SK, Baloji NR (2020) Automated quantitative subsurface evaluation of fiber reinforced polymers. Infrared Phys Technol 110:103456
15. Kiranyaz S, Ince T, Abdeljaber O, Avci O, Gabbouj M (2019) 1-d convolutional neural networks for signal processing applications. In: ICASSP 2019–2019 IEEE international conference on acoustics, speech and signal processing (ICASSP). IEEE, pp 8360–8364
16. Kim J-H (2019) Assessment of Electrocardiogram Rhythms by GoogLeNet deep neural network architecture. J Healthcare Eng
17. Li H, Huang J, Ji S (2019) Bearing fault diagnosis with a feature fusion method based on an ensemble convolutional neural network and deep neural network. Sensors 19(9):2034
18. Subhani S, Chandra Sekhar Yadav GVP, Ghali VS (2019) Defect characterization using pulse compression-based quadratic frequency modulated thermal wave imaging. IET Sci Measur Technol 14(2):165–172
19. Krizhevsky A, Sutskever I, Hinton GE (2012) Imagenet classification with deep convolutional neural networks. Adv Neural Inform Process Syst
20. Chung Y, Shrestha R, Lee S, Kim W (2020) Thermographic inspection of internal defects in steel structures: analysis of signal processing techniques in pulsed thermography. Sensors 20(21):6015

Omni-Directional Zeroth Order Resonator (ZOR) Antenna for L-Band Applications

Komal Roy, Rashmi Sinha, Chetan Barde, Sanjay Kumar, Prakash Ranjan, and Anubhav Jain

1 Introduction

Antennas are one of the useful components of communication devices which find its applications ranging from telecommunications to biomedical services, satellite to defenses applications, etc. [1]. As the antenna is used for higher frequency range, one must require larger bandwidth which increases the size and fabrication complexity of the antenna [2]. Additional to this signal received or transmitted by the antenna get faded due to lightning, rain, etc. [3]. Therefore, antenna designs for low frequency are very useful and cover almost all GPS services and satellite services [4]. The L band is one of the most important frequency band used in low frequency region which covers frequency range from 1 to 2 GHz and plays a virtual role in applications such as radars, GPS, radio, telecommunications use, terrestrial communications and telecommunications, and aircraft surveillance [5]. The L band is also a useful band because signals can easily penetrate through fog, rain, storm, clouds, and antennas used in this band can accurately receive data in all weather conditions, day, and night [6]. The antennas reported till date for L band applications are directional and have smaller beam width [7, 8]. To overcome this limitation, this paper presents an Omni-directional radiation pattern ZOR antenna which is one of the applications of CRLH-TL [9]. CRLH-TL is a combination of Right-handed Transmission Line (RH-TL) and Left-Handed Transmission Line (LH-TL). CRLH transmission line consists of series and parallel combination of inductor and capacitor that leads to the

K. Roy (✉) · R. Sinha · C. Barde · S. Kumar (✉)
National Institute of Technology, Jamshedpur, Jharkhand, India
e-mail: 2017rscs004@nitjsr.ac.in

P. Ranjan
Indian Institute of Information Technology, Bhagalpur, Bihar, India

A. Jain
Birla Institute of Technology, Jaipur, India

© The Author(s), under exclusive license to Springer Nature Singapore Pte Ltd. 2021   443
M. K. Bajpai et al. (eds.), *Machine Vision and Augmented Intelligence—Theory and Applications*, Lecture Notes in Electrical Engineering 796,
https://doi.org/10.1007/978-981-16-5078-9_37

Fig. 1 The equivalent
circuit of CRLH-TL (L_R =
Right handed inductor, C_L =
Left handed capacitor, C_R =
Right handed capacitor, L_L
= Left handed inductor

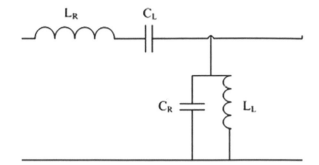

formation of the either series resonance or parallel resonance [10, 11]. So, it can be considered that ZOR can be operated in either series mode or in parallel mode [12] as shown in Fig. 1.

In series mode, resonant frequency depends on the effect of series elements (L_R and C_L), and in parallel mode, resonant frequency depends on the effect of parallel elements (C_R and L_L) as described in Eq. (1) [13].

$$\omega_{se} = \sqrt{L_R C_L} \tag{1}$$

$$\omega_{sh} = \sqrt{C_R L_L} \tag{2}$$

where ω_{se} = series resonant frequency and ω_{sh} = parallel resonant frequency. The antenna is termed as ZOR antenna because at operating frequency the value of relative permittivity (ε) and permeability (μ) are equal to zero, and at this particular frequency, Omni-directional radiation pattern is achieved [14].

This paper presents the Omni-directional ZOR antenna for L-Band applications. Antenna design is a combination of two SRR, in which outer ring is combination of circular shape and inner ring is a combination of a square shape. The unit cell of proposed structure comprises of metallic patch at the top of dielectric substrate FR4. The overall dimensions of the proposed antenna consist of 12 mm × 12 mm, and − 10 dB bandwidth of 20 MHz is achieved ranging from 1810 to 1830 GHz with respect to the center frequency of 1820 GHz. The results obtained in this paper is simulated using Ansys-HFSS 19.1v which is based on Finite Element Method (FEM). Mesh size is kept λ/20 mm so that results obtained are much pre-sized.

2   Antenna Design and Description

The antenna design proposed in this paper consists of three layers. Top and bottom layer are made up of copper ($\varepsilon_r = 1$, loss tangent $\delta = 0$) acting as a conducting material similarly, and the middle layer is made up of FR4 ($\varepsilon_r = 4.4$, loss tangent δ

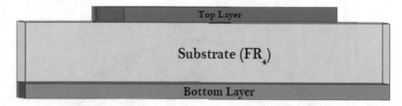

Fig. 2 Three layer structure of a proposed antenna

= 0.02) acting as a dielectric substrate. The structure is designed in such a manner so that dielectric substrate is jammed between the two copper layers as shown in Fig. 2.

The proposed antenna design is a combination of two SRR in which outer rings are combination of circular shape and inner ring is a combination of square shape. Different combinations of circular shape and square shapes are used by hit and trial method to obtain the ZOR behavior, but it is found that if a single circular shape SRR or single square shape SRR or combination of single circular shape and square shape outer most SRR or inner most SRR are used, then Omni-directional radiation pattern is not achieved and all the resonant frequency are available at high frequency with directional radiation pattern. Therefore, the combinations of two SRR of different shapes are used in order to achieve Omni- directional radiation at low frequency region.

The overall dimension of the proposed antenna is 12 mm × 12 mm. In order to feed the antenna gap, feeded line is used. The front view of antenna is shown in Fig. 3.

3 Results and Discussion

The proposed Omni-directional ZOR antenna is designed using hit and trial method and simulated using commercially available FEM solver ANSYS-HFSS 19.1v. The results obtained are discussed in detail.

3.1 Return Loss

The return loss of the proposed antenna obtained after simulation is −12 dB at center frequency of 1820 MHz. The −10 dB bandwidth achieved is 20 MHz ranging from 1810 to 1830 MHz as shown in Fig. 4.

The center frequency is acting as a ZOR frequency where the value of permittivity and permeability is zero, and it is proved by plotting beta vs. frequency plot as shown in Fig. 5.

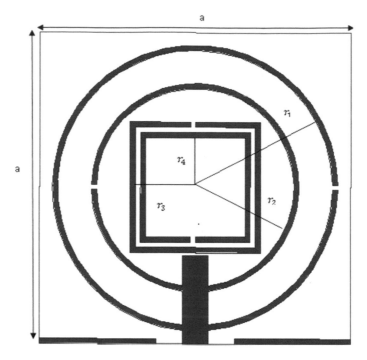

Fig. 3 Front view of proposed ZOR antenna (a $= 12$ mm, $r_1 = 5.5$ mm, $r_2 = 4$ mm, $r_3 = 2.5$ mm, $r_4 = 2$ mm)

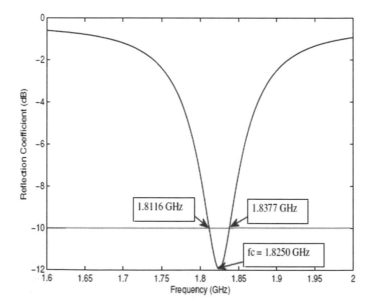

Fig. 4 The reflection coefficient of proposed ZOR antenna

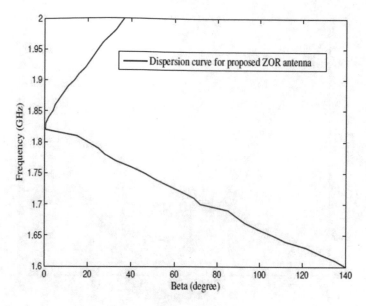

Fig. 5 Beta versus Frequency (Dispersion curve) plot of proposed ZOR antenna

3.2 Voltage Standing Wave Ratio (VSWR)

The VSWR of a simulated result obtain is 1.6766 at 1820 MHz center frequency which implies that proper impedance matching is done between the gap feed line and patch design as shown in Fig. 6.

3.3 Radiation Pattern

The radiation pattern achieved after simulation of the proposed antenna consists of 2-D radiation pattern which resembles almost as a dumbbell shape as shown in Fig. 7a. Figure 7b shows that the complete circle shape is obtained which confirms the Omni-direction radiation pattern.

Figure 8 shows the 3-D radiation pattern along with the proposed antenna, and it is acting as Omni- direction along Z-axis where maximum radiation is along X and Y direction at almost 360°.

3.4 Current Distribution

The current distribution obtained is non-uniform in case of directional antennas, whereas it is uniform in case of Omni-directional ZOR antenna. The current distribution obtained for the proposed antenna is uniform throughout the feed line and patch which confirms the presence of Omni-directional radiation pattern along the antenna as shown in Fig. 9.

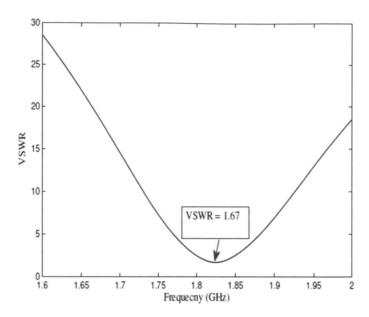

Fig. 6 VSWR plot of proposed ZOR antenna

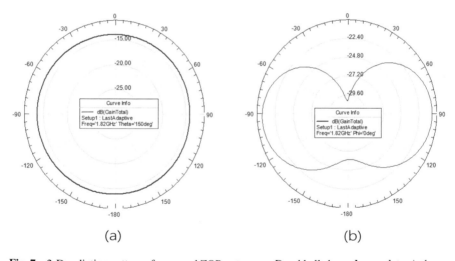

Fig. 7. 2-D radiation pattern of proposed ZOR antenna. **a** Dumbbell shape. **b** complete circle

4 Experimental Setup

The proposed Omni-directional ZOR antenna reflection coefficient is measured inside the Anechoic-Chamber with the help of Vector Network Analyzer (VNA). The experimental set inside the Anechoic-Chamber is shown in Fig. 10.

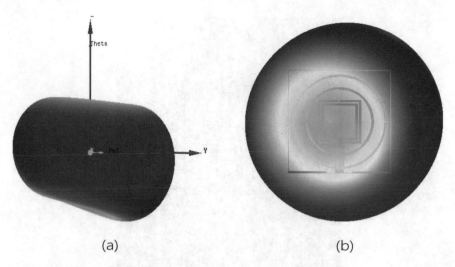

(a)   (b)

Fig. 8. 3-D radiation pattern of proposed ZOR antenna. **a** Omni-direction along Z axis. **b** Omni-direction along antenna

Fig. 9 Uniform current distribution of proposed ZOR antenna

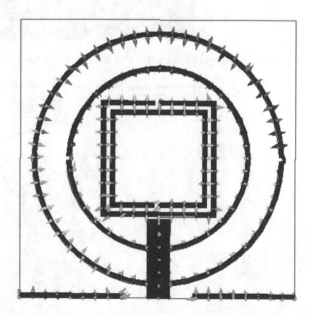

The measured result and simulated result plots are portrayed in Fig. 11, and it is observed that both the plots are almost similar to each other with little bit of variation due to setup.

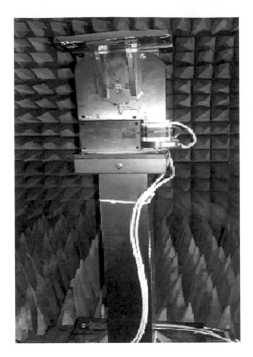

Fig. 10 The proposed ZOR antenna placed in a pedestal stand inside the Anechoic-Chamber

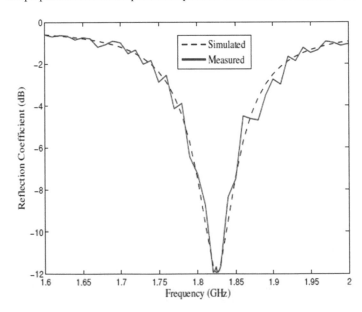

Fig. 11 The reflection coefficient of measured and simulated proposed ZOR antenna

5 Conclusion

The proposed Omni-directional ZOR antenna structure comprises of metallic patch at the top of dielectric substrate FR_4. The proposed antenna works at a center frequency of 1820 MHz with -10 dB bandwidth of 20 MHz ranging from 1810 to 1830 MHz. The antenna operates for L-Band applications especially for telecommunications services. The overall dimension of proposed antenna is 12 mm $\times$ 12 mm. The radiation pattern of proposed antenna is Omni-directional which is proved by current distribution plot, 2-D radiation and 3-D radiation plots. The current distribution obtains in uniform through the structure. The ZOR frequency is proved by beta vs. frequency plot. All the simulation is carried out through commercially available FEM solver ANSYS-HFSS 19.1v. The experimental result obtained is tested inside the Anechoic-Chamber. Mesh size is kept $\lambda/20$ mm so that results obtained are much pre-sized.

References

1. Johnson RC, Jasik H (194) Antenna engineering handbook. McGraw-Hill Book Company, New York, 1356 p. No individual items are abstracted in this volume (1984)
2. McAllister MW, Andrew Long S, Conway GL (1983) Rectangular dielectric resonator antenna. Electron Lett 19(6):218–219
3. Huff GH et al (2003) A novel radiation pattern and frequency reconfigurable single turn square spiral microstrip antenna. IEEE Microwave Wirel Components Lett 13(2):57–59
4. Thid B et al (2007) Utilization of photon orbital angular momentum in the low-frequency radio domain. Phys Rev Lett 99(8):087701
5. Karmakar NC, Bialkowski ME (1999) Circularly polarized aperture-coupled circular microstrip patch antennas for L-band applications. IEEE Trans Antennas Propag 47(5):933–940
6. Fu S et al (2009) Broadband circularly polarized slot antenna array fed by asymmetric CPW for L-band applications. IEEE Antennas Wirel Propag Lett 8:1014–1016
7. Cao B et al (2015) High-gain L-probe excited substrate integrated cavity antenna array with LTCC- based gap waveguide feeding network for W-band application. IEEE Trans Antennas Propag 63(12):5465–5474
8. Ali T, Biradar RC (2017) A compact hexagonal slot dual band frequency reconfigurable antenna for WLAN applications. Microwave Opt Technol Lett 59(4):958–964
9. Alibakhshi-Kenari M et al (2016) New compact antenna based on simplified CRLHTL for UWB wireless communication systems. Int J RF Microwave Comput Aided Eng 26(3):217–225
10. Huang C et al (2018) A planar multiband antenna based on CRLH-TL ZOR for 4G compact mobile terminal applications. In: 2018 international workshop on antenna technology (iWAT). IEEE
11. Luo Xin-Shuai et al (2018) Broadband and wide beamwidth circularly polarized antenna based on CRLHTL for navigation terminal applications. Microwave Opt Technol Lett 60(7):1638–1644
12. Ibrahim AA, Abdalla MA, Hu Z (2018) Compact ACS-fed CRLH MIMO antenna for wireless applications. IET Microwaves Antennas Propag 12(6):1021–1025
13. Nuthakki, Rajasekhar V, Dhamodharan SK (2018) Bandwidth enhancement of ZOR antenna by loading novel via-Less CRLH-TL unit cells. AEU-Int J Electron Commun 83:501–511
14. Huang C, Jiao Y-C, Weng Z (2018) Novel compact CRLHTL based triband MIMO antenna element for the 5G mobile handsets. Microwave Opt Technol Lett 60(10):2559–2564

Detection of Acute Lymphoblastic Leukemia by Utilizing Deep Learning Methods

Gundepudi V. Surya Sashank, Charu Jain, and N. Venkateswaran

1 Introduction

Leukemia is a type of cancer that spreads through the blood and lymph tissues to inhibit the blood-forming tissues' abilities to fight off infections. To be able to identify the presence of Leukemia, blood cell segmentation and identification is pivotal. However, an issue arises when a large amount of blood samples is required by hematologists to help detect this presence. White blood cells contain essential data that assists hematologists in distinguishing numerous diseases, including leukemia. In terms of modernization, analyzing the blood samples can help in screening leukemia.

To be able to detect the existence or non-existence of a certain illness in a patient, diagnosis must be performed by a human physician by inferring from a dataset which can consist of signs, symptoms, medical images, and exams [1]. An incorrect diagnostic report can bear hostile results, for instance, prescription of medication with undesirable side effects on the patient's health. Incorrect diagnosis may also complicate the treatment procedures, and this may lead to act as a financial burden on the patient [2]. To assist hematologists achieve a greater diagnostic accuracy, various number of assistant systems were recommended. Many diseases, including glaucoma [3], skin cancer [4], breast cancer [5], and leukemia [6], are already addressed by such systems. Employing such assistant systems may help yield accurate and rapid results which could effectively subside diagnostic and treatment costs, increase the chances of remission, or even prolong the patient's life [7]. Leukemia can arise

G. V. Surya Sashank (✉) · C. Jain · N. Venkateswaran
Sri Sivasubramanya Nadar College of Engineering, Kalavakkam, Chennai 603110, India
e-mail: gundepudi18047@mech.ssn.edu.in

C. Jain
e-mail: charu18033@ece.ssn.edu.in

N. Venkateswaran
e-mail: venkateswarann@ssn.edu.in

from several causes, such as exposure to radiation and certain chemicals, as well as family history [8]. A physician can diagnose leukemia via a number of tests, such as, inspecting for physical signs such as a pale skin from anemia or the inflammation of the lymph nodes. Leukemia can also be diagnosed with a blood test, by observing the images of the blood cells or by a bone marrow biopsy which uses a specialized test to reveal the presence or absence of Leukemia. However, such methods of diagnosis can be unreliable and also expensive. Since these diagnoses need to be performed by a human physician, it may also take time which could be used for treating the patient. Therefore, an automated, accurate, and affordable system that can distinguish between healthy and unhealthy blood smear images is a desideratum [1, 4, 6–10].

Since ALL diagnosis associates closely with morphological changes of WBCs and manual morphological analysis may experience the ill effects from several potential limitations [1, 4, 7], numerous automatic ALL diagnosis techniques have been proposed in recent years [1, 4, 6, 7, 9]. To accomplish robust and effective computerized diagnosis, distinguishing the attributes of healthy and blast cells is a crucial factor. Although many studies on the separation and recovery of the nucleus and cytoplasm or purely nuclei of the cells utilizing segmentation techniques are available, limited investigations have been led on the selection of significant discriminative attributes from the segmented regions to effectively benefit subsequent ALL diagnosis [1, 4, 6, 8–10].

This research plans to deal with the aforementioned challenges by proposing two classification systems using machine learning models. The dataset ALL-IDB2 [11] consists of 260 segmented lymphocytes of which 130 are ALL affected blood images and the remaining 130 belong to the healthy class. Using data augmentation, the dataset size was increased from 260 to 760 images.

For the Hybrid AlexNet and Machine Learning based ALL detection model, these images were pre-processed before feeding them to the pre-trained CNN, AlexNet for feature extraction, and subsequently different classifiers were used for efficaciously separating ALL positive blood images. Further on, the AlexNet based ALL detection model used AlexNet for feature extraction as well as classification after image pre-processing. The metrics of classifiers were then analyzed, and the most efficient algorithm among them was found. Promising results were obtained through the second detection model with an accuracy of 100%.

2 Literature Review

Maria et al. [7] predicted leukemia using Support Vector Machines, k-Nearest Neighbors, Neural Networks, Naïve Bayes, and Deep Learning and also compared their performances. For diagnosis of leukemia using blood images, Vogado et al. [1] utilized a Convolutional Neural Network, along with Support Vector Machine, Multilayer Perceptron, and Random Forest thereby introducing a new framework. This framework was different, requiring less processing time as it did not implement segmentation.

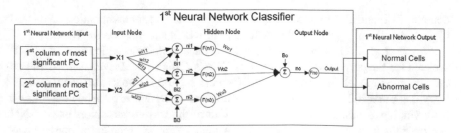

Fig. 1 A simple neural network classifier [8]

Laosai et al. [4] categorized lymphoid stem cells and myeloid stem by making use of K Means clustering in order to assess his new classifier framework. The features including shape and texture were extracted from the segmented cytoplasm and nucleus. SVM surpassed all the classifiers with 92% accuracy.

Subhan [9] analyzed cancerous cells using image processing algorithms to reduce the expense and also to increase the accuracy.

Supardi et al. [6] differentiated acute myelogenous leukemia (AML) and acute lymphocytic leukemia (ALL) by utilizing k-NN. 80% accuracy was achieved using cosine distance metric.

Vincent et al. [8] also segregated AML and ALL leukemia types using 100 blood smear images. After extracting GLCM and fractal features, 97.7% accuracy was reached utilizing neural network classifier.

Adjouadi et al. [10] utilized 220 blood samples and implemented ANN architecture to classify ALL and AML. This produced very high sensitivity results which increased with increased data set size.

Loey et al. [2] detected leukemia using transfer learning which solved many problems and also proposed two classification models set up on blood images (Fig. 1).

Gautam et al. [12] utilized Otsu thresholding for segmentation and Naïve Bayes for classification. At an average time of 22 s per image, 68 images were classified at an accuracy rate of 80.88%.

Chen et al. [3] proposed a new DL architecture consisting of four convolutional layers and two fully-connected layers utilizing ORIGA and SCES datasets. For detecting glaucoma, the area under the curve (AUC) for the two databases was found to be 0.831 and 0.887 in the receiver operating characteristic curve.

For skin lesion classification, Kawahara and Hamarneh [13] proposed a CNN architecture utilizing various images which would work for multi-resolution input. Wang et al. [5] obtained 0.7051 as a score for tumor localization task and AUC to be 0.925 image classification. This system was combined with a pathologist's analyses which resulted in an increased AUC of 0.995. Agaian et al. [14] proposed a method in which 80 blood images were utilized to obtain 98% accuracy for isolation from sub and complete images and also for localization of the lymphoblast cells.

Thanh et al. [15] made use of 1188 blood cell images which were used for segregating normal and abnormal blood cell images. 96.6% accuracy was achieved after implementing a CNN. A contour aware segmentation was proposed by Imran Razzak and Naz [16] and also used ML based on CNN features for classification on 64,000 blood cells. Results gave 94.71% accuracy for RBCs and 98.68% for WBCs.

Sajjad et al. [17] proposed a framework on a cellphone which is also cloud-assisted for the purpose of localization of WBCs. This was achieved using a trained classification model. In the end, the WBCs were separated into five different classes.

A computer aided ALL diagnosis system was introduced by Abdeldaim et al. [18] which was based on image analysis. Out of the various classifiers used, k-NN achieved the best classification accuracy. An automatic cell recognition system was proposed by Yu et al. [19] which was implemented by applying DL methods. The results obtained made it clear that the leukocytes were recognized with less hardware limitations and higher accuracy.

Pansombut et al. [20] executed a CNN classifier in order to distinguish lymphocytes and ALL subtypes. Classification was implemented using multilayer perceptron (MLP) and random forest. Automated image based ALL detection system was employed by Kumar et al. [21] using k-means clustering algorithm. The model accomplished an accuracy of 92.8% which was tested with kNN and Naïve Bayes Classifier on 60 samples. Madhukar et al. [22] utilized 50 images and demonstrated that the classification of blood smear images containing multiple nuclei can be completely automated. The correctly grouped cases were around 93.5% which stands as a testament that the technique yields good results.

Setiawan et al. [23] performed classification on 1710 cells which were derived from bone marrow. Eight cell types were utilized from three precursor cells. Classification was performed after segmentation and feature selection in a sequential manner.

In order to solve a similar problem, Rehman et al. [24] proposed a method which consisted of a CNN segmentation and DL techniques. He implemented the model in an attempt to train bone marrow images for classification and achieved an accuracy rate of 97.78%.

Another attempt at implementing a computer-aided diagnosis framework was made by Faiydullah et al. [25] in order to characterize leukemia from blood microscopic images.

Using Zack algorithm and histogram equalization, Patel and Mishra [26] made use of k-mean clustering approach for white blood cell detection. 93% accuracy was achieved by SVM for classification. Microarray gene expression profiles were used by Dwivedi [27] who devised a framework which was based on supervised machine learning for the diagnosis of ALL and AML. The Artificial neural network which was used for classification was evaluated using eight different classification metrics and achieved an accuracy rate of 98%. The only error was in the identification of AML on tenfold cross-validation and leave-one-out approach.

Krizhevsky et al. [28] came up with the CNN, Alexnet and explained its architecture and features. A review of computer-aided diagnosis systems was performed by Shafique and Tehsin [29] who differentiated them based on their methodologies that incorporated enhancement, segmentation, feature extraction, classification, and accuracy.

A summary of the literature survey can be seen in Table 1.

Table 1 Summary of literature survey

Authors	Method	Number of images	Classification	Performance (%)
Vogado et al. [1]	CNN	108	SVM, Multilayer Perceptron, Random Forest	100
Laosai and Chamnongthai [4]	Image processing	100	SVM	92
Subhan and Kaur [9]	Hough transform	–	kNN	93
Supardi et al. [6]	12 features manually extracted	1500	kNN	86
Vincent et al. [8]	CNN	100	Neural network	97.7
Adjaoudi et al. [10]	ANN	220	SVM, ANN	96.67
Loey et al. [2]	CNN	2820	CNN	100
Gautam et al. [12]	Image processing	88	Naïve Bayes	80.88
Chen et al. [3]	CNN	650	Soft-max classifier	88.7
Kawahara and Hamarneh [13]	CNN	–	CNN	–
Wang et al. [5]	CNN	400	GoogLeNet, AlexNet, VGG16	98.4
Agaian et al. [14]	Image processing	80	SVM	98
Thanh et al. [15]	CNN	1188	FC	96.6
Imaran Razzak and Naz [16]	CNN	108	Extreme Learning Machine	90.1
Sajjad et al. [17]	Mobile cloud computing	1030	SVM	94.3
Abdeldaim et al. [18]	ANN	260	k-NN	–
Yu et al. [19]	CNN	2000	CNN	88.5
Pansombut et al. [20]	CNN	363	FC	80
Kumar et al. [21]	Image processing	60	kNN, Naïve Bayes	92.8
Madhukar et al. [22]	Image processing	50	SVM	93.5
Setiawan et al. [23]	Image processing	105	SVM	98.67
Rehman et al. [24]	CNN	330	FC	97.78

(continued)

Table 1 (continued)

Authors	Method	Number of images	Classification	Performance (%)
Faivdullah et al. [25]	Image processing	100	–	79.38
Patel and Mishra [26]	Image processing	77	SVM	93.57
Dwivedi [27]	ANN	–	ANN	98%
Shafique and Tehsin [29]	CNN	260	FC	96.06

3 Methods

Deep transfer learning is adopted for the two systems in order to differentiate ALL lymphocytes from healthy ones in this paper. Transfer learning gives results faster, and the effort is also reduced in designing the models from scratch without compromising the efficacy (Figs. 2 and 3).

Both the models made use of a pre-trained convolutional neural network. One of the most observable features of leukemia disease is the uncontrollable proliferation of abnormal white blood cells inside human bone marrow. Due to this proven fact, it is understandable that normal and abnormal white blood cell images can be roughly classified based on the quantity of white blood cells that appear under one frame of peripheral blood smear image. As for leukemia type classification, it can be done by

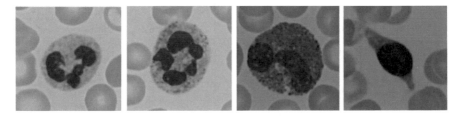

Fig. 2 Healthy Lymphocytes

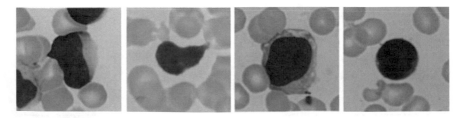

Fig. 3 ALL affected Lymphocytes

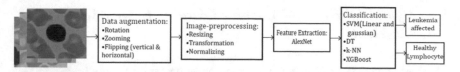

Fig. 4 Diagram representing the first detection model

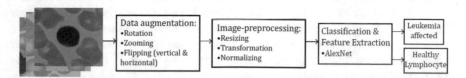

Fig. 5 Diagram to represent the second detection model

proper extraction of key differentiating features from each leukemia type. Figure 4 shows the Hybrid AlexNet and Machine Learning based ALL detection system which begins with data augmentation which includes rotation, zooming, and flipping (both horizontal and vertical). This is followed by resizing, transformation, and normalizing as a part of image pre-processing. Finally feature extraction and classification is implemented by AlexNet and five well-known classifiers, respectively. On the other hand, AlexNet is employed for both feature extraction and classification in the AlexNet based ALL detection model, which is visualized in Fig. 5.

3.1 Dataset Description

The ALL-IDB is a database containing images of blood cells and was released in two version ALL-IDB1 and ALL-IDB2. All images in the datasets have a typical resolution equal to 2592 × 1994, captured with a PowerShot G5 camera [1]. The version, ALL-IDB2 [11] comprises 260 segmented lymphocytes of which 130 are Acute Lymphoblastic Leukemia positive blood images and the remaining 130 are healthy lymphocytes. Figures 2 and 3 depict ALL free lymphocytes and ALL affected blood samples, respectively. Data Augmentation is adopted to increase the size of the data-set to create new training data from existing training data. After utilizing data augmentation, the dataset increased from containing 260 images to 760 images by trying to rotate the image by a certain angle, zooming into the images at different rates and flipping the images both horizontally and vertically.

3.2 Hybrid AlexNet and Machine Learning Based ALL Detection

This system consists of three steps: image pre-processing, feature extraction, and classification.

Image Pre-processing. Pre-processing of the 760 images was done to alter the data to a machine-readable format. Within this step the images are first resized into an image with a resolution of 256x256. The image is now transformed into a Tensor containing three values, the channel of the image, the height of the image, and the width of the image. The tensor is then normalized using the standard mean of [0.485, 0.456, 0.406], and a standard deviation of [0.229, 0.224, 0.225] for AlexNet to ensure all the data lies within the same range.

Feature Extraction. Feature extraction is choosing the best possible analytical features, depicting the picture by the mathematical qualities, and enabling the programmed framework to perform the recognition [4]. In computer vision and image processing, feature extraction is a procedure that reduces the images' data into a large set of features that holds information about the images' dimensions and colors. This process of elicitation of features from the input images *feature extraction*. Highlight determination significantly impacts the classifier execution; therefore, a right selection of highlights is a critical advance [14]. Generally, a considerable lot of the features use texture, geometrical, and statistical analyses of the image. This selection aims to eliminate unnecessary attributes and consequently simplify the prediction model, decreasing the computational expense, giving a superior comprehension of the outcomes discovered [4]. These features are considered to help the classifier execution [1]. As indicated by [26], feature determination frameworks are fundamentally utilized to distinguish significant properties and basic data.

An ideal choice of properties for classification issues requires a comprehensive search of every single imaginable subset of attributes [27], making it unrealistic when the quantity of characteristics is excessively high. For this reason, several researchers have created diverse attribute selection methods. Each of these techniques uses distinct selection criteria and search algorithms to assess and to discover heuristically the most suitable subset of attributes [4].

A CNN is a network formed by several layers that can be utilized in object recognition and image classification. Among these layers, we have the convolutional layers that can modify the representation of the data through filters. For the most part after a convolutional layer, an activation function is used, and these functions perform non-linear transformations in the data, in order to generate linearly separable outputs. One of the most common functions used with this purpose is the Rectified Linear units (ReLu), presented in Eq. (1), where x is the input to a neuron.

The pretrained AlexNet uses in-built functions to extract the features from the image by applying a convolution on the 2-dimensional plane and activating the rectified linear unit function element-wise. This helps us extract the required features of each and every image.

$$\text{Relu}(x) = \max(0, x) \tag{1}$$

Classification. Classification is a type of supervised learning that aims to categorize a given set of data into various classes. In this case, the classifiers were implemented to separate ALL lymphocytes from healthy ones by making use of the pre-processed images. 75% of the dataset was used to train the classifiers, and the remaining 25% was used to test it.

The different classifiers tested were k Nearest Neighbors, Support Vector Machine (linear and Gaussian), Decision Trees, and XGBoost.

Support Vector Machine (SVM). Support vector machines are one of broadly utilized algorithms for leukemia detection. This algorithm is utilized to output and optimize hyperplanes that characterizes the given information based on their features. The fundamental reason behind the selection of SVM for leukemia detection is that it is a binary classifier that can efficaciously classify between normal and affected cells. The goal of the support vector machine algorithm is to discover a hyperplane in an N-dimensional space that particularly orders the data points. To separate the two classes of data points, there are numerous conceivable hyperplanes that could be picked. The objective is to locate a plane that has the greatest distance between data points of the two classes. Maximizing the margin distance gives some support, so future information focuses can be characterized with more certainty.

K-Nearest Neighbor (KNN). The k-nearest neighbors' (KNN) algorithm is a basic supervised machine learning algorithm which categorizes a data point depending on the nearest neighboring data points. K-nearest neighbor is a generally utilized classification and regression technique that uses the nonparametric and lazy learning method to group diverse information. In k-nearest neighbor algorithm, classification is done by the voting from the nearest neighbors. In light of this voting, objects will be relegated to their applicable classes. For acute lymphoblastic leukemia cell classification, k-NN classifier is utilized to improve classification results for the normal and blast cells [29].

XGBoost. It is an optimized distributed gradient boosting library intended to be exceptionally proficient, adaptable, and versatile.

Decision Trees. It is a Supervised Machine Learning technique, i.e., it can explain what the input is and what the corresponding output is in the training data, where the data is continuously split indicated by a certain parameter. The tree can be explained by two elements, in particular, decision nodes and leaves. The leaves are the decisions or the ultimate results. And the decision nodes are the place where the data is split.

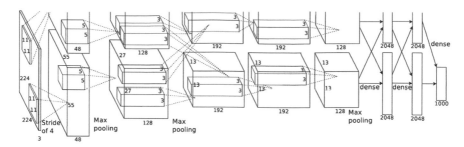

Fig. 6 AlexNet architecture [28]

3.3 AlexNet Based ALL Detection

In this system of detection, both feature extraction and classification were implemented using the pre-trained CNN, AlexNet after data augmentation, and image pre-processing.

AlexNet Architecture. The general architecture of the CNN, AlexNet was depicted by Krizhevsky et al. [28] which contained eight layers with weights. Out of these, the initial five are convolutional and the remaining are fully connected. When the output of the last fully-connected layer was fed to a 1000-way softmax, a distribution was created. This maximized the multinomial logistic regression objective, which was comparable to maximizing the average across training cases of the right label's log-probability under the prediction distribution.

The kernel maps of the previous layers of the second, fourth, and fifth convolutional layers are distinctly associated to each other since they reside on the same GPU (see Fig. 6). Also, the kernel maps of the second layer are connected to the kernels of the third convolutional. In this architecture, the first and second layers are followed by the response-normalization layers. And similarly, the fifth convolutional layer and the response normalization layer are followed by max-pooling layers. Finally, the output of each convolutional and fully-connected layer is obtained. The ReLU non-linearity is applied on the output obtained.

Feature Extraction and Classification. The pretrained AlexNet model which is based on CNN was implemented on the dataset which was divided into 75% for training and 25% for testing. The CNN was configured for the used data, and the final three layers were fine-tuned through transfer learning.

3.3.1 Performance Evaluation Metrics in Classification

In order to ensure the effectiveness of the presented system, we employed certain measures based on which decisions were made. Certain metrics that are used for the purpose of evaluating the classifiers are mentioned in this section. Some of the important terms to be noted are explained in the confusion matrix depicted in Table 2.

A confusion matrix is a table that is used to help visualize the performance of a classification algorithm on a dataset for which the number of true values is known. The columns in a confusion matrix represent the true values of the category, and the rows represent the predicted values of the same.

Precision. Precision is the ratio of the number of true positives to the sum of true positives and false positives. Therefore, it tells us how many of the classified items are relevant. With respect to our problem at hand, it gives us the proportion of the images which have been classified correctly, either as ALL affected or not, with respect to the total number of classified images.

$$Prescision = TP/(TP + FP) \tag{2}$$

Recall (Sensitivity). Recall quantifies the number of correctly predicted positive instances with respect to the total number of actually positive instances belonging to the dataset. Therefore, it gives us the proportion of images it has classified as ALL affected with respect to the total number of ALL affected images.

$$Recall = TP/(TP + FN) \tag{3}$$

Accuracy. It computes the ratio of the number of correctly predicted data points with respect to the total number of data-points present in the dataset. It includes the correctly classifying ALL affected and also healthy lymphocytes.

$$Accuracy = (TP + FN)/(TP + TN + FP + FN) \tag{4}$$

Specificity. Specificity is the fraction of leukemia patients without cancer who are tested negative. Specificity quantifies the number of negative class predictions made out of all negative examples in the data-set.

$$Specificity = TN/(TN + FP) \tag{5}$$

Table 2 Confusion matrix

	Actually positive (1)	Actually negative (0)
Predicted positive (1)	True Positive (TP) Lymphocyte images correctly predicted to be infected with ALL	False Positive (FP) Lymphocyte images wrongly predicted to be infected with ALL
Predicted negative (0)	False Negative (FN) Lymphocyte images wrongly predicted to be healthy	True Negative (TN) Lymphocyte images correctly predicted to be healthy

F-Measure. F-measure is a single score that can help balance the concerns of precision and recall. It is evaluated as the harmonic mean of Precision and Recall.

$$F\text{-Measure} = (2 \times \text{precision} \times \text{recall})/(\text{precision} + \text{recall}) \tag{6}$$

4 Experimental Results and Discussion

Jupyter Notebooks were utilized to implement both the classification systems. 760 microscopic lymphocyte images were considered for evaluation.

In the Hybrid AlexNet and Machine Learning based ALL detection model, after data pre-processing, the features were extracted to train the classifiers using AlexNet. Classification techniques k-NN, SVM, Decision trees, and XGBoost were employed on a dataset which was divided into 75% for training data and the rest for testing. Gaussian and linear kernel functions were used with the SVM classifier. The k-NN classifier was implemented by setting $k = 6$, and the maximum number of iterations was set to 30.

The performances of all classifiers were evaluated using Specificity, Accuracy, Recall and Accuracy. Table 3 shows the performance of each classifier which was implemented. Here, Recall takes into account the lymphocyte images that are wrongly predicted to be healthy, and since we are focusing on ALL affected images, recall scores are important. Similarly, as F1 score is the harmonic mean of Precision and Recall, both F1 score and Recall values were observed to evaluate the classifiers. Linear SVM gave the highest Recall and F1 scores.

According to the given data, the AlexNet based ALL detection system using AlexNet yielded accuracy of 100% on 1.00e-04 learning rate with 30 epochs and batch size set to 32 (Table 4).

Table 3 Results for classification for the CNN and other classifiers

Classification methods		Precision (%)	Recall (sensitivity) (%)	F1-measure (%)	Accuracy (%)	Specificity (%)
First system	SVM (Linear)	99	97	98	98.17	98.73
	SVM (Gaussian)	99	96	97	97.43	98.73
	Decision trees	87	92	88	87.82	83.50
	XGBoost	95	97	96	96.15	94.93
	k-NN	96	97	97	96.79	96.20
Second system	AlexNet	100	100	100	100	100

Table 4 Confusion matrix Values for employed classifiers

Classification methods		True Positives	False Positives	True Negatives	False Negatives
First system	SVM (Linear)	98	2	89	1
	SVM (Gaussian)	96	4	89	1
	Decision trees	86	14	81	9
	XGBoost	95	5	88	2
	k-NN	99	1	87	3
Second system	AlexNet	100	0	90	0

Good accuracy rate for all implementations was received even with low learning rate with a smaller number of epochs. Even for the second model, the dataset was divided into 75% training data and 25% test data, i.e., 97% and 98% respectively in the first system of detection. Nevertheless, AlexNet is the best classifier with 100% F1 and recall scores proving to be the better model out of the two models.

5 Conclusion

The proposed methods have been performed on 760 lymphocyte images from the ALL-IDB2 dataset of which 570 images are utilized for training, while 190 pictures are saved for testing. The early recognition of acute lymphoblastic leukemia can help adequately in its treatment. For the same reason, in this paper, we proposed two classification models recognizing sans leukemia and leukemia-affected blood lymphocyte images. The two models utilize transfer learning. In the Hybrid AlexNet and Machine Learning based ALL detection model, a pre-processed CNN known as AlexNet is utilized for feature extraction, and other notable classifiers, for example, Decision Tree, XGBoost, SVM (linear and Gaussian), and k-NN, were utilized for classification of the blood lymphocytes. Trials exhibited the predominance of the linear SVM classifier with the highest F1 score and Recall of 98.15% and 98% respectively. The AlexNet based ALL detection model utilizes AlexNet for both feature extraction and classification and outperforms all aforementioned classifiers with a 100% score for all metrics.

Acknowledgements We are thankful to Scotti [11] for providing us with a high-quality image database.

References

1. Vogado LHS, Veras RDMS, Andrade AR, De Araujo FHD, de Silva RRV, Aires KRT (2017) Diagnosing leukemia in blood smear images using an ensemble of classifiers and pre-trained convolutional neural networks. In: Proceedings of the 2017 IEEE 30th SIBGRAPI conference on graphics, patterns and images (SIBGRAPI), Niteroi, Brazil, 17–20 October 2017, pp 367–373
2. Loey M, Naman M, Zayed H (2020) Deep transfer learning in diagnosing leukemia in blood cells. Computers 9:29. https://doi.org/10.3390/computers9020029
3. Chen X, Xu Y, Wong DWK, Wong TY, Liu J (2015) Glaucoma detection based on deep convolutional neural network. In Proceedings of the 2015 37th annual international conference of the IEEE engineering in medicine and biology society (EMBC), Milan, Italy, 25–29 August 2015. IEEE, Piscataway, NJ, USA, pp 715–718
4. Laosai J, Chamnongthai K (2014) Acute leukemia classification by using SVM and K-Means clustering. In: 2014 IEEE international electrical engineering congress (iEECON), Chonburi, Thailand, 19–21 March 2014, pp 1–4
5. Wang D, Khosla A, Gargeya R, Irshad H, Beck AH (2020) Deep learning for identifying metastatic breast cancer. Computers 9:29, 11 of 12. arXiv arXiv:1606.05718
6. Supardi NZ, Mashor MY, Harun NH, Bakri FA, Hassan R (2012) Classification of blasts in acute leukemia blood samples using k-nearest neighbour. In: IEEE 8th international colloquium on signal processing and its applications, pp 461–65
7. Maria IJ, Devi T, Ravi D (2020) Machine learning algorithms for Diagnosis of Leukemia. Int J Sci Technol Res 9(1). ISSN 2277-8616
8. Vincent I, Kwon K-R, Lee S-H, Moon K-S (2015) Acute lymphoid leukemia classification using two-step neural network classifier. In: 21st Korea-Japan joint workshop on frontiers of computer vision (FCV), January 2015
9. Subhan KP (2015) Significant analysis of Leukemic Cells extraction and detection using KNN and Hough Transform Algorithm. Int J Comput Sci Trends Technol 3(1): 27–33
10. Adjouadi M, Ayala M, Cabrerizo M et al (2010) Classification of leukemia blood samples using neural networks. Ann Biomed Eng 38(4):1473–1482
11. Scotti F, Labati RD, Piuri V (2020) ALL-IDB (Acute Lymphoblastic leukaemia-International Database). IEEE Dataport, October 15, 2020
12. Gautam A, Singh P, Raman B, Bhadauria H (2016) Automatic classification of leukocytes using morphological features and Naïve Bayes classifier. IEEE Region 10 conference (TENCON), pp 1023–1027, November 2016
13. Kawahara J, Hamarneh G (2016) Multi-resolution-tract CNN with hybrid pretrained and skin-lesion trained layers. In: Proceedings of the international workshop on machine learning in medical imaging, Athens, Greece, 17 October 2016. Springer, Cham/Canton of Zug, Switzerland, pp 164–171
14. Agaian S, Madhukar M, Chronopoulos AT (2014) Automated screening system for acute myelogenous leukemia detection in blood microscopic images. IEEE Syst J 8:995–1004
15. Thanh TTP, Vununu C, Atoev S, Lee S-H, Kwon K-R (2018) Leukemia blood cell image classification using convolutional neural network. Int J Comput Theory Eng 10:54–58
16. Imran Razzak M, Naz S (2017) Microscopic blood smear segmentation and classification using deep contour aware CNN and extreme machine learning. Proceedings of the IEEE Conference on Computer Vision and Pattern Recognition Workshops, Honolulu, HI, USA 21–26:49–55
17. Sajjad M, Khan S, Jan Z, Muhammad K, Moon H, Kwak JT, Rho S, Baik SW, Mehmood I (2016) Leukocytes classification and segmentation in microscopic blood smear: A resource-aware healthcare service in smart cities. IEEE Access 5:3475–3489
18. Abdeldaim AM, Sahlol AT, Elhoseny M, Hassanien AE (2018) Computer-aided acute lymphoblastic leukemia diagnosis system based on image analysis. In: Advances in soft computing and machine learning in image processing. Springer, Berlin/Heidelberg, Germany, pp 131–147

19. Yu W, Chang J, Yang C, Zhang L, Shen H, Xia Y, Sha J (2017) Automatic classification of leukocytes using deep neural network. In: Proceedings of the 2017 IEEE 12th international conference on ASIC (ASICON), Guiyang, China, 25–28 October 2017. IEEE, Piscataway, NJ, USA, pp 1041–1044

20. Pansombut T, Wikaisuksakul S, Khongkraphan K, Phon-on A (2019) Convolutional neural networks for recognition of lymphoblast cell images. Comput Intell Neurosci 2019:7519603

21. Kumar S, Mishra S, Asthana P (2018) Automated detection of acute leukemia using k-mean clustering algorithm. In: Advances in computer and computational sciences. Springer, Berlin/Heidelberg, Germany, pp 655–670. Classification of Blasts in Acute Leukemia Blood Samples Using k-Nearest Neighbour—IEEE Conference Publication.

22. Madhukar M, Agaian S, Chronopoulos AT(2012) Deterministic model for acute myelogenous leukemia classification. In: Proceedings of the 2012 IEEE international conference on systems, man, and cybernetics (SMC), Seoul, Korea, 14–17 October 2012, pp 433–438

23. Setiawan A, Harjoko A, Ratnaningsih T, Suryani E, Palgunadi S (2018) Classification of cell types in Acute Myeloid Leukemia (AML) of M4, M5 and M7 subtypes with support vector machine classifier. In: Proceedings of the 2018 international conference on information and communications technology (ICOIACT), Yogyakarta, Indonesia, 6–7 March 2018, pp 45–49

24. Rehman A, Abbas N, Saba T, Ur Rahman SI, Mehmood Z, Kolivand H (2018) Classification of acute lymphoblastic leukemia using deep learning. Microsc Res Tech 81(11), 23 October 2018

25. Faivdullah L, Azahar F, Htike ZZ, Naing WN (2015) Leukemia detection from blood smears. J Med Bioeng 4:488–491

26. Patel N, Mishra A (2015) Automated leukaemia detection using microscopic images. Procedia Comput Sci 58:635–642

27. Dwivedi AK (2018) Artificial neural network model for effective cancer classification using microarray gene expression data. Neural Comput Appl 29:1545–1554

28. Krizhevsky A, Sutskever I, Hinton GE (2012) Imagenet classification with deep convolutional neural networks. In Proceedings of the advances in neural information processing systems, Lake Tahoe, CA, USA, 3–8 December 2012, pp 1097–1105

29. Shafique S, Tehsin S (2018) computer-aided diagnosis of Acute Lymphoblastic Leukaemia. In: Hindawi computational and mathematical methods in medicine, vol 2018, Article ID 6125289, 13 p

Feature Optimization of Digital Image Watermarking Using Machine Learning Algorithms

Manish Rai, Sachin Goyal, and Mahesh Pawar

1 Introduction

The transformation of the digital area of data needs security and copyright protection. The security and copyright protection process worked digital watermarking methods. The digital watermarking methods give the ownership of digital data over the communication network by the nature of digital watermarking deals in two different approaches, such as spatial domain and pixel-based domain [1–3]. The limited approach of pixel-based watermarking methods always tampered and lost the copyright protection and integrity of digital data. Over the pixel-based watermarking methods, the spatial process of digital watermarking had a large number of several algorithms and increased the security strength of digital watermarking. The continuous improvements of robustness of digital watermarking are based on transform function, the birth of feature based watermarking algorithms. Feature based watermarking algorithms used various transform-based function such as DCT ($Discrete\ Cosine\ Transforms$), DWT ($Discrete\ Wavelet\ Transforms$) FFT ($Fast\ Fourier\ Transform$), and scale invariant feature transform. The transform function contains two types of feature attribute; one is high content of features and other is lower content of features [4–7]. The high content of features is basically part of high frequency (HF) and cannot proceed for the mapping of features for the processing of watermarking. The most of authors and researchers used lower content of features; the lower content of features is part of low frequency (LF). The feature based watermarking algorithms are needed for the compactness of embedding using

M. Rai (✉) · S. Goyal · M. Pawar
RGPV University, Bhopal, Madhya Pradesh, India

S. Goyal
e-mail: Sachingoyal@rgtu.net

M. Pawar
e-mail: maheshpawar@rgtu.net

© The Author(s), under exclusive license to Springer Nature Singapore Pte Ltd. 2021   469
M. K. Bajpai et al. (eds.), *Machine Vision and Augmented Intelligence—Theory and Applications*, Lecture Notes in Electrical Engineering 796,
https://doi.org/10.1007/978-981-16-5078-9_39

ML algorithms. The machine learning algorithms provides the feature optimization and pattern optimization [8, 9]. The process of pattern generation and optimization enhance the imperceptibility and robustness of watermarking. Various authors used the machine learning based algorithms such as KNN, SVM, and PNN [10]. The process of machine learning approach describes in two manners such as supervised learning and unsupervised learning [11, 12]. Both approaches are used in various methods for the quality of digital watermarking algorithms. Supervised learning such as SVM (*Support Vector Machine*) and KNN algorithms is used for the prevention of security attacks such as geometrical and filter-based attacks. The process of attacks deformed the quality of digital image watermarking. Proposed ensemble-depended ML approach is used for the process of digital image watermarking. The proposed ensemble algorithms are based on the two classifier, support vector machine and back prorogation (BP) neural network [13, 14]. The proposed algorithms reduce the error between watermark image and source image. The reduced value of error indicates the great potential of digital image watermarking [15–17]. The existing technique of watermarking methods faced a problem of feature optimization and feature selection. Due to this issue, the process of watermarking suffered some problem mention here.

1. Less value of imperceptibility
2. Factor of robustness
3. The maximum amount of the pixel of the number of correlation (NC)
4. Less composite strength of features and easily tampered and loss their integrity of watermarking.

Overall limitation proposed feature optimization based on a machine learning algorithm for better feature optimization and feature selection. The proposed algorithm resists the geometrical attacks and increases the value of robustness. The rest part of paper describe as follows: part II describe the related work of transform function, machine learning, SVM, and DT (Decision Tree). Part III describes the process of proposed work. Part IV describe the parameters and result of our simulation. Part V describes the final concluding points in conclusion.

2 Related Work

Transform Function

Transform function implied very important role in digital image watermarking. The transform preprocesses the source image and symbol image. Various researcher used various transform function for the decomposition of image data in process of embedding. The family of transform function includes FFT, DCT, DWT, and LWT [18–20]. The LWT (lifting wavelet transform) function is more time efficient than conventional wavelet transform function. The lifting wavelet transform reduces the value of lower intensity of noise and produce integer value of transform function. In this paper we used LWT transform function for extraction of feature coefficient of source image and symbol image. In current trend of digital watermarking various authors used LWT transform function for coefficient selection in domain and increased the value of quality of watermark image [7, 11, 21]. The LWT function is also better feature extraction methods than DWT transform function. The processing of LWT function involves three steps for the decomposition of raw image, such as splitting, predication, and update. The process of function describes here (Figs. 1, 2, 3 and 4).

SPLIT: Divide the original signal $x[n]$ into non overlapping even and odd samples that is $x_e[n]$ (even samples) and $x_0[n]$ (odd samples),

$$x_e[n] = x[2n], x_0[n] = x[2n + 1] \tag{1}$$

PREDICT: If even samples and odd samples are correlated then one can be the predictor of other. To predict $x_0[n]$ we use $x_e[n]$ samples using:

$$d[n] = x_0[n] - P(x_e[n]) \tag{2}$$

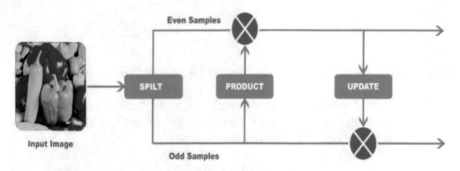

Fig. 1 Feature extraction process diagram

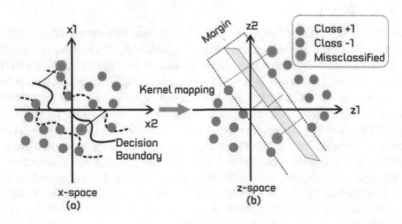

Fig. 2 Process block diagram of non-linear support vector machine

Fig. 3 Methods of boosting
and resample of data and
hypothesis

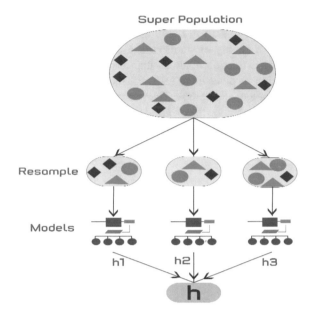

where $d[n]$ is the difference between the original sample and its predicted value
which is defined as high frequency component and $P(.)$ is the predictor operator.

UPDATE: With the help of update operator $U(.)$ and detail signal $d[n]$, we can
update the even samples. Then the low frequency components $l[n]$ which shows the
coarse shape to the original signal are got as follows:

$$l[n] = x_e[n] + U(d[n])$$ (3)

Machine Learning

Machine learning (ML) is the generation of process improvements and optimization
of results. Machine learning provides various algorithms for the process of regression,
classification, clustering, and time series prediction. Nowadays multiple authors used
machine learning algorithms in image preprocessing and post-processing, such as
image compression, image fusion, and biometric recognition [22–24]. The process of
machine learning algorithms enhances the predictability of the model and increases
the quality and security strength of image process data. In this paper, machine learning
algorithms are used for the process of digital image watermarking. The proposed
digital image watermarking algorithm is based on the ensemble-based classifier [25–
27]. The proposed ensemble-based classifier is the process of boosting and used two
well know classifiers, one is a SVM, and the other is a DT. Here the SVM used
as a base classifier and DT algorithm used as a feature selector of LWT transform
function based on sample selection on high entropy gain. The proposed algorithm is
very time efficient in compression of other machine learning algorithms.

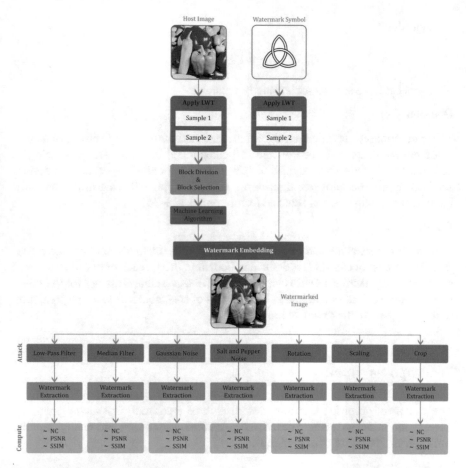

Fig. 4 Proposed algorithm model

Support Vector Machine (SVM)

The processing of support vector machine deals with hyperplane and lie data point on hyperplane. The non-separable plan act as vector point. The description of class definition describes as $x_i \in R^d$, $i = 1,......,l$, where x defines the data sample point and y defines the label of class as $y_i \in \{+1,-1\}$. the describe these class categorize the sample of feature matrix of watermark. Consider a hyper-plane $W^T x_i + b = 0$ that categorized the level of class as negative and positive [26]:

$$W^T x_i + b \geq +1 \, for \, all \, x_i \in P$$

$$W^T x_i + b \geq -1 \, for \, all \, x_i \in P \tag{4}$$

W^T is an adjustable weight vector, and x_i is the input vector and is the bias term.

Equivalently:

$$y_i . (W^T . x_i - b) \geq 1 \forall i, = 1 \ldots N \tag{5}$$

In this case, we say the set is linearly separable.

Decision Tree

The entropy-based classification algorithm. The maximum value of entropy of feature value represents as leaf node of tree and categorized the data. The processing of decision tree is with three algorithm ID3, C.4.5, and cart. The process of feature selection applied decision tree algorithm as ID3. The applied ID3 algorithm measures the maximum gain value of selected feature points [22–25].

Boosting

The process of machine learning algorithm derived the methods of ensemble classifier. The process of ensemble is defined as boosting. In approach of boosting we used support vector machine as base classifier and ID3 as variable classifier for the selection of feature of watermark image. The process of ensemble increases the prediction ratio of support vector machine [26–28].

3   Proposed Work

The process of proposed algorithm describes three section. In first section mapping of extracted in second section describe the feature optimization and finally describe embedding of watermark in section II.

Section I. Mapping of Features

The extracted feature coefficient is mapped with labeled data D and defined as the class of feature with c1, c3,....Ck. The relation of coefficient with class is Cr. These relations are non-overlapping feature coefficient of LWT. The regression of relation is

$$C_d \cap C_e = \emptyset \forall_{d \neq e} \tag{6}$$

Lemma 1 *The labelled features data D of vector D = vectors $D = \{v_1, v_2, \ldots \ldots . v_n\}$, where each $v_j = \{a_{j1}, a_{j2}, \ldots \ldots . a_{js}\}$ is a set of features and the user-defined classes $\{C_1, C_2, \ldots \ldots \ldots . C_k\}$ determine the non-overlapping partitions of D. The features of watermark image CW of class Cr.*

$$CS(C_r = \{a_j, a_k, \ldots \ldots . a_m\} \subseteq \{a_1, a_2, \ldots \ldots . a_s\} \tag{7}$$

Section II. Feature Optimization and Feature Selection

Lemma 2 *The selection of features points of real image and watermark image Pi and discriminate the feature subset as.*

$$P_{i+1}[CS'(C_g) = CS(C_g) \cup a_r] > P_i[CS(C_g)]$$

$$P_{i+1}[CS'(C_g) \cup a_r] > P_{i+1}[CS(C_g) \cup a_t] \forall t \neq r \tag{8}$$

Lemma 3 *The unclassified set of features points in the region of classification is*

$$unc_{cs'(c_r)} = DT(CS'(C_g)) \leq s \tag{9}$$

The function of DT is decision tree of feature select or of class of embedding.

Section III. Watermark Embedding

Input: feature data of source image $D = \{v_1, v_2, \ldots\ldots v_n\}$, where each $v_j = \{a_{j1}, a_{j2}, \ldots\ldots a_{js}\}$ is a set of features of mapped class $\{C_1, C_2, \ldots\ldots C_k\}$ and a watermark image labeled instances T.

Lemma 4

Output: watermark image
1. Mapped the class of watermark with original image for watermarking
2. Call lema-3 for classified region of image for the mapping
3. Measure the value of correlation of pattern
    $$pattern\ (P) = Dij - Vij \qquad (10)$$
    $\qquad\qquad$ the value of Dij matrix is refrence image and Vij
    $\qquad\qquad$ is watermark image
4. Measure value features difference of watermark image and reference image

    $$CS(C_i)' = CS(C_i) \cup a_{jh}$$
    $$f = f - a_{jh}$$
    $\qquad\qquad\qquad$ labe with
    $$\pi_{<CS'(C_i)>}(D) \quad (11)$$
    the class of CS is subst of features group of optimal
    and f is final set of feature with sum of label
    of watermark

5. determine the value of class of DT
    the process of decision Tee to make embedding of features component
    $measure\ f$(pattern of final region)
    if $Ff > BFf$(check the pattern strength)
    $BFf = F$
    $select = DT$
    $DT = DT + 1$
6. embedded process is done
7. exit

The process of applied attacks on the final watermark image checks the validation and robustness of digital watermarking algorithms. The used attacks in two categories, one is a low-intensity attack, are also called gaussian attacks such as low pass filter, noise, and paper salt. These types of attacks degraded the quality of the watermark image. In feature-based watermarking techniques, such types of aggression cannot deform the pixel position, and robustness of the watermark image remains. In the case of geometrical attacks such as scaling, rotation, and cropping, the embedding image's location is visible and break the imperceptibility of digital watermarking. The proposed algorithm defense this type of attack due to the process of optimized features for watermarking. The streamlined features reduce the pixel gap difference of reference image and watermark image.

4 Results

The watermarking algorithm is checked on 300 color images of size (512 ∗ 512). The different class of images such as man, follower, peppers, and other texture image. These images collected from CVG-UGR image dataset. All the analysis and experiment have been carried out in Windows − 10 based MATLAB13. The hardware used for the implementation process is a laptop with Intel core i7-processor and 8 GB-Ram. For the evaluation of analysis, the following formula was used (Figs. 5, 6, 7, 8, 9 and 10).

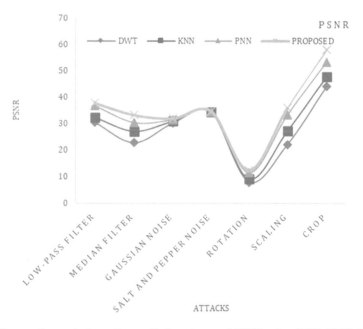

Fig. 5 Comparative analysis applies on Barbara image of PSNR using DWT, KNN, PNN and Proposed techniques with different attacks as low-pass-filter, median-filter, gaussian-noise, salt & pepper noise, rotation, scaling and crop. In all attack point of time proposed have a higher PSNR result respectively 37.91, 33.36, 32.11, 34.88, 12.47, 36.24, 58.06

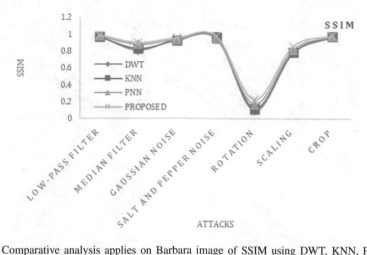

Fig. 6 Comparative analysis applies on Barbara image of SSIM using DWT, KNN, PNN and Proposed techniques with different attacks as low-pass-filter, median-filter, gaussian-noise, salt & pepper noise, rotation, scaling and crop. In all attack point of time proposed have a higher SSIM result respectively 0.99, 0.90, 0.96, 0.98, 0.23, 0.86, 0.99

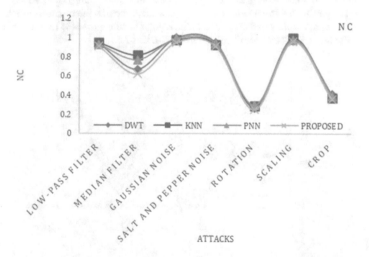

Fig. 7 Comparative analysis applies on Barbara image of NC using DWT, KNN, PNN and Proposed techniques with different attacks as low-pass-filter, median-filter, gaussian-noise, salt & pepper noise, rotation, scaling and crop. In all attack point of time proposed have a lower NC result respectively 0.91, 0.62, 0.95, 0.91, 0.25, 0.96, 0.36

The value of RMSE indicates the error difference value of real image and final watermark image. The lower value of RMSE shows the watermark image's good quality and enhance the value of PSNR (Tables 1, 2, 3, 4, 5 and 6).

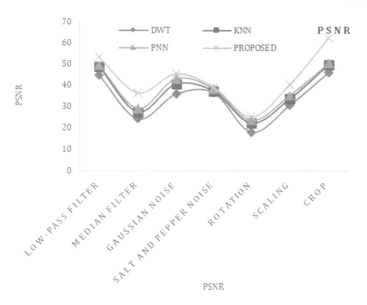

Fig. 8 Comparative analysis applies on Peppers image of PSNR using DWT, KNN, PNN and Proposed techniques with different attacks as low-pass-filter, median-filter, gaussian-noise, salt & pepper noise, rotation, scaling and crop. In all attack point of time proposed have a higher PSNR result respectively 53.32, 36.56, 45.67, 39.25, 25.34, 40.45, 62.55

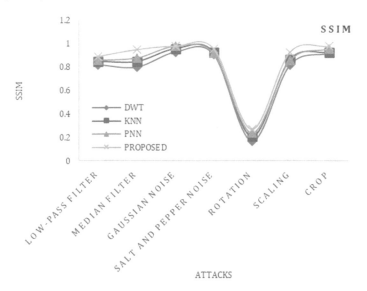

Fig. 9 Comparative analysis applies on Peppers image of SSIM using DWT, KNN, PNN and Proposed techniques with different attacks as low-pass-filter, median-filter, gaussian-noise, salt & pepper noise, rotation, scaling and crop. In all attack point of time proposed have a higher SSIM result respectively 0.89, 0.95, 0.98, 0.96, 0.27, 0.93, 0.98

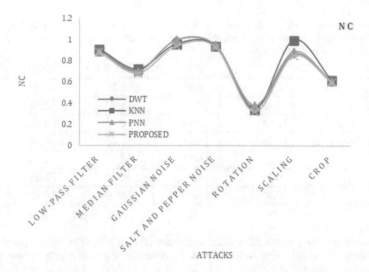

Fig. 10 Comparative analysis applies on Peppers image of NC using DWT, KNN, PNN and Proposed techniques with different attacks as low-pass-filter, median-filter, gaussian-noise, salt & pepper noise, rotation, scaling and crop. In all attack point of time proposed have a lower NC result respectively 0.88, 0.68, 0.94, 0.93, 0.32, 0.85, 0.60

Table 1 Comparative analysis of different techniques DWT, KNN, PNN and proposed for PSNR using different attacks as low–pass filter, median filter, Gaussian noise, salt & pepper noise, rotation, scaling and crop with BARBARA

ATTACK	DWT [12]	KNN [13]	PNN [14]	PROPOSED
Low-pass-filter	30.58	32.48	36.84	37.91
Median-filter	22.83	27.25	30.52	33.36
Gaussian-noise	30.30	31.07	31.58	32.11
Salt & pepper noise	34.27	34.53	34.58	34.88
Rotation	8.02	9.23	11.56	12.47
Scaling	22.27	27.46	33.55	36.24
Crop	44.31	47.99	53.51	58.06

$$RMSE = \sqrt{\frac{1}{m \times n} \sum_{i=0}^{m-1} \sum_{j=0}^{n-1} [O_{image}(i, j) - W_{image}(i, j)]^2} \qquad (12)$$

where $m \times n$ is the image's size, (i, j) is the pixel location, O_{image} is the real image, and W_{image} is the watermarked image. Then PSNR is defined as

$$PSNR = 20\log_{10} \frac{Max(O_{image})}{RMSE} \qquad (13)$$

Table 2 Comparative analysis of different techniques DWT, KNN, PNN and proposed for SSIM using different attacks as low-pass filter, median filter, Gaussian noise, salt & pepper noise, rotation, scaling and crop with BARBARA

ATTACK	DWT [12]	KNN [13]	PNN [14]	PROPOSED
Low-pass-filter	0.97	0.97	0.98	0.99
Median-filter	0.81	0.83	0.88	0.90
Gaussian-noise	0.94	0.93	0.94	0.96
Salt & pepper noise	0.96	0.97	0.95	0.98
Rotation	0.10	0.12	0.17	0.23
Scaling	0.78	0.79	0.82	0.86
Crop	0.97	0.98	0.98	0.99

Table 3 Comparative analysis of different techniques DWT, KNN, PNN and proposed for NC using different attacks as low-pass filter, median filter, Gaussian noise, salt & pepper noise, rotation, scaling and crop with BARBARA

ATTACK	DWT [12]	KNN [13]	PNN [14]	PROPOSED
Low-pass-filter	0.94	0.95	0.93	0.91
Median-filter	0.67	0.82	0.77	0.62
Gaussian-noise	1.00	0.98	0.99	0.95
Salt & pepper noise	0.95	0.93	0.94	0.91
Rotation	0.27	0.29	0.30	0.25
Scaling	0.97	1.00	0.98	0.96
Crop	0.41	0.38	0.39	0.36

Table 4 Comparative analysis of different techniques DWT, KNN, PNN and proposed for PSNR using different attacks as low-pass filter, median filter, Gaussian noise, salt & pepper noise, rotation, scaling and crop with peppers

ATTACK	DWT [12]	KNN [13]	PNN [14]	PROPOSED
Low-pass-filter	44.85	48.84	49.48	53.32
Median-filter	24.38	27.52	29.25	36.56
Gaussian-noise	36.03	40.70	43.26	45.67
Salt & pepper noise	36.72	37.35	38.43	39.25
Rotation	18.20	22.32	23.65	25.34
Scaling	30.72	33.64	35.25	40.45
Crop	46.13	49.72	50.34	62.55

The measure value of robustness used this numerical as

Table 5 Comparative analysis of different techniques DWT, KNN, PNN and proposed for SSIM using different attacks as low-pass filter, median filter, Gaussian noise, salt & pepper noise, rotation, scaling and crop with peppers

ATTACK	DWT [12]	KNN [13]	PNN [14]	PROPOSED
Low-pass-filter	0.82	0.85	0.86	0.89
Median-filter	0.80	0.85	0.88	0.95
Gaussian-noise	0.93	0.96	0.98	0.98
Salt & pepper noise	0.91	0.93	0.92	0.96
Rotation	0.17	0.21	0.24	0.27
Scaling	0.82	0.87	0.86	0.93
Crop	0.92	0.93	0.96	0.98

Table 6 Comparative analysis of different techniques DWT, KNN, PNN and proposed for NC using different attacks as low-pass filter, median filter, Gaussian noise, salt & pepper noise, rotation, scaling and crop with peppers

ATTACK	DWT [12]	KNN [13]	PNN [14]	PROPOSED
Low-pass-filter	0.90	0.91	0.88	0.88
Median-filter	0.71	0.72	0.70	0.68
Gaussian-noise	1.00	0.96	1.00	0.94
Salt & pepper noise	0.94	0.94	0.95	0.93
Rotation	0.36	0.34	0.38	0.32
Scaling	0.87	1.00	0.89	0.85
Crop	0.60	0.62	0.61	0.60

$$NC = (\frac{\sum_{i=0}^{m-1} \sum_{j=0}^{n-1} W_o(i,j) - W_E(i,j)}{\sqrt{\sum_{i=0}^{m-1} \sum_{j=0}^{n-1} W_o^2(i,j)} \times \sqrt{\sum_{i=0}^{m-1} \sum_{j=0}^{n-1} W_E^2(i,j)}}) \qquad (14)$$

where WO is the original watermark and WE is the extracted watermark.

ANALYSIS

Barbara and Peppers Image with their watermark image.

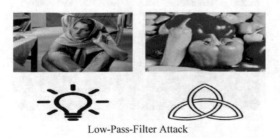

Low-Pass-Filter Attack

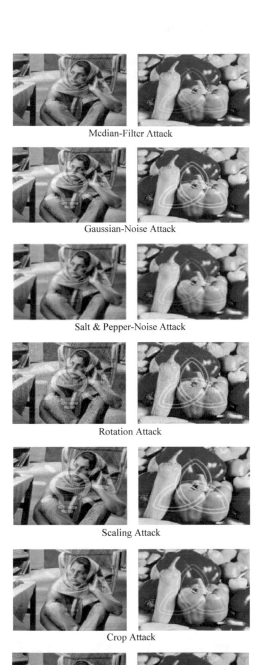

Median-Filter Attack

Gaussian-Noise Attack

Salt & Pepper-Noise Attack

Rotation Attack

Scaling Attack

Crop Attack

5   Conclusion

The proposed methods of digital image watermarking are very efficient and robust against different types of attacks. The proposed method is a combination of two processes: one is feature extraction, and the other is a machine learning-based watermark embedding. The LWT (lifting wavelet transform function) is a very efficient process of feature extraction in even and odd samples. The ensemble of support vector machine and decision tee produce a better watermark image. The decision tree algorithms used for the selection of features for the prediction of LWT transform function for the process of embedding. For the validation and strength measuring, apply different types of attacks, such as geometrical and conventional attacks of the watermark. In proposed algorithms predicts better value of SSIM and NC, the cost of SSIM indicates the strength of imperceptibility and value of NC suggests the robustness of watermark image. The proposed algorithms also focus on the quality of digital image watermarking, validation of a class of model used PSNR parameters; the high-end value of PSNR indicates the better quality of watermark image. The proposed algorithm compared with three other algorithms, DWT, KNN, and PNN. The DWT transform function is a well-known watermarking algorithm but faced a problem of security and quality of digital image watermarking. The other two algorithms KNN and PNN are machine learning algorithms that perform better results instead of DWT. But the proposed algorithms are better than PNN and KNN algorithms. In the future reduces the time complexity of proposed algorithms and used some real variant image data for the processing of watermarking.

References

1. Abdelhakim AM, Abdelhakim M (2018) A time-efficient optimization for robust image watermarking using machine learning. Expert Syst Appl 100:197–210
2. Subasi A, Kevric J, Canbaz MA (2019) Epileptic seizure detection using hybrid machine learning methods. Neural Comput Appl 31(1):317–325
3. Mehta R, Rajpal N, Vishwakarma VP (2018) Robust image watermarking scheme in lifting wavelet domain using GA-LSVR hybridization. Int J Mach Learn Cybern 9(1):145–161
4. Mishra A, Rajpal A, Bala R (2018) Bi-directional extreme learning machine for semi-blind watermarking of compressed images. J Inf Secur Appl 38:71–84
5. Erwin Q, Arp D, Rieck K (2018) Forgotten siblings: unifying attacks on machine learning and digital watermarking. In: 2018 IEEE European symposium on security and privacy (EuroS&P), pp 488–502. IEEE
6. Rouhani BD, Chen H, Koushanfar F (2018) DeepSigns: a generic watermarking framework for protecting the ownership of deep learning models
7. Adi Y, Baum C, Cisse M, Pinkas B, Keshet J (2018) Turning your weakness into a strength: watermarking deep neural networks by backdooring. In: 27th {USENIX} security symposium ({USENIX} Security 18), pp 1615–1631
8. Zear A, Singh AK, Kumar P (2018) Multiple watermarking for healthcare applications. J Intell Syst 27(1): 5–18

9. Zhou Xi, Cao C, Ma J, Wang L (2018) Adaptive digital watermarking scheme based on support vector machines and optimized genetic algorithm. Math Probl Eng 2018

10. Ghadi M, Laouamer L, Nana L, Pascu A (2018) Rough set theory based on robust image watermarking. In: Advances in soft computing and machine learning in image processing. Springer, Cham, pp 627–659

11. Huynh-The T, Cam-Hao H, Nguyen Anh Tu, Taeho Hur, Bang J, Kim D, Amin MB, Kang BH, Hyonwoo Seung, Lee S (2018) Selective bit embedding scheme for robust blind color image watermarking. Inf Sci 426:1–18

12. Saxena N, Mishra KK, Tripathi A (2018) DWT-SVD-based color image watermarking using dynamic-PSO. In: Advances in computer and computational sciences. Springer, Singapore, pp 343–351

13. Narayan CP, Bhagat KS, Chaudhari JP (2019) Watermarking based image authentication for secure color image retrieval in large scale image databases

14. Kusy M, Kowalski PA (2018) Weighted probabilistic neural network. Inf Sci 430:65–76

15. Zhou NR, Luo AW, Zou WP (2019) Secure and robust watermark scheme based on multiple transforms and particle swarm optimization algorithm. Multimed Tools Appl 78(2): 2507–2523

16. Behnam K, Moghaddam ME (2018) A predictive model-based image watermarking scheme using Regression Tree and Firefly algorithm. Soft Comput 22(12):4083–4098

17. Erwin Q, Rieck K (2018) Adversarial machine learning against digital watermarking. In: 2018 26th European signal processing conference (EUSIPCO), 519–523. IEEE

18. Kumar SA (2018) Introduction to the special issue on recent developments in multimedia watermarking using machine learning. Journal of Intelligent Systems 27(1): 1–3

19. Sharma V, Mir RN (2019) An enhanced time efficient technique for image watermarking using ant colony optimization and light gradient boosting algorithm. J King Saud Univ-Comput Inf Sci

20. Aditi Z, Singh AK, Kumar P (2018) A proposed secure multiple watermarking technique based on DWT, DCT and SVD for application in medicine. Multimed Tools Appl 77(4):4863–4882

21. Pathak Y, Arya KV, Tiwari S (2019) Feature selection for image steganalysis using levy flight-based grey wolf optimization. Multimed Tools Appl 78(2):1473–1494

22. Kumar P, Sharma AK (2019) A robust image watermarking technique using feature optimization and cascaded neural network. Int J Comput Sci Inf Secur (IJCSIS) 17(8)

23. Sun L, Xu J, Liu S, Zhang S, Li Y, Shen C (2018) A robust image watermarking scheme using Arnold transform and BP neural network. Neural Comput Appl 30(8):2425–2440

24. Sriti T, Singh AK, Ghrera SP, Elhoseny M (2019) Multi-layer security of medical data through watermarking and chaotic encryption for tele-health applications. Multimed Tools Appl 78(3):3457–3470

25. Kasorn G, Karnjana J, Aimmanee P, Unoki M (2018) Digital audio watermarking method based on singular spectrum analysis with automatic parameter estimation using a convolutional neural network. In: International conference on intelligent information hiding and multimedia signal processing. Springer, Cham, pp 63–73

26. Bui DK, Nguyen T, Chou JS, Nguyen-Xuan H, Tuan DN (2018) A modified firefly algorithm-artificial neural network expert system for predicting compressive and tensile strength of high-performance concrete. Constr Build Mater 180:320–333

27. Mishra A, Sharma L (2014) Video watermarking scheme using motion vectors with RBF neural network

28. Ahmed AS, Salah HA, Jameel JQ, Naoum RS (2019) A robust image watermarking based on particle swarm optimization and discrete wavelet transform

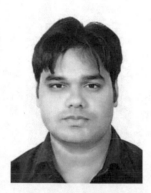

Manish Rai received his Bachelor's degree in Computer Science and Engineering, RGPV university Bhopal in 2009, M.Tech. in CSE from RGPV university, Bhopal in 2013 and he is currently a candidate for his Ph.D. degree in Computer science and engineering from RGPV university Bhopal His areas of interests are multimedia security, image encryption and digital watermarking, datasecurity, image processing, Computer nework.

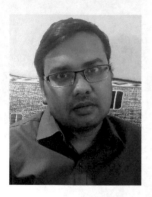

Sachin Goyal received his Bachelor's degree in Computer Science and Engineering, ITM, Gwalior, M.Tech. in Information Technology from Samrat Ashok Technological Institute, Vidisha, Bhopal, India and Ph.D. in Information Technology in 2013 from Rajiv Gandhi Proudyogiki Vishwavidyalaya, Bhopal, Madhya Pradesh, India. Currently he is working as an Assistant Professor, Department of Information Technology, University Institute of Technology, Rajiv Gandhi Proudyogiki Vishwavidyalaya, Bhopal (Madhya Pradesh), India. He has published more than 30 Research Papers in various International & National Journals & Conferences, including SCIE Journals & Scopus Journals. He is guiding 06 Students in PhD program. He is a Reviewer of Applied soft computing, Elsevier and IET Taylor and Francis and many other International Journals and conferences. He is also a member of IEEE. He was taking lecturer in National Law Institute University, Bhopal under M.S program in Cyber Law and Information Security.

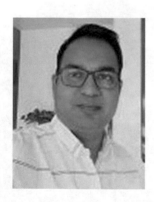

Mahesh Pawar received his Ph.D in CSE from RGPV University. Since 2007 he has served as one of the faculty members of Department of Information Technology, RGPV University, where he is currentlyworkingas a Associate Professor. He has published more than 40 Research Papers in various International & National Journals & Conferences, including SCIE Journals & Scopus Journals.

Diabetes Classification Using Machine Learning and Deep Learning Models

Lokesh Malviya, Sandip Mal, Praveen Lalwani, and Jasroop Singh Chadha

1 Introduction

Diabetes mellitus (DM) is also known as diabetes is a medical condition where the pancreas does not produce enough insulin, so blood sugar level rises and it affects various organs, in particular the eyes, kidneys, and nerves [1]. Three kinds of diabetes exist, namely, type I diabetes, type II diabetes, and gestational diabetes [2]. The pancreas produces very little insulin in the case of type I diabetes or even no insulin. Roughly 5–10% of all diabetes is type I and occurs not only in puberty or infancy but also in adulthood as well [3]. Type II diabetes occurs if insulin is not adequately released by the body. Approximately 90% of diabetic patients are of type II diabetes in the world. Type II is similar as third type of diabetes, i.e., gestational diabetes mellitus (GDM). In many ways, since it requires a mixture of comparatively inadequate secretions of insulin. Approximately 2–10% of all pregnant women is affected by gestational diabetes, after delivery, it can progress or disappear.

Early diagnosis of diabetes has always been one of the leading areas of research. Various machine learning methods are used for dealing with healthcare problems which are typical in nature. Most of the medical data contains non-linearity, non-normality, and an inherent correlation structure. Therefore, the conventional and

L. Malviya (✉) · S. Mal · P. Lalwani · J. S. Chadha
VIT Bhopal University, Bhopal, India
e-mail: lokesh.malviya2020@vitbhopal.ac.in

S. Mal
e-mail: sandip.mal@vitbhopal.ac.in

P. Lalwani
e-mail: praveen.lalwani@vitbhopal.ac.in

J. S. Chadha
e-mail: jasroop.singh2018@vitbhopal.ac.in

© The Author(s), under exclusive license to Springer Nature Singapore Pte Ltd. 2021   487
M. K. Bajpai et al. (eds.), *Machine Vision and Augmented Intelligence—Theory and Applications*, Lecture Notes in Electrical Engineering 796,
https://doi.org/10.1007/978-981-16-5078-9_40

extensively used classification techniques like logistic regression, naive Bayes, etc., cannot classify the data properly due to inefficient convergence.

1.1 Author's Contribution

List of author's contribution as follows:

- In this paper, review of various machine learning methods is presented and compared based on confusion matrix and AUC score on Pima Indian dataset.
- In addition, deep learning model ANN is also applied for the comparative analysis.
- It is observed obtained accuracy of extra tree classifier is better than other tested machine learning models as well as deep learning model (ANN).
- Performance of deep learning model is quite low as the data-set has less number of instances which causes inept learning (inefficient training or convergence).

1.2 Article Organization

Next section comprises all the suitable existing approaches of diabetes classification using machine learning. The proposed methodology is presented and discussed briefly in Sect. 3. The performance analysis of machine learning algorithms is shown in Sect. 4. Finally, Sect. 5, concludes the article and paves path for the future research direction.

2 Literature Review

Nowadays, diabetes is a chronic disease which poses a great threat to individual's physical well-being. The blood glucose is one of the major traits of diabetes, which is higher than the normal level, because of defective insulin secretion with special biological effects, [1, 4]. Diabetes results in persistent damage and dysfunction of different body tissues and organs, specially kidneys, eyes, heart, blood vessels, and nerves [2]. The common medical symptoms are increased thirst and regular urination, due high blood glucose level [3]. Diabetes cannot be treated successfully with medications alone and the patients are prescribed with insulin therapy.

With the modern life style, diabetes is becoming more and more prevalent in the everyday lives of people. Therefore, it has become one of the leading areas of research. In medicine, diabetes diagnosis is based on fasting blood glucose, glucose tolerance, and spontaneous levels of blood glucose [3, 5]. The earlier diagnosis helps medical professionals to cater the disease easily. Machine learning can assist medical professionals for early screening of patients in order to reduce the work load in hospitals. In addition, it can also be used as filter to classify potential of diabetes mellitus in patients with respect to their physical movement data and it can serve as a reference for doctors [6]. The most discussed and complex problems are selection of important features and the selection of best classifier.

In recent times, several algorithms are used to forecast diabetes, including the conventional machine learning methods [7], such as support vector machine (SVM), decision tree (DT), logistic regression, etc.

In [8], author has applied logistic regression model for the prediction of different onsets of type II diabetes, in order to deal with the high-dimensional datasets. In [9], authors concentrated on glucose as a parameter and used diabetes, which is a multivariate regression problem, to predict support vector regression (SVR). In addition, more and more studies have used ensemble techniques to enhance the accuracy [7]. A new ensemble method, Rotation Forest, which incorporates 30 machine learning techniques, was proposed in [10]. In [11], authors suggested a method of machine learning that modified the rules for the prediction of SVM. Machine learning approaches are commonly used to predict diabetes and produce preferred results. DT is one of the common methods of machine learning in the medical field, which has classifies with high precision. Many DTs are created by random forest (RF). The neural network is a common method of machine learning that has improved performance in many aspects recently. So we used DT, RF, and neural network to predict diabetes in this research.

3 Proposed Methodology

In this section, description of proposed work is presented in two subsections. Firstly, description of machine learning model on well-known dataset Pima is presented, thereafter, description of fine tuned ANN model on the same dataset is provided.

3.1 Proposed Methodology Based on Machine Learning

This section consists of system architecture and description of proposed algorithm.

System Architecture

In this subsection, pictorial representation of system architecture is shown in Fig. 1, which includes various phases, namely, data pre-processing and splitting of pre-processed data into train and test sets, training and testing of models, respectively.

Dataset Description

The review of machine learning methods is performed on the Pima Indian dataset [12, 13]. In particular, all patients are females of Pima Indian heritage who are at least 21 years old. The dataset comprises eight pregnancy features, plasma glucose concentration after a 2-h oral glucose tolerance test, diastolic blood pressure, skin

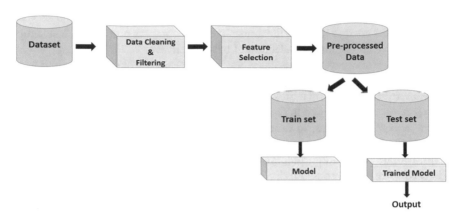

Fig. 1 System architecture

fold thickness of triceps 2-h serum insulin, body mass index, pedigree feature, and age of diabetes. This dataset contains 786 initial values of diabetic data including missing values which are removed, remaining dataset is 392.

Data pre-processing

Data pre-processing has been performed on the dataset to make it semantically strong, ensuring consistency throughout the dataset. The dataset has been checked for null values (NaN value). In total, 392 null values have been observed. Further, the potential outliers have been identified with respect to normal distribution. The patient with diabetes is labeled as 1 and non-diabetic patient as 0.

Cleaning & Filtering

After pre-processing the data and analyzing the inconsistencies. Then cleaning and filtering is performed which includes removal of outliers, encoding of categorical values, handling of missing values, substitution of NaN values (substituting mode for categorical variable and mean for continuous variable), etc. The outliers have been substituted with median values to enhance the consistency of each attribute some of them have been represented in Figs. 2, 3, 4, and 5, respectively.

Feature Selection

The important features are selected from the cleaned and filtered data. Exploratory data analysis (EDA) is used to analyze and understand the variable and their mutual relationships. The feature selection is done using correlation matrix. As all input variables should be independent of each other and this can be checked by calculating correlation of variables.

Fig. 2 Glucose before
filtering

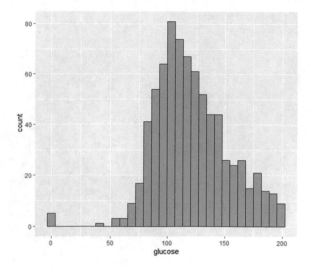

Fig. 3 Glucose after
filtering

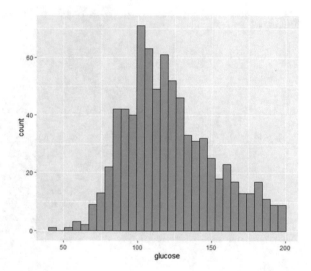

Description of ML Models

Firstly, the pre-processed data is split into two parts, train set and test set, with
composition of 80% and 20%, respectively. Then famous machine learning models,
namely, RF, DTs, extra trees (ET), etc., are applied.

Proposed Algorithm 1

The proposed algorithm for diabetes classification is shown in Algo.1, in which,
description of various feature label from × 1 to × 8 has been summarized in Table
1.

Fig. 4 Blood pressure
before filtering

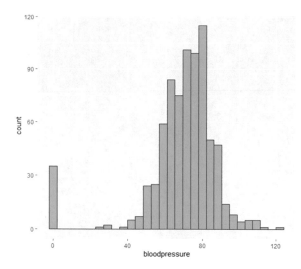

Fig. 5 Blood pressure after
filtering

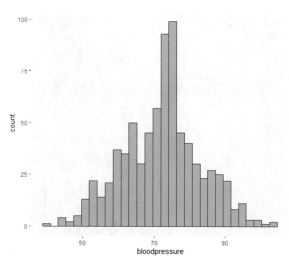

Table 1 Attributes of dataset

Attributes	Representation
Pregnancies	× 1
Glucose	× 2
Blood pressure	× 3
Skin thickness	× 4
Insulin	× 5
Bmi	× 6
Diabetic predigree function	× 7
Age	× 8

Algorithm 1: Proposed algorithm for diabetes.

  Result: Classifier labels for test instances
  Input: The train dataset consisting of input features such as x1, x2, x3, x4, x5, x6, x7, x8 and output label y;
  Output: Predicted Labels (0: non-diabetic and 1: diabetic);
  Procedure;

1. Dataset analysis to identify any anomalies;
2. Cleaning and Filtering (handling null and missing values);
3. Feature selection (using Correlation Matrix);
4. Application predictive models using DT, ETs, K-nearest neighbor, RF, SVM, and XGBoost;
5. Evaluation of results using Confusion matrix;

3.2 Proposed Methodology Based on Machine Learning

In this subsection, description of ANN architecture and composition of its layers is given.

Architecture of ANN

See Fig. 6.

Description of Layers

Artificial neural network (ANN) has been used, which is composed of five layers as shown in Fig. 6. In the first layer has 96 neurons, second layer has 48 neurons, third layer consists of 24 neurons, fourth layer has 12 neurons, and last layer 1 neuron.

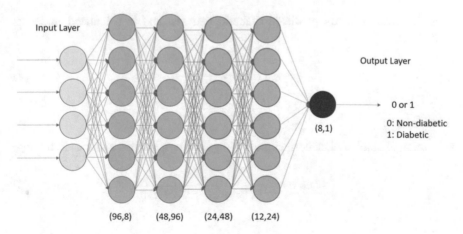

Fig. 6 ANN architecture

Description of Activation Function

All layers except last layer uses ReLu (Rectified Linear Unit) activation function, while last layer uses sigmoid activation function.

4 Performance Analysis

In the performance analysis, various indicators, namely, confusion matrix (Recall, F1-Score, and Accuracy and Precision) and AUC curves have been taken into the consideration and have been summarized in Table 2. The detailed description is given below.

4.1 Confusion Matrix

To evaluate the performance of applied machine learning models on test set [14], different metrics have been used which are mentioned below:

Recall.

It is the ratio of true positive (Tp) to the sum of Tp and false negative (Fn) and is calculated under as following:

$$Recall = \frac{Tp}{Tp + Fn} \tag{1}$$

Precision.

It is the ratio correctly predicted diabetic patients, and is calculated under as following:

$$Precision = \frac{Tp}{Tp + Fp} \tag{2}$$

Accuracy.

It is ration of number of all correct predictions, and is calculated under as following:

$$Accuracy = \frac{(Tp + Tn)}{(Tp + Fp + Tn + Fn)} \tag{3}$$

F1-Score.

It is the harmonic average of precision and recall, and it is calculated under as following:

$$F1 - Score = \frac{(2 * Precision * Recall)}{(Precision + Recall)} \tag{4}$$

where Tp: The number of patients that have diabetes and the predictive model has classified them correctly, true negative (Tn): The number of patients that do have diabetes and the predictive model has predicted them correctly, false positive (Fp): The number of patients that have diabetes but the predictive model has classified them in non-diabetic category, Fn: The number of patients do not have diabetes but the predictive model has labeled or identified them as diabetic patients.

Confusion matrix measures the ability of the predictive models for classifying the patients which are susceptible towards diabetes classification on Pima dataset.

4.2 Learning Curve of ANN

The learning curve of ANN has been shown in Fig. 7 and attains an accuracy of 73.85% on test set and 80.29% on train set. However, the accuracy of ANN is low as the dataset used for training is very small (Figs. 8, 9, 10, and 11).

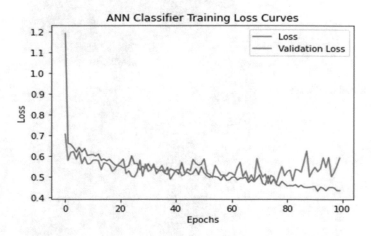

Fig. 7 Learning curve of ANN

Fig. 8 Accuracy on test set

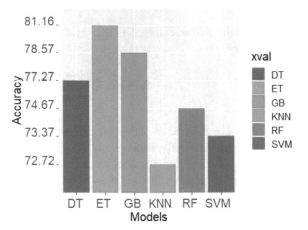

Fig. 9 Precision on test set

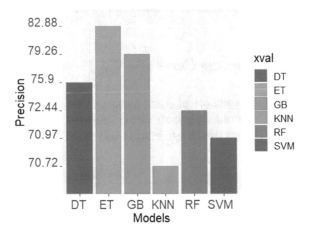

Fig. 10 Recall on test set

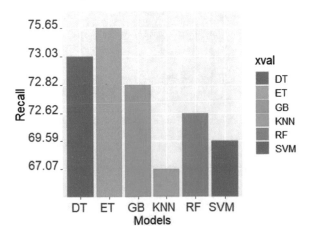

Fig. 11 F1-score on test set

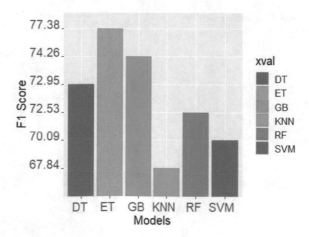

Table 2 Metrics showing combined results

Model		Precision	Recall	F1-Score	AUC score
RF	- - - - - -	72.44	72.62	72.53	83
DT	- - - - - -	75.90	73.03	72.95	77
KNN	- - - - - -	70.72	67.07	67.84	76
GB	- - - - - -	79.26	72.82	74.26	85
SVM	- - - - - -	70.97	69.59	70.09	82
ET	- - - - - -	82.88	75.65	77.38	81

4.3 AUC Curve Analysis

The measure and quantify the models performance on positive and negative classes AUC curve has been used. Higher the value of the AUC score, the better the model performs on both positive and negative classes [15].The AUC scores of different predictive models which are used to predict the target variable has been represented in Table 2 (Figs. 12 and 13) .

In accordance to AUC scores Adaboost classifier outperforms other respective algorithms on the test set. The graphical representation of AUC scores of models are shown in Figs. 14, 15, 16, 17, 18, and 19.

4.4 Performance in Terms of Recall

On the basis of recall, ET classifier out performs other algorithms having a recall of 75.65%. However, DTs have also achieved a subtle recall of 73.03%.

Fig. 12 Obtain result of
random forest

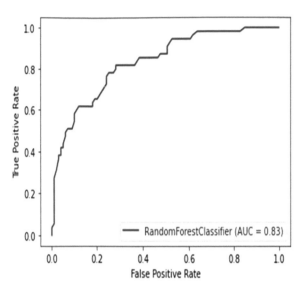

Fig. 13 Obtain result of
decision tree

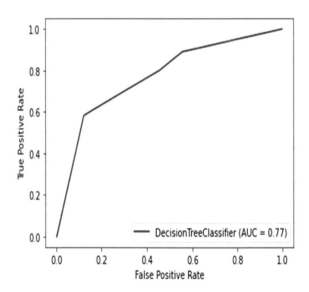

4.5 Performance in Terms of F1-Score

On the basis of F1 score, ET performs best over other algorithms achieving a F1-score
of 77.38%.

Fig. 14 Obtain result of
k-nearest neighbor

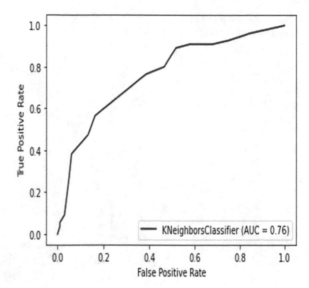

Fig. 15 Obtain result of
gradient boosting

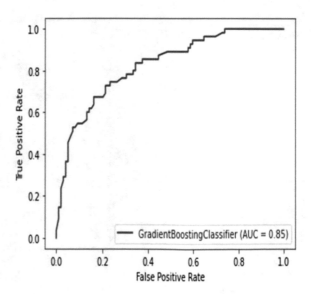

4.6 Performance in Terms of Precision

Again ET classifier out performs over other algorithms having a precision of 82.05%.

Fig. 16 Obtain result of
support vector machine

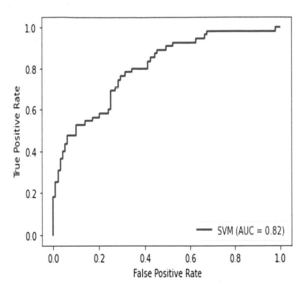

Fig. 17 Obtain result of
extra tree

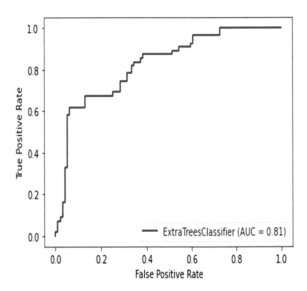

4.7 Performance in Terms of Accuracy

In terms of accuracy, ET classifier performs best with respect to other algorithms
having an accuracy of 81.16%.

Fig. 18 SVM

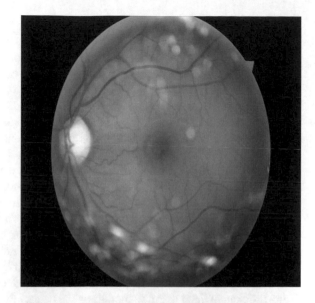

Fig. 19 ET

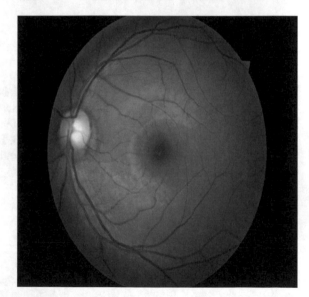

4.8 Performance in Terms of AUC Score

On the basis of AUC score, gradient boosting classifier performs best having an AUC score of 85%. However, RF, SVM, and ET also have achieved good AUC scores of 83%, 82%, and 81%, respectively.

5   Conclusion

Machine learning has been extended too many areas of medical health through the exponential advancement of machine learning. Lots of data mining and machine learning techniques have applied on diabetes dataset for risk prediction of disease. In this paper, review of machine learning techniques on Pima dataset was presented. Pima Indian diabetes dataset is taken as part of the study, which consists of 768 patients, of which 268 patients are diabetic and 500 patients are controls. In the performance analysis, we have tested six famous machine learning algorithms, namely, RF, DTs, K-nearest neighbor, gradient boosting, SVM, and ETs in terms of confusion matrix and AUC score. It was observed that the ET classifier outperforms over the other algorithms having an accuracy of 81.16% and an AUC score of 81%. In the future research direction, deep learning approaches can be applied for the further enhancement of accuracy and AUC score. Furthermore, we can combine the output of ML models on numerical data with deep learning model of image classification to make the prediction more precise (diabetic retinopathy). Genetic algorithms can also be used in future to enhance the accuracy and resample data to handle the over fitting problem of deep learning models as the dataset Pima is very small.

6   Future Research Directions

Diabetes mellitus is a common complication seen in diabetic patients on their retina as white spots which effects vision of a person. This symptom can be analyzed using OCT images of retina and can be classified using deep learning algorithms like CNN [16], Imagenets (VGG16, InceptionNet, ResNet, etc.). In the future work, we will be classifying diabetic patients on the basis of OCT retinal images and will try to enhance the classification accuracy so that it can be adopted in healthcare sector.

References

1. Lonappan A, Bindu G, Thomas V, Jacob J, Rajasekaran C, Mathew KT (2007) Diagnosis of diabetes mellitus using microwaves. J Electromagn Waves Appl 21(10):1393–1401
2. Krasteva A, Panov V, Krasteva A, Kisselova A, Krastev Z (2011) Oral cavity and systemic diseases—diabetes mellitus. Biotechnol Biotechnol Equip 25(1):2183–2186
3. Sorin BUZURA, Vasile DADARLAT, Bogdan IANCU, Adrian PECULEA, Emil CEBUC, Rudolf KOVACS et al. (2020) Logical, masking internal node. In: 2020 IEEE International conference on automation, quality and testing, robotics.
4. Mujumdar, Aishwarya, Vaidehi V (2019) Diabetes prediction using machine learning algorithms. Procedia Comput Sci 165:292–299
5. Cox ME, Edelman D (2009) Tests for screening and diagnosis of type 2 diabetes. Clin Diabetes 27(4):132–138

6. Polat K, Güneş S (2007) An expert system approach based on principal component analysis and adaptive neuro-fuzzy inference system to diagnosis of diabetes disease. Digit Signal Process 17(4):702–710
7. Çalişir D, Doğantekin E (2011) An automatic diabetes diagnosis system based on LDA-wavelet support vector machine classifier. Expert Syst Appl 38(7):8311–8315
8. Kavakiotis I, Tsave O, Salifoglou A, Maglaveras N, Vlahavas I, Chouvarda I (2017) Machine learning and data mining methods in diabetes research. Comput Struct Biotechnol J 15:104–116
9. Lee, Bum Ju, Jong Yeol Kim (2015) Identification of type 2 diabetes risk factors using phenotypes consisting of anthropometry and triglycerides based on machine learning. IEEE J Biomed Health Inform 20(1):39–46
10. Ozcift A, Gulten A (2011) Classifier ensemble construction with rotation forest to improve medical diagnosis performance of machine learning algorithms. Comput Methods Programs Biomed 104(3):443–451
11. Han L, Luo S, Jianmin Yu, Pan L, Chen S (2014) Rule extraction from support vector machines using ensemble learning approach: an application for diagnosis of diabetes. IEEE J Biomed Health Inform 19(2):728–734
12. Kumari V Anuja, Chitra R (2013) Classification of diabetes disease using support vector machine. Int J Eng Res Appl 3(2):1797–1801
13. .Zehra, Amatul, Tuty Asmawaty, Aznan M (2014) A comparative study on the pre-processing and mining of Pima Indian diabetes dataset. technical report. 80, 98, 99, 102, 106, 138, 141, 142
14. Marom, Nadav David, Lior Rokach, Armin Shmilovici (2010) Using the confusion matrix for improving ensemble classifiers. In 2010 IEEE 26th Convention of electrical and electronics engineers in Israel. 000555–000559. IEEE
15. Bradley AP (1997) The use of the area under the ROC curve in the evaluation of machine learning algorithms. Pattern Recogn 30(7):1145–1159
16. Alyoubi Wejdan L, Shalash Wafaa M, Abulkhair Maysoon F (2020) Diabetic retinopathy detection through deep learning techniques: a review. Inform Med Unlocked 100377

An Efficient Algorithm for Web Log Data Preprocessing

Vipin Jain and Kanchan Lata Kashyap

1 Introduction

World Wide Web is a huge resource of information. It consists of an enormous amount of information that is accessed by the users. It is a virtually infinite storage space that contains unlimited data in terms of text, picture, page, audio, and video. Web users can access and share information easily. Internet data is an unstructured format or dynamic in nature. Many times web user is unable to access the desired information. Sometimes user gets the wrong information also. Due to this, a web user spends a huge time on the Internet. Web data is increasing rapidly. So, an efficient solution is required to solve the user problem. The web log information is generated when the user accesses any website. This web log contains useful information regarding web user behavior [1]. Web log data contains unnecessary or irrelevant data. The web log information can be used to predict the user requirement in advance. The browsing time of the web user can also be reduced by web page predication and web mining techniques. A brief description of web mining taxonomy is given in subsequent subsections.

1.1 Web Mining

Web mining is the application of data mining techniques. The aim of web mining is to extract useful information from the web page. Various web mining techniques can

V. Jain (✉) · K. L. Kashyap
VIT University, Bhopal, Madhya Pradesh 466114, India
e-mail: vipin.jain2020@vitbhopal.ac.in

K. L. Kashyap
e-mail: kanchan.k@vitbhopal.ac.in

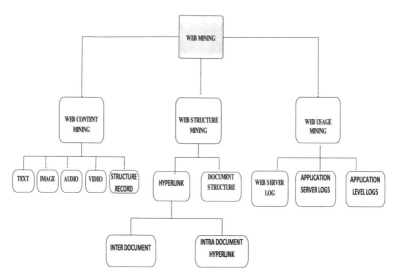

Fig.1 Web mining taxonomy

be applied to extract useful information from the World Wide Web. Useful patterns of user behavior can be obtained by web mining techniques. It provides a good web environment for the user. Two approaches can be applied in web mining: (a) data-based approach uses data mining technique and (b) process-based approaches to extract useful information from the web content such as Hyperlink and logs data. Web mining is classified into three categories: (a) web content mining, (b) web structure mining, and (c) web usage mining [2]. Web mining taxonomy is shown in Fig. 1

Web content mining is the process of extracting useful information from the contents of web documents. It may contain text, images, audio, video, or structured records such as lists and tables. Web structure mining is the process of discovering structured information also known as web graph. It consists of pages as a node and hyperlinks as edges for connecting the related pages. This can be further divided into two types according to the structure information: (a) a hyperlink may be a structural unit that connects a location during a website to a special location, either within an equivalent website or on a special website. A hyperlink that connects to a special part of an equivalent page is named an intra-document hyperlink, and a hyperlink that connects two different pages is known as an inter-document hyperlink [2].

(b) Document Structure is the content within an Internet page that can be organized into a tree-structured format supported by the various HTML and XML tags within the page. Web usage mining is the application of knowledge mining techniques to get interesting usage patterns from web usage data. Web usage data captures the identity or origin of web users along with user browsing behavior. Web mining consists of three steps: (a) web data preprocessing, (b) patterns discovery, and (c) patterns analysis. Web data prepossessing is used to reduce the web browsing time and to predict the user access behavior prediction.

Data cleaning is used in the preprocessing step to remove unnecessary or irrelevant data from the web logs. Data cleaning is required for better analysis of web user behavior and its prediction. In this work, an efficient algorithm has been proposed for data cleaning.

Contribution: Existing preprocessing works have used only a single parameter such as HTTP success status code for data cleaning [1]. In this work, hybrid algorithm is proposed for web log data preprocessing. Data cleaning is performed by filtering web log data by the HTTP request code, HTTP method, URL extension, and crawlers.

The structure of this paper is given as follows. Related work of the data cleaning is described in Sect. 2. Proposed algorithm is described in Sect. 3. Experimental result analysis is presented in Sect. 4 followed by the conclusion which is discussed in Sect. 5.

2 Literature Review

Many prepossessing techniques have been applied by various authors. Anand et al. proposed the algorithm for data extraction and cleaning [3]. In this work, all URL methods, all HTTP status codes with failed URL extensions are removed. The limitation of this work is that the robot entries in the log file are not removed by the proposed algorithm. Srivastava et al. described various heuristic and non-heuristic techniques for web log preprocessing [4]. Ryang et al. proposed a novel algorithm to find high utility patterns over a data stream based on a sliding window mode [5]. The limitation of this work is that the generation of web user patterns is not used. Anand et al. focus on the web usage mining process to explore data cleaning [3]. Zaarour et al. proposed an algorithm based on a refined time-out heuristic for session identification [6]. Singh et al. proposed a model that is based on the collaborative filtering (CF) technique for the web page recommendation system framework [7]. A modified version of the Rule Growth algorithm to find the sequential rules for the data cleaning is proposed by Erminer et al. [8]. An integrated framework of convolutional neural network and recurrent neural network is proposed by Chen et al. for data cleaning [9]. Parvatikar et al. applied Internet user routing patterns which are Apriori and FP-growth algorithm for pattern detection [10]. Logistic web page prediction using Biogeography Optimization Algorithm (LWPP-BOA) is proposed by Gangurde et al. Genetic algorithm is applied for predicting the web page in this work [11]. Tiwari et al. proposed a profile-based closed sequential pattern mining algorithm for user behavior patterns [12].

3 Proposed Model

Data preprocessing of the web log is performed in this work which consists of two steps: (a) data cleaning and (b) frequency of web page access counting. The block

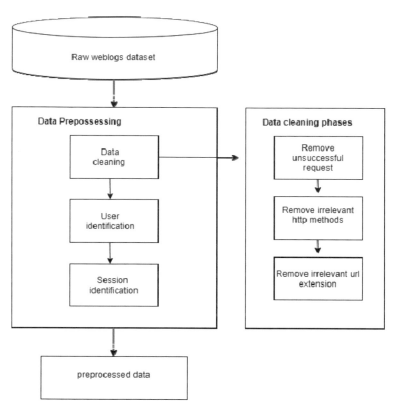

Fig. 2 Block diagram of data cleaning process

diagram of the proposed work is shown in Fig. 2. A brief description of each step of data preprocessing is given in a subsequent subsection.

3.1 Dataset

First, log data from the web log file is given as input in the proposed algorithm to remove unnecessary or irrelevant data from it. In this paper, a sample web log dataset is taken from NASA-HTTP (National Aeronautics and Space Administration) for validation of the proposed algorithm [17]. This dataset contains a total of 16,007 records and its file size is 1090 kb. The sample log which is in Internet Information Services (IIS) format is shown in Fig. 3. Each log file contains the hidden information of the web user.

Fig.3 Dataset information

```
Total Records 16007
<class 'pandas.core.frame.DataFrame'>
RangeIndex: 16007 entries, 0 to 16006
Data columns (total 1 columns):
 #   Column                 Non-Null Count  Dtype
---  ------                 --------------  -----
 0   IP,Time,URL,Staus  16007 non-null  object
dtypes: object(1)
memory usage: 125.2+ KB
```

Fig. 4 Sample web log data

```
1007949021.553    3089    192.168.201.11
TCP_HIT/200          12044          GET
http://www.computer.org              graeme
DIRECT/64.58.76.99 text/html

1292703446.102       2750   10.100.29.22
TCP_MISS/200         7676          GET
http://livescore.com/                 -
DEFAULT_PARENT/2001:d30:101:1::5
text/html

1293006348.196       1156   10.100.29.78
TCP_MISS/200         1003          GET
http://websms.starhub.com/websmsn/usr/chec
kNewMsg.do?                           -
DEFAULT_PARENT/2001:d30:101:1::5
text/html
```

3.2 Web Log

The footprint is automatically stored in a file known as a server web log data file while Internet surfing by the user. The web log is a text file that contains web user information in terms of IP address, date, time, HTTP methods, visiting URL, and HTTP request code [15]. A sample of the common log file is shown in Fig. 4.

3.3 Data Cleaning

Step-by-step algorithm for data cleaning is given as follows:

Algorithm 1: For Data Cleaning.

Input: Web server log data.
   Output: Filtered web log data.

1. Start.
2. Read Web server log data.

3.   Scan Web server data log file.
4.   While (status = = 200).
5.   Read IP and URL.
6.   If (URL extension = = (*.html ||*.php ||*.asp ||*.aspx ||*.jsp) 6.1 save URL and IP address.
7.   if resultant URL content = null value

   7.1 delete URL.

8.   if URL = spider.txt || robot.txt || crawler.txt

   8.1 delete URL.

9.   now if resultant data not contain Get method.
10. drop that URL and IP address.
11. Save the records.
12. Fetch next data.

   In this algorithm, first, web server log information is taken as input from the Nasa http_ access log file. Next, the successful hit of the URL is checked by its status code. The number of rows with successful hits is stored in a new database. Further, the data is removed based on the URL feature. If the URL extension consists of media format (images, audio, and video), then it is removed. The URLs with HTML, PHP, asp, jsp, and aspx web page extension are stored. Various machine-generated web robot files are removed. Further, the URLs and IP without GET method are removed. The null and missing values are removed from the web log dataset to get a preprocessed dataset for further use.

4   Experimental Results and Discussions

Proposed algorithm is implemented by using the Python programming language version 3.7. Raw data is taken from the Nasa_http_access_log web log file. Each column of each record is extracted from the dataset for cleaning. The result of datasets before and after the data cleaning is shown in Figs. 5 and 6, respectively. The number of records with HTTP request code, irrelevant URL extension, and a number of duplicate values of the various features before cleaning is presented in Fig. 5(a), (b) and (c) respectively. The number of records with HTTP request code, irrelevant URL extension, and a number of duplicate values of the various features after cleaning is presented in Fig. 6(a), (b) and (c) respectively.

   The total number of logs obtained after applying the proposed algorithm is presented in Fig. 7. It can be observed from Fig. 7 that the original 16,007 records are reduced into only unique 2868 records. Totally, 82.08% deduction is obtained in the original data (Table 1).

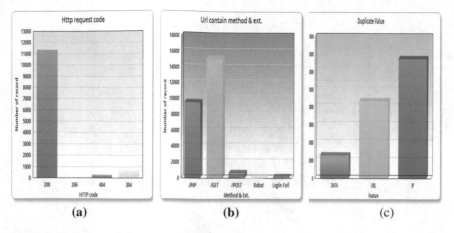

Fig. 5 Number of records before cleaning: **(a)** HTTP request code, **(b)** URL information, and **(c)** Duplicate values

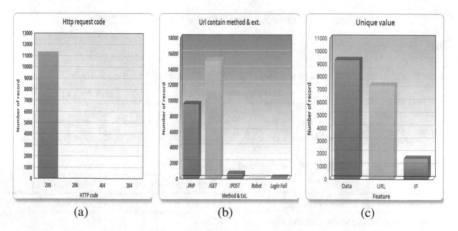

Fig. 6 Number of records after applying proposed algorithm: **(a)** HTTP request code, **(b)** URL information, **(c)** duplicate values

4.1 Comparison of the Proposed Algorithm with Existing Work

The comparative analysis of the proposed algorithm with an existing algorithm of Mehra et al. is also performed [1]. Data cleaning is done based on HTTP status code and the URL extension with *.txt, *.mpg, *.gif, *.css, and *.jpg. The comparative result is shown in Table 2 and Fig. 8. It can be observed that the proposed algorithm outperforms the existing algorithm [1].

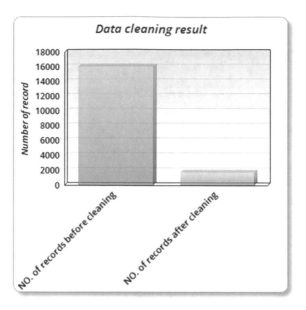

Fig.7 Data cleaning result

Table 1 Total number of records and size of the dataset before and after cleaning

–	Number of records	Size (in kb)
Before cleaning	16,007	1090
Unique records after cleaning	2868	211

Table.2 Comparative analysis of the proposed algorithm

–	Proposed algorithm	Mehra et al. [1]
Number of records before cleaning	16,007	2100
Number of unique records after cleaning and prepossessing	2868	416

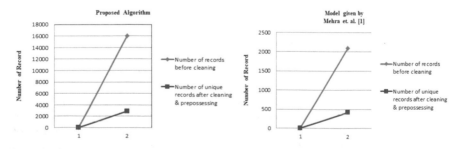

Fig. 8 The comparative analysis of the proposed algorithm with Mehra et al. [1]

5 Conclusions

Web usage mining is the better way to find out the web user behavior for its web prediction. For effective prediction, irrelevant data must be removed in preprocessing step by data cleaning algorithm. Data cleaning is the most important part of web usage mining. Therefore, data must be preprocessed before applying any mining technique for better web user behavior prediction with reduced time consumption. The data cleaning phase also required to obtain the good quality and accurate data. In this paper, an efficient algorithm is presented for data cleaning and obtained 82.08% data reduction. It can be observed from the result that the proposed algorithm cleans irrelevant, noisy, incomplete, and inconsistent data from the web logs. Various machine learning techniques will be applied for web user behavior prediction in future work.

References

1. Mehra J, Thakur RS (2018) An effective method for web log preprocessing and page access frequency using web usage mining. Int J Appl Eng Res 13:1227–1232
2. Etzioni O (1996) The world wide web: quagmire or gold mine? Appears in Comm ACM 1 motivation. 1–6
3. Anand S, Rani Aggarwal R (2012) An efficient algorithm for data cleaning of log file using file extensions. Int J Comput Appl 48:13–18. https://doi.org/10.5120/7367-0097
4. Srivastava M, Garg RK, Mishra PA (2014) Preprocessing techniques in web usage mining survey. Int J ComputAppl 97:1–9. https://doi.org/10.5120/17104-7737
5. Yun U, Lee G, Yoon E (2017) Efficient high utility pattern mining for establishing manufacturing plans with sliding window control. IEEE Trans Ind Electron 64:7239–7249. https://doi.org/10.1109/TIE.2017.2682782
6. Guerbas A, Addam O, Zaarour O, Nagi M, Elhajj A, Ridley M, Alhajj R (2013) Effective web log mining and online navigational pattern prediction. Knowl Based Syst 49:50–62. https://doi.org/10.1016/j.knosys.2013.04.014
7. Singh S, Aswal MS (2017) Towards a framework for web page recommendation system based on semantic web usage mining: a case study. In: Proceedings 2016 2nd International conference on next generation computing technologies (NGCT) 2016.329–334. https://doi.org/10.1109/NGCT.2016.7877436
8. Fournier-Viger P, Gueniche T, Zida S, Tseng VS (2014) ERMiner: sequential rule mining using equivalence classes. 108–119. https://doi.org/10.1007/978-3-319-12571-8_10
9. Chen X, Zhang Y, Ai Q, Xu H, Yan J, Qiny Z (2017) Personalized key frame recommendation. SIGIR 2017 Proceedings of the 40th international ACM SIGIR conference on research and development in information retrieval. 315–324. https://doi.org/10.1145/3077136.3080776
10. Parvatikar S (2014) Analysis of user behavior through web usage mining. Int J Comput Appl 27–31
11. Gangurde RA, Kumar B (2020) Biogeography optimization algorithm based next web page prediction using weblog and web content features. IAES Int J Artif Intell 9:327–335. https://doi.org/10.11591/ijai.v9.i2.pp327-335
12. Tiwari S, Gupta RK, Kashyap R (2019) To enhance web response time using agglomerative clustering technique for web navigation recommendation. Springer Singapore. https://doi.org/10.1007/978-981-10-8055-5

13. Nguyen TTS, Lu HY, Lu J (2014) Web-page recommendation based on web usage and domain knowledge. IEEE Trans Knowl Data Eng 26:2574–2587. https://doi.org/10.1109/TKDE.201 3.78

14. UmaMaheswari SK, Srivatsa S (2014) Algorithm for tracing visitors & apos; on-line behaviors for effective web usage mining. Int J ComputAppl 87:22–28. https://doi.org/10.5120/15189-3553

15. Deepa A, Raajan P (2015) An efficient preprocessing methodology of log file for web usage mining. Int J Comput Appl 13–16

16. Fournier-Viger P, Nkambou R, Tseng VSM (2011) Rule growth: mining sequential rules common to several sequences by pattern-growth. Proceedings of the 2011 ACM symposium on applied computing (SAC). 956–961. https://doi.org/10.1145/1982185.1982394

17. ftp://ita.ee.lbl.gov/html/contrib/NASA-HTTP.html

Classification of Idioms and Literals Using Support Vector Machine and Naïve Bayes Classifier

J. Briskilal and C. N. Subalalitha

1 Introduction

The process of labeling or organizing the text data into groups is called text classification. This is an integral part of Natural Language Processing (NLP). We are living in the digital era, where we are surrounded by the text on our social media pages, advertisements, blogs, e-books, etc. Most of this text data is unstructured, so classification can be extremely useful to identify this content. Text classification has the wide variety of applications; some of them are Spam detection, Sentiment Analysis, Topic labeling, Language detection, Tagging online content, Intent Detection, etc. In this paper text classification is done on idioms and literals, whereas this idiom and literal classification plays a major role in the NLP applications like Machine Translation and Information Retrieval (IR) systems.

Natural language is still being researched a lot due to the complexities that are inherent in the language interpretations. This gets even worse when the language interpretations are done automatically by the computers. This necessitates automatically disambiguating the text and extracting the intended meaning. This paper makes one such attempt by focusing on classifying the idioms and their literal counterparts. This has been perceived as a text classification task and has been implemented using two Machine Learning classification algorithms, namely, Support Vector Machine (SVM) and Naïve Bayes classifier.

An idiomatic phrase contains words that have a figurative, non-literal meaning while a literal phrase has words that match with an idiomatic phrase but means the direct meaning of the words [1, 2]. Example 1 shows a sentence that can act both as an idiom and a literal. Idioms generally exist in all languages, in English alone, there

J. Briskilal (✉) · C. N. Subalalitha
SRM Institute of Science and Technology, Potheri, Kattankulathur, Chengalpattu District, TamilNadu 603 203, India
e-mail: briskilj@srmist.edu.in

© The Author(s), under exclusive license to Springer Nature Singapore Pte Ltd. 2021   515
M. K. Bajpai et al. (eds.), *Machine Vision and Augmented Intelligence—Theory and Applications*, Lecture Notes in Electrical Engineering 796,
https://doi.org/10.1007/978-981-16-5078-9_42

are an approximate twenty-five thousand idiomatic phrases. This paper puts forth a binary text classification through which the idioms and literals are classified. Text classification proves to be one of the main preprocessing techniques in most of the NLP applications such as Machine Translations, IR, Summary Generation systems, and chatbots [3]

Example 1 Jaffy **kicked the bucket**

In this example, Jaffy literally kicked a true, actual bucket. However the idiomatic meaning for this sentence is "Jaffy has died".

The idiomatic phrases are disambiguated from their literal counter parts through the context they are used in [4]. This paper relies on a sentence-level context interpretation to classify the idioms and literals. This paper makes an initial experimentation toward this intent classification task.

In the existing works idioms are recognized using token-based, type-based [5] approach and idioms are detected as an outlier using Principal Component Analysis (PCA) [6].

Classification of idioms and literals is the biggest challenge and it is widely used in many NLP applications like Machine Translation (MT), Information Retrieval (IR), and Chatbots. By approaching this as a classification task, this paper has attempted to resolve this [7, 8]. In this paper we have used machine learning algorithms like Support Vector Machine (SVM) and Naïve Bayes (NB) classifier to classify idiom and literal sentences and observed that the probability-based classifiers like NB was not able to give better results when used in a small-sized dataset environment.

Rest of the paper is organized as follows Sect. 2 describes the Background, Sect. 3 describes Literature survey, Sect. 4 describes the Proposed Experimental setup for Idiom and Literal classification, Sect. 5 describes the Experimental results, and Sect. 6 gives the Conclusion and Future works.

2 Background

2.1 Support Vector Machine (SVM)

A Support Vector Machine (SVM) is a classification algorithm that is used to classify either binary or for multi-class classification. This paper uses SVM as a classifier to classify the idiom and literal texts.

SVM is a linear and maximum margin classifier. SVM finds a hyperplane to separate two classes namely idiom and literal.

Given the training data $(\mathbf{X_1}, \mathbf{Y_1})$, $(\mathbf{X_2}, \mathbf{Y_2})...$, where X_1 represents the category of context features that are used to classify the idiom which is represented by Y_1 and where X_2 represents the category of context features that are used to classify the literal which is represented by Y_2.

$$\mathbf{f}(\mathbf{X_i}) = < \mathbf{w} \cdot \mathbf{X_i} > +\mathbf{b} \tag{1}$$

In Eq. (1) [9], $\mathbf{f}(\mathbf{X_i})$ is a function that categories the test input text by taking the context features in it and predicts the appropriate class. $\mathbf{W}$ represents the weight of the feature vectors and $\mathbf{b}$ is the bias. If $\mathbf{f}(\mathbf{X_i}) \geq \mathbf{0}$, the test input is assigned to idiom class and if it is less than 0 it belongs to literal class.

If $f(X_i) \geq 0$, $Y_i =$ **idiom; else** $Y_i =$ **literal**

2.2 Naïve Bayes (NB)

Apart from SVM, Naïve Bayes Classifier is also used to classify the idioms and literals. Given a text during testing, the Naïve Bayes classifier finds if it is a literal or idiom by finding the posterior probability for each class using Eqs. (2) and (3).

$$P(Idiom|x) = \frac{P(x|Idiom)P(Idiom)}{P(x)} \tag{2}$$

$$P(Literal|x) = \frac{P(x|Literal)P(Literal)}{P(x)} \tag{3}$$

where X is the feature vectors that are context words,

$P(x|Idiom)$ and $P(x|Literal)$ refers the likelihood,

$P(Idiom)$ and $P(Literal)$ refer the prior probability, $P(x)$ refers the evidence probability.

Equations (2) and (3) shows the posterior probability of idioms/literal given a single feature, whereas, Eq. (4) shows the total posterior probability of an idiom or a literal class calculated for a set of features. Having calculated the posterior probabilities of each class, the maximum of the two is chosen by using Eq. (4)

The formal decision rule is given by

$$\hat{y} = \mathbf{argmax}_{k \in \{Idiom, Literal\}} p(C_k) \prod_{i=1}^{n} p(x_i|C_k). \tag{4}$$

where $P(C_k)$ refers to either probability of idiom or literal class. The next section gives the details of the state-of-the-art works done on text classification.

3 Literature Survey

Literature survey has been done in two dimensions. One is from the perspective of recognition of Idioms and the other one is from the perspective of classification of texts that are not idioms using machine learning algorithms. These two dimensions have given a broader perception of features and types of machine learning algorithms that are used in text classification and in idiom recognition.

3.1 Works Related to the Recognition of Idioms

Peng et al. have come with two approaches to identify idiom and literal texts. The first approach computes the inner product of context word vectors with the vector representing a target expression. Second method computes idiomatic and literal covariance matrices from local context in word vector space. VNC and COCO datasets have been used for classifying idioms and literals [5]. Fazly et al. have come up with two techniques, the first technique is type-based classification, in which the linguistic properties of idioms are captured and used as a statistical measure for the classification of idioms and literals. And in the second technique they have used a token-based classification, in which classification of idiom and literal has been done based upon the context words [10]. Feldman et al. have attempted to recognize idiom as an outlier using Principal Component Analysis (PCA) identify idiom and Three nearest neighbor classifiers to classify the idiom from its literal counterpart, and VNC dataset has been used [6]. Peng et al. attempted an idea to recognize idiom by using Latent Dirichlet Allocation (LDA) method. It was used to extract the topics from the paragraph which contain idiom and literal [11].

3.2 Works Related to the Classification of Text

Gurinder et al. have come up with two methodologies to classify the sentiment of the news article. One is the Multivariate Bernoulli method and the other is Multinomial Naïve Bayes method for classification of the sentiment which is present in the news article [12]. Liu et al. have attempted Parallel Naïve Bayes algorithm to classify the Chinese text data using Resilient Distributed Datasets (RDD) which has been used for classification [13]. Soumick et al. have proposed a multithreading approach using SVM to classify the blogs, tweets, and document. Multithreading approach has been used to reduce the preprocessing phase [14]. Said et al. have proposed Arabic text using SVM classification model, in which Chi-square technique was used to extract the features from Arabic document dataset which has been used and SVM is used for classification [15].

It can be observed that Sentence level idiom and literal classification have not been done in the existing works.

In this paper, we have attempted to classify the sentence-level classification of idiomatic phrases and literal phrases. And we have used our in house dataset for the classification.

The next section gives the explanation about the proposed experimental setup for idiom and literal classification.

4 Proposed Experimental Setup for Idiom and Literal Classification

In this paper, SVM and Naïve Bayes classifiers have been used for classifying idioms and literals present in the given input text. A dataset of 1471 sentences containing both idiomatic phrases and the literal usages. Figure 1 shows the proposed experimental setup for idiom and literal classification.

The input text is preprocessed and the features that are relevant for the text classification are extracted and then fed to the classifiers.

4.1 In-House Dataset Creation

In-house dataset contains 1471 sentences of Idiom and literal. 735 Idioms and 735 Literal sentences are present. Dataset has been annotated by three domain knowledge experts the author and verified by the experts. Figure 2 shows the count plot of the dataset.

In the above diagram, "neg" refers to literal sentences and "pos" refers to idioms.

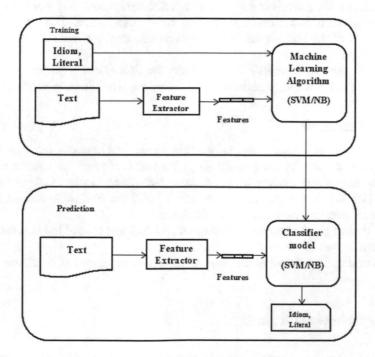

Fig. 1 Proposed framework of idiom and literal classification

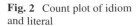
Fig. 2 Count plot of idiom and literal

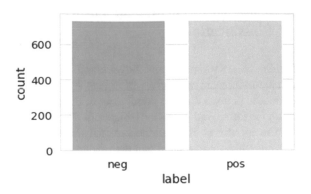

The data is preprocessed; features are extracted followed by feeding them to the classifiers.

4.2 Data Preprocessing Techniques

Data preprocessing involves duplicate removal, tokenization, stop word removing, converting text to lower cases, stemming, and lemmatization. This enhances the consistency of the training data and allows precise decision-making using NLTK Python library.

In this paper we have used NLTK library for data cleaning purpose, once the dataset is loaded we have performed the following data cleaning methods using NLTK library.

Feature Extraction:

Feature extraction is the process of extracting the required attributes from the dataset to train the machine learning model. Once the text is cleaned, we need to convert the text into vectors that are in an understandable form for the machine learning model [16, 17]. In this paper we have used TF-IDF transformer to convert text to vectors representing the frequency of the features.

The dataset is split into 80% training set and 20% test set and fed into the SVM and Naïve Bayes Classifiers.

The next section describes the observations on the experimental results obtained.

5 Experimental Results

The model has been tested using in-house dataset containing 1471 sentences comprising of 735 Idiom and 735 Literal sentences. Precision, Recall, and Accuracy were used as the performance metrics. Tables 1 and 2 show the results given SVM

Table 1 Evaluation metrics for SVM Classifier

Idiom/literal	Precision	Recall	F-Score
Literal	0.87	0.88	0.88
Idiom	0.87	0.87	0.87

Table 2 Evaluation metrics for Naïve Bayes classifier

Idiom/literal	Precision	Recall	F-Score
Literal	0.93	0.69	0.79
Idiom	0.76	0.95	0.84

and Naïve Bayes Classifiers. Precision and Recall metrics can be calculated using three factors, namely, True Positive (TP), False Positive (FP), and False Negative (FN). The equations for Precision and Recall are shown below.

$$Precision = \frac{TP}{(TP + FP)} \tag{5}$$

where the number of idioms correctly classified as idioms is expressed by TP and the number of literals incorrectly classified as idioms is represented by FP.

$$Recall = \frac{TP}{(TP + FN)} \tag{6}$$

The number of idioms wrongly reflected as literals is defined by FN.

For the factors of Precision and Recall, a confusion matrix is shown in Figs. 3 and 4.

Fig. 3 Confusion matrix for SVM classifier

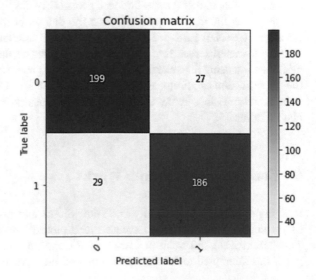

Fig. 4 Confusion matrix for
Naïve Bayes classifier

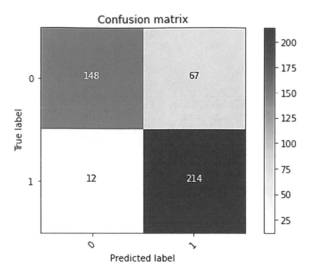

It can be observed from Tables 1 to 2 that SVM performs better. The reason for 0.76 percentage precision for the idiom class obtained by Naïve classifier is due to the fact that Naïve Bayes classifier classifies based on the frequency of the features. If the category is in the test dataset, was observed less frequently in the training dataset, then model will assign a less probability to it. This is due to the disadvantage of feature extraction. The reason for 0.69 percentages is due to the large feature dissimilarity in the testing and training datasets. This can also be alleviated by increasing the dataset or increasing the context span of feature extraction from sentence level to paragraph level. This can be explained using an example. Consider the test sentence of idiomatic phrase "The coach said I have to *pull my socks up* or I'll lose my spot on the team." here this feature had less probability despite being a potential feature in classifying the text. In general, when the dataset is small, the probability-based classifiers like Naïve Bayes are not a good choice compared to that of SVM.

Also it was observed that SVM performs better because it works well with text classification using linear kernel functions. In this paper we have used linear SVC for the classification of idioms and literals. Training a SVM with linear kernel is faster compared with other kernels. Also, SVM with linear kernel works well for the text classification.

6 Conclusion and Future Works

It is important to automatically spot the idioms and distinguish them from their literal equivalents in order to create more precise applications such as Machine Translation (MT), Information Retrieval (IR), and Question Answering systems. This paper has attempted to recognize idioms and literal texts. This has been perceived as a classification task using SVM and Naïve Bayes classifiers. This paper has used sentence-level feature extraction. The performance difference observed between the classifiers was mainly due to the features that contributed to the classification task. The Naïve Bayes classifier relies on the probability of the features and the size of the dataset was not capable enough to pull up the precision and recall scores. A paragraph-level feature extraction could have yielded more features in order to overcome the size of the dataset. Again there is a possibility of misclassification when an inappropriate feature has more frequency and could affect the performance. However, even in that case SVM might give a better performance. From the experiments done, SVM performs better compared to that of Naïve Bayes for the dataset used by us. This decision has to be reiterated by comparing with more datasets having varied contexts.

References

1. Fass D, Lesgold A, Patel V (1997) Processing metonymy and metaphor. Ablex Publishing Corporation, Greenwich, CO
2. Do Dinh E-L, Eger S, Gurevych I (2018) One size fits all? A simple LSTM for non-literal token and construction-level classification. In: Proceedings of the second joint SIGHUM workshop on computational linguistics for cultural heritage, social sciences, humanities and literature
3. Madankar M, Chandak MB, Chavhan N (2016) Information retrieval system and machine translation: a review. Proc Comput Sci 78:845–850
4. Sag IA et al (2002) Multiword expressions: a pain in the neck for NLP. In: International conference on intelligent text processing and computational linguistics. Springer, Berlin, Heidelberg
5. Peng J, Feldman A (2015) Automatic idiom recognition with word embeddings. In: Information management and big data. Springer, Cham, pp 17–29
6. Feldman A, Peng J (2013) Automatic detection of idiomatic clauses. In: International conference on intelligent text processing and computational linguistics. Springer, Berlin, Heidelberg
7. Cacciari C (1993) The place of idioms in a literal and metaphorical world. In: Teoksessa Cacciari C, Tabossi P (toim.) Idioms: processing, structure, and interpretation, pp 25–55
8. Cook P, Fazly A, Stevenson S (2007) Pulling their weight: exploiting syntactic forms for the automatic identification of idiomatic expressions in context. In: Proceedings of the workshop on a broader perspective on multiword expressions
9. Bennett K, Demiriz A (1998) Semi-supervised support vector machines. Adv Neural Inf Process Syst 11:368–374
10. Fazly A, Cook P, Stevenson S (2009) Unsupervised type and token identification of idiomatic expressions. Comput Linguist 35(1):61–103
11. Peng J, Feldman A, Vylomova E (2018) Classifying idiomatic and literal expressions using topic models and intensity of emotions. arXiv:1802.09961
12. Singh G et al (2019) Comparison between multinomial and Bernoulli Naïve Bayes for text classification. In 2019 International conference on automation, computational and technology management (ICACTM). IEEE
13. Liu P et al (2019) Parallel naive Bayes algorithm for large-scale Chinese text classification based on spark. J Central South Univ 26(1):1–12
14. Chatterjee S, Jose PG, Datta D (2019) Text classification using SVM enhanced by multi-threading and CUDA. Int J Mod Educ Comput Sci 11(1)
15. Bahassine S et al (2020) Feature selection using an improved Chi-square for Arabic text classification. J King Saud Univ-Comput Inf Sci 32(2):225–231

16. Birke J, Sarkar A (2006) A clustering approach for nearly unsupervised recognition of nonliteral language. In: 11th conference of the European chapter of the association for computational linguistics
17. Mason ZJ (2004) CorMet: a computational, corpus-based conventional metaphor extraction system. Comput Linguist 30(1):23–44

Modeling Indian Road Traffic Using Concepts of Fluid Flow and Reynold's Number for Anomaly Detection

V. Varun Kumar, Alankrita Kakati, Mousumi Das, Aarhisreshtha Mahanta, Puli Gangadhara, Chandrajit Choudhury, and Fazal A. Talukdar

1 Introduction

Automatic traffic video surveillance video analysis and detection problems are a mature field of research. They have been under continuous research and development for the last couple of decades. This has led to the development of many image processing methods that have been dedicatedly used for scene analysis and object detections in traffic scenarios. Simultaneously, with the advent of learning-based methods and various feature engineering techniques, the problem of detecting anomalies in different forms of data has also been of interest to researchers in the field of computer vision, data science, etc. Detecting or predicting anomalies in a traffic scenario has many extremely positive implications, like finding the root cause of traffic congestions, accidents, or even avert traffic congestions or mishaps. Every year, millions of dollars are wasted worldwide due to wastage of fuel, valuable time, damages to humans and properties, etc. These mishaps, resources, and time can be saved if the traffic congestions and accidents can be averted. This needs a thorough analysis of the traffic scenario. However, a humongous amount of surveillance video data generated along every route makes manual analysis of the surveillance videos a gigantic and near-impossible task. This needs automation of the process. Also, the increasing population of the globe and aggressive consumption of the limited stock of fossil fuel are gradually making the need for an automated expert system for analyzing traffic scenarios unavoidable.

V. V. Kumar (✉) · A. Kakati (✉) · M. Das (✉) · A. Mahanta (✉) · P. Gangadhara (✉) ·
C. Choudhury (✉) · F. A. Talukdar (✉)
Electronics and Communication Engineering Department, National Institute of Technology Silchar, Silchar, India
e-mail: chandrajit@ece.nits.ac.in

F. A. Talukdar
e-mail: fazal@ece.nits.ac.in

© The Author(s), under exclusive license to Springer Nature Singapore Pte Ltd. 2021   525
M. K. Bajpai et al. (eds.), *Machine Vision and Augmented Intelligence—Theory and Applications*, Lecture Notes in Electrical Engineering 796,
https://doi.org/10.1007/978-981-16-5078-9_43

In recent years with overall advancement in machine learning algorithms and befitting computational devices, many real-time problems including traffic scene analysis and accurate anomaly detection are possible to a great extent. However, in our initial research, we found that most of the datasets [1–9] that are being used in developing these algorithms are traffic video surveillance data that are taken in cities of different developed countries. In the scenarios of these datasets, the anomalies mostly are caused by heavy speeding or rash driving by a single or a few individuals. But someone who has visually sampled the traffic scenario of a thickly populated city in a developing country, like India, will clearly realize how different the scenarios are in these cities compared to the scenarios depicted by the databases. The traffic scenarios in these databases overall are quite disciplined compared to the Indian traffic scenario. In countries like India, the traffic scenario consists majorly of vehicles moving while being in close proximity to each other, vehicles of different types and sizes using the same road and even the same traffic lane, and while doing so the vehicles change their lane and overtake each other frequently. Factors like these make even segmentation of vehicles from the video surveillance video frames extremely difficult. As a result, the proposed methods that are developed on the databases like [1–9] don't fit into the situation faced in cities of countries like India.

In this work, we propose a simple and effective method to model the Indian traffic scenario as fluid flow and use the concept of Reynold's number to detect anomalies in the traffic scenario. There are no available databases as such so we have captured a few videos of the traffic condition and have used them for training and testing of our algorithm. If we compare the movement of vehicle traffic with the flow of fluid. Congestions and accidents, i.e., anomalies, as the turbulence in the flow, without these anomalies the flow can be considered streamline flow. One of the most popular ways to quantify the turbulence or streamline flow of fluids is Reynold's number [10]. In this work, we have mapped the concept of Reynold's number [10] into the road traffic scenario. We have devised a few parameters in the vehicle traffic scenario equivalent to the parameters in fluid dynamics needed for the computation of Reynold's number. We discuss these parameters and ways to compute them, followed by experimental results on real-time data to establish the efficiency of the proposed method in this article.

This paper is organized in the following manner: Sect. 2 gives a brief idea about the relevant works that have been reported in the last decade, Sect. 3 discusses the proposed method, Sect. 4 discusses the details of experimentation carried out and the results achieved and finally Sect. 5 discusses the conclusion of our work.

2 Relevant Works

There has been extensive work done in this field and there are numerous works reported in this field. To follow the existing works in this field, we found the survey works reported in [9, 11–18] very useful. These survey works present an analysis of the methods used in anomaly detection in general including the works dealing with vehicle traffic. Based on these surveys, the relevant works in this field can be summarized as follows.

Many feature engineering- and learning-based alarming systems have been reported. For these works, many combinations of features and learning methods have been used. A few of these mentionable methods are sub-trajectories along with Multi-instance learning [19], 3D spatio-temporal volumetric model using code-book model learning [20], MDTs from spatio-temporal models using Dynamic Texture model [20], Hybrid feature set consisting of HOS, HOG and PSO using SVM classifier [21], Handcrafted HOG + HOF features along with automatic CNN extracted features [22], histogram of optical flow [23] and more recently, code words of spatio-temporal regions [24], abnormality score from generator and critic in a GAN model [25], and size and motion parameters of the dynamic objects in the scene [26].

Among the supervised learning-based methods, [27, 28] used Hidden Markov Model (HMM) [27]-based model, [29] used One Class Support Vector Machine (OCSVM) [30–32] used Gaussian Regression (GR) [33–35] used Convolutional Neural Networks (CNN) [26, 36, 37] used Multiple Instance Learning (MIL), [35, 38] used Long Short-Term Memory (LSTM) networks, [39] used Fast Region-based CNN (Fast R-CNN), etc.

A few of the mentionable works based on unsupervised or semi-supervised learning are [40] using Latent Dirichlet Allocation (LDA), [41] using Probabilistic Latent Semantic Analysis (pLSA) [24, 42] using Hierarchical Dirichlet Process (HDP) [43–45] using Gaussian Mixture Model (GMM), [46] using Density-Based Spatial Clustering of Applications with Noise (DBSCAN) [47, 48] using Fisher Kernel Method, [25, 50] using Generative Adversarial Network (GAN) [51], and Ranking of Multi-instance-based learning model [26].

Besides these works, recently, methods have been reported [52] that consider vehicles in both static and dynamic states on or near the road edge to detect and even predict any upcoming anomalies. Also, deep learning-based real-time anomaly detection systems have been proposed [53].

The databases used for these above-discussed methods are NVIDIA AI City Database [1], CAVIAR [2], QMUL [3], UCSD [4], Bellview [5], NGSIM [6], AIRS [7], Car Accident [8] and i-lids [9].

3 Proposed Method

In general, Indian road traffic scenes are quite haphazard, in the sense; various kinds of static and dynamic objects are visible on the scene. Also, these objects are generally quite close to each other. This poses a great challenge, under changing illumination conditions, for computer vision problems like the one at hand. In our approach, we first try to segment and select only the relevant objects, i.e., the moving vehicles/humans on the road. First, we colorwise (RGB) segment the scene using mean shift segmentation [57]. But just depending on the color information for segmentation does not serve the purpose as segmentation only gives the partitions of the scene frame based on color information. It does not use the motion of the information. Also, as the scene is dynamic in nature, with changes in illumination conditions or different set of vehicles in the scene quality of the segmentation is going to vary. This is also the reason why did not prefer techniques like background subtraction for this purpose. Instead, we also calculate the optical flow of the scene w.r.t. the previous frame of the video stream. We use the gradient-based approach [61] for computing the optical flow. The horizontal and vertical velocities are used to compute the magnitude of 2D velocities at each pixel. The earlier segmentation method had given us a set of segments or, groups of adjacent pixels on the scene frame. The average magnitude of velocities of each of these segments is computed. A threshold (ϵ) is applied to avoid the segments that have negligible average velocity. This helps to avoid the effect of noise on the individually computed optical flow as well as image segmentation. For each segment, the mean and standard deviation of the pixel velocities is computed and the segment with low standard deviation was recognized as an individual vehicle. However, later it was found that if the initial threshold ϵ and the range bandwidth and spatial radius of mean shift segmentation are properly selected, thresholding on the standard deviation of velocities does not contribute much to the end result. So, this step was later discarded. Once we have obtained the segments that are in motion in the scene, we can treat these segments as particles in a flowing fluid.

Here, it might seem unacceptable that segments are considered as vehicles when we can clearly see that a vehicle's image can have multiple segments. We need not bother about a vehicle generating multiple segments and then creating multiple points in the fluid motion system. The reason is that even if multiple segments are created from a single vehicle in every frame, these segments will appear to be adjacent and have the same velocity. So, these adjacent segments will not create any problem in our model. That is because there is no question of any kind of turbulent interaction among them.

In our approach given these particles (of flowing fluid) and the information of their motion, we compute Reynold's number of the fluid to decide if the flow is turbulent or smooth. To do so, we need to correlate and convert various parameters for fluid dynamics, deciding Reynold's number, into the vehicle traffic scenario.

Reynold's number R was defined in [10] as

$$R = \frac{\rho V D}{\mu} \tag{1}$$

where ρ is the density of fluid, V is the velocity of flow, D is the diameter of the pipe and μ is the dynamic viscosity. Dynamic viscosity, μ, is in turn defined as

$$\mu = \frac{\tau}{\partial V / \partial y} \tag{2}$$

where τ is the shear stress defined as the tangential force per unit area. Also, $\partial V/\partial y$ is the rate of change in velocity of the fluid with change in the distance along the width of the pipe, i.e., as we move from the boundary to the center of the pipe. As a whole, Reynold's number can be stated as

$$R = \frac{\rho V D (\partial V/\partial y)}{\tau} \tag{3}$$

However, the calculation of Reynold's number, Eq. (3), requires the flowing fluid to be considered within a constrained region, like a pipe. To put this constraint, we partition the scene image into a predefined set of non-overlapping blocks. The vehicles located to be in motion within a block are considered the fluid particles flowing in that block, just like in a pipe.

The parameters of fluid motion considered in (3) can be mapped to the vehicle traffic scene's relevant parameters by finding the correlation of motion of vehicles in traffic with fluid motion. The density of fluid, ρ, here is the number of vehicles found in each block.

$$\rho_T = \frac{K}{Area\ of\ the\ Block} \tag{4}$$

K = Number of vehicles in the block;
Area of the Block = $w \times h$;
w = Width of the block;
h = Height of the block.
The velocity of flow, V, is the average velocity of the vehicles in a block.

$$V_T = [u_m, v_m]^T \tag{5}$$

where $u = \frac{1}{K} \sum_{i=1}^{K} u_i; v_m = \frac{1}{K} \sum_{i=1}^{K} v_i$.

$[u_i, v_i]^T$ is the average horizontal and vertical velocities of the pixels of the ith segment considered as a single particle or vehicle.

This parameter gives the information of the overall magnitude and direction of movement of vehicles located in a block. Diameter of the pipe D in Eq. (3) is the width of the flowing fluid or width that accommodates the flow of fluid, i.e., the maximum distance perpendicular to the direction of the flow. We calculate D as the width within the block, perpendicular to the direction of the average velocity of the vehicles. However, if the orientation of the camera is maintained such that the traffic direction is, on average, always horizontal or vertical in the recorded frames then we can very easily calculate D as

$$D_T = height\ or,\ width\ of\ the\ block. \tag{6}$$

The dynamic viscosity μ in fluids accounts for the interaction of various layers of the fluid under motion. As defined in (2), μ is a ratio of shear stress and the rate of change of velocity along the radius of the pipe. Shear stress arises due to cohesive force between, the layers of fluid and due to adhesion between the pipe's inner surface and fluid layer at the boundary of the pipe. The velocity of fluid changes along the radius of the pipe because the adhesion force at the pipe's inner surface is quite larger, in general, than the cohesion force fluid layers at the pipe's center. This ratio gives information about the resistance faced by the fluid layers in moving through the pipe, and this resistance is dependent on the position of the layer along the radius of the pipe. In vehicle traffic, the movement or behavior of a vehicle depends on the behavior of the neighboring vehicles. For example, if a moving vehicle takes a turn or gradually changes its lane or path, the nearby vehicles have to accordingly adjust their movement to avoid any collision. With more errand and drastic behavior of the individual vehicle, the movements of the nearby vehicles get more disturbed. This can be compared with the molecular cohesion and adhesion force seen in the case of the flow of fluids. In the case of vehicle traffic, we define the dynamic viscosity as

$$\mu_T = \frac{\tau_T}{\partial V_T / \partial y} \tag{7}$$

where τ_T is the equivalent of shear stress. τ_T is calculated as the average acceleration per unit area of the block. The average acceleration of the block is computed as the difference of average velocity of vehicles in the block, V_T computed at t^{th} frame from that computed at $(t-1)$th frame, i.e.,

$$\tau_T = \frac{|V_T^t - V_T^{t-1}|}{(w \times h)} \tag{8}$$

In Eq. (3) the rate of change of velocity $\partial V / \partial y$ is computed along the radius of the pipe. However, in the case of the vehicle traffic, the constraint on the velocity or possible changes in the velocity of the individual vehicles is far more lenient compared to that in the case of fluid motion, the reason of course being the free will of individual drivers. As a result, we model this rate of change of velocity along directions of the vehicle's position w.r.t. the mean of positions of all vehicles in that block.

$$\partial V_T / \partial y = \frac{\Delta V}{\Delta n} \tag{9}$$

where $\Delta V = \sum_{i=1}^{K} \sqrt{(u_i - u_m)^2 + (v_i - v_m)^2}$
$\Delta n = \sum_{i=1}^{K} \sqrt{(x_i - x_m)^2 + (y_i - y_m)^2}$
$x_m - \frac{1}{K} \sum_{i=1}^{K} x_i; \, y_m = \frac{1}{K} \sum_{i=1}^{K} y_i$

(x_i, y_i) is the centroid of a segment of pixels that is considered as a single point or vehicle. Thus, the ratio of Eq. (9) tells us about the variation in the velocities of different moving segments in the block, with the distance of their positions from the mean of positions of all the vehicles in that block. The mean position of vehicles (x_m, y_m) will be toward the crowded region in the block. Thus, if the vehicles remain in the same direction, the ratio in Eq. (9) remains constant. If the vehicles that are far away from the crowded region or that can be considered aloof in the block change their velocity compared to the mean velocity of all vehicles in the block, then also the effect is not significant. However, if the vehicles closer to crowded regions or vehicles with more vehicle(s) in their neighborhood change their velocity, then the ratio changes significantly. As a result, the computed Reynold's number changes. This modeling is befitting for the task at hand. The ratio of Eq. (9) gives us a sense of comparative randomness in the motion of those vehicles that can influence the overall traffic flow in the block, in a way that may lead to an anomaly. Again, τ_T captures the information of the change in average motion of vehicles in consecutive frames. The ratio in Eq. (7) thus is the change in average velocity of the block w.r.t. the change in the randomness of the vehicle motion in the block.

Combining Eqs. (1)–(9), we get Reynold's number for vehicle motion R_T as

$$
\begin{aligned}
R_T &= \frac{K}{w \times h} \times \frac{V_T^t D_T (w \times h)}{|V_T^t - V_T^{t-1}|} \times \frac{\Delta V}{\Delta n} \\
&= D_T K \times \frac{V_T^t}{|V_T^t - V_T^{t-1}|} \times \frac{\sum_{i=1}^{K} \sqrt[2]{(x_i - x_m)^2 + (y_i - y_m)^2}}{\sum_{i=1}^{K} \sqrt[2]{(u_i - u_m)^2 + (v_i - v_m)^2}}
\end{aligned}
\tag{10}
$$

While implementing, we have always added a small bias in the range of 10^{-3} to the denominator of the ratios so as to avoid any singularity.

We expect in this modeling that the computed equivalent Reynold's number will show considerable change in value during the occurrence of an anomaly. The proposed computational method is presented in the algorithmic form in Table 1.

During our initial experimentation, we found that Reynold's number increases by a large value in case of any anomalous movement of the vehicle(s).

We used a hard threshold-based method to just classify a few cases using the defined parameter Eq. (10). For this purpose, we computed a threshold for classifying anomalous situations from the normal ones. From the training video frames, we computed the maximum value of R_T in normal cases, let's denote it as $Normal\_R_T^{max}$, and from the anomaly cases we computed the minimum value of R_T, let's denote it as $Anomaly\_R_T^{min}$. Clearly, $Anomaly\_R_T^{min} \gg Normal\_R_T^{max}$. The threshold is taken to be the mid-point between $Anomaly\_R_T^{min}$ and $Normal\_R_T^{max}$.

$$
Th = \frac{1}{2}(Anomaly_{R_T}^{min} + Normal_{R_T}^{max})
\tag{11}
$$

Table 1 Algorithmic representation of the proposed method to find Reynold's number equivalent from the tth frame of a traffic video

Goal: Find the Reynold's number of the traffic as it appears in each block at the tth frame of the traffic video.

Given:

    a.   three consecutive frames, f_{t-2}, f_{t-1} and f_t from the video,

    b.   the number of non-overlapping blocks, each frame in that particular video is partitioned into, say N,

    c.   the details of the blocks $\{b_i\}_{i=1}^N$,

          where $b_i = \{(x,y)^i, w, h\}$, $(x,y)^i$ = coordinate of the top-left corner of the block,

          h = height, w = width of the ith block

    d.   a threshold value, $\in$

Initialize:

    a.   Equalize the histograms of the individual frames f_{t-2}, f_{t-1} and f_t

    b.   Compute the gradients of the frames $f_{t-2}, and f_{t-1}$ along x-direction, $\nabla_x f_{t-2}$ and $\nabla_x f_{t-1}$

    c.   Compute the gradients of the frames $f_{t-2}, and f_{t-1}$ along y-direction, $\nabla_y f_{t-2}$ and $\nabla_y f_{t-1}$

    d.   Compute the optical flow at the f_{t-1} and f_t: $[u_{t-1}, v_{t-1}]$ and $[u_t, v_t]$ using the gradient based equation: $u_t \times \nabla_x f_{t-1} + v_t \times \nabla_y f_{t-1} = f_t - f_{t-1}$ and similarly for $[u_{t-1}, v_{t-1}]$

    e.   Segment f_{t-1}, f_{t-2} and f_t using mean shift segmentation [60].

        f.   Calculate the average optical flow of all the pixels in each segment of f_{t-1}, f_{t-2} and f_t: $\left[u_{avg}^j, v_{avg}^j\right]$ for the jth segment in each frame.

    g.   Consider only the segments that have average of optical flow greater than a threshold $\left[u_{avg}^j, v_{avg}^j\right] > \in$

    h. $R_{seq} = [\ ]$, an empty array

    a.   for i = 1 to N, do:

    b.   extract the ith block from f_{t-2}, f_{t-1} and f_t, say B_{t-2}^i, B_{t-1}^i and B_t^i

    c.   calculate K for block B_t^i.

    d.   calculate V_T^t and V_T^{t-1} as in eqn. (5)

    e.   calculate D_T as in eqn.(6)

    f.   calculate $\frac{\Delta V}{\Delta n}$ as in eqn.(9)

    g.   calculate the Reynold's number, R_T, at the tth instance as in eqn. (10)

    h.   store the calculated Reynolds number: $R_{seq}[t, i] = R_T$

    i.   end

4 Experimentations

There are no available datasets on Indian scenarios that can be used for experimentation purposes in our work. We therefore recorded our own dataset of traffic video surveillance data. We have recorded almost 4 h of video data at different times of the day and at different weather conditions, thus considering changing traffic conditions under different illumination conditions in the day. We have also changed the

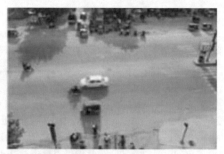

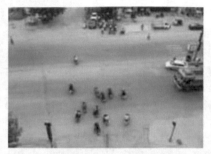

(a) frame of a video captured at noon with no shadow. Video is captured from greater height.

(b) frame of a video captured at afternoon with bright light and distinct shadows.

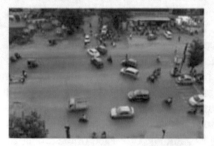

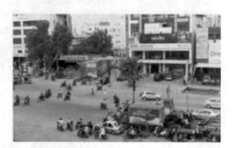

(c) frame of a video captured at dusk with poor illumination.

(d) frame of a video of the same road region is captured but from a different view point.

Fig. 1 The images depict the variations in captured videos in terms of illumination condition, camera perspective, camera elevation, traffic density and condition

perspective of the camera by changing the view angle, elevation, and also, we have also taken videos of different road regions. A few sample frames of the videos have been shown in Fig. 1.

For recording purposes, we have used a tripod-mounted Canon EOS 1200D DSLR camera. The videos captured were RGB color videos with a pixel resolution of 640×480 at a frame rate of 30 FPS (4:3). A couple of the videos were also captured with a pixel resolution of 1920×1080 at a frame rate of 24 FPS (16:9). We did so to experiment with the effect of spatio-temporal resolution of the video feed on the proposed method. We have taken 70% of the videos as train and the rest 30% as test cases.

We first visually inspected all the videos for any anomaly, and we labeled the frames and the corresponding blocks that were found to have anomalies. During manual labeling, we considered the blocks of frames, containing the following cases as anomalies:

a.   vehicles changing lanes with other vehicle(s) present in the neighborhood,
b.   vehicles moving way out the average flow direction,

c.   vehicles overtaking other vehicle(s),
d.   vehicles abruptly changing their velocities and
e.   vehicles getting close to each other tending to converge.

For implementation purposes, we manually decided the region on the frames of each video (for training as well testing purposes) that should be considered for the task at hand. Also, the relevant region on a video is further equally partitioned into a pre-decided number of blocks. We did this because in real-life scenarios, such algorithms run of video feed from surveillance cameras. Now, surveillance cameras' positions are pre-decided and fixed while capturing a video. Thus, we can always break the frames of a video feed from a particular camera fixed at a particular position. This is also generally done in real-life scenarios to avoid parts of the frames that are not relevant to road traffic information. For all the videos, in our experiments we have broken the region of the frame that covers traffic movement and to some extent its neighborhood into 2×3 or 3×2 blocks. The parameter equivalent to Reynold's number as described above (10) was computed for each block across all the frames in a video. Reynold's number equivalent parameters of a particular block from all the frames of the video are stacked to get the time sequence of these values. For each video, there are 6 such sequences. The threshold given in Eq. (11) was computed from the train case videos only. All the 6 sequences of Reynold's equivalent values from all the training videos were considered to compute the threshold as described in Eq. (11). Reynold's number Eq. (10) value was calculated for each of the blocks of all the test videos. The sequences from test videos were compared with the computed threshold. Values found above the threshold were considered anomaly cases. So, if the nth value of a sequence is found to have an anomaly, that means the nth frame of that particular video has an anomaly in the region of the block that the sequence is computed from.

In Figs. 2 and 3 example images are shown to demonstrate the reflection of occurrence of an anomaly in certain blocks of certain frames in the corresponding Reynold's number sequence. In Fig. 2, we can see that a scooter (marked in the image of Fig. 2b) is moving against the direction of the vehicles really close to it, which has caused a spike in computed Reynold's number sequence at frame 138. Here, the totally opposite direction of velocities of the marked scooter w.r.t. the nearest motorbike (just below, in the image Fig. 2b) and also the proximity of these two vehicles have caused the spike. Again, in Fig. 3 is an example of a pedestrian crossing the road when the vehicles still have the green signal to move. The frame is broken into 3×2 blocks and as a result, the marked pedestrian and the approaching vehicles on the right side of the pedestrian in the image lie in the same block. The huge difference in velocities of the pedestrian and the vehicles causes the spike in the sequence of Reynold's number.

In the plots shown in Figs. 2d and 3d, the obtained Reynold's values are seen to have a vast difference in range. This is due to the dependence of the computed value on the traffic conditions like density, velocity, etc. Here, a proper normalization method is required for automatic detection. At present, just for initial evaluation purposes, a simple hard thresholding-based method is used for detecting any spike

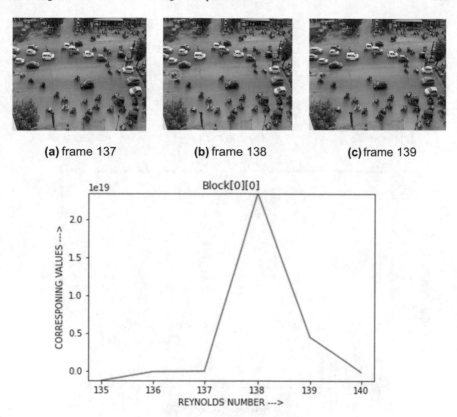

(a) frame 137   **(b)** frame 138   **(c)** frame 139

Fig. 2 Example case of the anomaly in vehicle movement causing a sharp rise in Reynold's number value

and hence anomaly. This is done without any normalization, and as a result the detection accuracy achieved till now is almost 50%. No quantitative comparison is presented for the proposed method because this work deals with only the modeling task, whose effectiveness is evaluated as to whether or not the occurrence of an anomaly causes a sharp change on the computed Reynold's number. For a fair and comprehensive comparison, the performance of the proposed model along with a time sequence anomaly detection technique has to be evaluated on a standard database. No such formal database is reported to exist till now, owing to which we had to capture our own video dataset for experimentation purposes. Moreover, to the best of our knowledge, there is no reported work in the detection of an anomaly for dense and haphazard traffic conditions as seen in Indian cities, which has been the focus of our work.

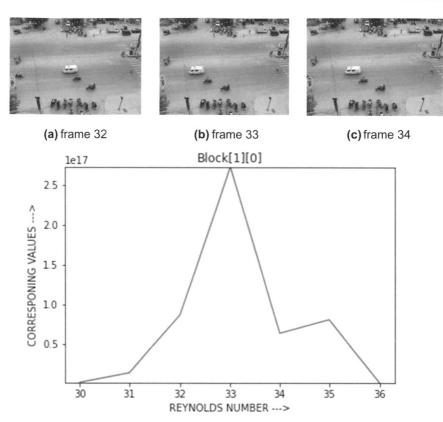

(a) frame 32   (b) frame 33   (c) frame 34

Fig. 3 Example of anomaly detection when a pedestrian crosses the road even when the signal to the vehicles is green

5   Conclusion

We have proposed a novel method for modeling the Indian road traffic scene similar to fluid motion. Using the concept of Reynold's number and its significance in fluid motion, an effective equivalent measure of streamline or turbulence flow has been derived in the case of dense traffic flow. The results achieved show the potential of this proposed model and formulation for anomaly detection in traffic movement. However, the derived measure of the turbulent or streamline motion of traffic shows huge variations in scale for different traffic videos, owing to the traffic conditions, which still remain a hurdle for accurate automatic anomaly detection. Devising a proper normalization scheme for the proposed Reynold's number equivalent formulation and a relevant time sequence analysis technique for the computed Reynold's number will be the course of our future work.

References

1. Naphade M, Tang Z, Chang M-C, Anastasiu DC, Sharma A, Chellappa R, Wang S, Chakraborty P, Huang T, Hwang J-N, Lyu S (2019) The 2019 AI city challenge. In: IEEE conference on computer vision and pattern recognition (CVPR) workshops, June, 2019, pp 452–460
2. Video dataset (2004) http://groups.inf.ed.ac.uk/vision/CAVIAR/CAVIARDATA1/. Accessed 20 Jan 2004
3. Hospedales T, Gong S, Xiang T (2012) Video behaviour mining using a dynamic topic model. Int J Comput Vision 98(3):303–323
4. Mahadevan V, Li W, Bhalodia V, Vasconcelos N (2010) Anomaly detection in crowded scenes. In: CVPR
5. Zaharescu A, Wildes R (2010) Anomalous behaviour detection using spatiotemporal oriented energies, subset inclusion histogram comparison and event-driven processing. In: ECCV
6. NGSIM. Next generation simulation community. https://ops.fhwa.dot.gov/trafficanalysistools/ngsim.htm
7. AIRS (2004) Traffic response and incident management assisting the river cities. http://groups.inf.ed.ac.uk/vision/CAVIAR/CAVIARDATA1/
8. Sultani W, Choi JY (2010) Abnormal traffic detection using intelligent driver model. In: ICPR
9. AVSS2007. i-lids. http://www.eecs.qmul.ac.uk/~andrea/avss2007d.html
10. Stokes G (1851) On the effect of the internal friction of fluids on the motion of pendulums. Trans Camb Philos Soc 9:8–106
11. Patil N, Biswas PK (2016) A survey of video datasets for anomaly detection in automated surveillance. In: ISED
12. Li Y, Xia R, Huang Q, Xie W, Li X (2017) Survey of spatio-temporal interest point detection algorithms in video. IEEE Access 5:10323–10331
13. Shirazi MS, Morris BT (2017) Looking at intersections: a survey of intersection monitoring, behavior and safety analysis of recent studies. IEEE Trans Intell Transp Syst 18(1):4–24
14. Ahmed SA, Dogra DP, Kar S, Roy PP (2018) Trajectory-based surveillance analysis: a survey. IEEE Trans Circuits Syst Video Technol 1–1
15. Lopez-Fuentes L, van de Weijer J, Gonzalez-Hidalgo M, Skinnemoen H, Bagdanov AD (2018) Review on computer vision techniques in emergency situations. Multimed Tools Appl 77(13):17069–17107
16. Mabrouk AB, Zagrouba E (2018) Abnormal behavior recognition for intelligent video surveillance systems: a review. Expert Syst Appl 91:480–491
17. Santhosh KK, Dogra DP, Roy PP (2019) Anomaly detection in road traffic using visual surveillance: a survey. arXiv:1901.08292
18. Ramachandra B, Jones MJ, Vatsavai RR (2020) A survey of single-scene video anomaly detection. arXiv:2004.05993
19. Yang W, Gao Y, Cao L (2013) Trasmil: A local anomaly detection framework based on trajectory segmentation and multi-instance learning. Comput Vis Image Underst 117(10):1273–1286
20. Roshtkhari MJ, Levine MD (2013) An on-line, real-time learning method for detecting anomalies in videos using spatio-temporal compositions. Comput Vis Image Underst 117(10):1436–1452
21. Kaltsa V, Briassouli A, Kompatsiaris I, Hadjileontiadis LJ, Strintzis MG (2015) Swarm intelligence for detecting interesting events in crowded environments. IEEE Trans Image Process 24(7):2153–2166
22. Hasan M, Choi J, Neumann J, Roy-Chowdhury AK, Davis LS (2016) Learning temporal regularity in video sequences. In: CVPR
23. Zhang Y, Lu H, Zhang L, Ruan X, Sakai S (2016) Video anomaly detection based on locality sensitive hashing filters. Pattern Recogn 59:302–311
24. Kaltsa V, Briassouli A, Kompatsiaris I, Strintzis MG (2018) Multiple hierarchical dirichlet processes for anomaly detection in traffic. Comput Vis Image Underst 169:28–39
25. Lee S, Kim HG, Ro YM (2018) Stan: spatio-temporal adversarial networks for abnormal event detection. In: ICASSP

26. Sultani W, Chen C, Shah M (2018) Real-world anomaly detection in surveillance videos. In: CVPR

27. Baum LE, Petrie T (1966) Statistical inference for probabilistic functions of finite state markov chains. Ann Math Stat 37(6):1554–1563

28. Biswas S, Babu RV (2014) Short local trajectory based moving anomaly detection. In: ICVGIP

29. Scholkopf B, Platt JC, Shawe-Taylor J, Smola AJ, Williamson RC (2001) Estimating the support of a high-dimensional distribution. Neural Comput 13(7):1443–1471

30. Hearst MA, Dumais ST, Osuna E, Platt J, Scholkopf B (1998) Support vector machines. IEEE Intell Syst Appl 13(4):18–28

31. Cheng K, Chen Y, Fang W (2015) Gaussian process regression-based video anomaly detection and localization with hierarchical feature representation. IEEE Trans Image Process 24(12):5288–5301

32. Sabokrou M, Fathy M, Hoseini M, Klette R (2015) Real-time anomaly detection and localization in crowded scenes. In: CVPRW

33. Rasmussen CE (2004) Gaussian processes in machine learning. In: Advanced lectures on machine learning. Springer, pp 63–71

34. Hu X, Hu S, Huang Y, Zhang H, Wu H (2016) Video anomaly detection using deep incremental slow feature analysis network. IET Comput Vision 10(4):258–265

35. Medel JR, Savakis A (2016) Anomaly detection in video using predictive convolutional long short-term memory networks. arXiv:1612.00390

36. Goodfellow I, Bengio Y, Courville A, Bengio Y (2016) Deep learning, vol 1. MIT press Cambridge

37. Burton A, Radford, J (1978) Thinking in perspective: critical essays in the study of thought processes. Routledge. ISBN 978-0-416-85840-2

38. Srivastava N, Mansimov F, Salakhudinov R (2015) Unsupervised learning of video representations using lstms. In: ICML

39. Hinami R, Mei T, Shin'ichi S (2017) Joint detection and recounting of abnormal events by learning deep generic knowledge. In: ICCV

40. Jeong H, Yoo Y, Yi KM, Choi JY (2014) Two-stage online inference model for traffic pattern analysis and anomaly detection. Mach Vis Appl 25(6):1501–1517

41. Kaviani R, Ahmadi P, Gholampour I (2015) Automatic accident detection using topic models. In: ICEE

42. Hofmann T (1999) Probabilistic latent semantic analysis. In: UAI

43. The YW, Jordan MI, Beal MJ, Blei DM (2005) Sharing clusters among related groups: hierarchical dirichlet processes. In: NIPS

44. Li Y, Liu W, Huang Q (2016) Traffic anomaly detection based on image descriptor in videos. Multimed Tools Appl 75(5):2487–2505

45. Wen J, Lai Z, Ming Z, Wong WK, Zhong Z (2017) Directional gaussian model for automatic speeding event detection. IEEE Trans Inf Forensics Secur 12(10):2292–2307

46. Ranjith R, Athanesious JJ, Vaidehi V (2015) Anomaly detection using dbscan clustering technique for traffic video surveillance. In: ICoAC

47. Ester M, Kriegel H-P, Sander J, Xu X et al (1996) A density-based algorithm for discovering clusters in large spatial databases with noise. In: Kdd

48. Wang J, Xia L, Hu X, Xiao Y (2018) Abnormal event detection with semi-supervised sparse topic model. Neural Comput Appl

49. Perronnin F, Sanchez J, Mensink T (2010) Improving the fisher kernel for large-scale image classification. In: ECCV

50. Goodfellow I, Pouget-Abadie J, Mirza M, Xu B, Warde-Farley D, Ozair S, Courville A, Bengio Y (2014) Generative adversarial nets. In: NIPS

51. Ravanbakhsh M, Nabi M, Sangineto E, Marcenaro L, Regazzoni C, Sebe N (2017) Abnormal event detection in videos using generative adversarial nets. In: ICIP

52. Raiyn J, Toledo T (2014) Real-time road traffic anomaly detection. J Trans Technol 04(03), Article ID:48351

53. Zhang M, Li T, Yu Y, Li Y, Hui P, Zheng Y (2020) Urban anomaly analytics: description, detection and prediction. IEEE Trans Big Data
54. Ullah W, Ullah A, Haq IU, Muhammad K, Sajjad M, Baik SW (2020) CNN features with bi-directional LSTM for real-time anomaly detection in surveillance networks. Multimed Tools Appl
55. Basharat A, Gritai A, Shah M (2008) Learning object motion patterns for anomaly detection and improved object detection. In: 2008 IEEE conference on computer vision and pattern recognition, pp 1–8
56. Benezeth Y, Jodoin P-M, Saligrama V, Rosenberger C (2009) Abnormal events detection based on spatio-temporal co-occurences. In: CVPR
57. Comaniciu D, Meer P (1999) Mean shift analysis and applications. In: Proceedings of the seventh IEEE international conference on computer vision, 1999, vol 2. IEEE, pp 1197–1203
58. Wang T, Qiao M, Deng Y, Zhou Y, Wang H, Lyu Q, Snoussi H (2018) Abnormal event detection based on analysis of movement information of video sequence. Optik-Int J Light Electron Opt 152:50–60
59. Xu Y, Ouyang X, Cheng Y, Yu S, Xiong L, Ng C-C, Pranata S, Shen S, Xing J (2018) Dual-mode vehicle motion pattern learning for high performance road traffic anomaly detection. In: Proceedings of the IEEE conference on computer vision and pattern recognition (CVPR) workshops, 2018, pp 145–152
60. Warren DH, Strelow ER (1985) Electronic spatial sensing for the blind: contributions from perception. Springer. ISBN 978-90-247-2689-9
61. Fleet DJ, Weiss Y (2006) Optical flow estimation. In: Handbook of mathematical models in computer vision. Springer, pp 237–257. ISBN 978-0-387-26371-7

Computer-Aided Malaria Detection Based on Computer Vision and Deep Learning Approach

Kartik Kumar, Gaurav Chandiramani, and Kanchan Lata Kashyap

1 Introduction

Malaria is a parasitic, deadly and infectious disease caused by the genus Plasmodium of unicellular eukaryotes. There are 5 parasitic species that are the cause of malaria in humans viz. *Plasmodium falciparum (P. falciparum), Plasmodium vivax (P. vivax), Plasmodium ovale (P. ovale), Plasmodium malariae (P. malariae), and Plasmodium knowlesi (P. knowlesi). Among all these, P. falciparum and P. vivax* are the most deadly. Malaria is typically transmitted through the bite of an infected Anopheles Mosquito. Bite of this mosquito releases the parasite into the vertebrate host's bloodstream. When health is concerned, early detection and treatment of ailment are foremost. Due to its deadly nature, a faster and scalable approach for detection of malaria is required. Current methodology includes manual examination of stained blood slides requiring proper classification and counting of parasitized and uninfected red blood corpuscles. This can be very detrimental in case of malaria related covid-like outbreak.

The aim of our work is to detect parasitized and uninfected corpuscles effectively and create a system that is less computationally expensive so that it can be deployed to web and end point devices easily. It also focuses on automation of the process and eliminates the need of tedious manual analysis by a trained professional to some extent.

K. Kumar (✉) · G. Chandiramani · K. L. Kashyap
VIT Bhopal University, Bhopal, Madhya Pradesh, India
e-mail: kartik.kumar2018@vitbhopal.ac.in

© The Author(s), under exclusive license to Springer Nature Singapore Pte Ltd. 2021   541
M. K. Bajpai et al. (eds.), *Machine Vision and Augmented Intelligence—Theory and Applications*, Lecture Notes in Electrical Engineering 796,
https://doi.org/10.1007/978-981-16-5078-9_44

1.1 Problem Statement and Major Contribution

This system employs image processing techniques for image preprocessing. The preprocessed images are fed into the trained convolutional neural network (CNN) model that classifies the image as to be parasitized with the malaria parasite or uninfected. Finally, performance of the system is compared with various other studies and traditional machine learning algorithms.

In Machine learning techniques, most of the applied features need to be identified by a domain expert in order to reduce the complexity of the data and make patterns more visible to learning algorithms to work. The biggest advantage of deep learning algorithms is that it learns high-level features from data in an incremental manner. This eliminates the need for domain expertise and hard core feature extraction. Another major difference between deep learning and machine learning is that machine learning models have limited tuning capability for hyperparameter tuning as compared to deep learning. Hyperparameter tuning in machine learning to achieve an optimal accuracy requires a lot of experimentation, it is comparatively more complex to find the optimal set of hyperparameters specific to a problem.

In this problem statement, 27,558 images of red blood cells with a dimension of 1024×1024 pixels, are taken as input. The machine learning model is computationally very expensive and time inefficient with 10,48,576 features. Even after resizing the image there is a high likelihood of losing crucial features. It takes hours to train the model and predict output for some set of input images. This type of model cannot be used for deployment so a deep learning approach is used in this work. However, to compare the accuracy of the machine learning approach, various machine learning algorithms are also implemented.

This work is structured in the following sections. The literature review is discussed in Sect. 2. The proposed model is described in Sect. 3. Experimental results are presented in Sect. 4. Conclusions are discussed in Sect. 5.

2 Literature Review

Vijayalakshmi et al. presented a study showing use of transfer learning for detecting malaria in microscopic images [1]. The proposed model in this study used a unified VGG (Visual Geometry Group) network and SVM (Support Vector Machine). The basic principle behind this unification is training top layers and freezing out the rest layers. Initially, k layers of pre-trained VGG are retained and (n–k) layers are replaced with SVM. For evaluating the VGG-SVM model performance malaria digital corpus was generated by acquiring blood smears images of malaria-infected and non-infected patients. Malaria digital corpus images were used to analyse the performance of VGG19-SVM, resulting in classification accuracy of 93.1% in identification of infected falciparum malaria. The main shortcoming of this study includes small dataset and is more computationally expensive.

Toha et al. presented a methodology involving the use of soft computing tools for malaria detection [2]. In this methodology, techniques like histogram, threshold and cluster analysis using Euclidean distance were applied to an image to detect and count the number of malaria parasites in thick blood smear. The drawbacks in this methodology included a tedious workflow that would require technicians to manually feed each and every image. This system will not work when testing mass amounts of samples.

Ross et al. performed a study involving automated image processing methods for the diagnosis and classification of malaria on thin blood smears obtained from a charge-coupled device camera connected to a light microscope [3]. This study used morphological and novel threshold techniques to identify the erythrocytes and possible parasites present on microscopic slides. Also, a two-stage tree classifier using backpropagation feedforward neural network was used to distinguish between true and false positives and was further used to identify the species of the infection. Proposed work in this study positively identified infected erythrocytes with a sensitivity of 85% and positive predictive value (PPV) of 81%. The drawbacks in this study included model capturing noise from the dataset as no noise removal image processing techniques were used. Additionally, the dataset taken into consideration was small which would result in model underfitting or overfitting depending on the number of epochs.

Reddy et al. explored transfer learning using ResNet-50 (Microsoft Residual Network) for Malaria cell image classification. Primarily, the study focussed on Microsoft's ResNet-50 neural network model for training and testing [4]. The selected model showed a training accuracy of 95.91% and validation accuracy of 95.4%. Also, in this study, base neural network models such as Google's Inception model and Oxford's VGG model alongside their architecture were discussed. This study concluded that transfer learning alongside convolution was extremely effective in predicting malaria-infected corpuscules. Additionally, use of Google's Inception model and Oxford's VGG model for the same dataset was suggested for possibly yielding better accuracy. Razzak et al. presented a case study exploring various strengths and weaknesses of deep learning for medical image processing [5]. In this case study, various algorithms related to deep learning such as CNNs, RNNs, LSTMs, ELMs and GANs alongside their architecture were discussed in detail. This study only focused on theoretical concepts of deep learning.

Litjens et al. demonstrated different approaches pertinent to medical image analysis which appeared in 2016 [6] Liang et al. demonstrated an approach that involved using Convolutional Neural Network-based image analysis for diagnosing malaria [7]. The approach shown in this work used 3-channel RGB images directly for convolution without any preprocessing which increased the computational complexity of the model. Additionally, the internal working structure of the defined model consists of very complex hidden layers that would add to the computational cost of the model by a significant amount. Proposed approach is also compared to transfer learning model using performance indicators such as average accuracy score of 97.37% obtained from ten-fold cross-validation based on the dataset, sensitivity of 96.99%, specificity of 97.75%, precision of 97.73%, F1 score of 97.36% and Matthews correlation coefficient of 94.75%.

Hung et al. presented a study involving use of Faster Region-based Convolutional Neural Network (Faster R-CNN) for Object Detection in Malaria Images [8]. In this approach, Faster R-CNN was fine-tuned with the available data and was compared with traditional baseline approach consisting of cell segmentation, extraction of several single-cell features and classification using random forests. Additionally, a less verbose two-stage approach involving AlexNet is demonstrated for assigning classes to objects. This approach gave an accuracy of 98% which is a significant improvement over the one-stage method that just involved using Faster R-CNN.

Das et al. performed a study involving use of machine learning approach for malaria parasite characterization and classification [9]. In this study, total ninety-four statistically significant features were obtained after segmentation of erythro-cytes using marker-controlled watershed transformation. Machine learning tech-niques namely Bayesian Learning and Support Vector Machine (SVM) were used for classification. The Bayesian approach showed the highest accuracy of 84%, sensi-tivity of 98.1% and specificity of 68.91% by selecting 19 most significant features. The SVM approach showed the highest accuracy of 83.5%, sensitivity of 96.62% and specificity of 88.51% using 9 most significant features.

Makkapati et al. presented a methodology involving segmentation of erythrocytes and chromatin dots in images taken from Lieshman-stained blood smear images [10]. This method was based on HSV color space that segmented RBCs and parasites by detecting dominant hue range and by calculating optimal saturation thresholds. Evaluation of the methodology was done with 55 annotated images showing the sensitivity and specificity of the proposed methods to be 83% and 98%, respectively.

Ruberto et al. presented a system for detecting and classifying malaria parasites [11]. This method used automatic thresholding based on a morphological approach to detect parasites in the blood. Here, grayscale granulometria based on opening with disk-shaped elements were used to segment cell images was proposed to preserve roundness and compactness of cells. This study proved the proposed methodology was more accurate compared to the classical watershed-based segmentation algo-rithm. Additionally, classification of parasites was done using a morphological skeleton which used endpoints as features for recognition. Study concluded that the proposed system achieved very good results and was only limited by its depen-dency on exposure and lighting conditions of the image. This study also gave way to newer research directives that could involve automated choice of morphological parameters in different exposure and magnification situations.

Ch et al. presented a study that involves coupling of Firefly Algorithm (FFA) and Support Vector Machine (SVM) to predict malaria incidences [12]. The performance of this coupling-based model is optimized by tuning the parameters of SVM which are determined by the FFA. FFA is based on the fact that luminosity created by the luminescent abdominal organ of one fly helps others fly to track the path of their movement to find their prey. FFA is a metaheuristic search algorithm. This study deals with the time series prediction, which seems irrelevant for us. Since we are more focused on malaria prediction not at what time malaria incidences can happen.

Quinn et al. proposed a methodology involving point of care diagnostics using microscopy and computer vision [13]. In this work, deep convolutional techniques are applied to three different microscopy workloads viz. diagnosis of malaria in thick blood smears, tuberculosis in sputum samples, and intestinal parasite eggs in stool samples. To overcome underfitting of the deep convolutional neural network model due to small size, it was trained for 500 epochs. This study concluded with the result of AUC = 1 for malaria dataset, showing that deep learning was extremely effective in managing such workloads.

3 Proposed Methodology

3.1 Dataset Details

The dataset is collected from a repository of segmented cells from the thin blood smear slide images from the Malaria Screener research activity [16]. To reduce the burden for microscopists in resource-constrained regions and improve diagnostic accuracy, researchers at the Lister Hill National Center for Biomedical Communications (LHNCBC), part of the National Library of Medicine (NLM), have developed a mobile application that runs on a standard Android smartphone attached to a conventional light microscope. Giemsa-stained thin blood smear slides from 150 P. falciparum-infected and 50 healthy patients were collected and photographed at Chittagong Medical College Hospital, Bangladesh. The dataset contains a total of 27,558 cell images with equal instances of parasitized and uninfected cells. Each image has a dimension of 1024×1024 pixels and 3 channels for RGB.

3.2 Image Preprocessing

An image is essentially a matrix of numbers that represent each and every pixel of the image. Image pre-processing is an integral part of this approach as it has been proven highly effective in improving time complexity and the performance of the model. In this work, the popular image processing framework OpenCV has been used to process the dataset images.

3.2.1 Applying Image Grayscale

Converting the image to grayscale is a very crucial part of the process. In OpenCV, transformations within RGB space like converting images to grayscale are supported by the cv::cvtColor function. Assuming 'A' as the pixel matrix of an image following function is applied:

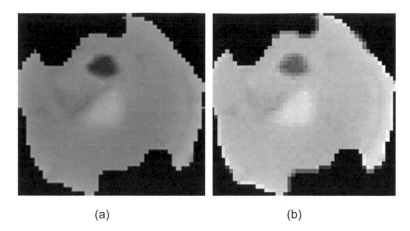

(a)   (b)

Fig. 1 Result obtained after applying RGB to gray conversion **a** Original giemsa-stained RBC image **b** Converted grayscale image

$$\text{RGB[A] to Gray} : Y \leftarrow 0.299 \cdot R + 0.587 \cdot G + 0.114 \cdot B \tag{1}$$

RGB to gray operation eliminates the RGB color channel in the image matrix and replaces it with a single color channel which reduces the time complexity of training the model by 3 folds. Image dimensions also change from $1024 \times 1024 \times 3$ to $1024 \times 1024 \times 1$ (Fig. 1).

3.2.2 Image Resizing

Image resizing is another known technique for reducing the time complexity while training the model. In this work, the giemsa-stained RBC image has been dimensionally reduced from 1024×1024 pixels to 48×48 pixels. OpenCV provides a cv::resize function which takes image, dimensions and interpolation as parameters. Image resizing in this work has been done using INTER_AREA interpolation method which does resampling using pixel area relation. It is the preferred method for image decimation, as it gives moire'-free results.

3.2.3 Image Blurring

Image blurring is a known technique that involves convolving the image with a low-pass filter kernel to eliminate high frequency content (noice, edges) from an image. Four different image blurring techniques viz. Averaging, Gaussian Blurring, Median Blurring, and Bilateral filtering can be applied for edge detection. The main purpose is to remove the noise from the image while keeping the edges sharp so that the anomaly can be detected clearly and more efficiently. In this work, the bilateral filter

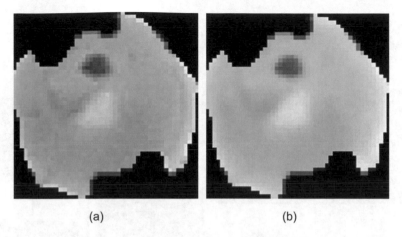

(a)　　　　　　　　　　　　　　　　(b)

Fig. 2 Grayscale image **a** showing anomaly and distortion nearby **b** Filtered image (After applying bilateral filter)

for blurring the images as it is highly effective in noise removal while keeping the edges sharp, is applied. This filter is very slow and hence the filter size (diameter of each pixel neighbourhood) and Sigma values (space, color—influence of other pixels) are assigned as 5 and 75, respectively. Specifically, lower values are chosen for these parameters as higher values showed increased time complexities while processing. Figure 2a shows the grayscale image, light distortion and noise can be seen which can hinder model training. Figure 3b. shows smoothened out image after the bilateral filter is applied. It can be analysed that the distortion in resultant image is minimal and smoothened alongside the border of the cell and the anomaly being preserved.

3.3　Proposed CNN Model

The CNN model is designed and trained from scratch for this work. The main reason behind designing a new CNN model other than using a pre-trained neural network is that for choosing a pre-trained neural network, we need to ensure that the chosen pre-trained network has been trained with the similar kind of images for which we are going to use in our scenario. Moreover, the dataset taken as input in the present work contains a substantial amount of images. Thus, training and designing of CNN are proposed from scratch. The architecture of proposed CNN is as follows: (i) Four convolutional layer (ii) Two max pooling layer (iii) Three dense or fully connected layer and (iv) One dropout layer

(i) **Convolutional layer**—This layer contains a certain number of filters whose parameters need to be learned. Each filter is convolved with the input volume of the image to compute an activation map made of neurons. In other words, the filter is slid

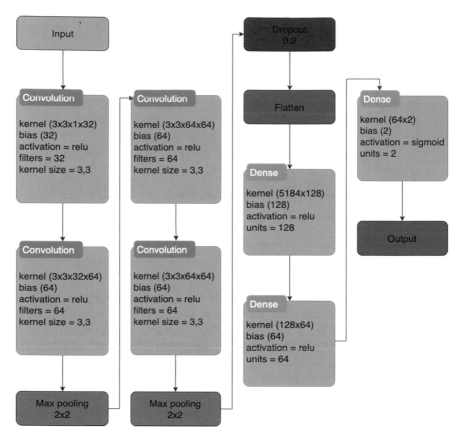

Fig. 3 Architecture of the proposed CNN model

across the width and height of the input and the dot products between the input and filter are computed at every spatial position. An optimal number of filters at every convolution layer is used to get better accuracy. The number of filters used at every convolution layer is presented in Fig. 3.

(ii) **Max pooling layer**—This layer is usually added after convolutional layers. The introduction of pooling layer after convolutional layers is a common pattern used for ordering layers in the CNN that may be repeated once or twice in the model. This layer replaces the output from the convolutional layer by deriving a summary statistic of the nearby outputs. This in turn reduces the output size, which decreases the computation time significantly. One pooling layer after two consecutive convolutional layers is introduced in the proposed model. The kernel size for max pooling used in the network is 2.

(iii) **Dense or fully connected layer**—The neurons have full connectivity with the neurons in the succeeding and preceding layer. Before the three-dimensional array output from convolutional and max pooling layers fed into a dense layer, it needs to be converted into a 1-dimensional array because the dense layer takes one-dimensional array as input. This conversion is done by the flatten operation on output from the convolutional layers. Total 3 dense layers and the number of neurons at each layer are given in Fig. 3.

(iv) **Dropout layer**—Due to large number of images there is a probability of overfitting in the proposed CNN model. This can result in a poor performance during testing on new data. The dropout layer is used to overcome the overfitting problem. At this layer, some number of outputs from a layer are dropped out or ignored at the time of training the model. The dropout layer is introduced before the dense layer in the proposed CNN model. Dropout parameter is set to 0.2 which means 20% of the input units will be dropped at this layer.

Each layer except the output layer uses an activation of rectified linear unit (ReLU). Considering experimental results in previous researches ReLU has shown extraordinary performance in terms of results for image processing tasks. ReLU basically rejects all the negative values coming from the neurons by converting them to zero. As compared to other activation functions ReLU has the lowest computational expense, which makes the model more efficient. The output layer has an activation of sigmoid that gives a binary value which is considered as the final output.

In the training phase Adam (Adaptive Moment Estimation) optimizer is used which is an algorithm to optimize the gradient descent at the time of backpropagation in a neural network. This algorithm is very efficient to handle large dataset which involves a lot of calculation with a large number of weights. Since the present problem is a two-class classification, so binary cross-entropy is used as the loss function. Binary cross entropy is the most fundamental function to deal with a binary classification problem. After a lot of experimentation, the value of batch size is obtained as 128. The model is trained for 20 epochs where the maxima in terms of accuracy is reached.

4 Experimental Results

The preprocessed images of 48×48 are given as input in the proposed CNN model. The model is trained with more than 27,000 images of red blood cells. After rigorous training and testing with various hyperparameters and preprocessing methodologies, optimal state is obtained where the accuracy of the model converges to a specific value. The performance of the trained model is analysed with various metrics: accuracy, sensitivity, specificity, precision, AUC, and F1_score. The output of the testing results are shown in Table 1. The average validation accuracy of 95.0% is obtained with the proposed CNN model. The ROC curve obtained from the proposed model is shown in Fig. 4. The highest 95% AUC is obtained which can be analysed from Fig. 4. The result of the proposed model is compared with traditional machine learning algorithms which are listed in Table 1. It can be analysed from the obtained results that the proposed model performs better than the traditional machine learning models.

Table 1 Validation results (in %) obtained from the proposed CNN model

Model	Sensitivity	Specificity	Precision	AUC	F1_score	Accuracy
Proposed Model	0.968	0.932	0.933	0.950	0.950	0.950
Logistic regression	–	–	–	–	–	0.669
Random forest	–			–	–	0.732
Decision tree	–	–	–	–	–	0.669
KNN	–	–	–	–	–	0.636
SVM	–	–	–	–	–	0.662

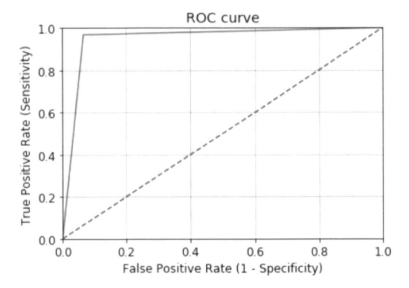

Fig. 4 ROC curve obtained from the proposed CNN model

5 Conclusions

In this work, a real-world medical imaging problem of malaria detection has been done. Malaria detection by itself is not an easy procedure and the availability of the right personnel across the globe is also a serious concern. A simple convolutional neural model is proposed in the present work. The bilateral image filtering technique has been applied for noise removal. The highest 95%, 93.2% and 96.8% of accuracy, sensitivity and specificity are obtained, respectively with the proposed model. The performance comparison of the proposed model with state-of-art machine learning techniques are also done. It is concluded that the performance of the proposed model is better than the traditional machine learning techniques. In future, the proposed model can be easily deployed on the web and endpoint devices for malaria detection.

References

1. Vijayalakshmi A, Rajesh Kanna B (2020) Deep learning approach to detect malaria from microscopic images. Multimed Tools Appl 79:15297–15317
2. Toha SF, Ngah UK (2007) Computer aided medical diagnosis for the identification of malaria parasites. In: IEEE-ICSCN, 22–24 Feb 2007, pp 521–522
3. Ross NE, Pritchard CJ, Rubin DM et al (2006) Automated image processing method for the diagnosis and classification of malaria on thin blood smears. Med Bio Eng Comput 44:427–436
4. Reddy ASB, Juliet DS (2019) Transfer learning with ResNet-50 for malaria cell-image classification. In: International conference on communication and signal processing, 4–6 Apr 2019, India
5. Razzak MI, Naz S, Zaib A (2018) Deep learning for medical image processing: overview, challenges and the future. In: Dey N, Ashour A, Borra S (eds) Classification in Bioapps. Lecture notes in computational vision and biomechanics, vol 26. Springer, Cham
6. Litjens G, Kooi T, Bejnordi BE, Setio AAA, Ciompi F, Ghafoorian M, van der Laak JAWM, Ginneken B, Sánchez CI (2017) A survey on deep learning in medical image analysis. Med Image Anal 42:60–88
7. Liang Z et al (2016) CNN-based image analysis for malaria diagnosis. In: 2016 IEEE international conference on bioinformatics and biomedicine (BIBM), Shenzhen, China, pp 493–496
8. Hung J, Goodman A, Ravel D et al (2020) Keras R-CNN: library for cell detection in biological images using deep neural networks. BMC Bioinform 21:300
9. Das DK, Ghosh M, Pal M, Maiti AK, Chakraborty C (2013) Machine learning approach for automated screening of malaria parasite using light microscopic images. Micron 45:97–106
10. Rao R, Makkapati V (2009) Segmentation of malaria parasites in peripheral blood smear images. IEEE international Conference on acoustics, speech, and signal processing, Taiwan Taipei, pp 1361–1364
11. Di Ruberto C, Dempster A, Khan S, Jarra B (2001) Morphological image processing for evaluating malaria disease. In: Arcelli C, Cordella LP, di Baja GS (eds) Visual Form 2001. IWVF 2001. Lecture notes in computer science, vol 2059
12. Sudheer Ch, Sohani SK, Kumar D, Malik A, Chahar BR, Nema AK, Panigrahi BK, Dhiman RC (2014) A support vector machine-firefly algorithm based forecasting model to determine malaria transmission. Neurocomputing 129:279–288
13. Quinn JA, Nakasi R, Mugagga PKB, Byanyima P, Lubega W, Andama A (2016) Deep convolutional neural networks for microscopy-based point of care diagnostics. In: Proceedings of the 1st machine learning for healthcare conference, in PMLR 56, pp 271–281
14. Bilateral Filter http://homepages.inf.ed.ac.uk/rbf/CVonline/LOCAL_COPIES/MANDUCHI1/Bilateral_Filtering.html
15. SciKit Learn Supervised Learning https://scikit-learn.org/stable/supervised_learning.html
16. Malaria dataset https://lhncbc.nlm.nih.gov/publication/pub9932

Embedded Vision-Based Intelligent Device for the Visually Impaired

Mohammad Farukh Hashmi, Sasweth C. Rajanarayanan, and Avinash G. Keskar

1 Introduction

Visually impaired people are several times as sharp as the average human being and have a unique alertness to sounds. While this holds true, vision holds the badge for being the most important sense that the human being is endowed with. A normal man's conversation with a person can convey a lot to him visually. Visual inferences are integral parts of a conversation. Though a visually impaired person draws deep insights from his or her society through other senses that they possess, it does not quite match the accuracy and speed that a visual contact has in inferring from a person's surroundings. This work aims to convey that part of the visual data to a visually impaired person that helps in adding more behaviour to his or her conversation. Conveying the emotion that a face shows to a visually impaired person makes him infer more during a conversation and makes him inch closer to what a person with a proper sight feels. This aims to augment the way a visually impaired person feels the world. Computer Vision has been making heavy strides in solving critical problems that abound in the society. Right from medical sciences to defence, there is literally no domain that computer vision has untouched. With a lot of algorithms being increasingly proposed in the domain of computer vision and deep learning, the selection of an algorithm to solve a particular problem has become dynamic. Face recognition algorithms like facenet by Google [1] have carved a pathway for facial recognition and can also be modified to add features that use the facial data and its features to predict

M. F. Hashmi (✉) · S. C. Rajanarayanan
Department of Electronics and Communication Engineering, National Institute of Technology, Warangal 506004, India
e-mail: mdfarukh@nitw.ac.in

A. G. Keskar
Department of Electronics and Communication Engineering, Visvesvaraya National Institute of Technology, Nagpur 440010, India
e-mail: agkeskar@ece.vnit.ac.in

© The Author(s), under exclusive license to Springer Nature Singapore Pte Ltd. 2021
M. K. Bajpai et al. (eds.), *Machine Vision and Augmented Intelligence—Theory and Applications*, Lecture Notes in Electrical Engineering 796,
https://doi.org/10.1007/978-981-16-5078-9_45

other parameters pertaining to a face like such as emotion, gender, age, etc. A few state-of-the-art deep learning models built with Neural Networks like the Residual Neural Networks can prove to be very helpful in this regard. Facial features are complex and therefore a face recognition model has to work upon multiple features that pertain to a face.

A Convolutional Neural Network can be used to achieve this end, but a CNN will not be able to deal with a lot of features. This is because more features demand more layers in the convolutional neural network. This causes problems like loss in gradient during backpropagation. To counter this, residual neural networks were introduced [2], which are capable of scaling up humongous amounts of layers present in a neural network and still show an improving performance. A RNN must therefore be used if there are a lot of features to work upon. This work uses a variant of ResNet called Wide ResNet. Problems like age and gender recognition solicit deep residual networks, residual networks that have huge number of layers. Diminishing reuse of features and therefore very slow training of these networks is an important problem to tackle in deep residual networks. The algorithm proposed in [3] presents a solution to this by reducing the depth of the network and increasing its width. These are called Wide Residual Networks or Wide ResNets in general. These networks are proven to show improved accuracy, besides improved efficiency when tested upon CIFAR and COCO datasets. This work uses a model built using Wide Residual Networks to classify the age and gender of a person using his or her facial data. A Convolutional Neural Network that had been trained upon the FER-2013 dataset to classify emotions was used. The dataset has the following classes of values: Happy, sad, angry, surprise, fear, disgust. This dataset had also been used in [4] to train a mini Xception Net to classify apparent emotions with a performance that is on par with humans. While there are models that guarantee a solid performance in classifying age, gender and emotions, performance results do not remain the same when these models are deployed on a hardware platform or a single board computer. This work is application-oriented and therefore uses a Raspberry Pi3, over which the models, along with its weights are deployed. The Raspberry Pi3 is interfaced with a Pi Camera that collects facial data. Resource allocation is a very important problem that needs to be acknowledged in embedded computing systems.

Face detection is an integral part of this work and is an important first step. The detected face is passed through the classifiers for classifying emotions, age and gender. The accuracy of the final result, be it emotion classification or age and gender classification depends heavily on the accuracy of the face detector, besides depending on the respective models' training and validation accuracies. Latency is a very important constraint for real-time embedded systems. Since an embedded system is proposed in this work the application is required to be working in real time. Face detectors show extensive levels of accuracy when implemented using neural networks, but demands heavy computational power. While a lot of work is going on to make deep learning models platform independent, there is no perfect algorithm that is completely resource aware. This is an important stake for real-time embedded systems and is very crucial to the system proposed in this work. The classifier built for detecting faces along with the emotion classifier's weights and the age and gender classifier's weights were stored locally on the Raspberry Pi. Raspbian OS, a real-time operating system that runs on the Raspberry Pi hosts the application software, which in this work is the proposed emotion, age and gender classifier. The Wide Residual Network was fine tuned to improve the accuracy of the age and gender classifier.

This paper is organized as follows: Sect. 2 talks about the work going on in this area. Section 3 throws light on the hardware setup that this work makes use of and Sect. 4 talks about the algorithms pertaining to its software counterpart. Section 5 is an explanation of how the prototype proposed works to convey the data that is estimated as emotion, age and gender to a visually impaired person. Section 6 is a take on results while Sect. 7 talks about the conclusions of this work, saving further scope for Sect. 8.

2 Related Work

There has been a lot of interesting and groundbreaking contributions to this important area. The work in [5] has used the IMDB-Wiki dataset for gender estimation from faces and has been an inspiration to this work. Computer Engineers are finding ways to make deep learning models platform independent. This makes way for easy deployments on a hardware platform. Deep learning has a lot of potential and making them available through application software on single board computers is difficult but truly helpful. Real-time embedded systems have a constraint on the resources that it can share among its hardware and software components. Deep learning algorithms need amendments to their core, as these algorithms are predominantly resource hungry. Computer Vision has therefore branched out into Embedded Vision, which is a positive step towards the future, as self-driving cars, robots and drones are all embedded systems with visual intelligence.

A lot of works are aiming to deploy deep learning models on mobile platforms and on single board computers [6] and a few others are working towards accelerating them on hardware platforms. On-device machine learning is therefore catching attention. This work is a step towards deploying deep learning models on single board computers to make embedded systems intelligent, yet functional in real time.

3 Hardware Setup

3.1 Raspberry Pi

This work uses a Raspberry Pi, over which the application software is run. The Raspberry Pi3 is a single board computer that houses an ARM Cortex M0 microprocessor and is one of the most popular single-board computing systems. The Raspberry Pi 3 comes with the Raspbian OS. The Raspbian OS is a real-time operating system,

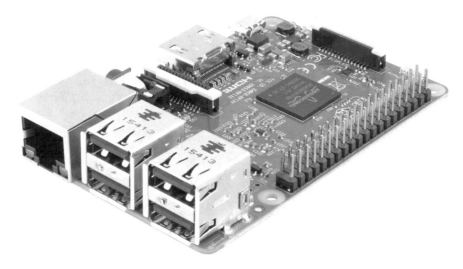

Fig. 1 The Hardware of Raspberry Pi 3 Board

which in this work would be hosting the application software. The Raspberry Pi comes with an Ethernet port, a USB-A port, a memory card on which the Raspbian OS has been mounted and a 3.5 mm headphone jack. The board solicits a 5 V power supply. It offers GPIO support with 40 GPIO headers which encompass pulse width modulation pins, SPI pins, I2C pins and Serial pins besides pins for power supply (5 V and 3.3 V). The Raspberry Pi 3 also contains the Wi-Fi and Bluetooth stack, making it suitable as a network edge device or a gateway device.

Figure 1 shows hardware of Raspberry Pi 3 board. The Raspberry Pi 3 has been interfaced with a Pi camera that has 8 megapixels and can shoot at 1080p. The camera here captures the facial data that the application software uses for achieving its end. Figure 2 shows the hardware of Pi camera that has been used in this work.

4 Algorithms Used

The software here refers to the application software that this work makes use of. The software development problem is seen as two sub problems- age and gender recognition and emotion classification.

4.1 Age and Gender Recognition

Age and gender are both estimated using a Wide Residual Network. The WideResNet is an improvement over the infamous ResNet or Residual Neural Network [3]. During

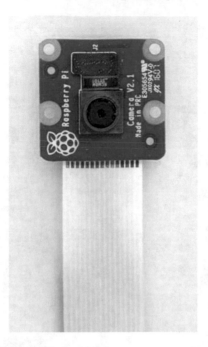

Fig. 2 The Hardware of Pi Camera

backpropagation in a convolutional neural network, repeated multiplications cause the gradient to vanish. The gradient thus becomes infinitely small. This leads to the saturation of the network and degradation in its performance. Resnet avoids this by skipping individual layers using a gateway connection. WideResNet or wide residual networks are obtained by widening a residual network, thus making the network shallow. To extract a good performance out of a CNN, WideResNet and Google Net make use of parallel network architectures [7]. WideResNet-16–8 has been used in this work to classify age and gender. WideResNet moreover is a parallelized version of the ResNet architecture [7]. Resnet-152 and WideResNet-16–8 have been shown in Fig. 3. WideResNets can be trained faster when compared to ResNets and have the same or improved accuracy as ResNets. Widening the network causes the number of parameters to increase which is a dismissive problem in this application. The network being shallow, allows for faster training. Parameters of the WideResNet have been shown in Fig. 4. The WideResNet was trained on the IMDB-Wiki dataset that has over 500,000 faces that are age and gender labeled. The model summary revealed a total number of parameters as 24,463,856, out of which 24,456,656 were trainable. The trained model along with its weights was deployed on the Raspberry Pi 3.

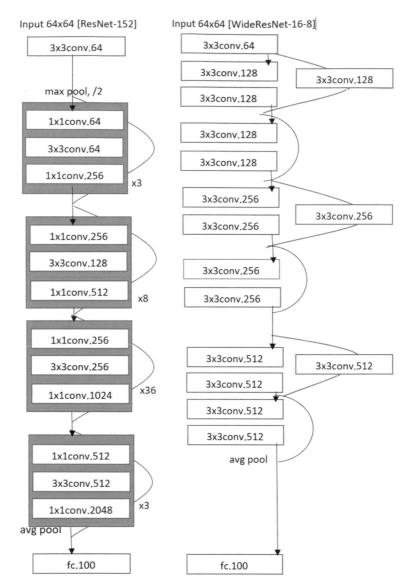

Fig. 3 The Architecture of ResNet-152; WideResNet-16–8

4.2 Emotion Recognition

The FER 2013 dataset has been used to train a mini Xception Net for emotion recognition. That dataset contain six types of emotions in the form of anger, happy, sad, fear, surprise and disgust. Figure 5 shows a few images from the FER-2013 dataset [8]. The dataset contains 547 images of the **Disgust** category, 4002 images of the **Surprise**

```
Total params: 24,463,856

Trainable params: 24,456,656

Non-trainable params: 7,200
```

Fig. 4 Parameters of the WideResNet

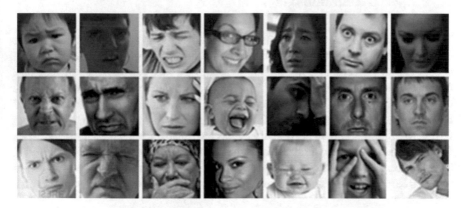

Fig. 5 A few images from the FER-2013 dataset

category, 5121 images of the **Fear** category, 4593 images of the **Angry** category, 6077 images of the **Sad** category, 6198 images of the **Neutral** category, 8989 images of the **Happy** category. While conventional machine learning approaches like Kneasrest neighbours and support vector machines can help with emotion classifications, a neural network achieves a bigger accuracy than the aforementioned algorithms [9]. The mini Xception Net was trained using the ImageNet dataset. The XceptionNet is an infamous architecture developed by Google and makes use of upgraded depthwise separable convolutions in its core. For the ImageNet dataset, the XceptionNet showed an accuracy of 94.5 percent, outperforming Inception-v3 and ResNet-152 and VGG-16 architectutres. Using the technique of transfer learning, the Xception Network was trained on the FER-2013 dataset in this work after freezing the body of the network that contains the ImageNet weights, to classify emotions and was able to achieve an accuracy of 66 percent on the FER-2013 dataset. The mini Xception network was so chosen, to work in real-time on embedded computing systems. The mini Xception Net along with its weights was deployed on the hardware. Parameters of the CNN built in this work have been shown in Fig. 6.

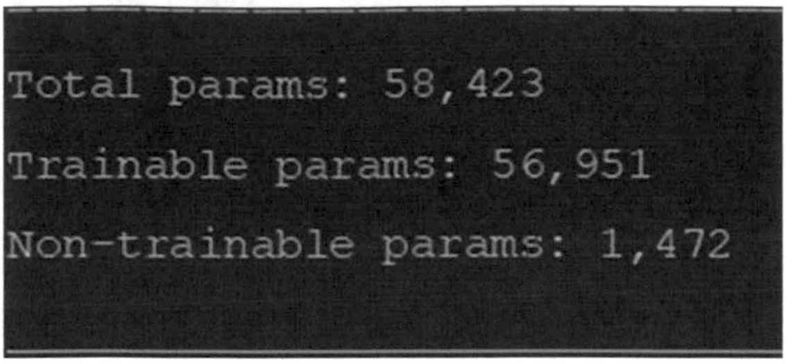

Fig. 6 Parameters of the
CNN built in this work

```
Total params: 58,423

Trainable params: 56,951

Non-trainable params: 1,472
```

5 Proposed Methodology

The Raspberry Pi 3 was interfaced with a Pi Camera to capture the facial data. Face detection is an important part of this work, as the device's overall accuracy is heavily dependent on the face detector's ability to detect a face properly. The Mutli-task Cascaded Convolutional Network (MTCNN) was initially used to implement a face detector [10]. The MTCNN is a deep learning algorithm and makes use of neural networks to achieve face detection. Orientation of faces did not prove to be a problem for the MTCNN. While this is true, there was a problem of resource allocation when the face detector was implemented on an ARM-based computer, the Raspberry Pi 3. This is often the problem with embedded computing systems. The algorithm proved to be resource hungry. Real-time performance of the system is very crucial for this application.

The MTCNN prevented the system from being real time. To counter this, a Haar-based cascade classifier, which uses Haar-based features to classify a face, was used. The Haar cascade classifiers are integral parts of the Viola-Jones Object detection algorithm. These cascade classifiers guaranteed a real-time performance on the Raspberry Pi 3 board. The Raspberry Pi offers support for the Raspbian OS. Raspbian OS is a Real-time Operating System (RTOS) and is a LINUX distribution. It therefore had support for XML files. The XML file of the Haar cascade classifier for detecting faces did not cause a problem when stored locally on the Raspberry Pi 3. The models for emotion and age and gender recognition, along with their weights were stored on the Raspberry Pi 3. A python script was written on the Raspbian OS that made use of the Haar-based cascade classifier to detect faces and the respective models and their weights to recognize the emotion, age and gender of the person in front of the camera. The detected labels were conveyed in real time as audio outputs to the visually impaired person using Google's text to speech library called gTTS, through a pair of earphones connected to the Raspberry Pi 3 board's 3.5 mm headphone jack. The proposed prototype has been sketched in Fig. 7. The performance of the system was observed to be in real time. Along with the conversation, other trait that can augment the way a conversation happens is also conveyed to a visually impaired person. This takes the experience of a visually impaired person to a whole new level and gives him more control over the conversation. Age detection helps the person with vision-based difficulties to decide the nature of the conversation which humans

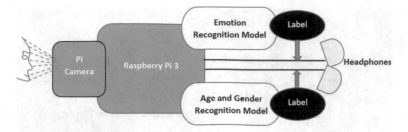

Fig. 7 The proposed system

have learnt and known doing. The age and gender detection model had to be fine-tuned to improve its accuracy in detecting a person's age. The system's real-time performance was achieved after due amendments were made to the models that were used like the one described above. Embedded Vision was thus implemented on a system. Machine Vision has been used to mimic human vision.

6 Experimental Results

The model when deployed on a Raspberry Pi 3 board was able to detect faces, classify the emotion it shows and estimate the age and gender of the person. Figs. 7, 8 and 9 show the results obtained in this work. The algorithm was tested on two

Fig. 8 Face that is Happy, 21 years old and Male (M)

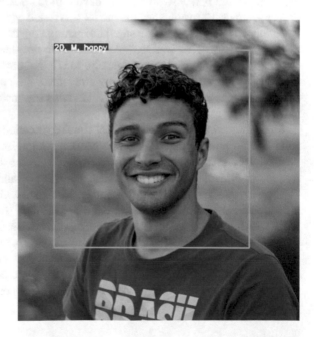

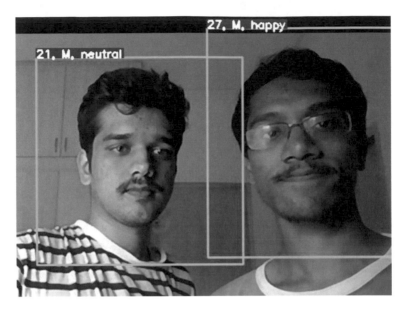

Fig. 9 Left: Neutral, 21 years old, M. Right: Happy, 27 years old, M

faces. In Fig. 8, the person on the right was 21 years old and a male, while the one on the right was 27 years old and a male. The faces are classified to be neutral and happy in Fig. 8 and were actually neutral and happy, respectively. The labels were conveyed to the person who had the device in his possession, as an audio output. Figure 9 shows the result when the model was tested against a video clip. The model had a tough time predicting the stipulated parameters for faces that were disoriented from the camera. This was because faces were not detected when they were not oriented towards the camera completely. MTCNN boosted the performance in this regard but was not deployable as it would make the application not work in real time. Faces that were oriented towards the camera showed a good performance, as indicated by Figs. 7, 8 and 9.

Since the work deals with a real-time application, latency is an important parameter to be considered. Age and gender recognition was performed using the WideResNet architecture and emotion recognition was done using an XceptionNet that was finetuned on the FER-2013 dataset, while retaining the ImageNet weights. The latency that the finetuned XceptionNet combined with the age and gender recognition model introduced averaged at **0.345613956451416** s. While the Xception Net, along with the age and gender recognition model introduced a latency that averaged at **0.28307580947875977** s. The Xception Net was able to outperform the CNN built in this work marginally by **0.06253814697** s. This latency calculation was made while using haar-based cascade classifiers for face detection and is an average of a total of seven readings of latency while running the models on a CPU. This latency also

Fig. 10 Face that is Neutral, 21 years old originally

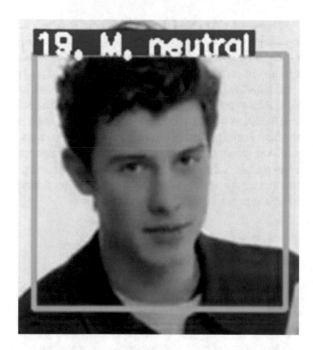

takes into consideration the time required for frame or image resizing and elementary image processing operations that are done before one forward passes through the network of the input is attempted.

7 Conclusions and Future Scope

The proposed system was able to classify emotions, age and gender with a good accuracy and acceptably low latency for a real-time system. Face detection did not take a hit and the application was able to run almost in real time which signifies an appropriate use of resources in the single board computer. There was a latency of about 0.28 s for classifying the age, gender and emotion of faces in a single frame, when Xception Net was used. The system did not perform extremely well with disoriented faces, classifying a wrong emotion that a disoriented face showed. This was because of the fact that haar-based cascade classifiers do not work good with disoriented faces. MTCNN on the other hand added accuracy while classifying emotions of faces that are disoriented from the camera but was causing the latency to increase to as high as 1.93 s. Age and gender were determined very accurately for most of the cases, with gender recognition being consistently accurate. Age recognition was faulty for a few faces, as shown above but by only a very narrow margin that is permissible for this application.

This work talks about the implementation of an embedded computing system that uses computer vision to classify emotions, age and gender and conveys the same as audio output to a visually impaired person. While this would augment the way visually impaired person perceives his peers and people who talk to him, it would be even helpful if this system is included with algorithms for real-time activity recognition. Real-time activity recognition along with the existing emotion, age and gender classification can itself become an eye to a visually impaired person by mimicking the human eye completely during a conversation with a person. Movements, actions, emotion, gender and age can be collectively recognized by a system and can be conveyed as audio outputs to the visually impaired person. This would sophisticate the system, make it robust and level it up to achieve the aim of helping visually impaired people at a sensitive level.

References

1. Schroff F, Kalenichenko D, Philbin J (2015) Facenet: a unified embedding for face recognition and clustering. In: Proceedings of the IEEE conference on computer vision and pattern recognition, pp. 815–823
2. He K, Zhang X, Ren S, Sun J (2016) Identity mappings in deep residual networks. In: Proceedings of the European conference on computer vision. Springer, Cham, pp. 630–645
3. Zagoruyko S, Komodakis N (2016) Wide residual networks. arXiv: 1605.07146
4. Minaee S, Abdolrashidi A (2019) Deep-emotion: facial expression recognition using attentional convolutional network. arXiv:1902.01019
5. Bhat SF, Dar TA (2019) Gender prediction from images using deep learning techniques. In: Proceedings of the 2019 IEEE international artificial intelligence and data processing symposium (IDAP), pp. 1–6
6. Wang J, Cao B, Yu P, Sun L, Bao W, Zhu X (2018) Deep learning towards mobile applications. In: Proceedings of the IEEE 2018 38th international conference on distributed computing systems (ICDCS), pp. 1385–1393
7. Ito HK, Okano T, Aoki T (2018) Age and gender prediction from face images using convolutional neural network. In: Proceedings of the IEEE 2018 Asia-Pacific signal and information processing association annual summit and conference (APSIPA ASC), pp. 7–11
8. Pramerdorfer C, Kampel M (2016) Facial expression recognition using convolutional neural networks: state of the art. arXiv:1612.02903
9. Singh D (2012) Human emotion recognition system. Int J Image, Graph Signal Process 4(8):50
10. Zhang K, Zhang Z, Li Z, Qiao Y (2016) Joint face detection and alignment using multitask cascaded convolutional networks. IEEE Signal Process Lett 23(10): 1499–1503

Genetic Algorithm Based Resident Load Scheduling for Electricity Cost Reduction

J. Jeyaranjani and D. Devaraj

1 Introduction

Smart electricity network is an emerging service that provides various solutions like reduction in peak demand, energy forecasting, cost-saving, security measures, quality improvement, theft detection, etc. Smart grid is the widespread area where the two-way communication makes the system smart. Demand Response is the major issue that requires dynamic regulation of electrical power. The consumers are categorized into two: residents and commercial. The targeted consumers could be residents for the reason of flexibility in altering power usage which is rather possible in commercial consumers. The consumers are being installed with smart metre that permits two-way communications between them and the utility. The utility companies might predict the consumption pattern of the consumers for near future and distribute the power accordingly. This could be achieved by using the historic consumption pattern of the consumers. This is one way of using prediction technique based on Demand Management. The solution initialization will be day ahead forecasting that picture out the future load requirement. The scenario may occur where the utility is insufficient with the supply of power for the expected period of time in dynamic time. The Management for the raised demand could be answered in such a way that the residents are impressed with the price scheme [1, 2]. The dynamic price value is proposed by the utility company who supplies electricity. The dynamic price is varying cost determined for every timeslot based on power availability at the slot. The timeslot is the split of 24 h time. It may differ from utility to utility (eg: per timeslot may be 30 min). If there is surplus power in specific timeslot, then the price is less in that timeslot, whereas the demand in power in specific timeslot will lead to an increase in price in the timeslot.

J. Jeyaranjani (✉) · D. Devaraj
Kalasalingam Academy of Research and Education, Anand Nagar, Krishnankoil, Virudhnagar, Tamilnadu 626126, India

© The Author(s), under exclusive license to Springer Nature Singapore Pte Ltd. 2021   565
M. K. Bajpai et al. (eds.), *Machine Vision and Augmented Intelligence—Theory and Applications*, Lecture Notes in Electrical Engineering 796,
https://doi.org/10.1007/978-981-16-5078-9_46

Utilizing the communication methodologies and prediction techniques, the utility may manage the power distribution. But to also satisfy it is the requirement to know the optimal power utilization strategy of their consumers. The expected utilization pattern of power by every consumer may be represented using the optimal algorithms.

1.1 Literature Survey

Various researches are carried out in Demand Response for the benefit of utility and the customers. Numbers of algorithms are experimented to provide solution where the optimization has played vital role in obtaining best solution out of all results. In this way, [3] uses the Genetic algorithm by proposing the combination of dynamic pricing scheme with the inclining block rate (IBR) model to address the nonlinear problem of peak reduction and cost–benefit. Baris Yuce et al. [4] explore the way of finding the best combination of load for the week using ANN and GA. Simon et al. [5] presented the finding of optimal energy storage system (ESS) schedule for peak demand reduction and load-leveling that uses simple heuristics to find possible optimal operation points for the ESS and improves the solutions found using genetic algorithm optimization. The optimization algorithm is implemented for ESS schedule for the distribution network operator at top level of the system architecture. This will be an extra managed burden to the utility which already works on managing the peak reduction using a consumption point of view [6]. [7–12] Proposes the predictive control frameworks where local Home Energy Management Systems are coordinated by the aggregator in order to come up with an agreement throughout negotiation iterations and provide a feasible solution to the centralized DR problem. This could involve in time consuming activity as there may be various levels of aggregation units [13]. This work also focuses on receiving the neighborhood power schedule and then scheduler is applied with the meta-heuristic cuckoo optimization algorithm for consumer's financial benefit. The demand response program implemented the residential load scheduling that include pricing schemes using the varieties of optimizations techniques [14–20]. The neighborhood scheduler strives with getting desired load curve such that it will provide a balanced consumption. GA-based DR scheme is presented in [21, 22] for appliance scheduling to minimize the electricity cost and Peak Average Ratio. [23] presents the stanford digital library metadata architecture used for the Demand Response Program.

1.2 Paper Outline

In Sect. 2, the mathematical formation of the identified problem is presented. Section 3 presents the purpose of optimization algorithm for the identified problem. In Sect. 4, the various constraints considered for finding the problem solution are explained. Section 5 presents the penalty module the represents the reduction in the penalty cost for the resident. Section 6 concludes the benefit of GA in reducing the electricity load during the peak time which is raised by the utility.

2 Mathematical Formulation of Problem

The load available in the home could be categorized into uninterruptible and shiftable. The scheduling of these variety of appliances is preferred by utility and implemented by the residents. The timestamp is considered as 24 timeslots per day. The uninterruptible load is provided with the priority for occupying the energy whereas the threshold energy value of the resident may not be a factor of consideration here. The threshold energy of the resident is verified for scheduling the remaining load such as shiftable loads. This type of scheduling operation may reduce the penalty for the resident.

The numbers of considered load are $N = 20$, where a resident may have more than one same type of load. Table 1 represents the 20 loads such as shiftable and uninterruptable. For our experiment, we considered that also as individual load eg: if a resident has two induction stove, then it will be listed as two loads. The reason behind the two load working timeslot may be varying. The 'N' loads itself include both uninterruptible and shiftable loads as represented in Eq. 1. Two vectors N_uninterruptable, (UL_n) and N_shiftable, (SL_n) are merged together to form the load vector 'N'.

$$N = \{UL_n \text{ and} SL_n\} = \{L_1, L_2, \ldots\ldots L_n\} \tag{1}$$

A matrix 'M1' represents the ON/OFF status of all loads for all timeslots. The status of the load for every time slot is specified as either 0 or 1. 0 is 'off' state and 1 is 'on' state. The representation is given by LS^t_n. Similarly, another matrix 'M2' represents the unit consumed by every load every time. The representation is shown as LE^t_n.

Table 1 The load details of the residents in terms of required energy, load category, timeslot

Name of the load	Total required energy (KWh)	Required energy per hour (KWh)	No of timeslots required	Timeslot window	Load category
Refrigerator	9	0.5	24	1–24	Uninterruptable
Inverter	1.6	0.5	15	5–20	Shiftable
Air condition	5.6	1	7	21–24, 1–4	Shiftable
Electric pump	1.0	0.75	2	6–7	Shiftable
Rice cooker	5.5	3	2	5–6	Shiftable

$$LS_n^t = \begin{cases} 1 & \text{If load is ON at time 't'} \\ 0 & \text{Otherwise} \end{cases} \quad (2)$$

The matrix 'M1'represnts the on/off status of all load and 'M2' represents the units consumed by every load in the resident

$$
\begin{array}{cc}
& \begin{matrix} t1\ t2\ t3......t24 \end{matrix} \\
M1 = \begin{matrix} L_1 \\ L_2 \\ . \\ . \\ L_{20} \end{matrix} & \begin{pmatrix} 0\,1\,1\,....................1 \\ ... \\ \\ ... \\ 1\,1\,0.....................0 \end{pmatrix}
\end{array}
\qquad
\begin{array}{cc}
& \begin{matrix} t1\ t2\ t3......t24 \end{matrix} \\
M2 = \begin{matrix} L_1 \\ L_2 \\ . \\ . \\ \end{matrix} & \begin{pmatrix} 0.4\,10\,3\,.............1.6 \\ 1\,4.1\,5\,.............0.3 \\ ..... \\ \\ 3.3\,2.1\,1.............6.2 \end{pmatrix}
\end{array}
$$

n—Loadswhere n=1,2....20

t—Time slotswhere t = 1,2,....24

LE_n^t—Units consumed by load 'n' at time t

E_t—Total energy consumed by all load at time t

C_t—Total cost at time t

LS_n^t—Load status (ON/OFF)

M—Matrix of Load status

As our experiments' main focus is on cost reduction, the cost of the resident's consumption is calculated specifically to time slot. The total energy consumed for every timeslot (E^t) is calculated by considering the Load which is in ON state and its units consumed. The unit of measurement of E^t is kWh. The status of the load (ON/OFF) is represented as LS_n^t, unit consumed is represented in KWh (Table 2).

In Automated Metering Infrastructure, the cost is not flat at all timeslot. The dynamic cost is proposed as the price plan by the utility with respect to the power availability is represented as C. The main aim is to minimize the cost for the consumed units without reducing the E_t.

Total energy consumed at timeslot 't':

Table 2 Parameters of GA

Parameters	Values
Population size	480
n	20
Number of iterations	5
P_c	0.9
P_m	0.1

$$E^t = \sum_{n=1}^{20} [LS_n^t * LE_n^t] \tag{3}$$

Cost of total energy consumed at timeslot 't':

$$C^t = \left[C * \sum_{n=1}^{20} [LS_n^t * LE_n^t] \right] \tag{4}$$

3 Genetic Algorithm

It is a stochastic population-based optimization algorithm capable for addressing linear and non-linear problem. It is inspired from natural science. The number of individuals is the population solution. The fitness value of the objective function is defined for each individual of the population. The population is evaluated to identify the better solution which has higher fitness for survival. Numbers of generations are provided for finding the best solution for the problem. The genetic operators' crossover and mutation are employed to fine-tune the obtained result. After number of generations, the population becomes stable with no further requirement for optimization. The binary-coded genetic algorithm uses the fixed decision parameter either 0 or 1. In this, the resolution is represented as the number of bits involved in the solution variable. In real-coded genetic algorithm, the solution variables are represented in its natural form (integer or floating point). In this paper, to solve the load optimization problem of the resident, the population solution variables are represented in its natural form. The Genetic representation of the individual solution (load) has 20 chromosomes (number of load) and genes are 24 (number of timeslots).

A random initial population is generated. The fitness of every individual is evaluated. The tournament selection method is used to select the fittest chromosome for next generation. In tournament selection, n individuals are selected at random from the population and the best of the n is inserted into the new population for further genetic processing. In the final solution, the selected good individuals will not survive with the same solution values. They cluster among themselves to find a better solution. The crossover is the genetic operator that combines the subset of parent chromosomes and produces the new children. In real-coded genetic algorithm, the Blended Crossover method is applied to the natural form representation of solution variable. Let P1 and P2 are the two parent chromosomes where P1 < P2. BLX create the children whose value is lying in the range {{P1 − α (P2 − P1)}......... {P2 − α (P2 − P1)}}, where α is a constant to be decided so that children solution do not come out of the range of domain of the said parameter.

Another parameter 'γ' has to be identified by utilizing the 'α' and a random number 'r' in the range of (0.0, 1.0) both exclusive.

$$\gamma = (1 + 2\alpha)r - \alpha \tag{5}$$

The children solutions C1 and C2 are determined from the parents as follows,

$$C1 = (1 - \gamma)P1 + \gamma P2 \tag{6}$$

$$C2 = (1 - \gamma)P2 + \gamma P1 \tag{7}$$

To avoid the repetition in the results after crossover, mutation is carried out. A random number is generated in the range of problem boundaries. Here the total timeslots are 24. So the random value range is between 0 and 24. The generated value is added to the children solution obtained from the crossover. Again the population is generated and evaluation of fitness is done. The new solutions are generated. After a number of iterations, it is judged whether the solution provided is optimal and the expected generation number of iteration is obtained.

4 Constraints for the Problem to be Satisfied

Constraint 1: Threshold Energy Monitor

To overcome the unplanned energy outage during the valley time of the utility and to prevent the resident from dumping the energy usage at a specific timeslot whose tariff is less, we propose a method of Threshold Energy Monitor. The load status and energy requirement of the load for every timeslot are known. The threshold energy for every timeslot is found by calculating Thres_E, which is the average of overall energy consumption. The load scheduling is proposed by calculating the energy required for the operation of uninterruptable load followed by shiftable load which may not exceed the threshold energy.

$$\text{Threshold Energy, } \text{Thres\_E} = \left\{ \sum_{t=1}^{24} \left\{ \sum_{n=1}^{20} [\text{LS}_n^t * \text{LS}_n^t]/20 \right\} /24 \right\} \tag{8}$$

Constraint 2: Uncompromised energy

The power demand rose in the utility, proposed price schemes or load schedule for the residents should not be affecting the Tot_E. The load scheduling pattern is proposed for every individual resident separately. This constraint is satisfied to provide uncompromised energy consumption of the resident. The total energy required for a resident per day is represented as

$$\text{Total required Energy, Tot\_E} = \sum_{t=1}^{24} \sum_{n=1}^{20} \left[LS_n^t * LS_n^t \right] \tag{9}$$

Constraint 3: shiftable load on peak.
Shiftable load is a vector which contains all shiftable loads represented as

$$SL_n = \{SL_1, SL_2, \ldots \ldots SL_n\}$$
$$\text{for all } n \in N\_\text{ shiftable} \tag{10}$$

The similarity between the planned operation timeslot of the shiftable load and peak timeslot will lead to the shift in operation time of the load. The shift could be performed either before the peak or after the peak based on the slot availability. Let the minimum and maximum Peak timeslot proposed by the utility be P_{min} and P_{max}. The required operation timeslot of shiftable load with the starting timeslot and ending timeslot is represented as OSL_n^{tmin} and OSL_n^{tmax}.

$$OSL_n^{tmax} < P_{min} \,||\, OSL_n^{tmin} > P_{max} \tag{11}$$
$$\text{for all } n \in N\_\text{shiftable}$$

Constraint 4: uninterruptable on peak

To address the peak demand the loads are scheduled in such a way that the peak slots are allocated with the uninterruptable load of the resident followed by the shiftable load. This constraint is the dependant of constraint 1. The energy required by the scheduled uninterruptable load of the resident during the peak timeslot is the definite energy requirement during the peak. The definite energy requirement is calculated for every timeslot in peak horizon (P_{min} and P_{max}). Total energy occupied by uninterruptable load at every timeslot 't' during peak horizon is represented as $Tot\_UL_n^t$. The timeslot 't' varies from P_{min} to P_{max}. The difference of Thres_E and every peak horizon timeslot's $Tot\_UL_n^t$ is calculated. The calculated peak_load value determines the penalty cost. If it is positive, then no penalty and the remaining energy are occupied by shiftable load. If it is negative, then the resident is added with penalty to the cost.

$$Tot\_UL_n^t = \sum_{n=1}^{n} \left[SUL_n^t * EUL_n^t \right] \tag{12}$$

$$\text{Peak\_load} = \text{Thres\_E} - Tot\_UL_n^t \tag{13}$$

$$\text{for all } t \in \text{Peak horizon}$$

Fig. 1 The penalty added to
the dynamic electricity cost

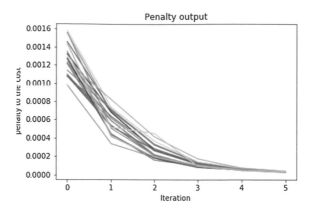

5   Reduction in Penalty Value

The objective of the work is to minimize the overall electricity cost of the resident per day and also to schedule the loads according to the dynamic pricing as proposed by the utility company. The appliances are scheduled where the average electricity usage of the resident is not compromised and also the uninterruptable loads are preferred to occupy the timeslots during peak time. On violating any of these constraints, penalty cost is added to the actual cost for the specific timeslot. The penalty is calculated as,

$$P = \sqrt{A} - Thres\_E \forall t \tag{14}$$

where A is the sum of all units of scheduled appliances at timeslot 't'. As this experiment has 24 timeslot per day, 24 penalty values are calculated and added to the dynamic cost of every timeslot. The genetic algorithm is implemented to find the optimal solution that produces less/no penalty. After number of iterations the penalty becomes neutral or zero. After obtaining this expected output, the generations are stopped.

Figure 1 represents the penalty value that is added to the dynamic electricity cost. This penalty value is getting reduced after each generation. The genetic algorithm is applied to identify the best individuals in each of the iteration and apply genetic operators to it. The new generation of population is generated. The penalty module is considered as the one of constrains that need to be evaluated in each generation.

6   Conclusion

The demand response strategy expects the reduction of electricity power usage at peak time. Load scheduling is the process of allocating the scheduled appliances with the required time for operation without any compromise in execution. To reduce the peak time electricity load usage, the appliances are rescheduled in its working time. The Genetic Algorithm is the optimization technique applied to schedule the load without any compromise in the usual load. It reduces the dynamic rate with the raised tariff for peak time load usage of customers.

References

1. Soares A, Gomes Á, Antunes CH, Cardoso H (2013) Domestic load scheduling using genetic algorithms. EvoApplications 2013, LNCS 7835. Springer, Berlin, Heidelberg, pp 142–151
2. Ullah I, Khitab Z, Khan MN, Hussain S (2019) An efficient energy management in office using bio-inspired energy optimization algorithms. MDPI Process 7:142. https://doi.org/10.3390/pr7 030142
3. Zhao Z, Lee WC, Shin Y, Song K-B (2013) An optimal power scheduling method for demand response in home energy management system. IEEE Trans Smart Grid 4(3)
4. Yuce B, Rezgui Y, Mourshed M (2016) ANN-GA smart appliance scheduling for optimised energy management in the domestic sector Energy Build 111:311–325. https://doi.org/10.1016/j.enbuild.2015.11.017
5. Agamah US, Ekonomou L (2017) Energy storage system scheduling for peak demand reduction using evolutionary combinatorial optimization. Sustain Energy Technol Assess 23:73–82
6. Paridari K, Parisio A, Sandberg H, Johansson KH (2015) Demand response for aggregated residential consumers with energy storage sharing. In: 015 IEEE 54th annual conference on decision and control (CDC) 15–18 Dec 2015. Osaka, Japan
7. Allerding F, Premm M, Shukla PK, Schmeck H (2012) Electrical load management in smart homes using evolutionary algorithms. In: Hao J-K, Middendorf M (eds) EvoCOP 2012. LNCS 7245. Springer Heidelberg, pp 99–110
8. Gao B, Liu X, Zhang W, Tang Y (2015) Autonomous household energy management based on a double cooperative game approach in the smart grid. Energies 8(7):7326–7343
9. Roy T, Das A, Ni Z (2017) Optimization in load scheduling of a residential community using dynamic pricing. In: 2017 IEEE power & energy society innovative smart grid technologies conference (ISGT) Washington, DC, 2017, pp 1–5
10. Elkazaz MH, Hoballah A, Azmy AM (2016) Artificial intelligentbased optimization of automated home energy management systems. Int Trans Electric Energy Syst
11. Tsui KM, Chan SC (2012) Demand response optimization for smart home scheduling under real-time pricing. IEEE Trans Smart Grid 3(4):1812–1821
12. Kim TT, Poor HV (2011) Scheduling power consumption with price uncertainty. IEEE Trans Smart Grid 2:519–527
13. Cakmak R, Altas IH (2016) Scheduling of domestic shiftable loads via cuckoo search optimization algorithm. IEEE Trans. ISBN 978-1-5090-0866-7/16
14. Javaid N, Ahmed F, Ullah I, Abid S, Abdul W, Alamri A, Almogren AS (2017) Towards cost and comfort based hybrid optimization for residential load scheduling in a smart grid. Energies
15. Vardakas JS, Zorba N, Verikoukis CV (2015) A survey on demand response programs in smart grids: Pricing methods and optimization algorithms. IEEE Commun Surv Tutor 17:152–178
16. Guerrero-Martinez MA, Milanes-Montero MI, Barrero-Gonzalez F, Miñambres-Marcos VM, Romero-Cadaval E, Gonzalez-Romera E (2017) A smart power electronic multiconverter for the residential. Sector Sens 17. https://doi.org/10.3390/s17061217
17. Xiong G, Chen C, Kishore S, Yener A (2011) Smart (In-home) power scheduling for demand response on the smart grid. In: Proceedings of IEEE PES conference on innovative smart grid technologies, Anaheim
18. Setlhaolo D, Xia X, Zhang J (2014) Optimal scheduling of household appliances for demand response. Electric Power Syst Res 116:24–28. https://doi.org/10.1016/j.epsr.2014.04.012

19. Yang C, Li H, Rezgui Y, Petri I, Yuce B, Chen B, Jayan B (2013) High throughput computing based distributed genetic algorithm for building energy consumption optimization. Energy Build 76:92–101. https://doi.org/10.1016/j.enbuild.2014.02.053

20. Yi P, Dong X, Iwayemi A, Zhou C, Li S (2013) Real-time opportunistic scheduling for residential demand response. IEEE Trans Smart Grid 4:227 234

21. Ahmed A, Manzoor A, Khan A, Zeb A, Ahmad H (2017) Performance measurement of energy management controller using heuristic techniques. In: Proceedings of the conference on complex, intelligent, and software intensive systems, Turin, 10–13 July 2017, pp 181–188

22. Mavrotas G, Karmellos M (2019) Multi-objective optimization and comparison framework for the design of distributed energy systems. Energy Conversation Management 180:473–495

23. Baldonado M, Chang C-CK, Gravano L, Paepcke A (1997) The stanford digital library metadata architecture. Int J Digit Libr 1:108–121S

CORO-NET: CNN Architecture to Diagnose COVID-19 Disease Using Chest X-ray Images

Rachi Jain and Devendra Kumar Medal

1 Introduction

Since December 2019, a novel coronavirus has spread from Wuhan to the whole of China, and many other countries. By December 6, more than 65 million confirmed cases, and more than 15,23,583 death cases were reported in the world according to WHO. Due to the unavailability of treatment or vaccine for novel COVID-19 disease, early diagnosis is important to provide the opportunity of immediate isolation of the suspected person and to decrease the chance of infection to a healthy population.

Reverse transcription-polymerase chain reaction (RT-PCR) [1] was introduced as the main screening method for COVID-19. However, the total positive rate of RT-PCR for throat swab samples is reported 30 to 60%, which accordingly yields to un-diagnosed patients, which may contagiously infect a huge population of healthy people. For this, Chest X-ray or computed tomography (CT) imaging as a routine tool for diagnosis is easy to perform. Chest CT has a high sensitivity for the diagnosis of COVID-19 and X-ray images show visual indexes correlated with COVID-19. Moreover, the X-ray images of the chest are given importance in the diagnosis of disease in the modern health care system. X-ray imaging systems are available in every hospital, thus the X-ray image-based approach is more convenient and easily available. Researchers are focusing on deep learning techniques to detect any specific features from x-ray images of COVID-19 patients. In recent times, deep learning has been very successful in various visual tasks which include medical image analysis as well. By accurately analyzing, identifying, and classifying patterns in medical images the deep learning has revolutionized automatic disease diagnosis. In the past, deep learning has led to success in disease classification using a chest X-ray image.

R. Jain · D. K. Medal (✉)
Department of Electronics and Communication Engineering, Jabalpur Engineering College, Jabalpur, Madhya Pradesh, India
e-mail: dmeda@jecjabalpur.ac.in

© The Author(s), under exclusive license to Springer Nature Singapore Pte Ltd. 2021   575
M. K. Bajpai et al. (eds.), *Machine Vision and Augmented Intelligence—Theory and Applications*, Lecture Notes in Electrical Engineering 796,
https://doi.org/10.1007/978-981-16-5078-9_47

The contributions of this research are summarized below:

1. To detect COVID-19, normal and pneumonia using chest X-ray dataset formed 3130 images and data augmentation is used.
2. Developing a deep CNN CORO-NET architecture to automatically assist the early diagnosis of patients of COVID-19, normal and pneumonia efficiently. Due to use of less number of parameters, this architecture becomes fast and less complex.
3. A detailed experimental analysis is provided in terms of accuracy, precision, Recall, F1-score, confusion matrix and receiver operating characteristic (ROC) using true positive rate (TPR) and false positive rate (FPR) to measure the performance of the proposed CORO-NET architecture.

The paper is organized as follows: Literature survey is provided in Sect. 2. About the dataset collection related to this study is described in Sect. 3. A description of the proposed architecture and dataset preparation are provided in Sect. 4. The experimental results and comparative analysis of the proposed CORO-NET architecture are provided in Sect. 5. Section 6 concludes the paper.

2 Literature Survey

There have been a few methods that have been tried in the past and recently in parallel with our work that aim to detect COVID-19.

Abbas et al. [2] developed a deep CNN, called Decompose, Transfer, and Compose (CNN) DeTraC-Net to identify Covid-19 cases from chest X-ray images. The model trained over 986 chest X-ray images. The accuracy obtained from this model was 95.12% a deep CNN, called Decompose, Transfer, and Compose (DeTraC), for the classification of COVID-19 chest X-ray images. Hemdan et al. [3] developed a COVIDX-Net for automatic detection of coronavirus infected lungs using chest X-ray images. The classification accuracy obtained from COVIDX-Net was 92.30%. Wang et al. [4] presented Covid-net for classification of COVID-19 from the chest X-ray images. Covid-net provided a classification accuracy of 93.30% than the compare Covid-net model to other deep convolutional neural networks. Quan et al. [5] utilized DenseNet and CapsNet fusion that is used to give their respective advantages and reduce the dependence on large data with accuracy of 95.70%. Sarker et al. [6] used a transfer learning technique for the detection of coronavirus patterns from the patient's chest X-ray. The developed model is named CovidDenseNet. The accuracy obtained from this model was 93.0% for binary class.

3 Available Dataset

Deep learning requires well-trained network to be exposed to at least thousands of images. As the emergence of pandemic COVID-19 is very recent, none of the repositories contain COVID-19 labeled data, thus requiring us to collect x-ray images from different sources of COVID-19, normal and pneumonia cases. First, 312 X-ray images of COVID-19 patient cases were collected from the following websites: GitHub [7, 8] and kaggle [9]. Then, 1471 images of normal cases and 1347 X-ray images of pneumonia cases were collected from the Github [7, 8] and Kaggle [9] repository, respectively. The objective of the dataset selection was to make it publically available so that it is extensible and accessible to many researchers. The number of X-ray images of each case in Table 1. The visualization of X-ray images of a different class in Fig. 1.

Table 1 Used dataset

Source Name	# Normal CXR	# Covid CXR	# Pneumonia CXR	Total
GitHub [7]	127	58	–	185
GitHub [8]	3	35	2	40
Kaggle [9]	1341	219	1345	2905
Total	**1471**	**312**	**1347**	**3310**

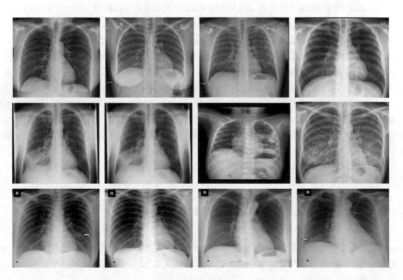

Fig. 1 The first row is for sample images of COVID-19 cases, second row is for sample of pneumonia cases and third row is for sample images of normal cases

Table 2 Utilized image augmentation parameter setting

Parameter	Rotation range	Width shift range	Height shift range	Zoom range	Shear range	Horizontal flip
Value	15	0.1	0.1	0.1	0.1	True

Table 3 Number of image per category

Category	# Normal CXR	# Covid CXR	# Pneumonia CXR
Training	1077	249	1175
Validation	136	32	149
Testing	134	31	147

4 Method

4.1 Data Preprocessing

The quality and quantity of the images hold importance in deep learning. In the image data, some of those images are not appropriate. Therefore, data pre-processing is necessary. We filtered them and resized all the images 224×224 in pixels. The method of generating new data from existing data, known as data augmentation [10]. In this Research paper, we use data augmentation to create a transformed version of the chest X-ray image to increase the number of data set. Table 2 represents the utilized image augmentation parameter setting. In data augmentation, we use the rotation of the actual image by 15%, zooming the image to 0.1, width shift range and height shift range are 0.1 for each and shear range is 0.1. The X-ray image was normalized by 1/225. We flip the image to create a mirror copy of original images along the horizontal axis. Horizontal axis flipping is much more useful than flipping the vertical axis. Also, we used one hot encoding for the label to assign a binary value corresponding to each class. The data is divided in the ratio of (8: 1: 1) as shown in Table 3.

4.2 Proposed CORO-NET Architecture

The proposed CORO-NET architecture used to detect Covid-19, normal and pneumonia patients from the X-ray images are in Fig. 2. The overall architecture is divided into three parts namely entry, middle, and exit flow.

The entry flow, the initial part of the architecture which accepts the X-ray image, extracts the features and passes to the middle part of the architecture. The entry flow is constructed from three 2D convolutional layers with a kernel size of 3×3 each, 2D max-pooling layers with kernel size and stride each of 1×1, and relu activation

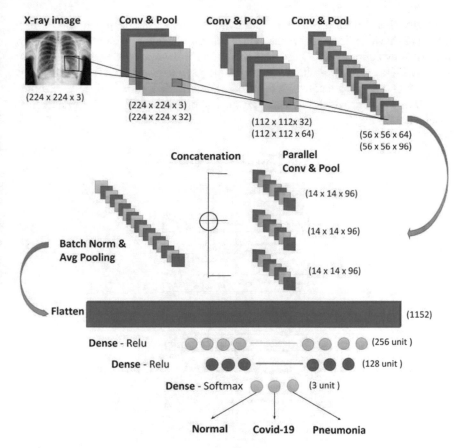

Fig. 2 Schematic diagram of the proposed CORO-NET

function. The input layer accepts 224 × 224 × 3 sized X-ray images and returns 28 × 28 × 96 features to the middle layer.

Middle part is divided into three parts to check the systematically categorical three classes (Covid-19, normal and pneumonia). It consists three 2D-convolutional layers which work parallelly, and then concatenation layer concatenates 3 layers and returns the 14 × 14 × 288 feature to exit flow.

The third part of the architecture is the exit flow. The exit part facilitates the classification of the feature. It takes input from the middle flow. Batch normalization and average polling used in it. After the dropout, it passes to the dense layer. The exit part is a combination of three dense layers of two relu and one the softmax activation function [11] of 256, 128 and 3 respectively. Exit part further classifies the feature acquired by classes that are Covid-19, normal and pneumonia. A Schematic diagram of CORO-NET is shown in Fig. 4.

The CORO-NET model has total 6,53,507 number of parameters which is comparatively less so that it takes relatively less time and its complexity is also small. The

CORO-NET architecture was built and evaluated using the deep learning library-Keras [12] having a TensorFlow backend. The CORO-NET has smooth gradient flow and fast convolution. The CORO-NET model implementation using deep 2D convolutions as it is easy to train it with more training samples, result in higher accuracy. Our CORO-NET architecture implementation available in this URL https://github.com/Rajsoni03/Coro_Net_Implementation. The proposed CORO-NET architecture is described in Fig. 3

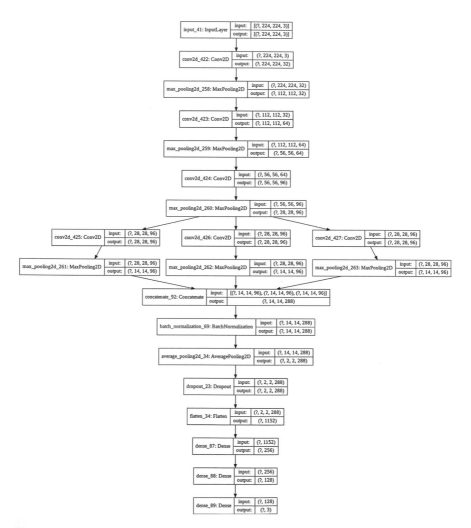

Fig. 3 CORO-NET architecture

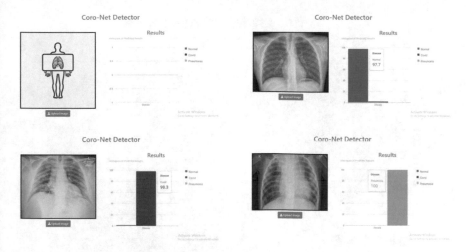

Fig. 4 Snapshots of graphical user interface (GUI)

4.3 Graphical User Interface (GUI)

In Deep Learning with Python, Application programming interface (API) like Tensor-Flow and Keras are allows us to develop a model programmatically. A GUI is a system, allows users to interact visually with computer programs or software. In this research, we used the Flask web framework to create a GUI and hosted it on cloud. The GUI helps all users to easily use the CORO-NET model and predict the Covid-19, normal and pneumonia disease by uploading their chest x-ray images. The URL of the GUI is https://coro-net.herokuapp.com Snapshots of GUI are shown in Fig. 4.

5 Result and Analysis

5.1 Experimental Analysis

Hyper-parameter optimization—For the hyper-parameter optimization, we use learning rate from 1e-5 to 1 and find the best point with the logarithm graph in Fig. 5. This graph is generated on different epochs with respect to find the best learning rate. Learning Rate Scheduler equation is shown in Eq. (1)

$$LR = 1e - 5 * 10^{(epoch/4)} \tag{1}$$

Training with optimized Hyper-parameter—The proposed CORO-NET was trained on a preprocessed dataset with optimized Hyper-parameter using Adam optimizer. The graph in Fig. 5 shows that the accuracy and loss fluctuate after the learning

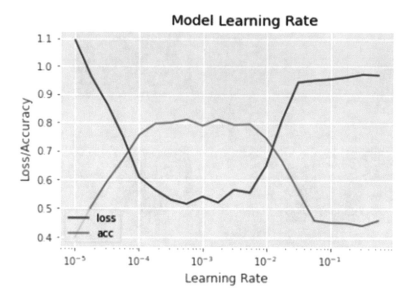

Fig. 5 Learning rate graph with accuracy/loss for hyper-parameter optimization

rate 1e-3. So given that learning rate 1e-3 is best for training with minimum loss and highest accuracy. Hyper-parameter used for training: epochs = 50, optimizer = Adam [13], loss = categorical cross-entropy, batch size = 32.

Fine-tuning—In this part, we freeze all the initial to middle layer (up-to concatenation layer) and train the rest model without augmented data (Raw data/actual data). In Fig. 6 the graph of accuracy and loss highly varies with the epoch but after the fine-tune of CORO-NET model, we get slightly stable graph with high accuracy and less loss which is shown in Fig. 7.

5.2 Quantitative Analysis

The following performance metrics are used to measure the performance of the CORO-NET architecture.

True Positive (TP) denotes the correctly predicted COVID-19 cases, False Positive (FP) denotes the normal or pneumonia cases that are misclassified as COVID-19 by the proposed system, True Negative (TN) denotes the normal or pneumonia cases that are correctly classified, and False Negative (FN) denote the COVID-19 cases that are misclassified as normal or pneumonia cases.

$$\text{Accuracy} = (\text{TP} + \text{TN}) / (\text{TN} + \text{FP} + \text{TP} + \text{FN}) \qquad (2)$$

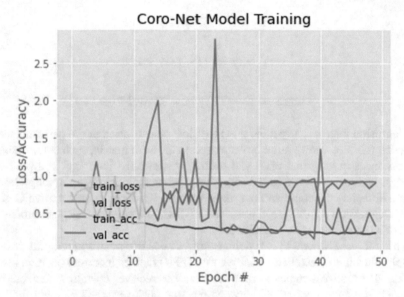

Fig. 6 Accuracy/Loss graph of CORO-NET model

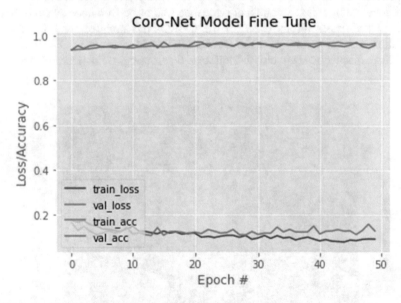

Fig. 7 Accuracy/Loss graph of CORO-NET model after fine-tune

$$\text{Specificity} = \text{TN} / (\text{TN} + \text{FP}) \tag{3}$$

$$\text{Sensitivity} = \text{TP} / (\text{TP} + \text{FN}) \tag{4}$$

$$\text{F1} - \text{score} = (2 * \text{TP}) / (2 * \text{TP} + \text{FP} + \text{FN}) \tag{5}$$

Confusion matrix is a specific table to allow visualization of the performance of a model. It is also known as an error matrix. In the error matrix, each column shows the instances in an actual class and each row shows the instances in a predicted class. It can make it easy to see the system when it is confusing among classes. Figure 8 depicts the confusion matrix of the test phase of the competitive CORO-NET architecture for disease classification (Covid-19, normal, and pneumonia). A total of 312 test images are classified.

The true positive rate (TPR) defines correct positive results among all positive samples during the test. False-positive rate (FPR) defines incorrect positive results among all negative samples during the test. The receiver operating characteristic curve (ROC) curves are added between the true positive rate (TPR) and the false positive rate (FPR). It is used to compare the overall performance in Fig. 9.

Moreover, Fig. 9 is the graphical representation of performance evaluation with accuracy and cross entropy (loss) of the CORO-NET architecture. The training, validation and test accuracy for the CORO-NET architecture is 99.0%, 95.9% and 96.15%, respectively, at epoch 50. Similarly, the training, validation and test loss is

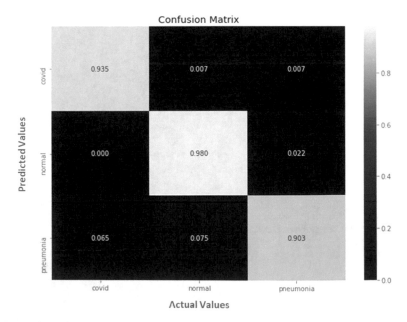

Fig. 8 Confusion matrix of the CORO-NET architecture

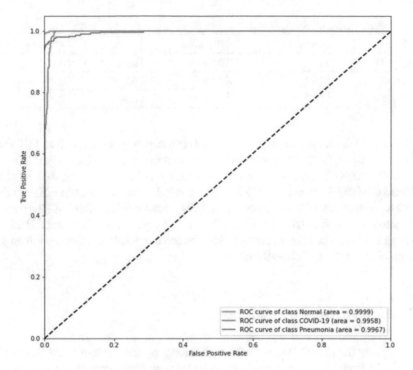

Fig. 9 ROC curve of the CORO-NET architecture

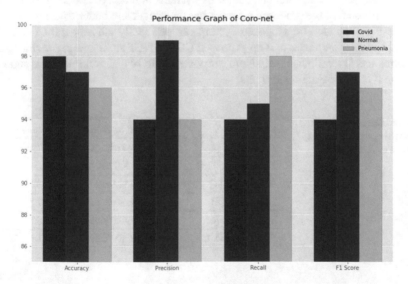

Fig. 10 The graphical representation of the results of the CORO-NET architecture

Table 4 Performance of the CORO-NET

Class	Accuracy (%)	Precision	Recall	F1-score
Covid-19	98.72	0.94	0.94	0.94
Normal	97.12	0.99	0.95	0.97
Pneumonia	96.47	0.94	0.98	0.96

0.31, 0.13 and 0.13, respectively. The overall accuracy, precision, recall and F1-score for each case of CORO-NET architecture are summarized in Table 4 (Fig. 10).

The CORO-NET architecture achieved accuracy of 98.72%, precision 0.94, recall 0.94 and 0.94 of F1-score for the COVID-19 cases. For the pneumonia classification, it recorded accuracy of 96.47%, precision 0.94, recall 0.98 and 0.96 of F1-score. In the normal cases, it obtained accuracy of 97.12%, precision 0.99, recall 0.95 and 0.97 of F1-score. The lowest accuracy was obtained in the normal cases while higher was obtained in the COVID-19 cases.

5.3 Architecture Comparison

By analyzing the results, it demonstrates that the proposed system could distinguish COVID-19 from pneumonia and normal cases with high accuracy. A comparison between our proposed system and existing systems in terms of accuracy is in Table 5. It was found that the proposed network has consistent and better true negative and true positive values. The proposed system can efficiently classify the COVID-19, normal and pneumonia cases. Our proposed CORO-NET architecture provides good performance. Overall, the result of our proposed CORO-NET architecture is superior compared to other existing systems.

Table 5 Comparison of the proposed system to existing in terms of Accuracy

Author	Architecture	Accuracy (%)
Abbas et al. [2]	DeTraC- Net	95.12
Hemdan et al. [3]	COVIDX-Net	92.30
Wang et al. [4]	Covid-net	93.30
Quan et al. [5]	DenseCapsNet	95.70
Sarker et al. [6]	CovidDenseNet	93.00
Rachi Jain, D. meda (Ours)	CORO-NET	**96.15**

6   Conclusion

During this health emergency, it is necessary to identify a single case of COVID-19 positive. We introduced a CORO-NET architecture for the detection of novel COVID-19 from X-ray images. Here, this architecture is used as a feature extractor as well as a classifier for the detection of coronavirus with less parameter. The performance of the proposed CORO-NET architecture is improved by selecting the best hyper-parameter and fine-tune the model that increases efficiency. The developed system obtained an accuracy of 96.15%. It is also small architecture than any approach and taking less time for training and testing which is proportionally faster.

References

1. Yang, Y, Yang M, Shen C et al (2020) Laboratory diagnosis and monitoring the viral shedding of 2019 nCoV infections. In: medRxiv
2. Abbas A et.al (2020) Classification of COVID-19 in chest X-ray images using DeTraC deep convolutional neural network. In: IEEE Press
3. Hemdan EED, Shouman MA, Karar ME (2020) Covidx-net: a framework of deep learning classifiiers to diagnose covid-19 in x-ray:arXiv preprint arXiv:2003.11055
4. Wang et al (2020) COVID-net: a tailored deep convolutional neural network design for detection of COVID-19 cases from chest x-ray images. arXiv:2003.09871
5. Quan H et al (2020) DenseCapsNet: detection of COVID-19 X-ray images using a capsule network. arXiv:2007.10785v3. [cs.LG]
6. Sarker L, Islam M, Hannan T, Zakaria A (2020) Covid-densenet:variability in covid-19 classifification using chest x-ray images. arXiv:2005.02167
7. https://github.com/agchung/Actualmed-COVID-chestxray-dataset
8. https://github.com/agchung/Figure1-COVID-chestxray-dataset
9. https://www.kaggle.com/tawsifurrahman/covid19-radiography-database
10. . Mikołajczyk A et al, Data augmentation for improving deep learning in image classification problem. In: International interdisciplinary PhD workshop (IIPhDW)]. https://doi.org/10.1109/IIPHDW.2018.8388338
11. Nwankpa C, Ijomah W, Gachagan A et al (2018) Activation functions:comparison trends in practice and research for deep learning. arXiv:1811.03378
12. Chollet F, Keras (2015) GitHub repository. https://github.com/fchollet/keras
13. Kingma PD, Jimmy B (2014) Adam: a method for stochastic optimization. arXiv:1412.6980. [cs.LG]

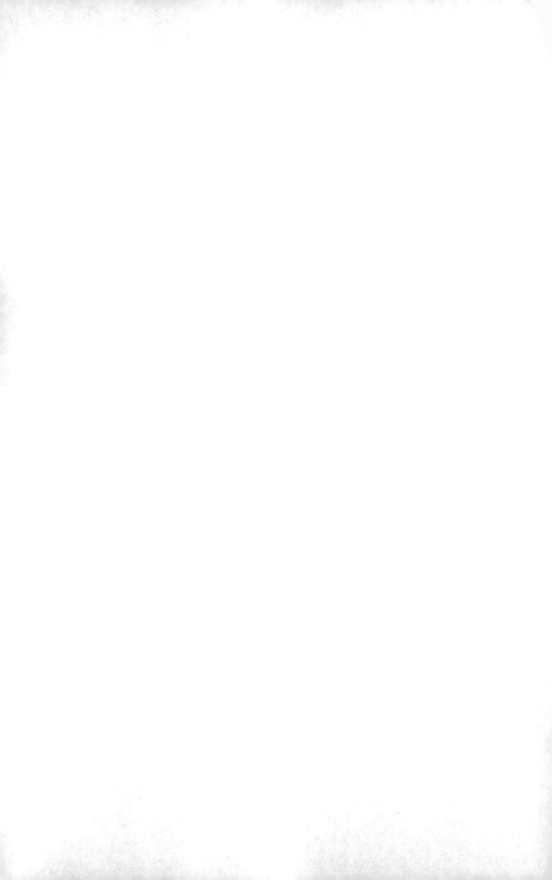

Stochastic Gradient Descent with Selfish Mining Attack Parameters on Dash Difficulty Adjustment Algorithm

Jeyasheela Rakkini and K. Geetha

1 Introduction

Dash is a more secure, fast, and affordable cryptocurrency. It is a scalable, user-friendly cryptocurrency. The Dash network has instant transaction confirmation. For a transaction to be irreversible, not liable to double spending, the other cryptocurrencies have to wait for 15 min to about one hour, Dash achieves instant transaction confirmation by a second layer of network nodes with 15 min and with 6 confirmations. The transaction that is confirmed to be valid has master nodes locking the input to the transactions. The master node broadcasts these transactions. The master nodes regularly form voting quorums to check whether these transactions are valid. This transaction will be included in blocks eventually with the inputs to the transaction being locked. When a valid solution is found when mining a block with the current mining difficulty, the miner creates new units of the Dash currency, which are the block rewards [1]. To avoid inflation the block rewards are reduced at regular intervals. The total coins in circulation are known as the coin emission rate. Dash has a decentralized governance and self-funding model. The scalability and mass adoption of Dash is due to the instant send feature of Dash with confirmation of two seconds. The InstaSend, PrivateSend transactions are the services that are facilitated by master nodes.

From the NIST dataset [8], the following parameters are considered, the number of past blocks that is considered in Dash difficulty adjustment algorithm is 24 blocks, there is off by one error bug present for Dash cryptocurrency, the number of simulations is 30, the alpha (which is the percentage of selfish miners) value ranges from 0.06 to 0.48 (their hash rate in increments of 2), the gamma (the percentage of honest miners who wants to switch to selfish mining strategy) value ranges from 0 to 0.9

J. Rakkini (✉) · K. Geetha
SASTRA Deemed University, Thirumalaisamudram, Thanjavur, Tamil Nadu-613401, India
e-mail: jeyasheelarakkini@cse.sastra.edu

© The Author(s), under exclusive license to Springer Nature Singapore Pte Ltd. 2021   589
M. K. Bajpai et al. (eds.), *Machine Vision and Augmented Intelligence—Theory and Applications*, Lecture Notes in Electrical Engineering 796,
https://doi.org/10.1007/978-981-16-5078-9_48

with an increment of 0.05 hash rate, the time warp is 0,3600 and 7200 s are considered, the number of blocks is 1000, the block time is 150 s, the win ratio with 7545 values, adjusted winning is the ratio of the time concerning win ratio, which is the ratio of selfish miner wins, the relative gain is (time adjusted relative revenue—alpha)/alpha, the adjusted relative gain is time adjusted relative revenue/(elapsed time/expected time), seconds per block is the average time taken by the selfish miner to mine a block, final height is the height of the blockchain, num of reorgs is the number of blocks reorganized, smwinreorgs is the number of times a fork occurred and the selfish miner has won. The metrics 'didbetternaive', 'didbettertimeadjust' are concerned with the time stamp manipulation of the blocks.

2   Related Work

Dash white paper [1] gives the technicality of Dash cryptocurrency with the quintessential features of decentralized governance, self-funding, and transaction locking. Bai et al. [2] gives the minimum hash rate and the minimum time needed for profitability and also the profitability of selfish mining with multiple mining pools. Bissias et al. [3] elaborates bonded mining, which is a proactive difficulty adjustment algorithm and this collects hash rate commitments from miners, secured with a bond from miners and the difficulty is set from these commitments got in bond. Those miners who deviate from this bond are penalized. Chicarino et al. [4] indicates the blockchain network is under the influence of selfish miners when the blockchain fork shows deviation in height. Davidson et al. [5] gives the profitability of selfish mining attacks with various cryptocurrencies such as bitcoin, bitcoin cash, dash, monero, and their difficulty adjustment algorithms. Grunspan et al. [6] gives the attraction of miners to mining pools, the time analysis of selfish mining attacks, the duration of the attack cycles using martingale's techniques, and the Doob stopping theorem. Heilman et al. [7] gives the profitability of selfish miners with a hash rate of 32% with all propagation advantages and the incentives for miners to adopt this strategy. Kwon et al. [8] gives a fork after withholding attack which is more rewarding that is up to four times more rewarding than the selfish mining attacks. Nayak et al. [9] combines network-level eclipse attacks with selfish mining attacks and also display the nonoptimality of selfish mining. Negy et al. [10] give intermittent selfish mining strategy that is more profitable than honest mining, especially when $\gamma = 0$, with selfish miners' hash rate greater than 37% and the profitability of selfish mining against various difficulty adjustment algorithms is also explored. Nicolas et al. [11] briefly compares the strategy type, advantages, and disadvantages of selfish mining attack's countermeasures. The GHOST protocol to mitigate selfish mining, infiltration of selfish miners, punishment on infiltration, truth state attribute in the transaction data structure, orphaned blocks withholding attack, broadcasting, withholding, detection, freshness preferred methodologies, zero block strategies are studied and surveyed. Niu et al. [12] have devised a two-dimensional Markov model, stationary distribution of that Markov model and calculated long-term mining rewards for both selfish and honest miners. Saad et al. [13] detects selfish mining by considering two parameters, transaction confirmation height and block publishing height. Selfish miners are disincentivized by a defense mechanism. The transaction's data structure is modified to obtain 'a truth state' for trapping selfish miners. Sapirshtein et al. [14] gives the profit threshold, minimal fraction of resources needed for an attacker to launch a profitable attack, and the bound below which the system is considered to be safe. The attackers with less than 25% of the computational resources gain from selfish mining as opposed to previous papers. The author also proves that the attacker launching a selfish mining attack can also perform a double-spending attack. Zhang et al. [15] omits blocks that are not published in time and it encourages blocks that have links to competing blocks of their predecessor. To our knowledge, we have found that none of the previous works have explored the machine learning model of selfish mining. The contributions of this work are (1) Implementation of linear regression model with gradient descent to find the best line of fit between gamma values and the relative gain values. (2) Mini-batch gradient descent and stochastic gradient descent for prediction of the relative gain with all the features of the dataset. It is crucial to find this metric, which will obviously give us the percentage of gamma miners who want to adapt selfish mining, switching from their honest mining strategy and their relative gain also.

3 Problem Definition

The prediction of the relative revenue of the selfish miners, which is the ratio of the blocks mined by the selfish miners with all the total number of blocks mined is not a trivial problem and it has to be dealt with and studied by machine learning models. The term, time-adjusted relative revenue is the ratio of the relative gain concerning (elapsed time/expected time) and the term time-adjusted relative gain is the ratio of (time adjusted relative gain—alpha) with alpha. Here alpha is the fraction of the honest miners who would like to adapt selfish mining owing to the successful reward earning trait of selfish mining. Hence the prediction of relative gain is explored here with linear regression and gradient descent with the attributes gamma and relative gain, mini-batch gradient descent, and stochastic gradient descent for the prediction of relative gain of selfish miners.

4 Results and Discussion

Linear regression using gradient descent depends on the standard formula for the line. The NIST dataset for selfish mining attacks is given on the website https://cat alog.data.gov/dataset/selfish-mining-simulator-for-cryptocurrencies and the JSON text file is converted to pandas data frame in python. The model is trained for a given NIST dataset with gamma and relative gain to predict the values of y for any given x. The best-fitting line that gives the minimum error for the given values of gamma and relative gain is implemented here. The gradient descent takes into account all the attributes multiplied by the weights and added with the bias factor for the calculation of 'y'. Now the root mean square error which is the difference between the predicted 'y' value and the real value of 'y' is considered for calculation. This is the cost function. The objective is to find the minimum value of 'm' and 'c'. The line corresponding to these values is the best fitting line or the line that gives the minimum error. Here 'm' is the slope and 'c' is the intercept. The cost function is differentiated concerning 'm' and 'c'. The value of 'm' is updated with the current value of 'm' subtracted from learning rate * differentiated value of the loss function concerning 'm'. The value of 'c' is updated with the current value of 'c' subtracted from learning rate * differentiated value of the loss function concerning 'c'.

4.1 Loss Function

The loss is the error in our predicted value of 'm' and 'c'. Our goal is to minimize this error and obtain the most accurate value of 'm' and 'c'. Mean squared error function is to calculate the loss, the two steps are given as,

1. For an x that is given, find the difference between actual 'y' and predicted 'y'.
2. The mean square error function is calculated which is the mean of the difference between actual 'y' values and predicted 'y' values.

   Gradient descent algorithm is an iterative optimization algorithm. The loss function is the function to be optimized, here in our case is the difference between the predicted y and the real value of y, which is the value of relative gain of selfish miners. The scatter plot of gamma concerning relative gain is plotted in Fig 1. The regression line of fit between the gamma values and the relative gain is shown in Fig 2.

Fig. 1 The scatter plot of gamma versus relative gain

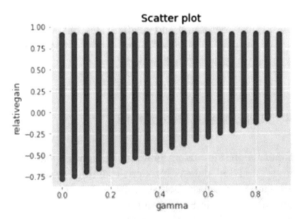

Fig. 2 The linear regression line of fit

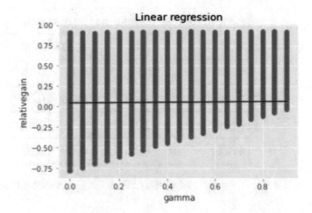

The epoch of 1000 is carried out for finding the minimum value of m and c for the best line of fit in gradient descent. The initial 'm' and 'c' values are 0.024731229061947763 0.043559816919804734 respectively. Thousand epochs are carried out with the initial values of 'm' and 'c' as 0, respectively and the tail of the epochs is shown in Fig. 3.

The head of the revised dataset with all the object variables such as name of the difficulty adjustment algorithm 'dash' and the offset error, the value of which is 'true' is removed is shown in Fig. 4. Now all the other attributes are considered for gradient descent and stochastic gradient descent.

The implementation is done in python for the gradient descent and stochastic gradient descent of the above dataset and is given in the GitHub link, https://git hub.com/jeyasheelarakkini344/StochasticGradientDescent-for-Dash-DAA-selfis hmining-profitabiltiy. Since the features are on a different scale, we have performed Scaling with Min-Max scaler function for the X that excludes 'relative gain' and for the 'y' that has the values of the column 'relative gain' only and is shown in Fig 5.

```
m 0.35474804777210417, b 0.08658856216828953, cost 0.13692592184375857 iteration 9983
m 0.35474804777210417, b 0.08658856216828953, cost 0.13692592184375857 iteration 9984
m 0.35474804777210417, b 0.08658856216828953, cost 0.13692592184375857 iteration 9985
m 0.35474804777210417, b 0.08658856216828953, cost 0.13692592184375857 iteration 9986
m 0.35474804777210417, b 0.08658856216828953, cost 0.13692592184375857 iteration 9987
m 0.35474804777210417, b 0.08658856216828953, cost 0.13692592184375857 iteration 9988
m 0.35474804777210417, b 0.08658856216828953, cost 0.13692592184375857 iteration 9989
m 0.35474804777210417, b 0.08658856216828953, cost 0.13692592184375857 iteration 9990
m 0.35474804777210417, b 0.08658856216828953, cost 0.13692592184375857 iteration 9991
m 0.35474804777210417, b 0.08658856216828953, cost 0.13692592184375857 iteration 9992
m 0.35474804777210417, b 0.08658856216828953, cost 0.13692592184375857 iteration 9993
m 0.35474804777210417, b 0.08658856216828953, cost 0.13692592184375857 iteration 9994
m 0.35474804777210417, b 0.08658856216828953, cost 0.13692592184375857 iteration 9995
m 0.35474804777210417, b 0.08658856216828953, cost 0.13692592184375857 iteration 9996
m 0.35474804777210417, b 0.08658856216828953, cost 0.13692592184375857 iteration 9997
m 0.35474804777210417, b 0.08658856216828953, cost 0.13692592184375857 iteration 9998
m 0.35474804777210417, b 0.08658856216828953, cost 0.13692592184375857 iteration 9999
```

Fig. 3 The tail of Epoch of 1000 iterations with 'm' and 'c' values

	npastblocks	numsims	alpha	gamma	timewarp	nur
0	24	30	0.06	0.00	0	10C
1	24	30	0.06	0.00	3600	10C
2	24	30	0.06	0.00	7200	10C
3	24	30	0.06	0.05	0	10C
4	24	30	0.06	0.05	3600	10C

Fig. 4 Head of the revised dataset of Dash DAA for selfish mining attack

```
array([[0.       , 0.       , 0.       , ..., 0.00712909, 0.       ,
        0.       ],
       [0.       , 0.       , 0.       , ..., 0.08143568, 0.       ,
        0.       ],
       [0.       , 0.       , 0.       , ..., 0.15221546, 0.       ,
        0.       ],
       ...,
       [0.06024096, 0.       , 1.       , ..., 0.63156367, 1.       ,
        1.       ],
       [0.06024096, 0.       , 1.       , ..., 0.699892  , 1.       ,
        1.       ],
       [0.06024096, 0.       , 1.       , ..., 0.78119513, 1.       ,
        1.       ]])
```

Fig. 5 Preprocessed X values of Dash dataset

In Fig 6, the target column which is 'relative gain' is shown as a one-dimensional array. The reshaped 'y' values are shown in Fig 7.

In Fig. 8, the weight which is multiplied with the 19 features and the bias to be added with the cost value is shown. The epoch versus cost graph is shown in Fig. 9. So as the number of epochs increases, the cost reduces. The predicted value of the relative gain is shown in Fig 10. for the

```
array([[0.00315664],
       [0.11179197],
       [0.20780369],
       ...,
       [0.9628732 ],
       [0.94094515],
       [0.96158514]])
```

Fig. 6 Preprocessed 'y' values of Dash dataset

```
array([0.00315664, 0.11179197, 0.20780369, ..., 0.9628732 , 0.94094515,
       0.96158514])
```

Fig. 7 The reshaped 'y' values

```
1 w, b, cost

(array([ 0.01894399,  1.         ,  0.14968947,  0.38459264,  0.1778896 ,
         1.         ,  1.         ,  0.29424759,  0.28740062,  1.05037929,
         0.46410234,  1.         ,  1.         ,  1.         ,  0.15286377,
         0.46153505,  0.35869449, -0.02869325, -0.01046175]),
 -0.7013018144130029,
 0.030703602187131265)
```

Fig. 8 The weight, bias, and cost values of mini-batch gradient descent

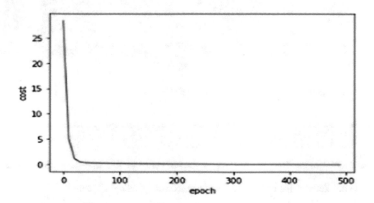

Fig. 9 Epoch versus cost graph of mini-batch gradient descent

```
1 predict(24,30,0.06,0,0,10000,150,0.013401937,0.01274954,11896.76315,-0.787507666,0,0,0,11000.03333,536.3,0.05911187,0,0,w,b)

-1.9794067748275297
```

Fig. 10 The predicted values of the relative gain attribute

given values of 24,30,0.06,0,0,10000,150,0.013401937,0.01274954,11896.76,
−0.78750766,0,0,0,11000.03333,536.3,0.05911187,0,0 is shown.

The Epoch versus cost graph of the stochastic gradient descent is shown in Fig 12 with 10000 epochs. The prediction value for the stochastic gradient descent is nearer to the original value than the mini-batch gradient descent and is shown in Fig 13.

```
(array([0.97200213, 1.        , 0.925644  , 0.93262439, 0.9300434 ,
        1.        , 1.        , 0.93923239, 0.93994549, 0.99557363,
        0.93904833, 1.        , 1.        , 1.        , 0.97687799,
        0.92407254, 0.93660731, 0.89156671, 0.89230224]),
 -0.12553496536683306,
 27.81069185041651)
```

Fig. 11 The weight, bias, and the cost of the stochastic gradient descent

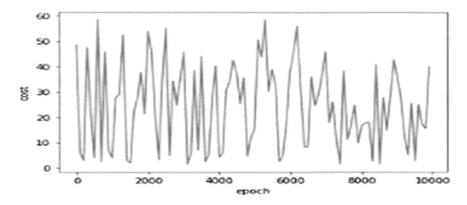

Fig. 12 Epoch versus cost graph of stochastic gradient descent

```
1 predict(24,30,0.06,0,0,10000,150,0.013401937,0.01274954,11096.76315,-0.787507666,0,0,0,11000.03333,536.3,0.05911187,0,0,w_sgd, b_sgd)

-0.9963587774532023
```

Fig. 13 The predicted value of relative gain in stochastic gradient descent

The gradient descent is for finding the local minimum in our dash difficulty adjustment algorithm for profitably of selfish mining is implemented. We have taken only the gamma values, which is the value of the honest miners and the relative gain attribute is taken for the gradient descent algorithm. Relative gain is the blocks mined by the selfish miners/total number of blocks mined in the main chain. The scatter plot of the above values with the regression line of best fit is implemented. Here the prediction of the values with mini-batch gradient descent and the stochastic gradient descent is implemented.

5 Conclusion

Thus, the gradient descent algorithm for the value of gamma and relative gain attributes in the dataset of the NIST dataset is implemented. The mini-batch gradient descent and stochastic gradient descent for all the attributes in the above dataset is implemented. Stochastic gradient descent is much faster than the mini-batch gradient descent. The high variance of the stochastic gradient descent causes the objective function to fluctuate. Both mini-batch and stochastic gradient descent algorithms are online learning algorithms. The future work can be deep learning models of the above problem definition.

References

1. Dash - Dash is digital cash you can spend anywhere. https://www.dash.org/
2. Bai Q et al (2019) A deep dive into blockchain selfish mining. In: IEEE international conference on communications vols. Institute of Electrical and Electronics Engineers Inc
3. Bissias G, Thibodeau D, Levine BN, Bonded mining: difficulty adjustment by miner commitment
4. Chicarino V, Albuquerque C, Jesus E, Rocha A (2020) On the detection of selfish mining and stalker attacks in blockchain networks. Ann des Telecommun Telecommun 75:143–152
5. Davidson M, Diamond T (2020) On the profitability of selfish mining against multiple difficulty adjustment algorithms, p 22
6. Grunspan C, Pérez-Marco R (2018) On profitability of selfish mining. arXiv
7. Heilman E, One weird trick to stop selfish miners: fresh bitcoins, a solution for the honest miner
8. Kwon Y, Kim D, Son Y, Vasserman E, Kim Y (2017) Be selfish and avoid dilemmas: fork after withholding (FAW) attacks on bitcoin. In: Proceedings of the ACM conference on computer and communications security. Association for Computing Machinery, pp 195–209. https://doi.org/10.1145/3133956.3134019
9. Nayak K, Kumar S, Miller A, Shi E, Stubborn mining: generalizing selfish mining and combining with an eclipse attack
10. Negy KA, Rizun PR, Sirer EG (2020) Selfish mining re-examined. In: Lecture notes in computer science (including subseries Lecture notes in artificial intelligence and lecture notes in bioinformatics), vol 12059 LNCS. Springer, Berlin, pp 61–78
11. Nicolas K, Wang Y, Giakos GC (2019) Comprehensive overview of selfish mining and double spending attack countermeasures. In: 2019 IEEE 40th Sarnoff symposium, Sarnoff 2019. Institute of Electrical and Electronics Engineers Inc. https://doi.org/10.1109/Sarnoff47838.2019.9067821
12. Niu J, Feng C (2019) Selfish mining in ethereum
13. Saad M, Njilla L, Kamhoua C, Mohaisen A (2019) Countering selfish mining in blockchains. In: 2019 international conference on computing, networking and communications, ICNC 2019. Institute of Electrical and Electronics Engineers Inc, pp 360–364. https://doi.org/10.1109/ICCNC.2019.8685577
14. Sapirshtein A, Sompolinsky Y, Zohar A (2017) Optimal selfish mining strategies in bitcoin. In Lecture notes in computer science (including subseries Lecture notes in artificial intelligence and lecture notes in bioinformatics, vol. 9603 LNCS. Springer, Berlin, pp 515–532
15. Zhang R, Preneel B (2017) Publish or perish: A backward-compatible defense against selfish mining in Bitcoin. In: Lecture notes in computer science (including subseries Lecture notes in artificial intelligence and lecture notes in bioinformatics), vol 10159. Springer, Berlin, pp 277–292

Visualizing and Computing Natural Language Expressions: Through a Typed Lambda Calculus λ

Harjit Singh

1 Introduction

Church introduced a Lambda operator λ in 1941 and it is a vital tool used in syntax and semantics. Since Montague's times, a typed formation of lambda abstraction has been popular in linguistics [1].[1] Sometimes, a lambda operator can be defined under lambda expressions to focus on a specific property in a context. It appears such as (a term = property) and fetching the predicate expressions in a second order logic and first order logic, respectively [2].[2] On the other hand, a lambda calculus is a set of expressions and rules that produce certain new expressions. In general, a single typed and monotyped lambda calculus is discussed many times in a literature [3].

However, it is a fact that the first order logic in contrast to a simple typed lambda calculus allows infinite types of expressions that fundamentally enumerate from the finite forms.[3] Secondly, typed lambda notations are standard in mathematics and

---

[1] It discusses a well-formed system in semantics through a systematic arrangement of typed mechanism in terms of natural language expressions that are semantically motivated. It represents the following

    (i) e is a type

    (ii) t is a type then

    (iii) both <e, t> is a type.

[2] See Allwood et al. [2, p. 156].

[3] Carpenter [4, p. 40] has pointed out that in a simple typed lambda calculus, each type either belong to a basic type or a functional type.

$$\text{Basic type} \leq \text{Typ}$$
$$(\sigma \rightarrow \tau) \,\epsilon\, \text{Typ if } \sigma, \tau \,\epsilon\, \text{Typ}$$

H. Singh (✉)

Indira Gandhi National Tribal University, Amarkantak, MP 484887, India

© The Author(s), under exclusive license to Springer Nature Singapore Pte Ltd. 2021   599

M. K. Bajpai et al. (eds.), *Machine Vision and Augmented Intelligence—Theory and Applications*, Lecture Notes in Electrical Engineering 796,

https://doi.org/10.1007/978-981-16-5078-9_49

computer science. At the same time, a single term calculus in itself has denoted a formal representation of syntactic structures that are somehow different from the first order and high order logic. On the other hand, we find three schemes when we seeing the axiomatic nature of a simple typed lambda calculus [4]. The following schemes are as

(a) α reduction
$$\vdash \lambda x.\alpha \rightarrow \lambda y.\ (\alpha\ [x \rightarrow y])$$

$[y \notin \text{Free}\ (\alpha)\ \&\ y \text{ is free for } x \text{ in } \alpha]$

(b) β reduction
$$\vdash (\lambda x.\alpha)\ (\beta) \rightarrow \alpha\ [x \rightarrow \beta]$$
$[\beta \text{ free for } x \text{ in } \alpha]$

(c) η reduction
$$\vdash \lambda x.(\alpha\ (x)) \rightarrow \alpha$$

$[x \notin \text{Free}\ (\alpha)]$

In the context of a natural language (i.e. English), lambda operator λ resolves passive and other cases within the propositional functions. It transforms such a function into one place predicate situation and binds the variables (x, y) in abstraction to define the expressions in the following way.[4]

(d) X kicked chaster $<e, t>$ type
      (kick' (chester')) (x)   Propositional Expression
      λ x [(kick' (chester')) (x)]   Lambda Expression

Here (d) shows that variable (x) is bound by the lambda operator and it is a well-formed expression for $<e, t>$ type [5, p. 116].

The paper has a total of five sections. The first section begins with the basic introduction of lambda calculus. The second section discusses the syntactic and semantic background of lambda calculus. The third section deals with the aims/objectives of the study. The fourth section analyzes the natural language expressions concerning lambda abstraction and application. The fifth section concludes the results and the future research.

---

[4] For more details see Cann [5, p. 116].

2   Related Works

As already has been pointed out lambda abstraction finds significant during Montague, and later many semanticists incorporated this into linguistics. It became a powerful tool to establish formal semantics. The following Fig. 1 shows the grammatical nature of a lambda expression.

Figure 1 interprets how lambda expression applies in relative clause, predicates and many other cases in a natural language. However, a classic instance of the lambda abstraction usually defines under 'the proper treatment of quantifiers in English'. See the Table 1.

Table 1 specifies that syntactic rules on the left handside translate into parallel with lambda symbol λ that directly controls the NP and VP constitutes [1, 6, p. 350].

In fact, lambda operator/abstraction operator λ is a kind of binder which denotes the infinite set of individuals in L_1. In that case, it shows the characteristic function of the set and sometimes, it shows the value description with the notation φ. On the other hand, when both lambda operator and value notation removes from the set, the left part is called β-reduction. Based on such function, almost many predicates like love, like, kill, eat, see, meet, etc., defines effortlessly [7, pp. 94–95].

Table 2 demonstrates that a predicate 'like' can be expressed with various names (i.e. Mary, John, Bill, Keat, etc.) bind with λ operator. It has a wide range here and may cover set of individual those who like m = Mary. Secondly, the value notation φ characterizes the set of individuals. And at last, both lambda operator λ and value notation φ can be removed from the set of individuals to form a β-reduction situation.

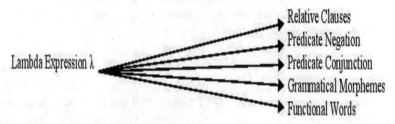

Fig. 1 Lambda expression λ with grammar

Table 1 Syntax (rules and interpretations)	Syntactic rules	Translation
	S → S and S	S'$_1$ & S'$_2$
	S → S or S	S'$_1$ ∨ S'$_2$
	VP → VP and VP	λx (VP'$_1$ (x) & VP'$_2$ (x))
	NP → NP or NP	λP. (NP'$_1$ (P) & NP'$_2$ (P))

Table 2 Syntax (categories and λ operator)

Syntactic categories	λ operator
Predicates and variables	λx. Likes (m, x)
Predicate (Likes) with set of individuals (D_e)	λx. Likes (x, m)
Value description	[λx. φ]
β-reduction	Loves (m, h)

3   Aims and Objectives

- To present a general survey on lambda operator λ
- To analysis natural language expressions in syntax and semantics through typed lambda calculus λ
- To compute results when typed lambda calculus switches from one natural language to another
- To propose an algorithm based on semantics of typed lambda calculus λ.

4   Analysis with Typed Lambda Calculus λ

We know that all objects around us identify with certain names, symbols, and terms, etc. Moreover, they are significant for a natural language considered English, Hindi, Punjabi, Marathi, Malayalam, etc. It is fascinating and challenging for us to develop any logical system for such languages. We take English as a formal language to understand the logical system for its expressions through typed lambda calculus. We begin with the following proposition.

(i)   Bill loves Elysha

It is a combination of Subject/NP and Predicate/VP where an individual constant Bill and Elysha respectively around the verb 'loves'. Here V denotes a verb that has binary relations and it is called a binary predicate. The 'loves' predicate attracts both arguments, but the first argument is an empty slot intituitvely. The following way defines this in L_1.

Loves (b, e)
Loves (_____, e)

We can compare the empty situation of 'loves' predicate with an abstraction that requires the formal representation to fill it up. See Table 3.

Table 3 Propositions with Lambda λ

Proposition	Explanation
P_1	Bill loves Elysha
Predicate (Binary)	Loves (b, e)
Intuition ground (Empty slot)	Loves (____ , e)
Abstraction field with λ	λ
λ with variable x	λx. Loves (x, e)

Table 4 Lambda abstraction

Lambda abstraction (syntax rule)	Lambda abstraction (semantics rule)
If α is an expression of type t and u variable of type σ then [λu] is an expression of type <σ, t>. We say σ and t as input type and output type of this expression	If α is an expression of type t and u variable of type σ then $[[λu\ α]]^{Mg}$ is that function f from Dσ into D_t such that for all objects o in Dσf (o) $= [[α]]^{Mg\ [u→o]}$

Adapted from Coppock and Champollion [6, p. 171]

Table 3 shows that a proposition 'Bill loves Elysha' has a binary predicate where the empty slot (____) is equal to abstraction. It fills up with a lambda operator λ under the name of a variable x.[5]

4.1 Lambda Abstraction (Syntax and Semantics)

Furthermore, we must discuss both syntax and semantics-based lambda abstraction rules.

Table 4, suggests that the input type goes to set of individuals and [λu. α] is the output expression. At the same time, the semantics rule gives $[[λu.\ α]]^{M,g}$ expression if there is an α and the domain of type must be under truth values.

4.2 Lambda Operator λ in Syntax

In syntax, individuals and their truth values and statements with conjunctions, disjunctions, quantifiers and formulas are TYPE only according to simply-typed lambda calculus. Thus, each expression carries at least one type of expression. Table 5 induces such expressions formally as.

Of these seven categories, the first is the basic level information about variables such as x, y, z in a constant form. The second application part deals with α and β; those also type expressions. The third part shows that α and β both represent similarity if

---

[5] Note that e denotes entity and t denotes truth values however both e, t used for functional types such as <e, t>. These functional types also called a set of infinites. They denote individuals and truth values under the domain. It is represented by $D_e =$ the domain of individuals and D_t expresses the truth values in the form of $D_t = \{1, 0\}$ Coppock and Champollion [6, pp. 167–68].

Table 5 Lambda and syntax

Basic expressions	Application	Equality	Negation	Binary	Quantification	Lambda abstraction
C_t, n (constant) V_t, n (variable)	For any types σ and t is an expression of type <σ, t> and β is an expression of type σ then [α] (β) is an expression of type t	If α and β are items, then α = β is an expression of type t	If φ is a formula, then so is ¬φ	If φ and Ψ are formulas then so are ¬φ, [φ ∧ Ψ], [φ ∨ Ψ], and [φ ↔ Ψ]	If φ is a formula and u is a variable of any type, then [∀ u φ] and [∃ u φ] are formulas	If α is an expression of type t and u is a variable of type σ then [λ u α] is an expression of type <σ, t>

Adapted from Coppock and Champollion [6, pp. 180–81]

they are terms. The negation part tells us that if φ is a formula then it can appear with ¬ also. Binary connectives mean that if any formula comes with φ ψ then it can be combined with ∨, ∧, ¬, ↔ like connectives. In quantification, a universal quantifier ∀ and existential quantifier ∃ exist with variables in a formula. On the other hand, in the lambda abstraction, any t expression binds with a lambda operator λ.

4.3 Lambda Operator λ in Semantics

Model and assignment function determine the natural language expressions by mapping the semantic values in $L_λ$. Further, we say that <D, I> both are necessary for M as a model that assigns the semantic values.[6] The following way describes this in L_1.

$$L_1 = M <D, I>$$
$$D = D_e \, D_t$$
$$I = \text{assignment function}$$
$$D = \text{Domain for individuals that represent through the types } e$$
$$D = \text{Domain for truth values } t$$

Table 6 shows that the first slot is for basic expressions with a non-logical constant and a variable. The second one is about the application of α and β expressions in the context of type. The third 'equality slot' discusses the truth value of α and β if they belong to the same type. The fourth 'negation slot' tell us that the φ formula translates into a ¬φ form. The fifth slot is the (negative, conjunctive, junction, etc.)

---

[6] Remember that in a model M = <D, I>, D is the domain for a set of individuals which interprets with D_e and D_t describes the truth values in the form of {0, 1}.

Table 6 Lambda and semantics

Basic expressions	Application	Equality	Negation	Binary connectives	Quantification	Lambda abstraction
If α is a non logical constant then $[[\alpha]]^{Mg=1\,(\alpha)}$	If α is an expression of type $<\sigma,$ $t>$ and β is an expression of type σ then $[[\alpha$ $([[\beta]]^{Mg} =$ $[[\alpha]]^{Mg} =$ $([[\beta]]^{Mg})$	If α and β related with same type then $[[\alpha$ $= \beta]]^{Mg}$ $= 1$	If ϕ is a formula, then $[[\neg\phi]]^{Mg} =$ 1 iff $[[\phi]]^{Mg} = 0$	If ϕ and Ψ are formulas, then $[[\phi \wedge \Psi]]^{Mg} = 1$ iff $[[\phi]]^{Mg}$ $= 1$ and $[[\Psi]]^{Mg} =$ 1	If ϕ is a formula and v is a variable the t type $[[\forall$ v. $\phi]]^{Mg} = 1$ iff for all o ϵ D: $[[\phi]]^{Mg\,[v\,\to\,o]}$	If α is an expression of type t and u us a variable of type σ then $[\lambda$ u $\alpha]^{Mg}$ is that function f from D_σ into D_t such that for all objets o in D_σ f (o) $=$ $[[\alpha]]^{Mg\,[\sigma\,\to\,o]}$

Adapted from Coppock and Champollion [6, pp. 187–88]

binary connectives formed by wffs. The sixth 'quantification slot' deals with universal and existential quantifiers, and the last seventh slot shows the lambda λ as a binder for types [7, 8, pp. 170–88].

5   Discussions and Results

Based on the above lambda abstraction λ in Tables 5 and 6, we take as input to compare two different languages to see the actual output. The first abstraction rule in syntax begins with usual expressions and ends with the lambda λ. It is sufficient to generalize the formal syntactic representations in both languages here. Secondly, abstraction rule in semantics has similar categorization and it computes such languages.

We see Tables 7 and 8 where both languages (English and Punjabi) have 1:1 correspondance in syntax and semantics of lambda calculus λ. Moreover, two natural languages are going to map in the same way. In other words, we argue that any 'y' kind of a natural language gets generated by formal language 'xs' . However, double complex and compound predicates, reduplicated forms and mainly addressing notes are typical instances that will discuss by following intention and intuition-based research and applications [8, 9].

Algorithm

Step 1: Start with assumption of type e, t for all objects

Step 2: Search the abstraction slots

Step 3: Fill up abstraction slots with a lambda operator λ

Step 4: Allow lambda operator λ as binder with variables x, y, and z

Step 5: Maintain model and assignment function in L_1

Table 7 Syntactic representations in English and Punjabi

Basic Expressions	Application	Equality	Negation	Binary Connectives	Quantification	Lambda Abstraction
English: e, t ∈ c, v	α, β ∈ t, σ α = s$_t$, β = P$_t$ English: α	α = β both languages (English and Punjabi) have same equal relations between α and β	Φ is a rule and ¬φ is also rule. English: predicates (likes, loves, kills and ¬) Punjabi: predicate (likes, loves, kills and ¬)	Φ ∨/∧ Ψ is a formula. English and Punjabi have also shown predicates with binary connectives P$_1$ ∧ P$_2$, P$_1$ ∨ P$_2$	Universal quantification [∀] and existential quantifier [∃]	α is t and λα Both English and Punjabi have α is bounded with λ
Punjabi: e, t ∈ c, v	[Subject] β = [predicate] Punjabi: α = [subject] β = [predicate]					
1:1	1:1	1:1	1:1	1:1	1:1	1:1

Table 8 Semantic representations in English and Punjabi

Basic expressions	Application	Equality	Negation	Binary connectives	Quantification	Lambda abstraction
English: α either a non-logical constant or α is a variable	α, β are type expressions in Model. Both English and Punjabi follow the type expression in the form of α and β	$\alpha = \beta$ then $[[\alpha = \beta]]^{Mg} = 1$ Both languages (English and Punjabi) have equal relations between α and β and if α is true then β must be true	ϕ is a rule and $\neg\phi$ is also a rule English and Punjabi have similar negative representations in the case of $[[\neg\phi]]^{Mg} = 1$ iff $[[\phi]]^{Mg} = 0$	$\Phi \vee/\wedge \Psi$ is a formula. English and Punjabi have also shown predicates with binary connectives $P_1 \wedge P_2$, $P_1 \vee P_2$ in M with assignment function	Universal quantification [∀] and existential quantifier [∃] Both quantifiers are part of set of individuals in D	α is t and $\lambda\alpha$ Both English and Punjabi have similar structure of D_σ and D_t
English: α either a non-logical constant or α is a variable						
1:1	1:1	1:1	1:1	1:1	1:1	1:1

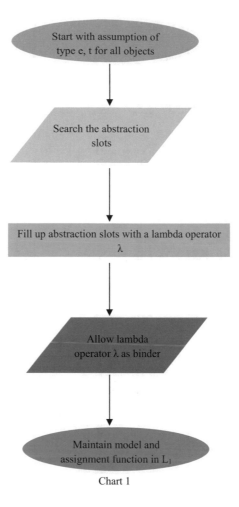

Chart 1

Step 1: Objects with <e, t/et>

Step 1: Objects with <e, t/et>

CN (AGR$_1$)	Predicate	CN (AGR$_2$)
Man	Loves	Woman
Woman	"	Man
Boy	"	Girl
Girl	"	Boy
Husband	"	Wife
Wife	"	Husband
Father	"	Mother
Mother	"	Father
Grandfather	"	Grandmother
Uncle	"	Aunt

$$e, t/et \left\{ \begin{array}{l} \text{CN (AGR}_1\text{): M}_x \ldots\ldots\text{U}_x \\ \text{CN (AGR}_2\text{): W}_x \ldots\ldots\text{A}_x \end{array} \right\}$$

PN (AGR$_1$)	Predicate	PN (AGR$_2$)
Sandeep	Loves	Kavita
Kala	"	Mala
Mehta	"	Kiran
Dalip	"	Deepa
Shamlal	"	Simran
Aman	"	Geeta
Sushil	"	Amita
Kuljeet	"	Sunita
Mahesh	"	Meena
Suresh	"	Sangeeta
Harmeet	"	Mamta
Amar	"	Sarita

$$e, t/et \left\{ \begin{array}{l} \text{PN (AGR}_1\text{): S}_x \ldots\ldots\text{S}_x \\ \text{PN (AGR}_2\text{): K}_x \ldots\ldots\text{S}_x \end{array} \right\}$$

Under step 1 we take two sets of common nouns (CNs) and proper nouns (PNs) with a single predicate 'loves'. AGR refers to another name such as arguments of both CNs and PNs that represent either e type or t type in a discourse [10, 11].

Step 2: Slots (_____)

CN (AGR$_d$)	PN (AGR$_d$)
Loves (_____, W)	Loves (_____, K)
Loves (_____, M)	Loves (_____, M)
Loves (_____, G)	Loves (_____, K)
Loves (_____, B)	Loves (_____, D)
Loves (_____, W)	Loves (_____, S)
Loves (_____, H)	Loves (_____, G)
Loves (_____, M)	Loves (_____, A)
Loves (_____, F)	Loves (_____, S)
Loves (_____, G)	Loves (_____, M)
Loves (_____, A)	Loves (_____, S)

According to step 2, it shows that an external or a front AGR place must be an empty slot in a predicate 'loves'. Such slot finds with CNs and PNs sets.

Step 3: Slots with lambda operator λ

Step 3: Slots with lambda operator λ

CN (AGR$_d$)	PN (AGR$_d$)
Loves (___, λ_W)	Loves (___, λ_K)
Loves (___, λ_M)	Loves (___, λ_M)
Loves (___, λ_G)	Loves (___, λ_K)
Loves (___, λ_B)	Loves (___, λ_D)
Loves (___, λ_W)	Loves (___, λ_S)
Loves (___, λ_H)	Loves (___, λ_G)
Loves (___, λ_M)	Loves (___, λ_A)
Loves (___, λ_F)	Loves (___, λ_S)
Loves (___, λ_G)	Loves (___, λ_M)
Loves (___, λ_A)	Loves (___, λ_S)

Step 3 determines that the empty slots in CNs and PNs are abstraction places that fills up with a lambda operator λ. We add this operator in front of each empty slot.

Step 4: Lambda operator λ as binder for variables x

$$\lambda x. \text{ Loves } (x, w\ldots\ldots\ldots A)$$
$$\lambda x. \text{ Loves } (x, k\ldots\ldots\ldots S)$$

In step 4, we argue that a lambda operator λ binds x variable in the same slot. Because it is difficult to select each name separately for the same function here.

Step 5: Model and assignment functions

$$M = \langle D, I \rangle \text{ and } g$$
$$M = D_e (\text{Any type } e, \, t/et \text{ in CN or PN in Step 1})$$
$$M = D_t (1, 0)$$

The step 5 defines the formal representation with a model (M) that contains (D) and (I) function assignment as g. Any set of individuals, as appears in step 1, is a part of e, t/et domain which directly links with truth values (1, 0).

6   Conclusion

We understand that a language like English has a formal representation. Small and simple statements in any natural language are expressions that are nothing but a set of finite or infinite types. We find that a lambda operator λ describes such infinite sets better because it takes all types of expressions (equality-based, negation-based, and so on) in the form of a type and binds them to avoid repeating any name. It also frames syntax and semantics of a natural language. Following such observations, a proposed algorithm helps us to analyze small CNs and PNs individual sets.

References

1. Partee BB, Ter Meulen AG, Wall R (2012) Mathematical methods in linguistics, vol 30. Springer, Dordrecht
2. Allwood J, Andersson GG, Andersson LG, Dahl O (1977) Logic in linguistics. Cambridge University Press, Cambridge
3. Gillon BS (2019) Natural language semantics: formation and valuation. MIT Press, Massachusetts
4. Carpenter B (1997) Type-logical semantics. MIT Press, Massachusetts

5. Cann R (1993) Formal semantics: an introduction. Cambridge University Press, Cambridge
6. Coppock E, Champollion L (2019) Invitation to formal semantics. Manuscript, Boston University and New York University. http://eecoppock.info/semantics-boot-camp.pdf
7. Barendregt HP (1984) The lambda calculus: its syntax and semantics. In: Studies in Logic, vol 103. NorthHolland Publishing Company, Netherlands
8. Moggi E (1988) Computational lambda-calculus and monads. University of Edinburgh, Department of Computer Science, Laboratory for Foundations of Computer Science
9. Lamping J (1989, December) An algorithm for optimal lambda calculus reduction. In: Proceedings of the 17th ACM SIGPLAN-SIGACT symposium on principles of programming languages, pp 16–30
10. Liang P (2013) Lambda dependency-based compositional semantics. Technical Report, arXiv: 1309.4408
11. Boudol G, Curien PL, Lavatelli C (1999) A semantics for lambda calculi with resources. Math Struct Comput Sci 9(4):437–482

Non-destructive Fusion Method for Image Enhancement of Eddy Current Sub-surface Defect Images

Anil Kumar Soni, Ranjeet Kumar, Shrawan Kumar Patel, and Aradhana Soni

1 Introduction

Non-destructive Evaluation (NDE) techniques are broadly used in various industries in order to assess the immaculacy and adequacy of materials and structure components without disturbing the functional properties and worth. The EC testing technique works in the principle of electromagnetic induction for inspection of the metallic materials. EC testing technique is used for detection and sizing of defects in the metallic material, but due to the skin effect phenomenon, penetration of eddy currents into the metallic material is limited and detection of sub-surface defects is challenging [1]. Use of large diameter EC probe and lower excitation frequency increase the detection sensitivity for sub-surface defects by increasing the deeper penetration of eddy current into the material [2–4]. However, the use of large diameter probe and lower excitation frequency cause the blurring or oversizing in defect images and also decrease in resolution as well as SNR [1]. In this regard, combining of defect information (image) from different excitation frequencies as well as different diameter probe are beneficial.

The process of combining two or more images containing complementary as well as redundant information into a single image is called image fusion. Image

A. K. Soni (✉) · S. K. Patel
Department of Electronics and Communication, SoS (E&T), Guru Ghasidas Vishwavidyalaya, Bilaspur, Chhattisgarh 495009, India
e-mail: anilsoni@ggu.ac.in

R. Kumar
School of Electronics Engineering, Vellore Institute of Technology, Chennai Campus, Chennai 600127, India

A. Soni
Department of Information Technologies, SoS (E&T), Guru Ghasidas Vishwavidyalaya, Bilaspur, Chhattisgarh 495009, India

© The Author(s), under exclusive license to Springer Nature Singapore Pte Ltd. 2021   613
M. K. Bajpai et al. (eds.), *Machine Vision and Augmented Intelligence—Theory and Applications*, Lecture Notes in Electrical Engineering 796,
https://doi.org/10.1007/978-981-16-5078-9_50

fusion maximizes the information content in the image [5]. Image fusion is gaining importance in NDE for image enhancement of the defect images and various fusion methodologies are successfully reported for different NDE defect detection techniques. Gros et al. used Bayesian analysis, Daubechie wavelet, steerable pyramid transform and multi-resolution mosaic-based image fusion methods to combine eddy current and infrared thermographic images from carbon fiber reinforced plastic (CFRP) composite panels. They observed that data fusion increased the knowledge about flaw location and size. They also reported that more advanced fusion techniques may be developed for a specific NDE application to reduce the uncertainty and increase the overall performance of NDE [6].

Multi-resolution-based image fusion techniques are proposed by various researchers and they have reported that by utilization of these transformation techniques removal of disturbing (noise) signal from defect images and retains the defect information are possible. They also reported that development of efficient algorithms is essential for dealing large amount of data from sensory, measurements and stored data [7–9]. Muduli et al. proposed a model for an efficient and reliable crack detection, which combines the best features of canny edge detection algorithm and Hyperbolic Tangent filtering technique using an efficient Max-Mean image fusion rule. They found that the fused images have high value of PSNR and an optimized edge detection technique [10]. A detailed survey is carried out by Arun et al. to identify the research challenges and the achievements till in the field of crack detection in NDE [11].

Apart of NDE, various image fusion methods are reported in different application. Wang et al. proposed a fractional Fourier transform-based image fusion method and found that the fractional Fourier transform develops the signal analysis into fractional domain and can reflect the signal information in the time domain and the frequency domain simultaneously and also provides more detailed information and higher spatial resolution [12]. Yi-Fei et al. develop the fractional differential masks for image enhancement and reported that the fraction differential-based techniques are more efficient for the images contains nonlinear behavior of information [13]. Images of sub-surface defects of metallic material are nonlinear in behavior; because the presence of various parameters effects the sub-surface defect images. From the above literature it is found that the fraction derivative-based image fusion methodology can improve the defect information and resolution. In this paper, factional derivative-based image fusion methodology is studied for improving the quality and information of the defect images and the performance of the proposed fusion algorithm is compared with the commonly used NDT fusion algorithms by using the image metrics such as SNR and entropy.

2 Theoretical Background

Proposed fusion method used the fractional derivative-based approach for combination of EC images. The proposed fusion method generates the derivative of the input images, which are used as input images for wavelet transform-based image fusion. Fractional derivative has three popular definitions by Griinwald–Letnikov (G–L), Riemann–Liouville (R–L), and Caputo, which is used in image processing and they are equivalent in initial condition. The R–L definition of derivative of fractional order $\alpha > 0$ is defined as [12, 14]:

$$_aD_t^\alpha = \frac{1}{\Gamma(n-\alpha)} \left(\frac{d}{dt}\right)^n \int_a^t \frac{f(\tau)}{(t-\tau)^{\alpha-n+1}} d\tau \, (n-1 < \alpha < n) \tag{1}$$

where $\Gamma(.)$ is a gamma function:

$$\Gamma(n) = \int_0^\infty t^{n-1} e^{-t} dt \tag{2}$$

Define the generalization of the factorial in the following form:

$$\Gamma(n) = (n-1)! \tag{3}$$

Proposed fractional derivative-based image fusion method is hybrid in nature which is the combination of fractional derivative and wavelet transform. Proposed image fusion method used the R–L definition of derivative and discrete wavelet transform. In this process, α order (0–1) derivative of input images is generated first and after that the wavelet transform-based image fusion is performed. For wavelet-based image fusion 3-level decomposition process is taken for the derivative of the input images. For reconstruction of the fused image inverse fraction derivative is generated by fraction order $(-\alpha)$. The algorithm flow diagram of the proposed fusion process is shown in Fig. 1.

3 Generation of Eddy Current Images

For generation of EC images of sub-surface defects, EC instrument is developed which comprising of low-frequency, high current excitation and high sensitive lock-in-based phase angle measurement blocks. Photograph of the experimental setup is shown in Fig. 2. Developed system generates the sine wave signal which has variable excitation current (up to 3A) and frequency ranging from 500 Hz to 80 kHz. Using NI PCI-7330 motion control card through LabVIEW program, an automated line scanning of EC probe over SS plate is realized. The excitation source signal and receiver coil response are acquired simultaneously using NI PCI-6220 data acquisition card (DAQ) for generation of sub-surface defect images [3].

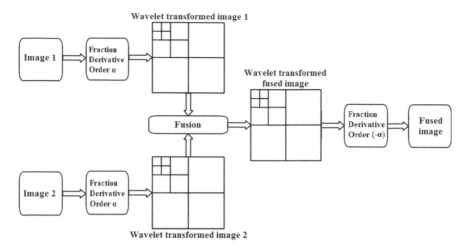

Fig. 1 Algorithm flow diagram for the proposed image fusion process

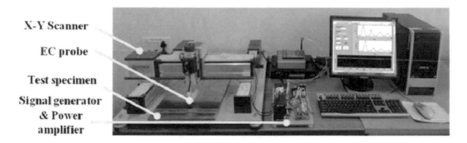

Fig. 2 Photograph of the experimental setup

For performance analysis of proposed image fusion methodology, phase angle images of a sub-surface defect located 8.0 mm below the surface at frequency 5 and 7 kHz have been generated using the developed ECT instrument and cup-core probe. Generated EC images of sub-surface defect have dimension as length 30.0 mm, width 2.5 mm and the depth 8.0 mm below the surface of a 12.0 mm thick stainless steel plate. These generated images have been used for evaluation of the proposed image fusion methodology. Generated input images are shown in Fig. 3.

4   Performance Analysis Metrics

For performance analysis of proposed fusion methodologies SNR, entropy and standard deviation have been used. The SNR is defined as the ratio of mean or expected value of flaw signal (μ_{Signal}) to the standard deviation of the noise (σ_{noise}) in the

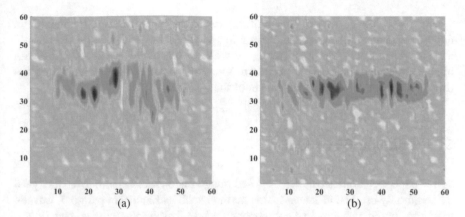

Fig. 3 EC defect images with frequency (a) 5 kHz (b) 7 kHz

image and define as [5]:

$$SNR = 10\log_{10}\frac{\mu_{Signal}}{\sigma_{noise}} \tag{4}$$

The SNR will tend to infinity when the flaw image is free from noise. Image with high SNR provides the better quality image.

The entropy of an image describes the amount of information present in the image. The entropy (H) of the image is defined as [5]:

$$H = -\sum_{i=1}^{M}\sum_{j=1}^{N} P(i, j)\log_2 P(i, j) \tag{5}$$

where P is the probability of pixel-level image intensity. Entropy is sensitive to noise and other unwanted rapid fluctuations in the image. Low entropy images have very little contrast and large number of redundant data. But the higher value of entropy shows the contrast in images and higher information content.

Standard deviation is a statistical quantity, which is used to measure the amount of variability or dispersion around the mean of the image. It is a measure of the image contrast and is defined as [5]:

$$Standard\ deviation(\sigma) = \sqrt{\sum_{i=0}^{M}\sum_{j=0}^{N}\frac{(I(i, j) - \mu)^2}{MN}} \tag{6}$$

$$\mu = \frac{1}{MN}\sum_{i=0}^{M}\sum_{j=0}^{N} I(i, j) \tag{7}$$

where I is the image, μ is the mean of the image, M and N refers to the maximum number of pixels in the image in horizontal and vertical direction respectively and i and j are the indices which refers to the individual pixels of the image. An image with high contrast would have a high standard deviation, because of the higher dispersion (higher range of data) around the mean of the image.

5 Result and Discussion

In this paper performance of the proposed image fusion method have been analyzed by commonly used NDE image fusion method such as Laplacian pyramid, wavelet transform-based and principal component analysis-based image fusion techniques. Process of implementation of this NDE image fusion method have been discussed by Thirunavukkarasu et al. [5]. From Fig. 3 it is clearly visible that the information contains in input image of sub-surface defect is not sufficient for characterization of defect. A good improvement in defect images have been found after the various fusion methods were applied. Figure 4 shows the fused images generated by using various NDE techniques and proposed image fusion method.

Table 1 and Fig. 5 shows the performance analysis matrices for the analysis of fused images. From the result, it is clearly seen that the proposed method has improved the quality of fused images. Laplacian pyramid and PCA-based image fusion approaches have improved the visibility of the defect in images but the SNR and SD have not improved. However, the wavelet transform-based fusion method show the improvement in SNR, standard deviation and entropy also. The proposed fusion method shows good improvement in performance matrices as well as the visibility of the defect image. A 13.64 dB SNR has been determined for the proposed methodology.

6 Conclusion

Laplacian pyramid, wavelet transform and principal component analysis-based image fusion techniques are compared with the proposed fractional derivative-based image fusion method. For this, the eddy current sub-surface defects images are utilized for enhancement which is generated by the developed eddy current instrument. The performance of image fusion techniques has been analyzed by SNR, standard deviation and entropy. The proposed fusion method showed highest improvement in SNR (13.64 dB), standard deviation (0.0085) and entropy (0.65) and found to be superior as compared to the other fusion methodologies. Hybrid nature of the image fusion method makes the proposed method more superior as compared to the direct wavelet transform.

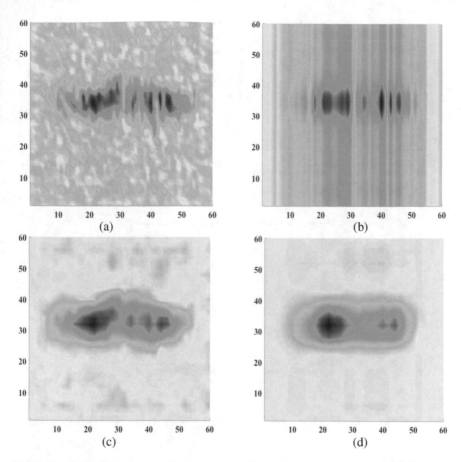

Fig. 4 Fused EC defect images. **a** Laplacian Pyramid. **b** Principal component analysis. **c** Wavelet transform. **d** Proposed Fusion method

Table 1 Performance Analysis Metrics of fused image

S. no	Fusion Method	Entropy	SNR	Standard deviation
1	Input Image 1 (5 kHz)	0.2242	5.62	0.0007
2	Input Image 2 (7 kHz)	0.2899	5.32	0.0014
3	Laplacian pyramid	0.3241	6.02	0.0015
4	PCA	0.369	10.43	0.0023
5	Wavelet Transform	0.5536	11.32	0.0047
6	Proposed Method	0.6461	13.64	0.0085

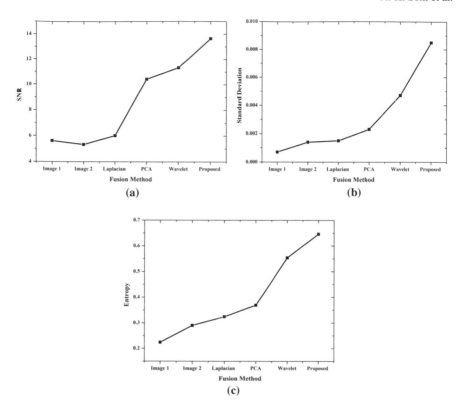

Fig. 5 Performance Analysis Metrics of fused image. **a** SNR. **b** Standard deviation. **c** Entropy

References

1. Rao BPC (2007) Practical eddy current testing. Narosa Publishing House, India
2. Soni AK, Sasi B, Thirunavukkarasu S, Rao BPC (2015) Development of eddy current probe for detection of deep sub-surface defects. IETE Tech Rev 33:386–395
3. Soni AK, Thirunavukkarasu S, Sasi B, Rao BPC, Jayakumar T (2015) Development of a high sensitivity eddy current instrument for detection of sub-surface defects in stainless steel plates. Insight Non-Destr Test Cond Monit 57:508–512
4. Soni AK, Rao BPC (2018) Lock-in amplifier based eddy current instrument for detection of sub-surface defect in stainless steel plates. Sens Imaging 19. https://doi.org/10.1007/s11220-018-0217-8
5. Thirunavukkarasu S, Rao BPC, Soni AK, Shuaib Ahmed S, Jayakumar T (2012) Comparative performance of image fusion methodologies in eddy current testing. Res J Appl Sci Eng Technol 4:5548–5551
6. Gros XE, Liu Z, Tsukada K, Hanasaki K (2000) Experimenting with Pixel-level NDT Data Fusion Techniques. IEEE Trans Instrum Meas 49
7. Liu Z, Forsyth DS, Komorowski JP, Hanasaki K, Kirubarajan T (2007) Survey: state of the art in NDE data fusion techniques. IEEE Trans Instrum Meas 56:2435–2451
8. Algarni ASM (2009) Image fusion based enhancement of electromagnetic nondestructive evaluation, King Saud University, PhD dissertation

9. Balakrishnan S, Cacciola M, Udpa L, Rao BP, Jayakumar T, Raj B (2012) Development of image fusion methodology using discrete wavelet transform for eddy current images. NDT&E Int 51:51–57
10. Muduli PR, Pati UC (2013) A novel technique for wall crack detection using image fusion. In: International conference on computer communication and informatics
11. Mohan A, Poobal S (2018) Crack detection using image processing: a critical review and analysis. Alex Eng J 57:787–798
12. Wang P, Tian H, Zheng W (2013) A novel image fusion method based on FRFT-NSCT. Math Probl Eng
13. Yi-Fei Pu, Zhou J-L, Yuan X (2009) Fractional differential mask: a fractional differential-based approach for multiscale texture enhancement. IEEE Trans Image Process 19:491–511
14. Yang Q, Chen D, Zhao T, Chen YQ (2016) Fractional calculus in image processing: a review. Fract Calc Appl Anal 19

Histogram-Based Image Enhancement and Analysis for Steel Surface and Defects Images

Ranjeet Kumar, Anil Kumar Soni, Aradhana Soni, and Saurav Gupta

1 Introduction

Product quality, it indicates the strength of the product that serves to the customer/consumer in all the field. In industrial production like steel plates and rods that essential for the infrastructure strength; here, quality assurance is a key aspect for the steel sheets or rods. To ensure quality and strength, different methods or systems are followed by industries like visual inspection [1, 2] and non-destructive testing [3–6], etc. Nowadays, visual inspection of surface and defect are in practice for steel sheets and rods due to its effectiveness and cost-effective process [7]. However, the quality of video or images also plays a key role in visual inspection. During the visual inspection, exposure of light or surrounding luminance can affect image quality. therefore, a robust image or video processing tools/image enhancement technique is needed to retain the image quality [7, 8].

In the production of steel at a larger scale, the rolling affects the surface microstructure of the steel sheets or rods [8, 9], which in turn impacts the mechanical properties in terms of quality and strength. Visual inspection methods or technology based on image processing has been widely used in various fields, such as electronics

R. Kumar (✉) · S. Gupta
School of Electronics Engineering, Vellore Institute of Technology, Chennai,
Tamilnadu 600127, India

A. K. Soni
Department of Electronics and Communication Engineering, SoS(E&T), Guru Ghasidas
Vishwavidyalaya, Bilaspur, Chattisgarh 495009, India
e-mail: anilsoni@ggu.ac.in

A. Soni
Department of Information Technologies, SoS(E&T), Guru Ghasidas Vishwavidyalaya, Bilaspur,
Chattisgarh 495009, India
e-mail: soni.aradhana@ggu.ac.in

© The Author(s), under exclusive license to Springer Nature Singapore Pte Ltd. 2021   623
M. K. Bajpai et al. (eds.), *Machine Vision and Augmented Intelligence—Theory
and Applications*, Lecture Notes in Electrical Engineering 796,
https://doi.org/10.1007/978-981-16-5078-9_51

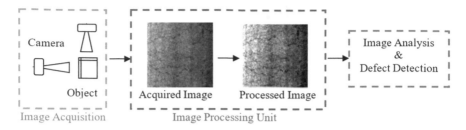

Fig. 1 Industrial visual inspection setup based on images and its analysis

chip, healthcare, the manufacturing industry, the textile industry, and the automobile industry, media and art industries for its exclusive advantages of perception, precision, and suitability [10]. Here, several techniques are developed for visual quality enhancement of steel surface images that help to analysis in defect identification by automated or semiautomated inspection system [11]. These techniques are followed several operations like morphological filtering, noise filtering, processing in the transform domain, data compression, histogram equalization for images even for the industrial application like product surface and defect inspection [12–16].

Indeed, the number of researches related to defect detection has grown rapidly over the past decade due to the rapid advance of the computing system, the improvement of sensor performance, and the progress of image processing technology. The basic components of a typical visual system are an image acquisition unit/camera, an image processing unit, and a control execution/analysis unit as illustrated in Fig. 1.

Here, visual inspection plays a key role for the detection of surface defects in real time; if image quality is suitable for human vision or computer vision system in different applications like defect segmentation and detection, defect classification, etc. [17, 18]. The objective of this paper is to evaluate different enhancement techniques based on histogram processing of surface images of steel plates and rods.

In this paper, the contrast control image enhancement technique has been exploited based on histogram processing. Here, the different histogram equalization process is also evaluated for the grayscale steel surface defect images. The performance measures with approximation quality metrices like peak signal-to-noise ratio (PSNR), mean square error (MSE), maximum error (ME) and ratio of l_2-norm values. Further enhanced images are very important inputs for automated system like classifiers or other operation.

In this context, this paper is organized as follows: a brief introduction of visual inspection and its importance discussed for steel surfaces in section *one*; further, section *two* explained the image enhancement with histogram techniques. In section *three*, detailed result analysis is elaborated with a brief of steel surface image dataset followed by the conclusion and references for the presented work.

2 Image Enhancement with Histogram

A grayscale image is one in which the value of each pixel is a single illustration of an amount of light, that is, it brings only intensity information [19]. Where low or high intensity of light or information may lead to poor visual quality of image, which may not use for information extraction by humans or machines. Therefore, the visual quality of images is further corrected by the different techniques in several application fields [16, 20]. Particular, in industrial applications like steel surface images are captured in grayscale by the system for visual inspection. Here, image enhancement techniques help a lot to maintain the visual image quality. As light intensity concern, images are explained with histogram analysis that represents the number of pixels in an image at each different intensity value found in that image.

In Fig. 2, two different histogram representations are shown for an image in original and processed form as illustrated in Fig. 1. Here, the original image histogram represents the frequency of pixel intensity in the range of 20–200; whereas processed image histogram represents the frequency of pixel intensity in the range of 10–255 that outcome is better visual quality of image. It's clearly illustrated enhanced visual image quality achieved with histogram processing as shown in Figs. 1 and 2. In this paper, three different histogram processing methods are exploited for steel surface grayscale images for better visualization of defects. These are as follows: histogram adjustment, histogram equalization and adaptive histogram equalization. The detail of these techniques is well explained by the researcher in the very rich reference database of image processing [17].

2.1 Histogram Analysis

Image histograms are broadly used in several fields of image processing, due to its low computational cost and many other advantages, such as image translation, rotation, and scale invariance, specifically in the fields of threshold segmentation of grayscale images, image retrieval and image classification based on the color scale. Here, histogram or contrast adjustment refers to the redistribution of the histogram of image over the entire scale of intensity [17, 21]. In this process, a linear mapping of a subgroup of pixel values to the entire range of display intensities (dynamic range). This outcome is a higher contrast image by less bright pixels whose value is below a specified value and high bright pixels whose value is above a specified value.

The process of regulating intensity values can be done inevitably using histogram equalization. Histogram equalization involves transforming the intensity values so that the histogram of the output image approximately matches a specified histogram. The equalization process referred to the cumulative distribution of histogram or image pixel values that produces better contrast and brightness as compared to the original image [18, 19].

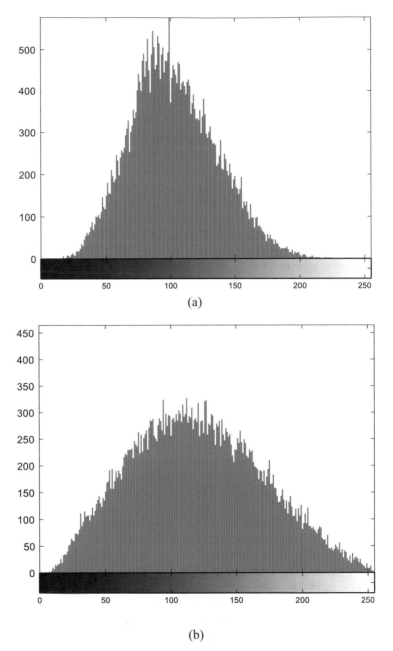

Fig. 2 Histogram representation for **a** original/acquired image, and **b** approximated/processed image of images shown in Fig. 1

Further, the HE technique is improved for the better visual quality of images. It varies from ordinary histogram equalization in the respect that the adaptive method computes multiple histograms, each corresponding to a distinct section or block of the image, and uses them to redistribute the brightness values of the image. It is, therefore, fit for refining the local contrast and enhancing the definitions of edges in each region of an image [20]. Still, AHE inclines to overamplify noise in relatively homogeneous regions of an image.

In this paper, these techniques are introduced in brief to enrich the feasibility of image processing techniques and tools in industrial applications like metal surface image processing. A rich literature is available in the field of image processing and applications; however, some of the suitable references are included for the detail information of techniques.

3 Results and Discussion

In this paper, steel surface defect images are obtained from the Northeastern University (NEU) surface defect database. The database contained 1800 grayscale images of 6 different kinds of surface defects of hot-rolled steel strip as follow: rolled-in scale (RS), patches (Pa), crazing (Cr), pitted surface (PS), inclusion (In) and scratches (Sc) [9, 22]. Figure 3 shows the 12 different images of pixel size 200×200 for 6 kinds of database defect subjects as discussed. With these images, histogram-based image enhancement techniques were analyzed with different quality metrics such as peak signal-to-noise ratio (PSNR), mean square error (MSE), maximum error (ME) and ratio of l_2-norm values of original and processed image. These metrics are especially prescribed and widely used in assessment or qualitative analysis of processed/approximated signals, images and video [15, 23–27]. These are defined as follows:

- Peak Signal to Noise Ratio (PSNR): $20 \log\left(\frac{2^B - 1}{\sqrt{\text{MSE}}}\right)$
  where MSE represents the mean square error and B represent the bit/pixel value of image.
- Mean Square Error (MSE): $\frac{\|X - Y\|^2}{N}$
  where X and Y represent the original and processed/approximated image and N is the total number of image pixels/elements.
- Maximum error (ME): $\max|X - Y|$
- l_2-norm ratio: $\frac{\|X - Y\|^2}{\|X\|^2}$

In this section, a qualitative and visual analysis are illustrated for different defect subject images in Figs. 4 and 5, respectively. In Fig. 4a, PSNR value is compared for presented techniques such as histogram/contrast adjustment (HA), histogram equalization (HE) and adaptive histogram equalization (AHE) with 12 different images of 6 surface defects. Where, AHE technique *PSNR* value is better with respect to other both techniques for the images except the patch defect images. Similarly, Figs. 4b,

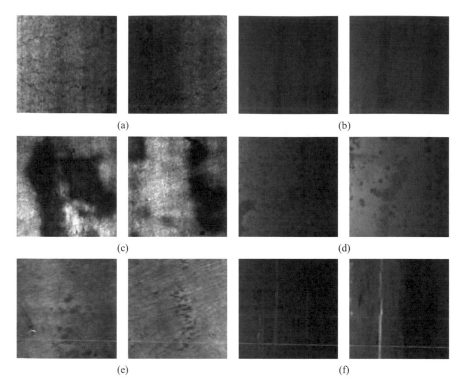

Fig. 3 Sample Steel Surface Defect Images: **a** crazing, **b** inclusion, **c** patches, **d** pitted surface, **e** rolled-in scale, **f** scratches [11]

c illustrate the comparative analysis of *MSE* for the techniques with sample surface defect image. It is clearly shown that the *MSE* of AHE processed images are less compared to other techniques for the images except the patch defect images.

In Fig. 4d, the l_2-norm ratio of difference of original and processed image with original image. It indicates the original pixel intensity deviation with respect to processed image value. Here, AHE technique scored less deviation as ratio as compared to others for all the sample images. With this analysis, AHE technique is more suitable for the steel surface images. Further, visual analysis was carried out for better interpretation or annotations of images.

Figure 5 illustrates the visual quality comparison of HA, HE and AHE techniques for 6 sample images of 6 kinds of surface defects from database. As discussed, based on quality metrices analysis AHE is better for the enhancement as compared to other techniques. Here, also observed enhanced image with HA or HE contains over or under brightness level that moves towards image quality degradation in some area of image. Whereas, AHE-based enhanced images are uniformly enhanced with balanced brightness levels that help to recognize the surface defect as per human vision system (HVS).

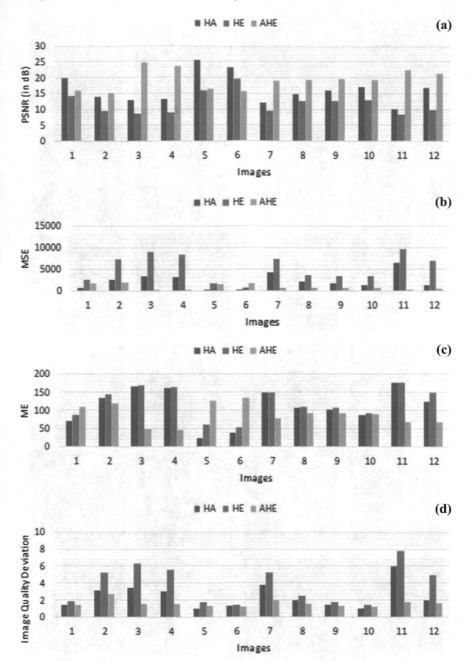

Fig. 4 Approximation quality analysis of different enhanced surface defect images using HA, HE and AHE technique based on different metrics such as **a** PSNR, **b** MSE, **c** ME and **d** Image Quality Deviation

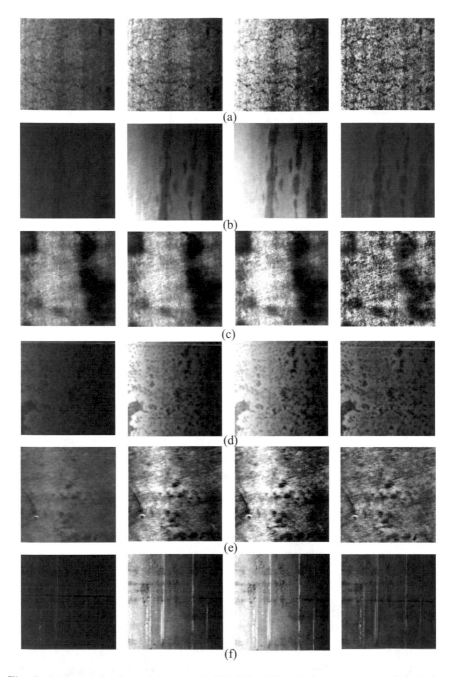

Fig. 5 Original and enhanced image with HA, HE, AHE techniques: **a** crazing, **b** inclusion, **c** patches, **d** pitted surface, **e** rolled-in scale, **f** scratches

Overall, quality metric and visual analysis indicate the histogram processing-based adaptive equalization method is more suitable for enhancement of grayscale steel surface defect images.

4 Conclusion

In this paper, histogram-based image enhancement techniques are studies for the grayscale steel surface defect images of different subjects. Here, results and its analysis are clearly recommended for the suitable technique based on quality metric and visual analysis that may be further evaluated with other annotation procedures. The texture scale of steel sheet or rod surface is uniformed that results in acquired images having uniform texture grayscale. However, poor visual quality of images may hide the defects like scratches, craze, etc. Here, adaptive histogram equalization (AHE) technique enhances the visual quality of image with balanced brightness, texture features as compared to HA and HE techniques. The enhanced image may be helpful for present and future semiautomated or fully automated visual inspection system in industrial applications.

References

1. Shapiro LG, Stockman GC (2001) Computer vision: theory and applications. Prentice Hall
2. Win M, Bushroa AR, Hassan MA, Hilman NM, Ide-Ektessabi A (2015) A contrast adjustment thresholding method for surface defect detection based on mesoscopy. IEEE Trans Ind Inform 11:642–649. https://doi.org/10.1109/TII.2015.2417676
3. Soni AK, Thirunavukkarasu S, Sasi B, Rao BPC, Jayakumar T (2015) Development of a high-sensitivity eddy current instrument for the detection of sub-surface defects in stainless steel plates. Insight Non-Destr Test Cond Monit 57. https://doi.org/10.1784/insi.2015.57.9.508
4. Thirunavukkarasu S, Rao B, Kumar Soni A, Shuaib Ahmed S, Jayakumar T (2012) Comparative performance of image fusion methodologies in eddy current testing. Res J Appl Sci Eng Technol 4:5548–5551
5. Soni AK, Sasi B, Thirunavukkarasu S, Rao BPC (2016) Development of eddy current probe for detection of deep sub-surface defects. IETE Tech Rev 33. https://doi.org/10.1080/02564602.2015.1113145
6. Soni AK, Rao BP (2018) Lock-in amplifier based eddy current instrument for detection of sub-surface defect in stainless steel plates. Sens Imaging 19:32. https://doi.org/10.1007/s11220-018-0217-8
7. Sun X, Gu J, Tang S, Li J (2018) research progress of visual inspection technology of steel products—a review. Appl Sci 8. https://doi.org/10.3390/app8112195
8. Ghorai S, Mukherjee A, Gangadaran M, Dutta PK (2013) automatic defect detection on hot-rolled flat steel products. IEEE Trans Instrum Meas 62:612–621. https://doi.org/10.1109/TIM.2012.2218677
9. Song K, Yan Y (2013) A noise robust method based on completed local binary patterns for hot-rolled steel strip surface defects. Appl Surf Sci 285. https://doi.org/10.1016/j.apsusc.2013.09.002
10. Shirvaikar M (2006) Trends in automated visual inspection. J Real-Time Image Process 1. https://doi.org/10.1007/s11554-006-0009-6

11. Ghatnekar S (2018) Use machine learning to detect defects on the steel surface. https://sof tware.intel.com/content/www/us/en/develop/articles/use-machine-learning-to-detect-defects-on-the-steel-surface.html
12. Kumar S, Sen Yadav J, Manoj K, Rajsekaran S, Kumar R (2019) Object localization and tracking using background subtraction and dual-tree complex wavelet transform. Int J Eng Adv Technol 8
13. Li W, Lu C, Zhang J (2012) A local annular contrast based real-time inspection algorithm for steel bar surface defects. Appl Surf Sci 258. https://doi.org/10.1016/j.apsusc.2012.03.007
14. Donoho DL, Huo X (2002) Beamlets and multiscale image analysis
15. Kumar R, Patbhaje U, Kumar A (2019) An efficient technique for image compression and quality retrieval using matrix completion. J King Saud Univ Comput Inf Sci. https://doi.org/10.1016/j.jksuci.2019.08.002
16. Blackledge J, Dubovitskiy D (2008) A surface inspection machine vision system that includes fractal texture analysis. https://doi.org/10.21427/D7QS5J
17. Gonzalez RC, Woods RE (2008) Digital image processing, 3rd ed. Prentice Hall
18. Luo Q, Fang X, Su J, Zhou J, Zhou B, Yang C, Liu L, Gui W, Tian L (2020) Automated visual defect classification for flat steel surface: a survey. IEEE Trans Instrum Meas 69. https://doi.org/10.1109/TIM.2020.3030167
19. Jain AK (1981) Image data compression: a review. Proc IEEE 69:349–389. https://doi.org/10.1109/PROC.1981.11971
20. Hummel R (1977) Image enhancement by histogram transformation. Comput Graph Image Process 6. https://doi.org/10.1016/S0146-664X(77)80011-7
21. Gonzalez RC, Woods RE (2010) Wavelets. Digital image processing, 2nd ed. Tata MacGraw-Hills
22. He Y, Song K, Dong H, Yan Y (2019) Semi-supervised defect classification of steel surface based on multi-training and generative adversarial network. Opt Lasers Eng 122. https://doi.org/10.1016/j.optlaseng.2019.06.020
23. Kumar R, Kumar A, Singh GK (2016) Electrocardiogram signal compression based on 2D-transforms: a research overview. J Med Imaging Heal Informatics 6. https://doi.org/10.1166/jmihi.2016.1698
24. Kumar A (2011) Wavelet based electrocardiogram compression at different quantization levels
25. Kumar A, Singh GK, Rajesh G, Ranjeet K (2013) The optimized wavelet filters for speech compression. Int J Speech Technol 16. https://doi.org/10.1007/s10772-012-9173-1
26. Patbhaje U, Kumar R, Kumar A, Lee H-N (2017) Compression of medical image using wavelet based sparsification and coding. In: 2017 4th international conference on signal processing and integrated networks, SPIN 2017
27. Huynh-Thu Q, Ghanbari M (2008) Scope of validity of PSNR in image/video quality assessment. Electron Lett 44. https://doi.org/10.1049/el:20080522

Predicting Depression by Analysing User Tweets

Abhay Kumar, Vaibhav Pratihar, Sheshank Kumar, and Kumar Abhishek

1 Introduction

Depression is a psychiatric disorder, and more than sadness [1]. It is a common psychiatric disorder, but a severe one. Depression often characterises feelings of being unmotivated, sad, and hopeless, discouraged, lack of interest in life. Depression comes with symptoms of anxiety, and sometimes Depression can lead to suicide [2]. For every person who attempts suicide, as per WHO report, 20 or more will attempt to end their life (WHO, 2012). Depression now becomes a global burden of disease and affects people across the globe. Depressive disorders (mood disorders) are of three types (1) Major depression (2) Persistent depressive disorder, (3) Bipolar disorder. Depression may cause due to a combination of biological, genetic, psychological and environmental, factors.

More than 300 million people of all ages suffer from this disorder globally. Supporting and treating this disorder have been considered insufficient, and there is still no reliable test for diagnosing this order. CES-D (Center for Epidemiologic Studies Depression Scale) designed some tests in the form of Questionnaires such as screening test, but they are not easily attainable.

To tackle these issues, we take the aid of social media as a tool for predicting Depression. People are increasingly using social media platforms to share their feelings with their contacts. Social media provides a means for capturing behavioural attributes like thinking, mood, communication and socialisation. The tweets or posts

A. Kumar (✉) · V. Pratihar · S. Kumar · K. Abhishek
Department of CSE, NIT Patna, Patna, Bihar, India
e-mail: abhay.kumar@nitp.ac.in

K. Abhishek
e-mail: kumar.abhishek@nitp.ac.in

used in social media may indicate feelings which characterise Depression. This paper proposes the hypothesis that a constant language activity expressing negativity in sentiment over a period of time may be a sign of Depression.

Significant contributions in this paper are as follows:

- We use Twitter for data mining for assessment for thousands of tweets with potential signs of Depression. Twitter seems to be a viable option for selection among all the other platforms since it provides user status access without any hassle.
- A lot of steps involving filtering and pre-processing are applied to generate data into a more structural and usable format for further stages. A tweet is then reduced to score (or vector) based on the expression of sentiment on a scaled basis, certain word count and overall word count. This score is then fed to a trained classifier model that compares depressed user class behaviour and standard user class.
- A potential list of depressed users is generated from the above step. This list comprises various Twitter handles—username of the person suspected of suffering from Depression. These handles are then used to retrieve the recent most tweets for further assessment which yields a list of people suffering from Depression.

The rest of the paper is organised as follows: Sect. 2 contains Related Work, Sect. 3 contains the Proposed Method for the model, Sect. 4 details the results obtained by the model and some Limitations. Section 5 concludes the research on our end, and the potential future work to improve or overcome major hurdles to optimise the results further.

2   Related Work

There has been much work in the past which focuses on text filtering and sentiment analysis. The various works include data mining from Twitter, blogs and other social media.

In 2010 Pak and Paroubek [3] showed that Twitter could be used to create a corpus for training a model for sentiment analysis. In 2012 Gokulakrishnan and Priyanthan [4] analysed the problem of sentiment analysis. They provided guidelines on how we can pre-process Twitter tweets to organise an enriched training set. In 2007 Godbole et al. [5] worked on identification of sentiment for news and blogs. There have also been many works that have proved that microblogs such as Twitter and the social activities present on the internet help recognise users' sentiment. In 2012 Kotikalapudi et al. [6] used real-time internet data to associate Depression and its signs in college students with internet usage. Similarly, Moreno et al. [7] showed that Facebook status updates might help analyse the user's mental health. The tendency to share their Depression and the treatment of Depression on Twitter was exposed by Park et al. [8]. In 2008 Pang and Lee [9] surveyed and described the techniques available for opinion-oriented information retrieval. Yang et al. [10] constructed a corpus for sentiment analysis after analysing the web blogs. He used SVM and CRF learners to classify sentiments of each sentence. Go et al. [11] created training data with Twitter and then perform sentiment search based on emoticons. He divided the tweets in 'positive' and 'negative' class and implemented Naïve Bayes classifier to training purpose. It worked well for two-class classification, but as the 'neutral' class was included, the classifier model could not give satisfactory results.

Kumar et al. [12] proposed a method to handle the Depression. The model is trained using Naïve Bayes, gradient boosting and random forest. A sample of 100 users is taken for analysis. The proposed model achieves a classification accuracy of 85.09%.

De Choudhury and Gamon [13] proposed a method to identify Depression using Twitter. Authors crowdsourced method to compile a list of Twitter users and Bag of Words approach to quantify each tweet. Their method recorded an accuracy of 81%, with a precision score of 0.86.

Early Detection of Depression was proposed by Hutto and Gilbert [14]. Authors used Rando Forest classifier to diagnose the disease. In their paper, authors used a dual model which performs better than singleton by more than 10%.

All the work that had been done till now focuses on determining the written statements or sentences' sentiment as either 'positive' or 'negative'. They have focused on microblogs and Twitter, which have significantly less text per user. Still, the work done so far establishes a platform that allows us to extract sentiment even from a single statement said by the user. The use of SVM and Naïve Bayes classifier has proved that they can be used for classification purposes of the text to find their sentiment. The textual data and the use of emoticons in the sentiment analysis have been proven very helpful. What is lacking is that none of the research so far has used these microblogs for determining the existence of Depression in the statement of the use.

3 Proposed Solution

The main issue for which a detailed model will be presented in this paper is threefold. (1) Extract the textual part of the tweet from different user accounts using API. (2) Create a dataset that contains the Twitter users' tweets. This dataset should be processed and ready to train on a required training model. (3) Given the dataset, every entry of that dataset has to be classified in one out of two desired classes, i.e. either the tweet is depressed or not depressed. To accomplish this task, a training model is required which will efficiently perform in the classification. Once any tweet is classified as depressed, the tweeting user can be judged based on his previous tweets, whether he had been showing the same sentiment in his past tweets or not. Judging on that it has to be predicted if that user is suffering from Depression or not.

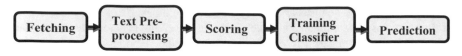

Fig. 1 Proposed methodology

It is done because one depressed behaviour or action does not qualify for the criteria to say that the person is depressed. He might be having a bad day. So, to know more accurately, past behaviour monitoring is also required.

3.1 Proposed Method

The proposed method of this paper shown in Fig. 1 is presented in four stages: (1) Data mining (2) Dataset Creation (3) Scoring of the tweets (4) Training of the classifier model and prediction of tweets.

Stage I: Data Collection

Tweets from are fetched using Tweepy API based on certain words that resemble the sentiment of Depression or grief in general. The mentioned API is capable of handling O-Authentication and also provides a streaming API. The streaming API provides tweets in real-time. Different Parameters can be used along with the API such as language constraints, geographical constraints, inclusion or exclusion of media entities (GIFs, Images, videos, etc.), re-tweeted status, etc., for better results. In addition to the above features, Tweepy can also retrieve recent-most tweets from a particular account with just the user's screen name.

A total of 3223 tweets was taken from @depressionarmy, @depressingmsgs, @depressionnote, @RethinkDep, and other similar Twitter handles that quote depressing thoughts often re-tweeted by people suffering from Depression. These tweets fetched were strictly of 'English' language without any media entities.

Algorithm: Fetch Tweets based on keywords
INPUT: Keywords which sound sad or depressed
OUTPUT: Tweets with username

---

1. Con Key = "************"
2. Con_SECRET = "***********************"
3. ACC_TOKEN = "*******************"
4. ACC_TOKEN_SECRET = "******************************"
5. auth = API.OauthHandler(CONSUMER_KEY,CONSUMER_SECRET)
6. auth.setAccess(ACCESS_TOKEN,ACCESS_TOKEN_SECRET)
7. api = API.Cursor
8. tweets = { }
9. **for** tweets in api.search(Depressed Keywords):
10.   **if** 'retweeted' **then**
11.   Add (tweet.user_name+tweet.retweeted.text) to tweets
12.   **else**
13. Add(tweet.user_name+tweet.text) to tweets
14.   **END if**
15. **END for**
16. **return** tweets

Stage II: Dataset Creation

All the tweets fetched from the Tweepy API come in XML format. There is a set of key-value pair for each tweet where keys refer to various attributes related to the tweets. The ones relevant for this study are the textual part of the tweet and the user id. So they are separated from the format, and a separate dataset is created using those. The tweets now gathered still have so many noises in it, and it has to be reduced in order to proceed further with our classification. Several methods have been applied to pre-process the tweets. They are discussed in the following paragraphs.

Filtering Phase

There are various overheads that will be unrecognisable by the model and will not possess any general significance. These entities need to be filtered out as they will create an exception error in further stages. Since the data is present in textual format, *regular expressions* are used extensively to achieve this task. Entities are matched and replaced with *white-spaces*. Different procedures are applied on top of each other. Some of these tasks are:

1. Hashtag removal ('#')
2. Mentions removal ('@')
3. Removal of URLs ('http://').

Algorithm: Filter Tweets
INPUT: Unfiltered Tweets retrieved using API, Regular Expression of unwanted entities
OUTPUT: Filtered Tweets
1.   filtered_tweets = { }
2.   **for** each tweet in unfiltered_tweets:
3.   **for** each word in tweet:
4.   **If** word matches with regular_expression **then**
5.   Remove that word
6.   **END If**
7.   **END for**
8.   filtered_tweed.append(tweet)
9.   **END for**

Preprocessing Phase

The output of the filtering phase contains data consisting of slangs, emoticons, abbreviations, etc. Furthermore, the data are not of relevant use yet. Several mechanisms are applied to make the data more structured and suitable for use. First, with the help of *regular expressions* abbreviations such as 'LOL' signifying 'Laughing Out Loud', 'rn' signifying 'right now', and slangs such as 'booooooooring' meaning 'boring', 'happppppy' instead of 'happy' are handled. Similarly, emoticons are turned to relevant words carrying the same meaning, for ex: ':-)' is converted to 'happy' while ':-(' is converted to 'sad'. Once the data is present in a regular English format, it can be brought down to a structural format for different phases.

The concepts of NLP are then applied to the dataset. Each tweet is *tokenised,* i.e. split into words, using the **NLTK** module library. These *tokenised* words still contain insignificant words which only increase computational overhead without providing any useful information. These words are usually 'prepositions','conjunctions' or 'Interjections', for ex. The words 'the', 'is', 'a', etc., will not convey any sentiment. A set of these kinds of words is already present in the **NLTK** library stored as *stop-words.* They are filtered out while handling each tweet in the tokenised set. Furthermore, the data present may contain different tense forms of some words, higher vocabulary words, etc. To handle this anomaly, *lemmatisation* [15], which is an advanced form of *stemming,* is used. The process of lemmatisation returns a word in its *root* form, which will be present in the lexicon. Note that the word returned from the lemmatisation process will be a dictionary word, a dictionary of the language of *corpora* over which the lexicon was trained. This process is quite vital and preferred over *stemming* since it is necessary to bring down each word to its correct root form so that the lexicon may utilise it for scoring the sentiments.

To generate a significant feature from each tweet, it is vital to understand the context of each and every word present in it. Hence, it is vital to determine what is the *part-of-speech* tag of each word is. Each and every word of the tokenised tweets are tagged using the *Hunpos tagger* of NLTK library. The tags generated are of excessive, unnecessary detail and needs to be further merged together to make the data more structured. A *chunking* phase is then applied, which takes word pos tags as input and provides a chunk of word-tags as output. Mainly after chunking only 5 tags remain—*noun(n), verb(v), adverb(adv), adjective(adj)* and pronoun*(pro)*. The data present at this stage is in word-tag format and can be directly fed to a lexicon to generate a numerical value which signifies a meaning resembling sentiment and henceforth carrying the same required information.

Since the primary task remains to determine sentiment in terms of some mathematical form, a set of attributes needs to be proposed which can be used to categorise the difference in behaviours of users of two types—the first type being the targeted type, i.e. person whose tweets indicate they might be suffering from Depression or deviating from natural behaviour and the second one being the regular people with no depressive episodes.

Stage III: Scoring

Now that a filtered dataset is created, some features are defined and derived from the tweets so that they can be fed as inputs to our classifier model. Various thinking processes have given the following scores for each tweet.

Depression Language

A person suffering from Depression exhibits a different vocabulary which is likely to consist of words such as 'stressed', 'down', 'upset', etc. [16]. Along with this, a particular set of keywords is also used by people, irrespective of their mental health state, to express a negative sentiment. Note that this negative sentiment is broadly defined. A good example would be the use of the word 'sad' which can be adopted in various ways ranging in different domains such as movie reviews, a sports post-match analysis, and criticism of a higher authority act and our targeted domain. These words can be vital for depression prediction only if found in a particular linguistic way. To express these two categories of words in terms of features, we define three attributes.

Lexicon Score

A lexicon, in vague terms 'the vocabulary of a person, language or branch of language', is a collection of information about the words of a language along with which lexical category of the class they belong to. These tedious tasks can be solved via a domain-specific lexicon which can be selected from various open-source lexicon resources developed for NLP purposes. A popular choice is Sentiwordnet [17] developed by Stanford. The selection for lexicon depends remarkably on the *corpora* over which it was trained. VADER [14, 14], developed by MIT, is attuned for analysing textual data present over social media, which stands on shoulders of NLTK and pattern matching. Each tweet is fed to the lexicon to retrieve a *compound score* in the range of -1.0 to 1.0 where -1.0 indicates an extremely negative sentiment and $+1.0$ indicates an extremely positive statement. Usually, for threshold values to classify sentiments, a range of -0.5 to 0.5 is used to embody neutral sentences, whereas the remaining region depicts negative and positive sentiments accordingly. This numerical representation of sentiment in a specific range can be considered vital for the partition of behavioural differences between depressed and non-depressed users.

Depressed Word Count

Since it has been already established via studies that a person suffering from Depression is exhibiting a strong use of specific keywords, a sentence containing those words would foreshadow depressive behaviour. A higher count of these words in a *tweet* would simply convey a more depressive behaviour.

Word Count

A general norm established in various studies for NLP purposes proposes that textual data comprising more words carries more information. This, in general, also makes more sense as a sentence with more words will carry more details, and hence the information, about the domain for which it was targeted. Hence, a tab on the count of relevant words is taken as a feature.

Each tweet in the initial dataset is now reduced to a tuple—a feature vector of three attributes—*lexicon score, depressed word count* and *total word count*. The data is highly structured as it exists in numerical form in the form of tuples.

Algorithm: Scoring of Tweets **INPUT:** Text of filtered and pre-processed Tweet, list of words which are often used by people suffering from Depression **OUTPUT:** A tuple of 3 elements where 1st, 2nd and 3rd element is lexicon score, count of depressed words, i.e. words often used by people suffering from Depression and total word count respectively.
1. Score = { } 2. Lexicon score = 0 3. Depressed Word Count = 0 4. Word Count = 0 5. **for** each word in tweet: 6. **If** word in depressed_words **THEN** 7.   Increment Depressed Word Count 8.   **END if** 9. Increment Word Count 10.   Lexicon score = lexicon Score + Lexicon Score of (word) 11. **END for** 12. Score = {Lexicon Score, Depressed Word Count, Total Word Count} 13. **return** score

Stage IV: Training and Prediction

The total tweets present in the initial dataset were manually classified into two classes—*depressed* and *non-depressed*. This classification was done by careful observation. The data present in the form of tuples of 3 attributes were modified to add a new attribute, where new attribute was the class tag of each tweet. This additional attribute is basically the desired output for the input set of the dataset.

These feature vectors and the labelled tag were fed to different binary classifiers, under the aid of supervised learning, to obtain a suitable prediction framework that could identify a tweet indicating sentiment of someone suffering from Depression.

The training of these classifiers was done in *K-fold cross-validation* to obtain better accurate results and reduce overfitting. These classifier models included *Naïve Bayes* classifier, *LSTM* classifier, and SVM with different kernels. The best performing classifier was *Support Vector Machine* which could solve the problem compared with the same accuracy as *Bayes* classifier while being computationally faster.

Different *kernels* of SVM were tried and tested for optimal selection of support vectors; including *linear* and non-linear kernels such as *polynomial* and *sigmoid*, where *radial basis function (RBF)* was found to be the most accurate with an accuracy of 93–94%.

Pseudocode to Find People Suffering from Depression

Algorithm: Classification of tweets
INPUT: Feature vector of a tweet consisting of lexicon score, word count, depressed word count
OUTPUT: Single output for each tweet to denoting whether it is depressed or not.

```
1.   Tweets[ ] = FetchTweets(KeyWords)
2.   Filter(Tweets)
3.   Preprocess(Tweets)
4.   Score[ ] = ScoreEvaluvation(Tweets)
5.   Potential Users[ ] = { }
6.   for itr in Score:
7.           UserName = itr[0]
8.           Features = itr[1]
9.   if (identifyDepressedTweet(Features) == True)
10.                          PotentialUsers.append(UserName)
11.  END if
12.  END for
13.  for User in PotentialUsers:
14.          Set[ ] = RecentTweets(User)
15.          RiskCount = 0
16.          For tweet in Set:
17.  if (identifyDepressedTweet(tweet) == True):
18.                          RiskCount = RiskCount+1
19.  END if
20.  if (RiskCount > 0.6 * sizeOf(Set)):
21.                          Notify()
```

4   Results and Discussion

In this model, the main work which has to be done is to predict the class to which the filtered tweet belongs. After implementing the classifier model, a prediction can be made for a tweet that signifies the sentiments of a tweet belonging to a depressed person or not.

The results of various classifiers are shown below in Figs. 2 and 3 for SVM and Naïve Bayes LSTM respectively. The Receiver Operating Characteristics (ROC) curve and the statistics such as accuracy and F1-Score are shown. Figure 4 shows the spread of dataset in the feature spac.

Another classifier used was LSTM which gave accuracy around 68%. LSTM used the relation between the words coming in whole sentences with each other. A separate library 'glove' has been used to find the relationship between the words. 'glove' is a pre-defined dictionary with the set relationship score of different words.

Apart from the results, there are some limitations to this approach. The scope of observation is solely limited to the Twitter users only, also the language used in the tweets must be English; otherwise, the tweet's score cannot be calculated. Sources other than text such as images, emoticons, gifs and videos are excluded from the input.

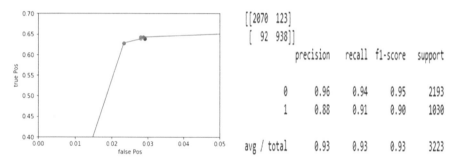

Fig. 2 ROC Curve and various scores of the SVM classifier

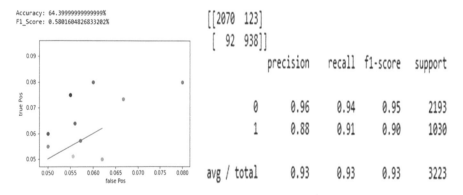

Fig. 3 ROC Curve and various scores of the Naïve Bayes Classifier

Fig. 4 Data visualisation on feature space projected as 2D

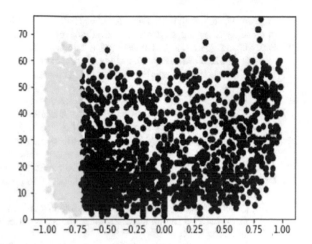

5 Conclusion and Future Work

In this work, it has been shown that social media and microblogs such as Twitter help determine the sentiment and further in this case whether the user is depressed or not. The proposed model successfully fetched raw tweets, filtered the noisy part and trimmed the tweet for text pre-processing. Further, the tweet's evaluation based on the lexicon is done, which provided each tweet's score. The classifier model present takes the tweet and the score vector and classifies the tweets in one of the two present classes, i.e. 'depressed' or 'non-depressed'.

Among future directions, we hope to understand how social media behaviour analysis can lead to the development of scalable methods to come out from depressing thoughts. Also, the tweet classification can be used to analyse the past tweets of a particular user to predict his depressive state.

References

1. The Anxiety and Depression Association of America (ADAA), www.adaa.org
2. https://www.who.int/mental_health/management/depression/who_paper_depression_wfmh_2012.pdf
3. Pak A, Paroubek P (2010) Twitter as a corpus for sentiment analysis and opinion mining. University of Paris
4. Gokulakrishnan B, Priyanthan P (2012) Opinion mining and sentiment analysis on a twitter data stream. In: IEEE conference, Colombo, Sri Lanka, INSPEC Accession Number 13285683
5. Godbole N, Srinivasaiah M, Skiena S (2007) Large scale sentiment analysis for news and blogs. Stony Brook University
6. Kotikalapudi R, Chellappan S, Montgomery F, Wunsch D, Lutzen K (2012) Associating depressive symptoms in college students with internet usage using real Internet data. IEEE Technol Soc Mag

7. Moreno M, Jelenchick L, Egan K, Cox E (2011) Feeling bad on facebook: depression disclosures by college students on a social networking site. Depress Anxiety 28(6):447–455

8. Park M, Cha C, Cha M (2012) Depressive moods of users captured in twitter. In: Proceedings of ACM SIGKDD workshop on healthcare informatics (HI-KDD)

9. Pang B, Lee L (2008) Opinion mining and sentiment analysis. Found Trends Inf Retr 2(1–2):1–135

10. Yang C, Lin KH-Y, Chen HH (2007) Emotion classification using web blog corpora. In: WI '07: Proceedings of the IEEE/WIC/ACM international conference on web intelligence, Washington, DC, USA. IEEE Computer Society, pp 275–278

11. Go A, Huang L, Bhayani R (2009) Twitter sentiment analysis. Final Projects from CS224N for Spring 2008/2009 at The Stanford Natural Language Processing Group

12. Katam S (2014) The Porter Stemmer. Indiana State University

13. De Choudhury M, Gamon M (2013) Predicting depression via social media. Microsoft Research, Redmond, WA, 98052

14. Hutto C, Gilbert E (2014) VADER: a parsimonious rule-based model for sentimentanalysis of social media text. In: Eighth international conference on weblogs and social media (ICWSM-14), Ann Arbor, MI

15. Gaurav D, Tiwari SM, Goyal A, Gandhi N, Abraham A (2019) Machine intelligence-based algorithms for spam filtering on document labelling. Soft Comput, 1–14

16. Rahul M, Kohli N, Agarwal R, Mishra S (2019) Facial expression recognition using geometric features and modified hidden Markov model. Int J Grid Util Comput 10(5):488–496

17. Cacheda F, Fernandez D, Novoa FJ, Carneiro V (2019) Early detection of depression: social network analysis and random forest techniques. J Med Internet Res 21(6):e12554

Alzheimer's Disease Diagnosis Using Structural MRI and Machine Learning Techniques

Samir Shrihari Yadav and Sanjay Raghunath Sutar

1 Introduction

Alzheimer's disease (AD) is the well-known neurodegenerative dementia in older adults, concerning 55% of all cases [1–3]. AD patients concert with premature inhibitors of cholinesterase [4, 5] and therefore be diagnosed with AD immediately and correctly. The initial symptoms of AD have been widely studied in recent years, approaching the idea of an amnestic mild cognitive impairment (MCI) [6, 7]. However, in the prospect of subsequent treatments, the urgent and accurate investigation of AD is not only demanding but also crucial. Clinical examination and neuropsychological assessment are two clinical diagnostic criteria with the diagnosis of dementia and after of the Alzheimer's phenotype [8]. Structural visualization is often used as part of neuropsychological studies to endorse AD diagnoses. Studies have shown that the medial temporal lobe(MTL) starts with neurodegeneration in AD, then passes entorhinal cortex, hippocampus, and limbic system, extending to the neocortical regions [9]. Therefore, there was considerable effort and research for discovering medial temporal lobe atrophy (MTA), particularly in entorhinal cortex and hippocampus and the amygdala [10]. MTA was measured using linear or volumetric measures, visual rating scales, and voxel based methods. In general, the specificity and sensitivity of hippocampus measures for classifying patients of AD from healthy old patients have been estimated to classify from 80 to 95% [11–15]. However, there are limitations to use evaluation of MTA for diagnosis of AD. MTA measurements in pre-dementia states like amnestic MCI are much less successful [11, 16–18]. Atrophy is not limited to the entorhinal cortex or the hippocampus in the initial stages of AD. In MCI patients as well as in AD patients other regions are affected [19]. Whole-brain methods to classify brain atrophy may therefore be

S. S. Yadav (✉) · S. R. Sutar
Dr. Babasaheb Ambedkar Technological University, Lonere, Raigad 402103, India
e-mail: ssyadav@dbatu.ac.in

© The Author(s), under exclusive license to Springer Nature Singapore Pte Ltd. 2021   645
M. K. Bajpai et al. (eds.), *Machine Vision and Augmented Intelligence—Theory and Applications*, Lecture Notes in Electrical Engineering 796,
https://doi.org/10.1007/978-981-16-5078-9_53

more effective in distinguishing AD and MCI patients from healthy patients that will emerge to AD. Researches suggest that volumetric measures of regions in the brain help to identify AD patients, classifying them from healthy elderly individuals [20]. When AD progresses, the ventricles, brain chambers containing cerebrospinal fluid, become progressively swollen, and the brain tissue begins shrinking. Patients in the final stages can lose the ability to identify others, feed themselves, communicate, and regulate body functions. Remembrance worsens and can almost become inexistent. By average, AD patients are treated for eight to ten years time, although this condition will continue for as long as twenty years.

The early identification and treatment of AD has been thoroughly studied over the last few years. Machine learning algorithms are very helpful in medical disease diagnosis [21–31]. In addition, progress in computational learning with the introduction of modern machine learning techniques which can handle high-dimensional data, including the support vector machine (SVM), has helped to build modern diagnostic methods focused on T1-weighted MRI to detect AD with high precision based on volumetric measurement of different brain regions [32].

The main objectives of this paper are:

1. Usage of a whole-brain MRI study for the individual assessment of ADpatients and the monitoring of stable elderly.
2. To compare different classifiers in AD diagnosis using the same study population.

For classification, we parcellate the patient's brain MRI into ROIs. And then focus only on a few different features like white matter (WM), gray matter (GM), and cerebrospinal fluid (CSF). Because these features make sense intuitively when dealing with neurodegenerative diseases like AD. The parcellation result is used to train the machine learning classifiers and then perform prediction on unseen data. The reminder of this paper is organized as: Sect. 2 gives methods and data used in this study. Section 3 discusses about the analysis of the data and experimental design. Subsequently results are discussed in Sect. 4. Finally conclusions are drawn in Sect. 5.

2 Materials and Methods

2.1 Dataset Exploration

In this study, we have used the Open Access Series of Imaging Studies (OASIS) database. The OASIS database consists of a series of MRI images. The first part of the database includes a cross-sectional collection of 416 patients aged between 18 and 96. Hundreds of those patients medically diagnosed with very mild to moderate AD are older than 60 years. The patients contain both men and women who are all right-handed. For each patient 3 or 4 individual T1-weighted MRI scans were obtained in

Table 1 Patient's level of dementia and Scores

Sr. No.	Dementia level	Score
1	Normal	0
2	Very mild	0.5
3	Mild	1
4	Moderate	2
5	Severe	3

single image sessions. Multiple in-session acquisitions provide a very high contrast-to-noise ratio, which allows the data to respond to a wide variety of analytical approaches, consisting of machine-controlled computational test. Dementia status is established using the clinical dementia rating (CDR) Scale. The CDR scale is a five-point scale used to distinguish six domains of functional and cognitive performance applicable to AD and similar dementias. The details required to include each ranking obtained by a semi-structured questionnaire and a collateral source (e.g., family member). Addition to this rating for each domain, an overall clinical dementia rating (CDR) score may be calculated through the use of an algorithm. This score is helpful in characterizing and recording the stage of impairment/dementia in a patient as seen in Table 1 In a single imaging session for each subject, three to four in dividual T1-weighted magnetization prepared rapid gradient-echo (MP-RAGE) images acquired on a 1.5-T Vision scanner (Siemens, Erlangen, Germany), which is shown in Fig. 1 for one random subject. Averaged motion-corrected images are then produced using the T1-weighted MP-RAGE images for each subject to improve the signal-to-noise ratio, which is shown in Fig. 2.

2.2 Data Preprocessing

To retrieve volumetric information of different parts of the brain, we have to perform several preprocessing stages, a few of which are mentioned below:

- Motion Correction and Conform
- Non-parametric Non-uniform intensity Normalization (N3)
- Talairach Transformation
- Normalization of Intensities
- Skull Strip
- EM Register (linear volumetric registration)
- CA Intensity Normalization
- CA Non-linear Volumetric Registration
- LTA with Skull
- Remove Neck

With the FreeSurfer image analysis package, which is recorded and freely available online for download, 31 preprocessing stages are performed on each

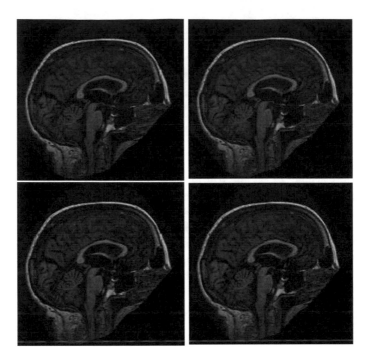

Fig. 1 The T1-weighted magnetization prepared rapid gradient-echo (MP-RAGE) images of one random subject

Fig. 2 Averaged motion-corrected image of a random subject acquired from images in Fig. 1

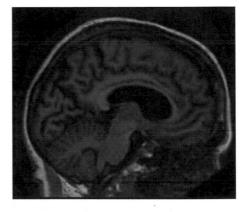

image (http://surfer.nmr.mgh.harvard.edu/) [33]. Details of each step are described in free-surfer documentation. The result of preprocessing is shown in Fig. 3 from a sagittal, coronal, and transverse view. The preprocessed images are visualized using FSL software, an extensive library of brain imaging data vi- sualization applications for FMRI, MRI, and DTI. Figure 3 shows how perfectly the skull is stripped, the neck is removed, etc.

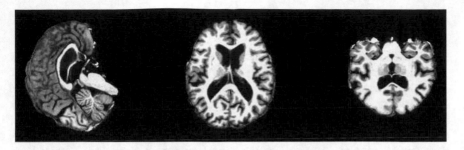

Fig. 3 Preprocessed image of the subject shown in Fig. 2 in sagittal, transverse, and coronal views (left to right)

Out of 416 subjects MRI images, 199 images successfully preprocessed. Other images failed because of the noise present in original image or poor quality of the image or CDR label is not known.

2.3 Feature Extraction

In the preprocessed images, the brain is parcellated into ROIs, and then the volume of different regions of the brain is extracted using the FreeSurfer tools. The features are obtained of brain segmentation and parcellation from both left and right hemisphere. 139 features related to the volume of different regions of interest are extracted in total, some of which are mentioned as follows:

1. Cerebrospinal fluid (CSF)
2. Left and right lateral ventricle
3. Left and right hippocampus
4. Left and right cerebellum white matter
5. left and right hemisphere cortex
6. left and right hemisphere surface holes
7. Estimated total intracranial (eTIV).

Finally, as the objective of the classification is to diagnose AD, the subjects with CDR greater than 0 are labeled as 1 (patient), and others (CDR = 0) are labeled as 0 (a control subject). Table 2 shows the outline of the OASIS dataset.

Table 2 OASIS dataset

Classes	2
Total samples	199
Samples per class	86(1), 113(0)
Dimensionality	139
Features	Real values

2.4 Visualization

The dataset is almost balanced, i.e., the number of samples of patients and controlled subjects is balanced. Figure 4 shows the dataset balance. The growing age is the most significant risk factor for Alzheimer's. Most individuals with the disease are 65 and older. This is shown in Fig. 5 as the distribution of age in the dataset for patients and controlled patients. As AD progresses, brain tissue shrinks. As an example, the brain mask volume and eTIV features extracted after preprocessing are shown in Figs. 6 and 7, respectively. From figures, it can be seen that patients are likely to have smaller eTIV and brain mask, which can be effectively used in the identification of AD. Cerebral white matter and cortex volume are plotted in Fig. 8. The figure shows that the two features tend to have smaller value in the patient compared to controlled subjects. It can be seen that patients and controlled subjects are relatively separable. In contrast, the ventricles, chambers within the brain that contain CSF, are noticeably enlarged in AD patients. This is shown in Fig. 9 by plotting the CSF volume versus age.

Plotting more important features in terms of how important they are in separating patients from control subjects, helps to achieve a better visualization. Therefore, we first calculate the features importance using random forest. The result is shown for the five most important features in Fig. 10.

A 3D visualization of three most important features namely Right-Amygdala, Left-Hippocampus, and Right-Inf-Lat-Vent is shown in Fig. 11. It can be clearly seen that the patient and controlled subjects have become more separable compared to the Figs. 8 and 9.

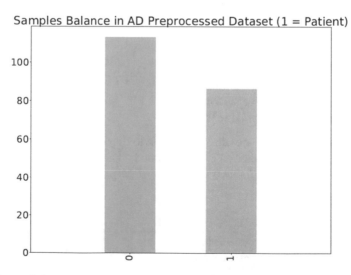

Fig. 4 Dataset balance

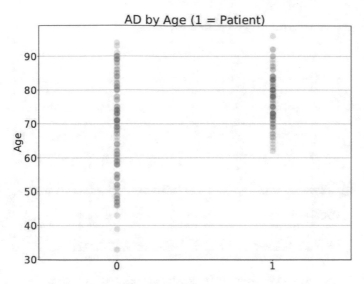

Fig. 5 Distribution of AD with age

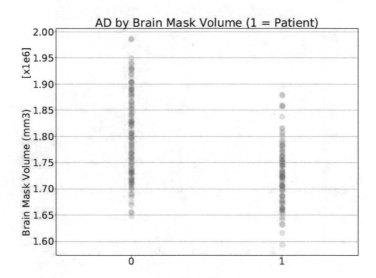

Fig. 6 Brain mask shrinkage in AD patients and controlled subjects

Therefore, classification by using all the 139 volumetric features extracted after preprocessing helps to achieve a high accuracy in AD identification.

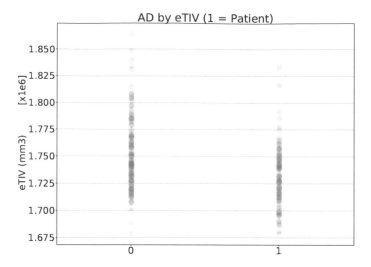

Fig. 7 eTIV shrinkage in AD patients and contorlled subjects

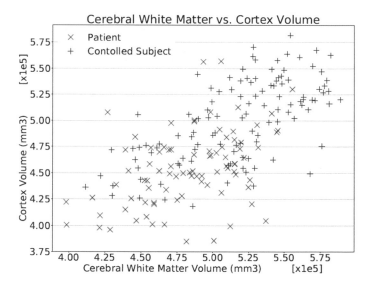

Fig. 8 Cerebral white matter volume versus cortex volume in AD patients and controlled subjects

3   Data Analysis

Data Analysis is done using the following supervised machine learning techniques:

– Logistic Regression: Logistic Regression is a statistical classification model to
determine the probabilities of the outcomes based on the occurrence of certain

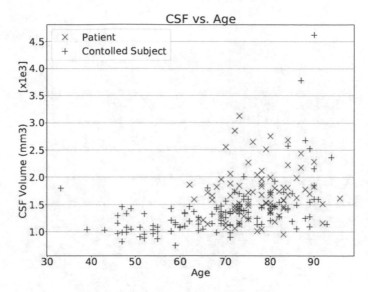

Fig. 9 CSF versus age in AD patients and controlled subjects

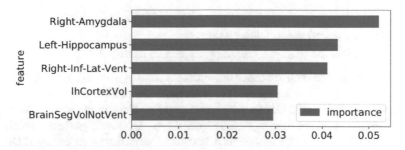

Fig. 10 Five most important features

features. The process of deriving this model is called training the model. This process finds weights for the features such that their linear combination can be used to determine the "most probable" outcome. However, linear models are unbounded and thus, they cannot be directly used to calculate the probabilities, which are bounded between 0 and 1. To achieve these bounds this process uses a squashing function which reduces the range of the linear function to be between 0 and 1.

To train this model a data set is used, which contains various observations of an experiment. Each observation of the experiment consists of the features and the outcome. For example, let us consider an observation of the data set for gender classification. Each observation of this data set consists of 800 features and their values for a person. It also contains a label to identify the person as male or female. This label acts as the outcome of the experiment.

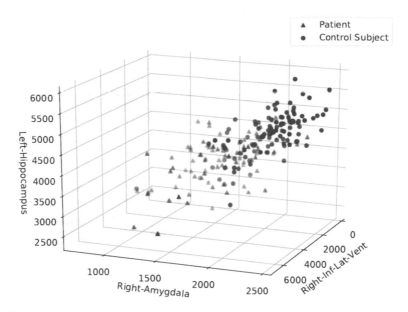

Fig. 11 Right-Amygdala, Left-Hippocampus, and Right-Inf-Lat-Vent 3D visualization

Why is it interesting and important?

Why is it hard? (E.g., why do naive approaches fail?)

The data can be used to deduce the optimal values of the weights for the features by solving a system of non-linear equations in 800 variables. However, achieving this by mathematical methods may be intractable. Thus, numerical methods like Gradient Descent are used to find optimal values. However, gradient descent for large data sets tend to be slow. This is because it has a time complexity of O(n2d) [3] where n is the number of observations and d is the number of dimensions. Thus, we use other numerical methods like Stochastic Gradient Descent (SGD) and L-BFGS which are less accurate but are faster.

Although, numerical methods make hard mathematical problems tractable, their convergence is dependent on a number of parameters. These parameters are called hyperparameters. Better hyperparameters can result in better results (global optima), faster convergence and less over-fitting (by using regularization). Unfortunately, trial and error is the only way to determine them. Determination of hyper parameter by trial and error is called grid search. To reduce the time taken to determine the best hyperparameters, we increase them in geometric progression.

What are the key components of my approach and results? Also include any specific limitations. In addition, this algorithm deals with the dilemma by using a logarithmic transformation on the outcome variable, which permits us to create a nonlinear association linearly. Therefore, logistic regression is chosen here to evaluate linear classifiers in the OASIS dataset classification task.

– Random Forests: Random Forests (rf) are ensembles of decision trees, proposed by Leo Breiman in the early 2000s [34] to ameliorate the instability of decision trees. In RF each tree is grown on a bootstrap sample from the training data, typically to its maximum depth. To increase robustness to noise and diversity among the trees, each node is split using the best split among a subset of features randomly chosen at that node. The number of features on which the trees are grown is one of the free parameters of the model. The final prediction is made by aggregating the prediction of M trees, either by a majority vote in the case of classification problems, or by averaging predictions in the case of regression problems. Another important free parameter of the model is the number of trees in the ensemble. RF is a bagging approach, which works on the assumption that the variance of individual decision trees can be reduced by averaging trees built on many uncorrelated subsamples. Moreover, increasing the number of trees in the ensemble, RF does not overfit the data. Therefore, this parameter is typically chosen to be as large as possible, consistently with the available hardware and computational time [34]. By contrast, boosted decision trees are made by building an iterative collection of decision trees, trained by giving more importance to training examples that were incorrectly classified by the previous trees.

RF can provide several measures of feature importance, computed by looking at the increase in prediction error when data for a feature is permuted while all other features remain unchanged. Feature selection based on RF if most often performed using one of these measures. However, several techniques for applying regularization to random forests have been proposed. These techniques broadly fall under two categories:

1. Cost-complexity pruning, which consists in limiting tree depth, resulting in less complex models;
2. Gini index penalization [35, 36].

In addition, [37] proposed to use a '1-norm to reduce the space-complexity of RF.

RF naturally handles numerical, ordinal and categorical variables, multiple scales and non-linearities. They also require little parameter tuning. This makes them popular for the analysis of diverse types of biological data, such as gene expression, Genome-wide Association Studies data or mass spectrometry [38]. In practice, feature selection schemes that rely on RF may be unstable [39], therefore feature selection stability measures must be adopted to avoid drawing inconsistent conclusions.

This algorithm performs feature selection implicitly as well as provides a pretty good indicator of feature importance. As the number of features is relatively high, using random forest can help us to try considering only essential features.

– Support Vector Machine (SVM): SVMs are broadly useful for problems in classification and regression, and they are part of a family of techniques known as margin methods. The defining goal of margin methods, and SVMs specifically, is to put as much distance as possible between data points and decision boundaries. We will dig deeper into what exactly this means over the course of the chapter.

One of the most appealing aspects of SVMs is that they decompose into convex optimization problems, for which we can find a global optimum with relative ease. We will explore the mathematical underpinnings of SVMs, which can be slightly more challenging than our previous topics, as well as their typical use cases. The theory behind SVMs has been around for quite some time (since 1963), and prior to the rise of neural networks and other more computationally intensive techniques, SVMs were used quite extensively for image recognition, object categorization, and other typical machine learning tasks. In particular, SVMs were and still are widely used for a subset of classification problems known as anomaly detection. The purpose of anomaly detection is to identify unusual data points. For example, if we are manufacturing widgets, we may wish to inspect and flag any widget that seems atypical with respect to the rest of the widgets we produce. Anomaly detection can be as simple as a binary classification problem where the data set is comprised of anomalous and non-anomalous data points.

As we will see, an SVM can be constructed from this data set to identify future anomalous points very efficiently. SVMs continue to be competitive in many real-world situations where we can define good features for our data. The kernel trick in SVM is to transform data, and then the optimal boundary within the possible outputs found based on these transformations. Naturally, some incredibly complex data transformations take place, and then figure out how to distinguish data on the basis of the labels or outputs specified. The benefit is that we can collect complex connections within data points without having to build complicated transformations of our own. The drawback is that the time of training is much longer as complexity is much more intensive.

3.1 Metrics

Evaluation of classifier is done by using either a graphical representation of performance, such as a receiver operating characteristic (ROC) curve or a numeric metric such as accuracy [40]. A straightforward choice to evaluate learning algorithms is the score, which is the percentage of patients correctly predicted, which is known simply as "accuracy." Other metrics, such as the area under the curve (AUC), recall, and precision, are also considered. It can be obtained from the confusion matrix and the ROC curve. A recall is an important metric as it can be more detrimental to predict a patient is not sick, If they are sick (False Negative), which results in a decision not to run further diagnostics and so to cause serious complications from not treating the illness. K-fold and leave-one-out cross-validation are two standard methods for measuring a model's performance on a dataset. In order to determine the accuracy of classification models, k-fold cross-validation should be used on a large volume of data as the accuracy of the classification model is usually too optimistic. The best example of cross-validation of k-fold is cross-validation leave-one-out. In this case of validation, the number of folds equals the number of instances. Nonetheless, in the case of a limited amount of data set or class value, e.g., gene sequence data, a

Table 3 System configurations	Dell PowerEdge T110 II Server	CPU : Intel Core2 Quad @ 2.6 GHz OS : Windows 7 Total Memory (RAM) : 8 GB No. of Cores: 4
	Dell Alienware X1	CPU: Intel Core i5 @ 2.8 GHz OS: Windows 10 Total Memory (RAM): 16 GB No. of Cores: 4

cross-validation can be used to achieve a fair approximation of the accuracy of the classification model. In this paper, since the number of instances is large enough, we have used k-fold cross-validation. After that, we applied significant statistical tests on the outcomes obtained from k-fold cross-validation. The following tests will be applied to compare different classifiers performance:

- Student's t-test (the simplest statistical test)
- Paired tests.

3.2 Software and Hardware Implementation

We manage the data files on the cluster and use two system for the designing of both our systems (Table 3).

3.3 Languages and Software Used

In this section we enumerate the software tools and languages used for the experiments.

1. Matlab (2016a, 2015b): To make the patches in both experiment • To max- pool the data in patch pooling and down-sampling the patches in (SCC)
2. C ++: To pool the learned dictionary • Sparse Coding, the code is taken from [41] and modified to fit our needs.
3. Python (2.7.12): For classification and file management
4. Shell: for scripting the above listed.
5. Software: SPM To preprocess the FDG-PET scans • InkScape for diagrams • Micron: for visualizing NiFTI files • MobaXterm/WinSCP/Putty: For accessing the cluster
6. Libraries: Python/2.7.12 (sklearn) for classifiers.

Visualization: Visualizations of graphs and data is done by using matplotlib library.

Features Importance Tree-based estimators can be used to calculate the sig- nificance of the feature, which can help to discard irrelevant features. Using feature

importance with forests of trees, we can draw the importance of features to see
if feature selection is necessary or not. The importance of features received from
Random Forest model is shown in Fig. 10.

4 Experimental Results

The three algorithms mentioned in Sect. 3 are implemented to classify titanic dataset.
The three algorithms are:

- Logistic regression
- Random Forests
- SVM classification

4.1 Hyperparameters Tuning

There are parameters for each classifier which have to be adjusted in order to have a
meaningful comparison. The hyperparameters that are adjusted here is as follows:

- Logistic Regression

    - Regularization Parameter

        [0.10, 0.01, 0.001, 0.0001, 0.00001]
    - Tolerance
        [0.1, 0.01, 0.001, 0.0001, 0.00001]

- Random Forests

    - Number of estimators

        5, 10, 15, 20, 25
    - Max depth
        [2, 3, 42–60]

- Support Vector Machine

    - C (l2 Regularization Coefficient)

        [0.1, 1, 10, 100, 1000]
    - Gamma (Free parameter of the Gaussian radial basis function)
        [10, 1, 0.1, 0.01, 0.001, 0.0001]
    - Kernel type
        [Linear, Poly, rbf]

The algorithms were run over 199 samples with 139 features. Cross-validation is applied internally and externally by $K = 10$ for externals and by $k = 5$ for internal (cross-validation tuning parameters).

The results for logistic regression, random forests, and SVM are shown in Tables 4, 5, and 6, respectively.

The metrics are as follows:

- Accuracy
- Confusion matrix

  - Recall
  - Precision

- AUC (Area Under ROC Curve)

Table 4 Logistic regression performance

Logit	Train accuracy	Test accuracy	TN	FP	FN	TP	AUC	Recall	Precision
K_0	0.8202	0.7143	10	2	4	5	0.6944	0.5556	0.7143
K_1	0.809	0.8571	11	1	2	7	0.8472	0.7778	0.875
K_2	0.809	0.5238	8	4	6	3	0.5	0.3333	0.4286
K_3	0.7989	0.85	11	0	3	6	0.8333	0.6667	1
K_4	0.7933	0.8	9	2	2	7	0.798	0.7778	0.7778
K_5	0.8045	0.9	10	1	1	8	0.899	0.8889	0.8889
K_6	0.7667	0.7895	11	0	4	4	0.75	0.5	1
K_7	0.8222	0.6842	8	3	3	5	0.6761	0.625	0.625
K_8	0.8278	0.5789	6	5	3	5	0.5852	0.625	0.5
K_9	0.7833	0.8421	10	1	2	6	0.8295	0.75	0.8571

Table 5 Random forests performance

Random forest	Train accuracy	Test accuracy	TN	FP	FN	TP	AUC	Recall	Precision
K_0	0.8652	0.5714	9	3	6	3	0.5417	0.3333	0.5
K_1	0.9101	0.8095	8	4	0	9	0.8333	1	0.6923
K_2	0.8933	0.7143	10	2	4	5	0.6944	0.5556	0.7143
K_3	0.8994	0.75	9	2	3	6	0.7424	0.6667	0.75
K_4	0.8827	1	11	0	0	9	1	1	1
K_5	0.8436	0.7	8	3	3	6	0.697	0.6667	0.6667
K_6	0.8722	0.7368	8	3	2	6	0.7386	0.75	0.6667
K_7	0.8722	0.7368	7	4	1	7	0.7557	0.875	0.6364
K_8	0.8833	0.7895	9	2	2	6	0.7841	0.75	0.75
K_9	0.8778	0.8421	10	1	2	6	0.8295	0.75	0.8571

Table 6 Support vector machine performance

SVM	Train accuracy	Test accuracy	TN	FP	FN	TP	AUC	Recall	Precision
K$_0$	0.8539	0.619	8	4	4	5	0.6111	0.5556	0.5556
K$_1$	0.8652	0.9048	11	1	1	8	0.9028	0.8889	0.8889
K$_2$	0.8764	0.6667	6	6	1	8	0.6944	0.8889	0.5714
K$_3$	0.8771	0.85	11	0	3	6	0.8333	0.6667	1
K$_4$	0.8603	0.7	7	4	2	7	0.7071	0.7778	0.6364
K$_5$	0.8547	0.65	7	4	3	6	0.6515	0.6667	0.6
K$_6$	0.8889	0.7368	10	1	4	4	0.7045	0.5	0.8
K$_7$	0.8389	0.9474	10	1	0	8	0.9545	1	0.8889
K$_8$	0.85	0.7368	9	2	3	5	0.7216	0.625	0.7143
K$_9$	0.8667	0.7368	9	2	3	5	0.7216	0.625	0.7143

In order to determine whether there is a substantial difference between the mean of the three methods, a variance analysis (ANOVA) evaluation was conducted for each of the metrics (accuracy, recall, precision, AUC). The null and alternate hypotheses are as follows:

- Null hypothesis: The true mean of all the three algorithms are the same.
- Alternate hypothesis: The true mean of the three algorithms is different.

4.2 ANOVA Test

ANOVA uses a statistical method to assess whether or not the outcomes of multiple groups are equal and thus generalizes the t-test to more than two groups. ANOVA is useful for checking for statistical significance by three or more methods (groups or variables). In order to ensure the associated p-value is valid, the ANOVA test has an essential assumption:

- The population standard deviations of the groups are all equal. This property is known as homoscedasticity.

For that reason, we have to first calculate the standard deviation of the three groups of accuracy. The results are shown in Table 7.

Table 7 Standard deviation on different criterion

std	Logit	RF	SVM
Test accuracy	0.1258	0.1105	0.1105
AUC	0.1268	0.1179	0.1104
Precision	0.1978	0.1336	0.1526
Recall	0.1609	0.2010	0.1626

Table 8 ANOVA test on different criterion

Test/Criterion	ANOVA
Test accuracy	0.9720
AUC	0.9679
Precision	0.9690
Recall	0.9785

As the standard deviation values are almost equal, we can perform ANOVA test. The results of ANOVA test is shown in Table 8.

The ANOVA test results demonstrate that the three classifiers are not significantly different and the null hypothesis can not be rejected. If the ANOVA test on any of the metrics was almost less than 0.1, we could go further and perform t-test to detect statistically different pairs of classifiers. Nevertheless, we have performed Welch t-test in the next section to further prove that the classifiers are not significantly different.

4.3 T-Test

For the means of two separate pairs of tests, i.e., the scores obtained for the algorithms, we calculate the T-test. The test checks whether the average (expected) value varies considerably between samples. If, for example, we find a significant p-value greater than 0.05 or 0.1, then we can not dismiss the null hypothesis of equal average scores. They dismiss the null hypothesis, that is, if the p-value is less than the threshold, e.g. 1%, 5% or 10%. When the data size and variances are unequal for groups, then Welch's t-test outperforms the Student's t-test. Both t-tests perform similarly when data size and variances are equals. We use Welch's t-test for this work. We also provide the results of and standard t-test. The results for both tests, Welch and standard t-test, are shown in Tables 9 and 10, respectively. The results show the fact that when the variances are almost equal, Welch's t-test and standard t-test give similar results. Considering the results of Welch's t-test, Table 9, we demonstrate that the null hypothesis cannot be rejected as the p-value is greater than 0.1 for any pair of algorithms and any metrics.

Table 9 Welch t-test

Standard	Test accuracy	AUC	Precision	Recall
Logit–SVM	0.987514558976	0.867896239608	0.711422776649	0.349726225454
RF–SVM	0.838589915295	0.825444904011	0.83410950904	0.85392449793
RF–Logit	0.837006408275	0.71377011516	0.573150893663	0.311849231929

Table 10 Standard t-test

Standard	Test accuracy	AUC	Precision	Recall
Logit–SVM	0.987517448177	0.867931453192	0.711703149617	0.349727624359
RF–SVM	0.83858991532	0.825455591706	0.834150603644	0.854014868845
RF–Logit	0.837045132973	0.713792872878	0.574128015242	0.312499517608

5 Conclusion

In this work, different classifiers models that can diagnose patients with an early AD and control subjects based on the volumetric measurements of MRI images are developed and evaluated. Our results indicate that machine learning techniques can aid the clinical diagnosis of AD. The results confirm that the volumetric measurements of different regions of the brain can be effectively used in AD identification and provide a potential for early diagnosis of Alzheimer's disease. The experimental results also show that the original hypothesis that done on one of the algorithms chosen would not perform better than the other. In terms of the metrics chosen for comparison, the three algorithms performed similarly. However, it should be noted that the run time of SVM is significantly higher than the other two, which is a benefit for logistic regression and random forests. The data preprocessing part also plays an essential role in the quality of final results and accuracy. It may also affect the final results of classifier differently and therefore, should be taken into account. As a result, Further work on preprocessing data can be considered as an essential step in future work.

For future work, collecting more data of both controlled subjects and patients can help to achieve higher accuracy. Combining OASIS with Alzheimer's Disease Neuroimaging Initiative (ADNI) dataset, which is another famous dataset in Alzheimer's disease, might help. Nevertheless, we should be aware of different scanning procedures and scaling as well as applying the same preprocessing and feature extraction on both datasets. Applying outliers detection can also be helpful, thereby detecting wrong labeled data to remove them from the training set and finally, diagnosis accuracy improvement. It is also beneficial to consider the CDR label as the output class. Moreover, evaluate the methods incorrectly, which differentiates between different forms of dementia, which is more challenging than only AD diagnosis.

References

1. Brookmeyer R, Gray S, Kawas C (1998) Projections of Alzheimer's disease in the united states and the public health impact of delaying disease onset. Am J Public Health 88(9):1337–1342
2. Ferri CP, Prince M, Brayne C, Brodaty H, Fratiglioni L, Ganguli M, Hall K, Hasegawa K, Hendrie H, Huang Y et al (2006) Global prevalence of dementia: a delphi consensus study. Lancet 366(9503):2112–2117

3. Ramaroson H, Helmer C, Barberger-Gateau P, Letenneur L, Dartigues J (2003) Prevalence of dementia and Alzheimer's disease among subjects aged 75 years or over: updated results of the Paquid cohort. Revue neurologique, vol. 159, no. 4, pp. 405–411, 2003

4. Winblad B, Wimo A (1999) Assessing the societal impact of acetylcholinesterase inhibitor therapies. Alzheimer Disease & Associated Disorders, vol 13, pp S9–S19

5. DeKosky ST, Marek K (2003) Looking backward to move forward: early detection of neurodegenerative disorders. Science 302(5646):830–834

6. Petersen RC (2004) Mild cognitive impairment as a diagnostic entity. J Intern Med 256(3):183–194

7. Winblad B, Palmer K, Kivipelto M, Jelic V, Fratiglioni L, Wahlund L-O, Nordberg A, Backman L, Albert M, Almkvist O et al (2004) Mild cognitive impairment–beyond controversies, towards a consensus: report of the international working group on mild cognitive impairment. J Intern Med 256(3):240–246

8. Glodzik L, Mosconi L, Tsui W, de Santi S, Zinkowski R, Pirraglia E, Rich KE, McHugh P, Li Y, Williams S et al (2012) Alzheimer's disease markers, hypertension, and gray matter damage in normal elderly. Neurobiol Aging 33(7):1215–1227

9. Braak H, Braak E (1995) Staging of Alzheimer's disease-related neurofibrillary changes. Neurobiol Aging 16(3):271–278

10. Leite AJB, Scheltens P, Barkhof F (2004) Pathological aging of the brain: an overview. Top Magn. Reson Imaging 15(6):369–389

11. Xu Y, Jack C, O'brien P, Kokmen E, Smith GE, Ivnik RJ, Boeve BF, Tangalos R, Petersen RC (2000) Usefulness of mri measures of entorhinal cortex versus hippocampus in ad. Neurology 54(9):1760–1767

12. Frisoni G, Laakso M, Beltramello A, Geroldi C, Bianchetti A, Soininen H, Trabucchi M (1999) Hippocampal and entorhinal cortex atrophy in frontotemporal dementia and Alzheimer's disease. Neurology 52(1):91–91

13. Laakso M, Soininen H, Partanen K, Lehtovirta M, Hallikainen M, Hanninen T, Helkala E-L, Vainio P, Riekkinen P (1998) Mri of the hippocampus in Alzheimer's disease: sensitivity, specificity, and analysis of the incorrectly classified subjects. Neurobiol Aging 19(1):23–31

14. Lehericy S, Baulac M, Chiras J, Pierot L, Martin N, Pillon B, Deweer B, Dubois B, Marsault C (1994) Amygdalohippocampal mr volume measurements in the early stages of Alzheimer disease. Am J Neuroradiol 15(5):929–937

15. Jack CR, Petersen RC, O'brien PC, Tangalos EG (1992) Mr-based hippocampal volumetry in the diagnosis of Alzheimer's disease. Neurology 42(1):183–183

16. Pennanen C, Kivipelto M, Tuomainen S, Hartikainen P, Hanninen T, Laakso MP, Hallikainen M, Vanhanen M, Nissinen A, Helkala E-L et al (2004) Hippocampus and entorhinal cortex in mild cognitive impairment and early ad. Neurobiol Aging 25(3):303–310

17. De Santi S, de Leon MJ, Rusinek H, Convit A, Tarshish CY, Roche A, Tsui WH, Kandil E, Boppana M, Daisley K et al (2001) Hippocampal formation glucose metabolism and volume losses in mci and ad. Neurobiol Aging 22(4):529–539

18. Convit A, De Leon M, Tarshish C, De Santi S, Tsui W, Rusinek H, George A (1997) Specific hippocampal volume reductions in individuals at risk for Alzheimer's disease. Neurobiol Aging 18(2):131–138

19. A"el Chetelat G, Baron J-C (2003) Early diagnosis of Alzheimer's disease: contribution of structural neuroimaging. Neuroimage 18(2):525–541

20. Bottino CM, Castro CC, Gomes RL, Buchpiguel CA, Marchetti RL, Neto MRL (2002) Volumetric mri measurements can differentiate Alzheimer's disease, mild cognitive impairment, and normal aging. Int Psychogeriatr 14(1):59–72

21. Yadav SS, Jadhav SM (2019) Deep convolutional neural network based medical image classification for disease diagnosis. J Big Data 6(1):113

22. Kadam VJ, Yadav SS, Jadhav SM (2018) Soft-margin svm incorporating feature selection using improved elitist ga for arrhythmia classification. In: International conference on intelligent systems design and applications, Springer, pp 965–976

23. Yadav SS, Jadhav SM (2019) Machine learning algorithms for disease prediction using iot environment. Int J Eng Adv Technol 8(6):4303–4307
24. Kadam V, Jadhav S, Yadav S (2020) Bagging based ensemble of support vector machines with improved elitist ga-svm features selection for cardiac arrhythmia classification. Int J Hybrid Intell Syst 16(1):25–33
25. Yadav SS, Kadam VJ, Jadhav SM (2019) Comparative analysis of ensemble classifier and single base classifier in medical disease diagnosis. In: International conference on communication and intelligent systems, Springer, pp 475–489
26. Yadav SS, Jadhav SM, Bonde RG, Chaudhari ST (2020) Automated cardiac disease diagnosis using support vector machine. In: 2020 3rd International conference on communication system, computing and IT applications (CSCITA), IEEE, pp 56–61
27. Yadav SS, Jadhav SM, Nagrale S, Patil N (2020) Application of machine learning for the detection of heart disease. In: 2020 2nd International conference on innovative mechanisms for industry applications (ICIMIA), IEEE, pp 165–172
28. Yadav SS, Jadhav SM (2020) Detection of common risk factors for diagnosis of cardiac arrhythmia using machine learning algorithm. In: Expert systems with applications, p 113807
29. Semwal VB, Mondal K, Nandi GC (2017) Robust and accurate feature selection for humanoid push recovery and classification: deep learning approach. Neural Comput Appl 28(3):565–574. (Springer, 2017)
30. Semwal VB, Singha J, Sharma PK, Chauhan A, Behera B (2017) An optimized feature selection technique based on incremental feature analysis for bio-metric gait data classification. Multimed Tools Appl 76(22):24457–24475. (Springer, 2017)
31. Semwal VB, Gaud N, Nandi GC (2019) Human gait state prediction using cellular automata and classification using ELM. Mach Intell Signal Anal 135–145. (Springer, 2019)
32. Cuingnet R, Gerardin E, Tessieras J, Auzias G, Leh'ericy S, Habert M-O, Chupin M, Benali H, Colliot O, Initiative ADN et al (2011) Automatic classification of patients with Alzheimer's disease from structural mri: a comparison of ten methods using the adni database. Neuroimage 56(2):766–781
33. Baumgartner T, Saulin A, Hein G, Knoch D (2016) Structural differences in insular cortex reflect vicarious injustice sensitivity. PloS one 11(12): e0167538
34. Breiman L (2001) Random Fofests. In: Machine learning, vol 45, pp 5–32. (Oct 2001)
35. Deng H, Runger G (2013) Gene selection with guided regularized random forest. Pattern Recogn 46:3483–3489. (Dec 2013)
36. Liu S, Dissanayake S, Patel S, Dang X, Mlsna T, Chen Y, Wilkins D (2014) Learning accurate and interpretable models based on regularized random forests regression. BMC Syst Biol 8(3):S5
37. Joly A, Schnitzler F, Geurts P, Wehenkel L (2012) L1-based compression of random forest models. In: 20th European symposium on artificial neural networks, 2012
38. Qi Y (2012) Random forest for bioinformatics. In: Ensemble machine learning, Springer, pp 307–323
39. Kursa MB (2014) Robustness of Random Forest-based gene selection methods. BMC Bioinf 15:8
40. Lever J, Krzywinski M, Altman N (2016) Points of significance: classification evaluation
41. Lin B, Li Q, Sun Q, Lai M-J, Davidson I, Fan W, Ye J (2014) Stochastic coordinate coding and its application for drosophila gene expression pattern annotation. arXiv:1407.8147
42. Burns D-A, Iliffe S (2009) Enfermedad de Alzheimer, pp 338, b158
43. Weiner MW, Veitch DP, Aisen PS, Beckett LA, Cairns NJ, Green RC, Harvey D, Jack CR, Jagust W, Liu E et al (2013) The Alzheimer's disease neuroimaging initiative: a review of papers published since its inception. Alzheimer's & Dement. 9(5):e111–e194
44. Langbaum JB, Fleisher AS, Chen K, Ayutyanont N, Lopera F, Quiroz YT, Caselli RJ, Tariot PN, Reiman EM ()2013 Ushering in the study and treatment of preclinical Alzheimer disease. Nat Rev Neurol 9(7):371–381
45. Kakimoto A, Kamekawa Y, Ito S, Yoshikawa E, Okada H, Nishizawa S, Minoshima S, Ouchi Y (2011) New computer-aided diagnosis of dementia using positron emission tomography: brain regional sensitivity-mapping method. PloS one 6(9):e25033

46. Lu S, Xia Y, Cai W, Fulham M, Feng DD, Initiative ADN et al (2017) Early identification of mild cognitive impairment using incomplete random forest-robust support vector machine and fdg-pet imaging. Comput Med Imaging Graph
47. Liu H, Motoda H (2007) Computational methods of feature selection. CRC Press
48. Friedman J, Hastie T, Tibshirani R (2001) The elements of statistical learning, vol 1. Springer series in statistics. Springer, Berlin
49. Jain A, Zongker D (1997) Feature selection: evaluation, application, and small sample performance. IEEE Trans Pattern Anal Mach Intell 19(2):153–158
50. Tang J, Alelyani S, Liu H (2014) Feature selection for classification: a review. In: Data classification: algorithms and applications, p 37
51. Guyon I, Gunn S, Nikravesh M, Zadeh LA (2008) Feature extraction: foundations and applications, vol 207. Springer
52. Jolliffe I (2002) Principal component analysis. Wiley Online Library
53. Mika S, Ratsch G, Weston G, Scholkopf B, Mullers K-R (1999) Fisher discriminant analysis with kernels. In: Neural networks for signal processing IX, 1999. Proceedings of the 1999 IEEE signal processing society workshop. IEEE, pp 41–48
54. Masaeli M, Dy JG, Fung GM (2010) From transformation-based dimensionality reduction to feature selection. In: Proceedings of the 27th International Conference on Machine Learning (ICML-10), pp 751–758
55. Schnass K, Vandergheynst P (2008) Dictionary learning based dimensionality reduction for classification. In: 3rd international symposium on communications, control and signal processing, 2008. ISCCSP 2008. IEEE, pp 780–785
56. Mairal J, Bach F, Ponce J, Sapiro G (2009) Online dictionary learning for sparse coding. In: Proceedings of the 26th annual international conference on machine learning. ACM, pp 689–696
57. Yin W, Osher S, Goldfarb D, Darbon J (2008) Bregman iterative algorithms for l_1-minimization with applications to compressed sensing. SIAM J Imaging Sci 1(1):143–168
58. Lv J, Jiang X, Li X, Zhu D, Zhang S, Zhao S, Chen H, Zhang T, Hu X, Han J et al (2015) Holistic atlases of functional networks and interactions reveal reciprocal organizational architecture of cortical function. IEEE Trans Biomed Eng 62(4):1120–1131
59. Lv J, Lin B, Zhang W, Jiang X, Hu X, Han J, Guo L, Ye J, Liu T (2015) Modeling task fmri data via supervised stochastic coordinate coding. In: International conference on medical image computing and computer-assisted intervention, Springer, pp. 239–246
60. Moody DI, Brumby SP, Rowland JC, Gangodagamage C (2012) Unsupervised land cover classification in multispectral imagery with sparse representations on learned dictionaries. In: Applied imagery pattern recognition workshop (AIPR), 2012 IEEE, pp 1–10

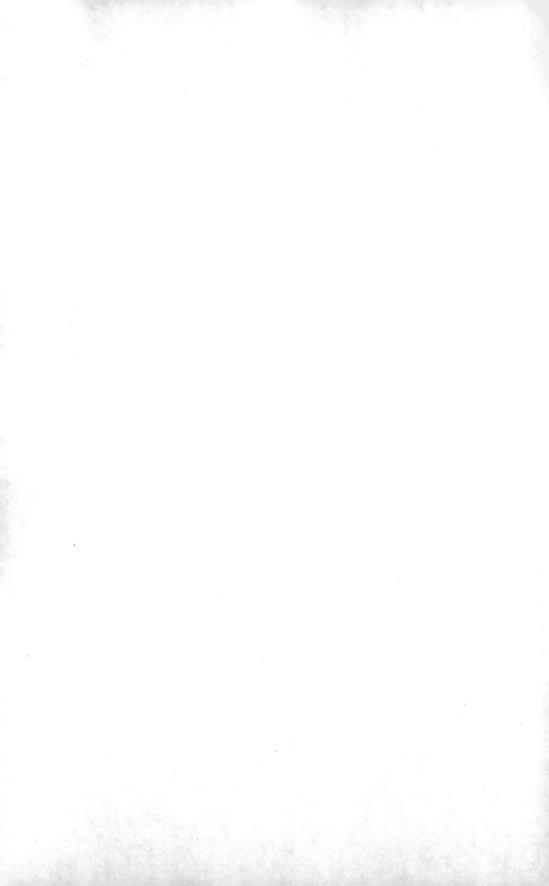

Supervised Machine Learning-Based DDoS Defense System for Software-Defined Network

Gufran Siddiqui and Sandeep K. Shukla

1 Introduction

Distributed Denial of Service (DDoS) is a cyber-attack in which an adversary controls a large number of machines (botnets) to make network resource(s) or machine unavailable for the intended users. Recently, multinational organizations like Amazon, Github, etc., were struck with DDoS attacks and suffered monetary and reputation damages. With the extensive growth in the number of vulnerable network devices and readily available attack tools, the volume, size, and complexity of DDoS attacks are likely to increase in the future. SDN in contrast to the traditional network separates the control plane from the data plane allowing fine-grained centralized control of networking devices. This network architecture allows innovations and programmability in computer networks. The important components of SDN infrastructure are as follows: the control plane, data plane, and control channel [1]. The control and data planes communicate through protocols such as Openflow [2].

Routing in Openflow enabled switches is performed based on the match action paradigm, where the processed packet's header is matched against the rules in the flow table. If there exists a match then the defined rule's action(s) (e.g., drop, forward to an out port, etc.) is performed on that packet. Routing in SDN is mainly categorized into proactive or reactive routing.

In reactive routing, a switch processes packets based on a flow table, if there exists a set of rule in switch table that matches the processed packet's headers, switch select the highest priority rule to forward the packet, Otherwise switch triggers a table-miss. Upon a table miss the switch will encapsulate the packet header with metadata such as

G. Siddiqui (✉) · S. K. Shukla
Indian Institute of Technology Kanpur, Kanpur, India
e-mail: Gufran@cse.iitk.ac.in

S. K. Shukla
e-mail: sandeeps@cse.iitk.ac.in

© The Author(s), under exclusive license to Springer Nature Singapore Pte Ltd. 2021   667
M. K. Bajpai et al. (eds.), *Machine Vision and Augmented Intelligence—Theory and Applications*, Lecture Notes in Electrical Engineering 796,
https://doi.org/10.1007/978-981-16-5078-9_54

ingress port, etc., into a control packet named $packet_{in}$ and forward it to the controller using a secure control channel. Whereas in proactive routing, all the possible sets of network flow rules are pre-installed in switches before the network communication begins and a table miss results in the dropping of the packet in the data plane.

After receiving the message, the controller computes a new rule using the global routing information of the network devices it has. It then encapsulates the rule into a control packet named $flow_{mod}$ and forwards it to the Openflow switches resulting in the installation of a new rule or if the controller finds the destination address to be broadcast or unknown, then the controller will send a $packet_{out}$ message to switches. Upon receiving $packet_{out}$, a switch will simply flood the packet in the network.

This reactive routing scheme allows SDN to rapidly adapt with changing network topologies, however, it also introduces new vulnerabilities at different layers of the SDN infrastructure where an adversary could use multiple bots to craft packets in such a way that doesn't match with any existing entries in flow tables resulting in overwhelming the controller with massive events causing saturation at the controller end. The table miss events will implicitly result in the exchanges of messages in between a controller and switch, therefore degrading the control channel bandwidth. The messages will results in the installation of a new rule, therefore occupying flow table space until the flow timeout is expired causing saturation at the data plane level. Also, these malicious packets may cause the replacement of an active benign connection(s) due to the limited size of the flow table (e.g., CISCO Openflow switches supports 2 K flows), thus degrading the network performance (e.g., increased delay can minimize the throughput of a flow) of the legitimate connection(s). The impact of these saturation attacks is thus cascading and could degrade the network performance or even worse, bring down the whole network.

Our main contributions are (i) Design a system to detect the saturation attacks (ii) Design a module that models the system's false positive rate to minimize the effect of the system's response towards benign traffic. (iii) Evaluate the system's performance using benchmark data sets provided by the Canadian Institute for Cybersecurity against standard performance metrics.

We organized the rest of the paper as follows: we review the previous work related to the DDoS attack defense framework in SDN in Sect. 2. We discuss the design of our proposed system in Sect. 3. Section 4 describes the implementation and evaluation details of our proposed system. We discuss the experimental results in Sect. 5. Finally, Sect. 6 concludes the paper with potential future work.

2 Related Works

In this section, we discussed a few machine learning-based DDoS defense and mitigation systems in SDN environment briefly [1, 3–5].

2.1 Machine Learning-Based Mechanism

Quamar et al. [6] implemented a Stacked Auto Encoder-based DDoS detection system. Their DDoS detection system consists of the following modules such as Traffic Collector and Flow installer (TCFI), Feature Extractor (FE), and Traffic Classifier (TC). TCFI module is triggered using a timer function every 60 s. TCFI module extracts the various header fields of packets that arrive at the controller either because of an installed rule or due to a table miss.

The FE module extracts a list of features from the packets list populated by the TCFI module. The FE module triggers the TC module which uses the Stack Auto Encoder to classify the traffic feature into normal and attack class. Their system offers a detection accuracy of 99.82% for binary classification, whereas for multiclass classification the system's accuracy is about 95.65% with a false positive rate lower than 5%. However, their proposed system suffers from processing capabilities as every packet traversing the network reaches the controller, secondly, the detection module triggers periodically at 60 s which will hinder the system from early detection, and mitigation of an attack.

Hu et al. [7] designed a light weighted DDOS detection system (ADM) composing of detection and mitigation modules. The system collects the flow stats information at the controller end using S-Flow or Controller-based method depending on the network environment such as Small Office/Home Office (SOHO) (where normal background traffic rate is a low) or large enterprise network (where normal background traffic rate is high). It then uses an entropy-based method for evaluating the traffic feature vector. Finally, the Support Vector Machine (SVM) classifies the traffic vector into normal or attack. Their experimental result shows that when the background traffic is set to 10 Mbps and the attacker flooding rate is set to 400 packets per second (PPS), the proposed system offers a 60 and < 60% attack detection rate with a control-based and s-flow-based method, respectively. However, when the attack rate is >= 850 PPS, the attack detection rate is found to be 100%.

In [8], a framework named ATLANTIC is designed to detect DDoS-based attacks. The framework composes of two steps to detect DDOS attacks, in the first step, entropy-based analysis is used to detect the variation in traffic feature(s) observed along with consecutive traffic snapshots. In the second step, the Support Vector Machine (SVM) classifier or k means clustering is used to classify the traffic flows into malicious or benign. The proposed framework obtained an accuracy of 88.7 with 82.3% precision using the SVM classifier.

Ye et al. [9] proposed a framework consisting of modules such as flow status collection, features extraction, and classification for TCP, UDP, and ICMP-based DDoS attacks detection. The framework uses the SVM for classification and offers a detection accuracy of 95.24% with a false positive rate of 1.26%.

In [10], a defense system is proposed named Floodlight Gaurd (FL-Gaurd). FL-Gaurd first prevents IP spoofing by monitoring the DHCP response/release message between the secure DHCP server and the client. Secondly, it uses the C-SVM classifier for detecting attacks. The proposed system offered an accuracy of 96.55%.

Chen et al. [11] proposed a defense system that collects packets at the controller end using the Tcpdump. It then uses the Extreme Gradient Boosting (XGBoost) method for DDoS detection from the collected packets. The proposed method shows high accuracy of 98.53% and a low false rate of 0.8%.

In [12], Mousavi et al. proposed a system that calculates the entropy of the extracted features from the traffic flows. For certain features, its entropy values are checked against the predefined threshold value to detect attacks. Threshold value selected after performing several experiments. Their approach is lightweight and offers high accuracy. However, may not be reliable as the threshold value may vary from scenario to scenario.

In contrast to the previous works, we propose a system that detects attacks with high accuracy and a low false-positive rate. We use a set of 30 features extracted from flow tables and $packet_{in}$ events to classify the traffic flows into normal or attack. We also model the system's false positive rate to minimize the interruption of the normal connection(s) by the system's response module without making the whole system's process cumbersome.

3   System Design

In this section, we discuss the overall architecture of our proposed system with a detailed description of its modules.

3.1   System Architecture

Our designed framework is composed of five modules that are as follows: traffic collector, feature extractor, traffic classifier, traffic state, and response as depicted in Fig. 1. We implemented these modules on top of the python-based POX controller.

Traffic Collector. The Traffic Collector module's task is to collect the traffic information at the controller end. Firstly, this module uses a timer function to periodically (e.g. T = 5 s) pull the existing flow table stats from the switches using the stats request and stats reply messages. Secondly, this module collects the information related to the number of events that occurred during an interval T.

The traffic collector module then groups the flow entries based on the source IP address and Ingress port. This module passes grouped flows to the feature extractor module. A network administrator can choose a lower time interval which will frequently trigger this module increasing the control-data plane communication and CPU cycle of the controller. Hence, an optimal value must be chosen depending on the load on the controller and the available bandwidth of the control-data channel.

Feature Extractor. For each group of flows obtained from the traffic collector module, this module extracts the features mentioned in Tables 1, 2, and 3 forming a feature vector of dimension 30×1.

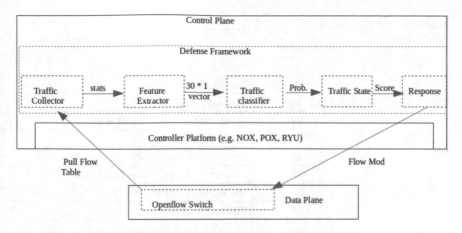

Fig. 1 System architecture

Table 1 Feature description of TCP flows

#	Feature description
1	Mean of flow duration
2	Standard deviation of flow duration
3	Median of flow duration
4	Mean of packet count
5	Standard deviation of packet count
6	Median of packet count
7	Mean of flow byte count
8	Standard deviation of flow byte count
9	Median of flow byte count
10	Distinct # source port
11	Distinct # destination port
12	Arrival rate of SYN packets
13	Arrival rate of ACK packets
14	Fraction of symmetric flow over total flows
15	Mean packet length

To increase the detection accuracy of the system, we normalized the traffic features using the min–max normalization with range [0, 1].

$$x_{norm}^{kth} = \frac{\left(x^{kth} - x_{min}^{kth}\right)}{\left(x_{max}^{kth} - x_{min}^{kth}\right)}$$

x_{norm}^{kth} = Normalize value for the kth feature

Table 2 Feature description of UDP flows

#	Feature description
16	Mean of flow duration
17	Standard deviation of flow duration
18	Median of flow duration
19	Mean of packet count
20	Standard deviation of packet count
21	Median of packet count
22	Mean of flow byte count
23	Standard deviation of flow byte count
24	Median of flow byte count
25	Distinct # source port
26	Distinct # destination port
27	Fraction of symmetric flow over total flows
28	Mean packet length

Table 3 Other feature descriptions

#	Feature description
29	Fraction of *packet_in* event for a host over total *packet_in* events happened in T interval
30	Inter arrival rate of flows

$$x_{\min}^{kth} = \text{Smallest value in } kth \text{ feature}$$

$$x_{\max}^{kth} = \text{Largest value in } kth \text{ feature}$$

Traffic Classifier. The normalized feature vector provides input to this module that consists of a simple classifier or a deep learning model. It output the probability (or confidence that a feature vector belongs to a particular class) and the class itself (e.g. in the case of binary classification, the class is either normal or attack).

Traffic State. Based on the output of the traffic classifier module, we could adopt a zero-tolerance response to the threat that is to prevent the host from occupying any network resources. However, the classifier module doesn't yield zero false-positive rates which could lead to the interruption of normal connections. One approach is to manually examine the threat by the network administrator which is tedious. To handle this issue, we implemented this module that maintains a score for every host within the network dynamically depending on the classifier module output, if a traffic feature vector for a given host a belongs to normal then its score is updated at an instant i in a linear fashion as per Eq. (1), otherwise the score is decreased by a factor of β as per Eq. (2)

$$S_a^i = (1 - \alpha) * S_a^{i-1} + prob * \alpha \tag{1}$$

$$S_a^i = \frac{S_a^{i-1}}{\beta^{prob}} \tag{2}$$

where, $\alpha \varepsilon [0, 1]$, $\beta > 1$, $prob$ is the traffic class probability return by the supervised classifier, and $threshold \varepsilon [0, 1]$.

Response. If the score of a host is found lower than a $threshold$, then this module installs a blocking rule of highest priority in Openflow switches matching the attacker IP and ingress port and also eliminates any existing rules that belong to the attacker's network location (i.e., Source IP and Ingress port), protecting the SDN infrastructure from the DDoS attacks.

4 Implementation and Evaluation

The implementation of the designed framework meets the OpenFlow policy. The implemented system is deployed on pox controller without making any hardware changes making it easily deployable.

4.1 Experimental Setup

We considered a simple tree topology consisting of 7 Openflow switches, 3 normal host, and 1 attacker host, as shown in Fig. 2. We emulate the network on Mininet and uses POX as a centralized controller. The hardware setting for running Mininet (OVSSwitch) [13] and POX controller [14] in Intel(R) Core (TM)-i5 -8300 CPU (2.30 GHz) with 3 GB RAM and set all links bandwidth to 1 Gbps, queuing delay to 10 ms, the maximum size of flow table to 2000 and switches are configured with least recently used (LRU) policy to replace an existing entry with a new rule [2] when the flow table is full.

4.2 Dataset

In this work, we use CICIDS2017 [15], and CICDDOS2019 [16] benchmark datasets containing benign and the new common attacks (e.g., UDP lag) to evaluate the performance of our system. However, in this work, we focus on DDoS attack traces based on TCP and UDP protocol only (note that the dataset CICDDOS2019 doesn't have ICMP protocol-based attack). We use the benign trace of CICIDS2017 and

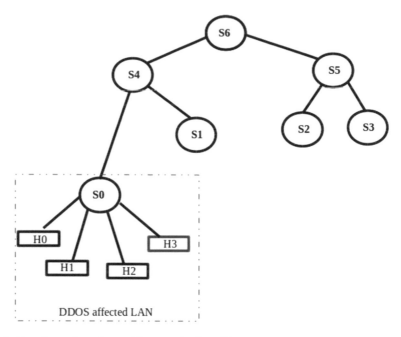

Fig. 2 Experimental topology with an attacker host H3

attack trace of the CICIDS2019 dataset for training and testing of various classifiers and Deep learning models.

We processed the datasets to obtain normal and attack traces containing TCP or UDP or TCP-UDP both protocols-based packets. We used tcpreplay [17] to replay the normal and attack traces of the same kind (e.g., TCP or UDP or TCP-UDP) at a rate of 100, 200, and 400 PPS, one at a time for about 2 h. The obtained records after processing datasets are shown in Table 4.

Table 4 #Records in the training and testing of models

	Protocol	Normal records	Attack records
Training	TCP	4313	4232
	UDP	193	3707
	TCP-UDP	3587	5298
Testing	TCP	4123	4231
	UDP	598	3707
	TCP-UDP	2472	5297

4.3 Supervised Machine Learning Classifier

In this section, we discuss a range of classifiers and deep learning (DL) models, their implementation, along with the optimal value of hyper-parameters used to train them, as shown in Table 5.

Gaussian Naive Bayes. Gaussian Naive Bayes is a variant of Naive Bayes classification with an assumption that the likelihood of the feature to be Gaussian distribution that is:

$$P(x_i|y) = \frac{1}{\sqrt{2\pi\sigma_y^2}}\exp\left(-\frac{(x_i - \mu_y)^2}{2\sigma_y^2}\right)$$

where the parameter μ_y and σ_y are estimated using the maximum likelihood, $x_i \in R^d$, and $y \in \{0,1\}$.

Decision Tree. Decision Trees is a supervised learning method where decision rules are learned from the data features. The test data is then classified using these learned decision rules taken at each node starting from the root, where a leaf node represents the predicted class label for a test data instance. However, this can lead to the over-fitting issue.

Random Forest. Random Forest is an ensemble learning classifier that is obtained by leaning several different decision tree classifiers on a training dataset. For testing data instance, it output the class that is the mode of the classes. This approach increases the prediction accuracy by controlling the over-fitting issue of the decision tree.

Adaboost. AdaBoost is a boosting ensemble model consisting of weak classifiers where the first classifier fits the original dataset with equal weights assigned to all data instances.

During each iteration, incorrectly classified instances' weights are adjusted so that the subsequent classifier fits the same dataset while focusing more on these incorrectly classified data instances. The final classifier thus combines each learned weak classifier prediction in the weighted form to output the final predicted class label of a data instance. In the implementation of the Adaboost classifier, the decision tree is taken as the weak classifier.

Category	Classifier	Library
Simple classifier	Gaussian Naïve Bayes (GNB)	Scikit learn
	Decision tree (DT)	
	Random forest (RF)	
	Adaboost (ADA)	
Deep learning model	LSTM	Tensorflow
	GRU	

Table 5 Implemented supervised ML classifiers

LSTM. Long short-term memory (LSTM) that having feedback connections can learn complex structures/patterns in the datasets. LSTM [18] is composed of three gates in each cell which are as follows: input, output gate and forget, these are calculated as follows:

$$i_t = \sigma\left(W_i.[h_{t-1}, x_t] + b_i\right), \; c_t^- = \tanh\left(W_c.[h_{t-1}, x_t] + b_c\right)$$

$$f_t = \sigma\left(W_f.[h_{t-1}, x_t] + b_f\right), c_t = f_t.c_{t-1} + i_t.c_t^-$$

$$o_t = \sigma\left(W_o.[h_{t-1}, x_t] + b_o\right), h_t = o_t.\tanh(c_t)$$

where x_t is the input at time t, W_i, Wc, and W_f are the weight matrices, b_i, b_c, b_f and b_o are biases, c_t and c_t^- are the new and candidate state of the cell respectively, f_t is forget gate and o_t is output gate, h_t is output vector, and $\sigma(z) = \frac{1}{(1+e^{-z})}$.

Gated Recurrent Unit. Gated Recurrent Unit (GRU) is equally effective variant of LSTM that does not maintain an internal cell state. GRU consisted of updated gate z_t, reset gate r and current memory gate h_t^-, they are calculated as follows:

$$z_t = \sigma(W_z.x_t + U_z.h_{t-1} + b_z), r_t = \sigma(W_r.x_t + U_r.h_{t-1} + b_r)$$

$$h_t^- = \tanh\left(W.x_t + r_t^\circ h_{t-1} + b_n\right), h_t = (1 - z_t)^\circ h_{t-1} + z_t^\circ h_t^-$$

where x_t, h_t is input vector and output vector, W_z, W_r, U_z, U_r, b_z, b_r are parametric matrices and vector, operator $^\circ$ is the hadamard product.

5   Experiments and Results

In this section, we evaluate the system's performance on the benchmark datasets using the following parameters: accuracy, precision, recall, F1 score, false alarm rate, and detection rate. In order to accurately detect attacks, the hyperparameters mentioned in Table 6 should be tuned well to achieve the best performance. In the experiment, we manually tuned the hyperparameter instead of the grid search as it is computationally expensive. We achieved the highest accuracy of 98.54%, low false alarm rate of 2.2% with zero false-negative using a random forest classifier. A detailed description of the performance of all the implemented supervised classifiers, is shown in Table 7. Performance parameters are calculated using the confusion matrix.

A confusion matrix, M, is a $n * n$ matrix that indicates how successful a classifier's predictions were, where n is the number of classes. For binary classification, the confusion matrix is $2 * 2$. The columns of the matrix are labeled as true classes and rows are labeled as predicted classes of all records as depicted in Fig. 3. The element

Table 6 Hyperparameters

Hyperparameters	RF	DT	ADA	LSTM	GRU
n_estimators	100	–	100	–	–
Criterion	Entropy	Entropy	Gini	–	–
Optimizer	–	–	–	Adam	Adam
Learning rate	–	–	–	$1e^{-4}$	$1e^{-4}$
Batch size	–	–	–	32	32
Epoch	–	–	–	50	100
Input layer unit	–	–	–	32	32
Hidden layer unit	–	–	–	16,8	16,8
Activation	–	–	–	tanh	tanh

Table 7 Performance metrics of all implemented classifiers

Classifier	AR	PR	RL	FS	FA	DR
GNB	96.68	97	97	97	4.85	99.98
RF	98.54	99	99	99	2.2	100
DT	96.61	97	96	96	2.42	97.67
ADA	97.4	98	97	97	3.85	100
LSTM	96.73	97	97	97	4.5	99.48
GRU	96.27	96	96	96	4.38	98.77

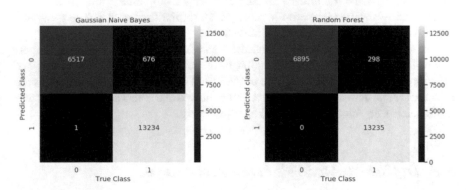

Fig. 3 Confusion Matrix for Gaussian NB and Random Forest classifier

at the zeroth row and zeroth column M[0][0] of the $2*2$ matrix represent the value of true-positive (TP), whereas element M[0][1] represents the false-positive (FP). The element at M[1][0] represents a value of false-negative (FN), whereas the element at M[2][1] represents true negative (TN) records. The performance metrics are defined as follows:

Table 8 Testing dataset under different traffic rate

Records	Packet per seconds (PPS)					
	600	800	1000	1200	1400	1600
#	2397	2025	1943	2121	1582	1612

$$Accuracy(AR) = \frac{TP + TN}{TP + TN + FP + FN}, Precision(PR) = \frac{TP}{TP + FP}$$

$$Recall(RL) = \frac{TP}{TP + FN}, F1score(FS) = 2\frac{PR * RL}{PR + RL}$$

$$False\ Alarm\ Rate(FA) = \frac{FP}{TN + FP}, Detection\ Rate(DR) = \frac{TP}{TP + FN}$$

Precision and *Recall* are calculated using the weighted average provided by sci-kit-learn API. True positive is the normal data records that are correctly classified as benign, where, the true negative is an attack data records that are correctly classified as an attack. Whereas, false positives are benign records that are wrongly classified as an attack, false negatives are attack records that are wrongly classified as benign.

As mentioned in Sect. 4.2, the training and testing dataset are generated when the normal and attack traffic traces are replayed at a rate of 100, 200, and 400 PPS, therefore we conducted an experiment intended to verify how well these trained classifiers perform when the normal and attack rate is higher than 400 PPS. In this experiment, we used the already trained classifiers from Table 7 and obtained the testing dataset for the higher traffic rates (PPS), similar to Sect. 4.2. The generated testing dataset records are shown in Table 8.

The experimental result shows that the Gaussian Naive Bayes classifier outperforms the other classifiers for the higher traffic rates with an average accuracy of 98.76% and an average detection rate of 99.79%. The performance comparison such as accuracy and detection rate of all the implemented classifiers against the different traffic rates is depicted in Figs. 4 and 5, respectively.

5.1 Traffic State Module's Parameters Analysis

In this section, we briefly analyze the system Traffic State module's parameters which minimize the effects of the response module on benign connections. We thus conducted an experiment to find a suitable value of the *threshold* while causing minimum delay to handle such cases. In this experiment, we use 5 min traffic traces from the testing dataset and already trained supervised classifier from Table 7 whereas the network is consisting of one normal and one attacker host. Other experimental settings are similar to the ones mentioned in Sect. 4.1.

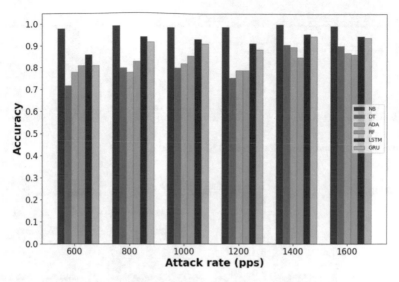

Fig. 4 Accuracy of all implemented classifiers under different traffic rates

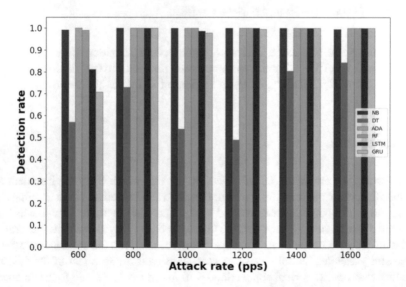

Fig. 5 Detection Rate of all implemented classifiers under different traffic rates

We replayed the traffic traces at a rate of 400 PPS and used Gaussian Naive Bayes classifier for calculating traffic class probability *prob* at every 5 s. We observed the score assigned by the traffic state module for each host (normal or attacker) over 5 min, as shown in Figs. 6 and 7 with different choices of α and β. A high value of β indicates low tolerance toward false-positive cases, whereas a high value of α meant that the current updated score at instant *i* is highly dependent on the Traffic Classifier

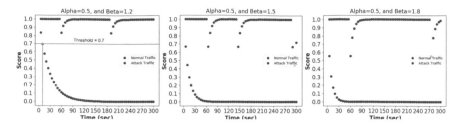

Fig. 6 Depict the score versus time graph for $\alpha = 0.5$

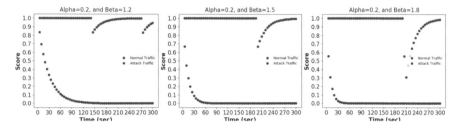

Fig. 7 Depict the score versus time graph for $\alpha = 0.2$

module, less on the past score. Therefore, by observing the pattern in Fig. 6, we could choose $\alpha = 0.5$ and $\beta = 1.2$ and thus we could set *threshold* to 0.7 (depicted in Fig. 6) causing a delay of 5 s for triggering the response toward the attacker traffics.

6 Conclusion

In this work, we propose a DDoS detection system on the SDN environment and evaluate the performance of different implemented supervised machine learning classifiers and models on datasets provided by the Canadian Institute for cybersecurity. The experimental results show that the Gaussian Naive Bayes classifier generalizes well with different traffic rates. The experiment result shows the score-based scheme successfully handles the false positive cases thus causing no effect of the system's response towards the normal connection(s). In future work, we will focus on attacks based on ICMP protocol, and multi-class classification so that the response module installs the filtering rule on the ingress switch to block the particular protocol-based attack, instead of blocking all types of connections originating from an attacker to the victim(s).

References

1. Zhang M, Bi J, Bai J, Li G (2018) FloodShield: securing the SDN infrastructure against denial-of-service attacks. In: Proceedings of the 2018 17th IEEE international conference on trust, security and privacy in computing and communications/ 12th IEEE international conference on big data science and engineering (TrustCom/BigDataSE). New York, NY
2. Openflow Specification https://www.opennetworking.org/wp-content/uploads/2014/10/openflow-switch-v1.5.1.pdf Accessed 10 Oct 2020
3. Swami R, Dave M, Ranga V Software defined networking-based DDoS defense mechanisms. ACM Comput Surv 52(2)
4. Peng H, Sun Z, Zhao X, Tan S, Sun Z (2018) A detection method for anomaly flow in software defined network. IEEE Access 6:27809–27817
5. Lee S, Kim J, Shin S, Porras P, Yegneswaran V Athena: a framework for scalable anomaly detection in software-defined networks. In Proceedings of the 2017 47th annual IEEE/IFIP international conference on dependable systems and networks (DSN'17)
6. Niyaz Q, Sun W, Javaid AY A deep learning based DDoS detection system in software-defined networking (SDN). arXi: 1611.07400
7. Hu D, Hong P, Chen Y ADM: DDoS flooding attack detection and mitigation system in software-defined Networking. In: Proceedings of the 2017 IEEE global communications conference (GLOBECOM'17)
8. Santos da Silva A, Wickboldt JA, Granville LZ, Schaeffer-Filho A ATLANTIC: a framework for anomaly traffic detection, classification, and mitigation in SDN. In: Proceedings of the 2016 IEEE/IFIP network operations and management symposium (NOMS'16)
9. Ye J, Cheng X, Zhu J, Feng L, Song L (2018) A DDoS attack detection method based on SVM in software defined network. Sec Commun Netw
10. Jing Liu, Yingxu Lai, and Shixuan Zhang, FL-GUARD: A detection and defense system for DDoS attack in SDN, in Proceedings of the 2017 International Conference on Cryptography, Security and Privacy (ICCSP'17)
11. Chen Z, Jiang F, Cheng Y, Gu X, Liu W, Peng J XGBoost classifier for DDoS attack detection and analysis in SDN-Based cloud. In: Proceedings of the 2018 IEEE international conference on big data and smart computing (BigComp'18). IEEE, pp 251–256
12. Mousavi SM, & St-Hilaire M Early detection of DDoS attacks against SDN controllers. In: Proceedings of the 2015 international conference on computing, networking and communication (ICNC'15)
13. Open vSwitch http://www.openvswitch.org Accessed 10 Oct 2020
14. Pox Wiki https://openflow.stanford.edu/display/ONL/POX+Wiki Accessed 10 Oct 2020.
15. CICIDS 2017 dataset https://www.unb.ca/cic/datasets/ids-2017.html Accessed 10 Oct 2020
16. CICDDOS 2019 dataset https://www.unb.ca/cic/datasets/ddos-2019.html
17. TcpReplay http://tcpreplay.synfin.net Accessed 10 Oct 2020
18. Hochreiter S, Schmidhuber J (1997) Long short-term memory. Neural Comput 9(8):1735–1780

A Pluggable System to Enable Fractal Compression as the Primary Content Type for World Wide Web

Bejoy Varghese and S. Krishnakumar

1 Introduction

Content delivery network (CDN) is a distributed network of different data services [1] to serve the data to clients in such a way that the spatial distance between the server and client is minimum. It is a distributed resource service, used as part of the internet to reduce the delivery time of the content from a URL to the client. Since the CDN provider has multiple data centers across the globe, the servers are load balanced and the resources are replicated to the data center servers using a distributed file system. As per the request from a client, a proxy server or name resolving service forwards the request to the spatially nearest server. Depending upon the CDN provider, the replication and load balancing technology may be changed, and these algorithms are proprietary in nature. A small amount of data reduction in a CDN can have an impact on a large number of clients.

One of the important aspects of CDN is that the majority of operations are data download and its frequency is very less in comparison with the data upload. When an image is uploaded in a CDN, a large number of clients access the same depending on the traffic to the website. So, the key aspect of reducing the data transfer is the mechanism used to compress the uploaded image. There are many image compression techniques available in the context of network data transfer. Widely used methods include Tagged Image File Format (TIFF), WEBP, Portable Network Graphics (PNG)

B. Varghese (✉)
Federal Institute of Science And Technology, Angamaly, Kerala 683577, India
e-mail: bejoyvarghese@fisat.ac.in

S. Krishnakumar
M G University Research Centre, Kottayam, Kerala 683001, India

and JPEG. All these methods take comparatively less time to compress and decompress the images. But in the CDN, compression can be occurred only once, while uploading the image to the CDN server, and decompression may be occurred many times depending on the access of the image from client side.

Even if Fractal-based Image Compression (FIC) offers a superior performance in terms of PSNR and Compression ratio, developers of internet-based applications don't prefer fractal-based techniques. This is because of the high execution time of FIC to find the affine transformations during the compression phase. But in the case of CDN, reduction in a bit of network traffic can impact millions of users as the download operation occurs multiple times at the user end. It is also noted that a large amount of data traffic on the Internet is handled by CDNs during the last few years.

Even though delivery speed of the CDN completely depends on the technology and backbone network of the provider, the ultimate objective is to increase the speed of data download for static assets. The main static assets which can be found in the CDN networks are the images and videos. So, the major traffic to any CDN network is the download request to these assets. The asset upload to the CDN network occurs only once. The backbone network of the CDN provider helps to replicate the uploaded assets to all the servers in the CDN [2]. Once the resource replication is completed worldwide, the URL gets registered in the URL registry of the CDN proxy and name resolvers. After completing the registration process, the client requests for the resource to be forwarded to the server which is spatially close to the client. In the case of a company that uses CDN to deliver the static asset such as the logo of the company everywhere on the internet. If the company uses the same logo URL in their mobile application, the data traffic may be high depending on the size of the image and the user base. So, the file format or the compression method used in the image can affect the data consumption on both server and client.

2   Methodology

Present system architecture uses a plugin system that can be connected to any CDN provider as shown in Fig.1. The plugin system handles the request for image upload from the user end. It accepts both raw image data and compression system specifications. If the client requests for fractal image compression, the plugin system runs an RL-based adaptive compression technique. This plugin includes the transformation predictor for the fractal compression. The learned weights for the pre-trained network are used in the system to achieve a faster compression process.

RL techniques are very efficient to interact with the environment which utilizes the Bellman equation to update the Q-function [3]. It always tries to increase the cumulative rewards by interacting with an environment that is not familiar earlier. The environment relies over a specific model which forms a control policy from its experience. The Q learning network uses another neural network, called target network to form an un-biased network of Bellman mean squared error. This target network in alignment with the QL network helps to couple the outputs of both main

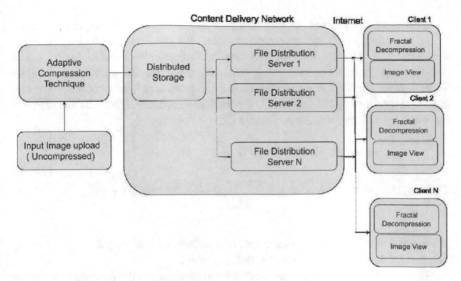

Fig. 1 Overview of system architecture

and target networks after each iterative period. Here the target network is fixed to give more focus on updating the Q network, leading to a better convergence factor.

Q learning in discrete domain is a tuple (W, S, A, F, R) where W is a stochastic width with state space S and action space A, T: S X A→ S, F is the state transition function, and R: S X A X S→ R is the cumulative reward function [4]. The reward function R and state transition function F are considered to be unknown and static throughout the convergence process. The policy tends π: → A is a PDF against the actions of each state. The Q-function $Q\pi$(S, A) for policy π is the reward to the agent for considering all the states Ɛ S, taking action Ɛ A, and then following policy π. The Q learning network always tries to achieve maximum rewards, and hence to predict the decisions with less time.

Deep Reinforcement Learning (DRL) is basically a Machine Learning algorithm, usually allows the agent to work on the environment, and hence to maximize the reward. Agent is capable to observe the environment and to align its actions more toward the positive rewards [5]. Adaptive fractal-based image compression is capable of finding out the affine transformations with much lesser time in comparison to classical FIC and its variants [6]. Initially, the system follows exhaustive search procedures as follows.

- The input image is partitioned into non-overlapping nxn range blocks, which form a range pool.
- Compute the affine transformations by finding the relation between range blocks and overlapping 2nx2n domain blocks.
- These transformation sequences are stored as the compressed image.

The Mean Squared Error (MSE) between range and domain blocks can be obtained by pre-calculating the luminance/chrominance offset and contrast scaling values as shown in Eq. 1. This can be used to determine the strength of a domain block. The computational cost can be reduced by eliminating the domain blocks with the Root Mean Square (RMS) values less than a pre-fixed threshold. The speed can be further improved by adopting the modified HV partitioning scheme, where the variable size partitions up to four splits are preferable [5].

$$min_D c \in \Omega MSE(R, D^c)$$

$$= min_{D \in \Omega} min_{S,0 \in R} \sum_{j=0}^{r-1} \sum_{j=0}^{r-1} (rij - (s \cdot \Psi(dij) + 0))^2 \qquad (1)$$

where s and o are the scaling parameter and luminance offset respectively. d_{ij} and r_{ij} are pixel intensities of domain block and range block.

When the compression process is completed as shown in the flow chart of upload plugin in Fig. 2, transformations are stored in the CDN file system and send the request for registration in the central registry of CDN. The plugin collects URL and sends it back to the client when the registration process is completed. If the client selects a compression technique such as JPEG or PNG, the plugin system sends the conversion request to standard Operating System (OS) utility and completes the process. The major advantage of using the plugin system is to port into any CDN using a standard HTTP REST Application programming Interface for file upload and registration process. So, the performance of the system can be measured across different CDN providers and different file types.

At the resource downloading end, the client side process requests the image using the URL given by the upload plugin system as shown in the process flow diagram of client application in Fig. 3. This request gets forward to the spatially nearest server by the CDN proxy or Name resolvers. Then the system sends the compressed image with the corresponding headers to indicate the compression technique. If the retrieved file uses a fractal-based method, the client uses a custom rendering method to convert it into bitmap format and fit to an image view of the User Interface (UI). If it is not a non-fractal method, the client uses the native image view available in the system to display the image. In both cases, the time for download and rendering is noted by a separate timer process. PSNR of the uncompressed image is also calculated by the measurement system.

3   Experimental Setup

Client side experimental setup includes android OS and custom application developed using android software development kit [6–8]. Figure 4 shows a demo android client application developed to test the present system. The server side plugin system

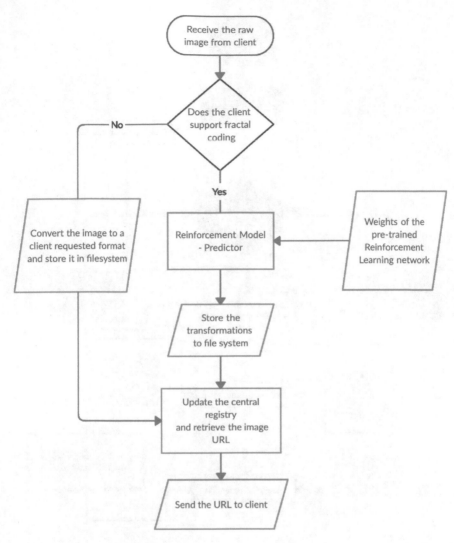

Fig. 2 Flow chart of upload plugin

is developed using Python language with support of Django web application development kit. Server side system uses HTTP REST Application programming Interface to establish the communication between the CDN provider and the plugin system [9]. The plugin system is designed to be modular to establish the communication to well-known CDN providers. The CDN providers include Amazon cloud front [9, 10], Cloudflare [11], Google cloud [12], Akamai [2]. Experiment conducted by uploading different size and varying texture images that are in raw format to the CDN and choose fractal based, JPEG or PNG as the compression as file format. The testing images include the same image with varying size by downsampling the number pixels. Each

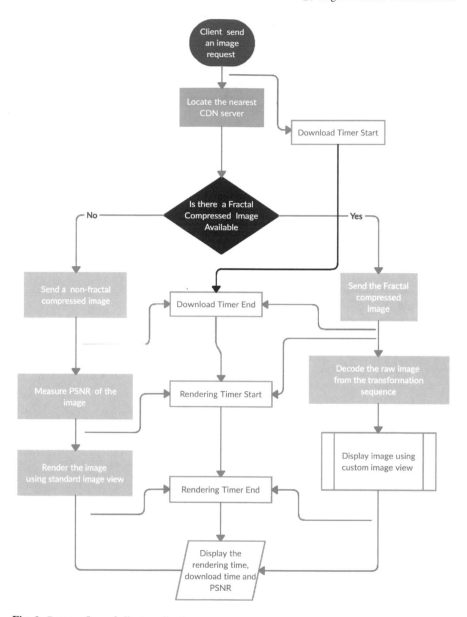

Fig. 3 Process flow of client application

Fig. 4 Output screen of the client application

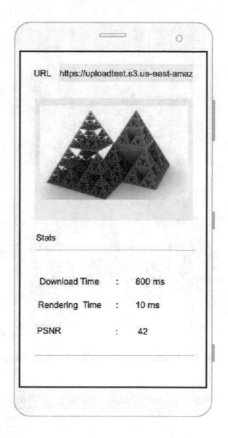

time the test is repeated with the above-mentioned CDN providers for image size of 100 KB to 100 MB. The test includes 10 different texture images, 20 different sizes of each and 4 CDN providers. The download time and sampling time for each test image are recorded in the mobile application.

4 Results and Discussion

The experiment shows that Fractal Image Compression based on RL technique is a clear winner compared to the JPEG and PNG compression methods. Figure 5 shows the PSNR comparison between these three methods with varying sizes of different images from Akamai CDN. The chosen images are the standard image set with varying texture patterns (a, b, c, d). The RL system is pre-trained using the ImageNet data set to ensure a better compression of the test images. The empirical analysis shows that the PSNR values of FIC are better than JPEG and PNG.

Akamai is chosen as the best provider in the test, based on the download speed comparison chart given in Table 1. The Table lists the download and rendering time

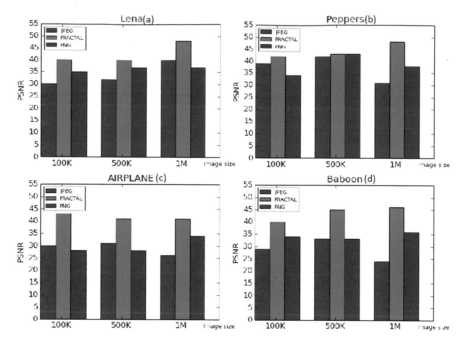

Fig. 5 Comparison of PSNR for different compression methods using different textures a, b, c, and d

Table 1 Download and rendering time for different compression methods in various CDNs

CDN Provider	Compression method	download time (ms)	Rendering time (ms)
Cloudflare	JPEG	1252	22
Google cloud [13]	JPEG	1200	
Amazon cloud front [12]	JPEG	1000	
Akamai	JPEG	800	
Cloudflare [14]	PNG	1100	30
Google cloud	PNG	985	
Amazon cloud front	PNG	900	
Akamai	PNG	852	
Cloudflare	FIC	874	11
Google cloud	FIC	800	
Amazon cloud front	FIC	822	
Akamai	FIC	500	

for different file compression techniques. The compressed images are generated from a distributed texture image of size 100 MB. The input image is in raw format and is compressed and uploaded to the CDN using this plugin system. The same procedure is followed for 10 texture images and 20 different sizes. The table lists a sample data for the image of size 100 M, and for all the combinations FIC method shows lesser download time compared to Wang et al. [15].

5 Conclusion

This paper adopts the fractal-based image compression as the primary image format for the CDNs and uses a plugin-based mechanism to upload the images to CDN. The present upload mechanism is compatible with different CDN providers. In the current scenario of the internet, there are no providers or the client software's support a fractal compressed image as a content type. Therefore, in order to test out the suggestion to use FIC as the primary image format, a plugin system has been developed for compression and also developed a mobile application to decompress, render and display the image. There are different fractal-based techniques available to develop a plugin system for compression. But the RL-based fractal compression is the fastest one available today. Hence, it is proved that the present system can drastically reduce the network load, power consumption and carbon footprint of the internet.

References

1. Dilley J, Maggs B, Parikh J, Prokop H, Sitaraman R, Weihl B (2002) Globally distributed content delivery. IEEE Internet Comput 6(5):50–58
2. Nygren E, Sitaraman RK, Sun J (2010) The Akamai network. ACM SIGOPS Operat Syst Rev 44(3):2–19
3. Li F, Qin J, Zheng WX (2020) Distributed Q–learning-based online optimization algorithm for unit commitment and dispatch in smart Grid. IEEE Trans Cybern 50(9):4146–4156
4. Jin C, Allen-Zhu Z, Bubeck S, Jordan MI (2018) Is Q-learning provably efficient? Adv Neural Inform Process Syst 4863–4873
5. Dong H, Ding Z, Zhang S (2020) Deep reinforcement learning: fundamentals, research and applications. Springer Nat
6. Varghese B, Krishnakumar S (2019) A novel fast fractal image compression based on reinforcement learning. Int J Comput Vis Robot 9(6):559
7. Roy SK, Kumar S, Chanda B, Chaudhuri BB, Banerjee S (2018) Fractal image compression using upper bound on scaling parameter. Chaos Solit Fract 106:16–22
8. Google: Android SDK (2015) Wearable Android^{TM}. pp 87–109
9. Lancaster A, Webster G (2019) Getting started with python. Python Life Sci 1–12
10. Cohen R, Wang T, et al (2014) The Android OS. Android application development for the Intel®{} platform. 131–190
11. Rubio D (2017) REST services with Django. Beginning Django, pp 549–566
12. Shaik B, Vallarapu A (2018) Amazon cloud
13. Google: Overview of Google Cloud Platform (2019) Google cloud certified associate cloud engineer study guide. pp 1–14

14. Cloudflare C (2020) The web performance. Security Company
15. Wang J, Chen P, Xi B, Liu J, Zhang Y, Yu S (2017) Fast sparse fractal image compression. PLoS One 12(9):e0184408

Printed in the United States
by Baker & Taylor Publisher Services